AF394588

Clinical Epidemiology

Practice and Methods

Second Edition

Edited by

Patrick S. Parfrey

Memorial University of Newfoundland, St. John's, NL, Canada

Brendan J. Barrett

Memorial University of Newfoundland, St. John's, NL, Canada

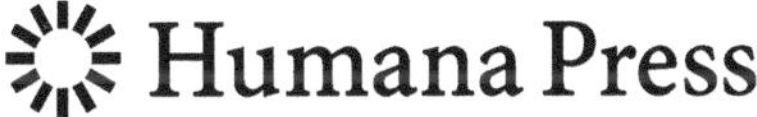

Editors
Patrick S. Parfrey
Memorial University of Newfoundland
St. John's, NL, Canada

Brendan J. Barrett
Memorial University of Newfoundland
St. John's, NL, Canada

ISSN 1064-3745   ISSN 1940-6029 (electronic)
Methods in Molecular Biology
ISBN 978-1-4939-2427-1   ISBN 978-1-4939-2428-8 (eBook)
DOI 10.1007/978-1-4939-2428-8

Library of Congress Control Number: 2015930615

Springer New York Heidelberg Dordrecht London

Humana Press is a brand of Springer
Springer Science+Business Media LLC New York is part of Springer Science+Business Media (www.springer.com)

Preface

Clinical epidemiology provides the scientific basis for the practice of medicine, because it focuses on the diagnosis, prognosis, and management of human disease. Therefore, issues of research design, measurement, and evaluation are critical to clinical epidemiology. This volume, *Clinical Epidemiology: Practice and Methods*, is intended to educate researchers on how to undertake clinical research and should be helpful not only to medical practitioners but also to basic scientists who want to extend their work to humans, to allied health professionals interested in scientific evaluation, and to trainees in clinical epidemiology.

This book is divided into six parts. The first three introductory chapters focus on how to frame a clinical research question, the ethics associated with doing a research project in humans, and the definition of various biases that occur in clinical research. Parts II–IV examine issues of design, measurement, and analysis associated with various research designs, including determination of risk in longitudinal studies, assessment of therapy in randomized controlled clinical trials, and evaluation of diagnostic tests. Part V focuses on the more specialized area of clinical genetic research. Part VI provides the basic methods used in evidence-based decision making including critical appraisal, aggregation of multiple studies using meta-analysis, health technology assessment, clinical practice guidelines, development of health policy, translational research, how to utilize administrative databases, and knowledge translation.

This collection provides advice on framing the research question and choosing the most appropriate research design, often the most difficult part in performing a research project that could change clinical practice. It discusses not only the basics of clinical epidemiology but also the use of biomarkers and surrogates, patient-reported outcomes, and qualitative research. It provides examples of bias in clinical studies, methods of sample size estimation, and an analytic framework for various research designs, including the scientific basis for multivariate modeling. Finally, practical chapters on research ethics, budgeting, funding, and managing clinical research projects may be useful.

The content of this book can be divided into two categories: The basics of clinical epidemiology and more advanced chapters examining the analysis of longitudinal studies (Chapters 5–8) and randomized controlled trials (Chapters 13–15). Examples and case studies have been encouraged.

All the contributors to this volume are practicing clinical epidemiologists, who hope the reader will join them in doing research focused on improving clinical outcomes.

St. John's, NL, Canada   *Patrick S. Parfrey*
                                                               Brendan J. Barrett

Contents

Preface.. *v*

Contributors.. *xi*

PART I   INTRODUCTION

1   On Framing the Research Question and Choosing the Appropriate
    Research Design 3
    Patrick S. Parfrey and Pietro Ravani

2   Research Ethics for Clinical Researchers 19
    John D. Harnett and Richard Neuman

3   Definitions of Bias in Clinical Research 31
    Geoffrey Warden

PART II   LONGITUDINAL STUDIES

4   Longitudinal Studies 1: Determination of Risk 51
    Sean W. Murphy

5   Longitudinal Studies 2: Modeling Data Using Multivariate Analysis 71
    Pietro Ravani, Brendan J. Barrett, and Patrick S. Parfrey

6   Longitudinal Studies 3: Data Modeling Using Standard Regression
    Models and Extensions 93
    Pietro Ravani, Brendan J. Barrett, and Patrick S. Parfrey

7   Longitudinal Studies 4: Matching Strategies to Evaluate Risk 133
    Matthew T. James

8   Longitudinal Studies 5: Development of Risk Prediction Models
    for Patients with Chronic Disease 145
    Navdeep Tangri and Claudio Rigatto

PART III   RANDOMIZED CONTROLLED CLINICAL TRIALS

9   Randomized Controlled Trials 1: Design................................. 159
    Bryan M. Curtis, Brendan J. Barrett, and Patrick S. Parfrey

10   Randomized Controlled Trials 2: Analysis 177
     Robert N. Foley

11   Randomized Controlled Trials 3: Measurement and Analysis
     of Patient-Reported Outcomes 191
     Michelle M. Richardson, Megan E. Grobert, and Klemens B. Meyer

12   Randomized Controlled Trials 4: Biomarkers and Surrogate Outcomes...... 207
     Claudio Rigatto and Brendan J. Barrett

13   Randomized Controlled Trials 5: Determining the Sample Size
and Power for Clinical Trials and Cohort Studies........................ 225
Tom Greene

14   Randomized Controlled Trials 6: On Contamination and Estimating
the Actual Treatment Effect 249
Patrick S. Parfrey

15   Randomized Controlled Trials 7: Analysis and Interpretation
of Quality-of-Life Scores... 261
Robert N. Foley and Patrick S. Parfrey

16   Randomized Controlled Trials: Planning, Monitoring, and Execution........ 273
Elizabeth Hatfield, Elizabeth Dicks, and Patrick S. Parfrey

Part IV   The Basics for Other Clinical Epidemiology Methods

17   Evaluation of Diagnostic Tests 289
John M. Fardy and Brendan J. Barrett

18   Qualitative Research in Clinical Epidemiology......................... 301
Deborah M. Gregory and Christine Y. Way

19   Health Economics in Clinical Research 315
Braden J. Manns

Part V   Clinical Genetic Research

20   Clinical Genetic Research 1: Bias................................. 333
Susan Stuckless and Patrick S. Parfrey

21   Clinical Genetic Research 2: Genetic Epidemiology
of Complex Phenotypes 349
Darren D. O'Rielly and Proton Rahman

22   Clinical Genetic Research 3: Genetics ELSI (Ethical, Legal,
and Social Issues) Research 369
Daryl Pullman and Holly Etchegary

Part VI   Methods in Evidence-Based Decision Making

23   Evidence-Based Decision-Making 1: Critical Appraisal.................. 385
Laurie K. Twells

24   Evidence-Based Decision-Making 2: Systematic Reviews and Meta-analysis 397
Aminu Bello, Natasha Wiebe, Amit Garg, and Marcello Tonelli

25   Evidence-Based Decision-Making 3: Health Technology Assessment........ 417
*Daria O'Reilly, Kaitryn Campbell, Meredith Vanstone,
James M. Bowen, Lisa Schwartz, Nazila Assasi, and Ron Goeree*

26   Evidence-Based Decision-Making 4: Development and Limitations
of Clinical Practice Guidelines..................................... 443
Bruce Culleton

27   Evidence-Based Decision-Making 5: Translational Research 455
Deborah M. Gregory and Laurie K. Twells

28 Evidence-Based Decision-Making 6: Utilization of Administrative
    Databases for Health Services Research   469
    Tanvir Turin Chowdhury and Brenda Hemmelgarn

29 Evidence-Based Decision-Making 7: Knowledge Translation   485
    Braden J. Manns

30 Evidence-Based Decision-Making 8: Health Policy, a Primer
    for Researchers   501
    Victor Maddalena

Index *519*

Contributors

NAZILA ASSASI • *Program for Assessment of Technology in Health (PATH), St. Joseph's Healthcare Hamilton, Hamilton, ON, Canada; Department of Clinical Epidemiology and Biostatistics, Faculty of Health Sciences, McMaster University, Hamilton, ON, Canada*

BRENDAN J. BARRETT • *Department of Medicine, Memorial University of Newfoundland, St. John's, NL, Canada*

AMINU BELLO • *Division of Nephrology, Faculty of Medicine and Dentistry, University of Alberta, Edmonton, AB, Canada*

JAMES M. BOWEN • *Program for Assessment of Technology in Health (PATH), St. Joseph's Healthcare Hamilton, Hamilton, ON, Canada; Department of Clinical Epidemiology and Biostatistics, Faculty of Health Sciences, McMaster University, Hamilton, ON, Canada*

KAITRYN CAMPBELL • *Program for Assessment of Technology in Health (PATH), St. Joseph's Healthcare Hamilton, Hamilton, ON, Canada; Department of Clinical Epidemiology and Biostatistics, Faculty of Health Sciences, McMaster University, Hamilton, ON, Canada*

TANVIR TURIN CHOWDHURY • *Department of Family Medicine, University of Calgary, Calgary, AL, Canada*

BRUCE CULLETON • *Renal Therapeutic Area, Baxter Healthcare, Deerfield, IL, USA*

BRYAN M. CURTIS • *Department of Medicine, Memorial University of Newfoundland, St. John's, NL, Canada*

ELIZABETH DICKS • *Eastern Health, St. John's, NL, Canada*

HOLLY ETCHEGARY • *Eastern Health, Memorial University, St. John's, NL, Canada; Clinical Epidemiology, Faculty of Medicine, Memorial University, St. John's, NL, Canada*

JOHN M. FARDY • *Department of Medicine, Memorial University of Newfoundland, St. John's, NL, Canada*

ROBERT N. FOLEY • *Division of Renal Diseases and Hypertension, University of Minnesota, Minneapolis, MN, USA; Department of Medicine, University of Minnesota, Minneapolis, MN, USA*

AMIT GARG • *Department of Medicine and Epidemiology, University of Western Ontario, London, ON, Canada*

RON GOEREE • *Program for Assessment of Technology in Health (PATH), St. Joseph's Healthcare Hamilton, Hamilton, ON, Canada; Department of Clinical Epidemiology and Biostatistics, Faculty of Health Sciences, McMaster University, Hamilton, ON, Canada*

TOM GREENE • *Internal Medicine, School of Medicine, University of Utah, Salt Lake City, UT, USA*

DEBORAH M. GREGORY • *Faculty of Medicine (Clinical Epidemiology), Memorial University of Newfoundland, St. John's, NL, Canada*

MEGAN E. GROBERT • *Outcomes Monitoring Program, Dialysis Clinic, Inc., Boston, MA, USA*

JOHN D. HARNETT • *Department of Medicine, Memorial University of Newfoundland, St. John's, NL, Canada*

ELIZABETH HATFIELD • *Clinical Epidemiology, Faculty of Medicine, Memorial University of Newfoundland, St. John's, NL, Canada*

BRENDA HEMMELGARN • *Department of Medicine, University of Calgary, Calgary, AL, Canada; Department of Community Health Sciences, University of Calgary, Calgary, AL, Canada*

MATTHEW T. JAMES • *Department of Medicine, University of Calgary, Calgary, AL, Canada; Department of Health Sciences, University of Calgary, Calgary, AL, Canada*

VICTOR MADDALENA • *Community Health and Humanities, Faculty of Medicine, Memorial University of Newfoundland, St. John's, NL, Canada*

BRADEN J. MANNS • *University of Calgary, Calgary, AB, Canada*

KLEMENS B. MEYER • *Division of Nephrology, Tufts Medical Center, Boston, MA, USA; Outcomes Monitoring Program, Dialysis Clinic, Inc., Boston, MA, USA*

SEAN W. MURPHY • *Department of Medicine, Memorial University of Newfoundland, St. John's, NL, Canada*

RICHARD NEUMAN • *Pharmacology, Faculty of Medicine, Memorial University of Newfoundland, St. John's, NL, Canada*

DARIA O'REILLY • *Program for Assessment of Technology in Health (PATH), St. Joseph's Healthcare Hamilton, Hamilton, ON, Canada; Department of Clinical Epidemiology and Biostatistics, Faculty of Health Sciences, McMaster University, Hamilton, ON, Canada*

DARREN D. O'RIELLY • *Faculty of Medicine, Memorial University of Newfoundland, St. John's, NL, Canada*

PATRICK S. PARFREY • *Faculty of Medicine, Memorial University of Newfoundland, St. John's, NL, Canada*

DARYL PULLMAN • *Medical Ethics, Division of Community Health and Humanities, Faculty of Medicine, Memorial University of Newfoundland, St. John's, NL, Canada*

PROTON RAHMAN • *Rheumatology, Memorial University of Newfoundland, St. John's, NL, Canada*

PIETRO RAVANI • *Department of Medicine, University of Calgary, Calgary, AB, Canada*

MICHELLE M. RICHARDSON • *Division of Nephrology, Tufts Medical Center, Boston, MA, USA; Outcomes Monitoring Program, Dialysis Clinic, Inc., Boston, MA, USA; Tufts University School of Medicine, Boston, MA, USA*

CLAUDIO RIGATTO • *Department of Medicine, Seven Oaks General Hospital, University of Manitoba, Winnipeg, MB, Canada; Department of Community Health Sciences, Seven Oaks General Hospital, University of Manitoba, Winnipeg, MB, Canada*

LISA SCHWARTZ • *Department of Clinical Epidemiology and Biostatistics, Faculty of Health Sciences, McMaster University, Hamilton, ON, Canada; Centre for Health Economics and Policy Analysis (CHEPA), McMaster University, Hamilton, ON, Canada*

SUSAN STUCKLESS • *Clinical Epidemiology Unit, Faculty of Medicine, Memorial University of Newfoundland, St. John's, NL, Canada*

NAVDEEP TANGRI • *Department of Medicine, Seven Oaks General Hospital, University of Manitoba, Winnipeg, MB, Canada; Department of Community Health Sciences, Seven Oaks General Hospital, University of Manitoba, Winnipeg, MB, Canada*

MARCELLO TONELLI • *Nephrology, University of Calgary, Calgary, AB, Canada; Department of Medicine, Cumming School of Medicine, University of Calgary, Calgary, AB, Canada*

LAURIE K. TWELLS • *Faculty of Medicine and School of Pharmacy, Memorial University of Newfoundland, St. John's, NL, Canada*

MEREDITH VANSTONE • *Department of Clinical Epidemiology and Biostatistics, Faculty of Health Sciences, McMaster University, Hamilton, ON, Canada; Centre for Health Economics and Policy Analysis (CHEPA), McMaster University, Hamilton, ON, Canada*

GEOFFREY WARDEN • *Faculty of Medicine, Memorial University of Newfoundland, St. John's, NL, Canada*

CHRISTINE Y. WAY • *School of Nursing and Clinical Epidemiology, Memorial University of Newfoundland, St. John's, NL, Canada*

NATASHA WIEBE • *Kidney Health Research Group, Department of Medicine, University of Alberta, Edmonton, AB, Canada*

Part I

Introduction

Chapter 1

On Framing the Research Question and Choosing the Appropriate Research Design

Patrick S. Parfrey and Pietro Ravani

Abstract

Clinical epidemiology is the science of human disease investigation with a focus on diagnosis, prognosis, and treatment. The generation of a reasonable question requires definition of patients, interventions, controls, and outcomes. The goal of research design is to minimize error, to ensure adequate samples, to measure input and output variables appropriately, to consider external and internal validities, to limit bias, and to address clinical as well as statistical relevance. The hierarchy of evidence for clinical decision-making places randomized controlled trials (RCT) or systematic review of good quality RCTs at the top of the evidence pyramid. Prognostic and etiologic questions are best addressed with longitudinal cohort studies.

Key words Clinical epidemiology, Methodology, Research design, Evidence-based medicine, Randomized controlled trials, Longitudinal studies

1 Introduction

Clinical epidemiology is the science of human disease investigation, with a focus on problems of most interest to patients: diagnosis, prognosis, and management.

Articles are included in this book on the design and analysis of cohort studies and randomized controlled trials. Methodological issues involved with studies of biomarkers, quality of life, genetic diseases, and qualitative research are evaluated. In addition, chapters are presented on the methodology associated with aggregation of multiple studies such as meta-analysis, pharmacoeconomics, health technology assessment, and clinical practice guidelines. Finally, important issues involved in the practice of clinical epidemiology such as ethical approval and management of studies are discussed. In this chapter we consider how to frame the research question, error definition, measurement, sampling, the choice of research design, and the difference between clinical relevance and statistical significance. In addition, here we provide an overview of principles and concepts that are discussed in more detail in subsequent chapters.

Patrick S. Parfrey and Brendan J. Barrett (eds.), *Clinical Epidemiology: Practice and Methods*, Methods in Molecular Biology, vol. 1281, DOI 10.1007/978-1-4939-2428-8_1, © Springer Science+Business Media New York 2015

2   Framing the Clinical Research Question

The research process usually starts with a general idea or initial problem.

Research ideas may originate from practical clinical problems, request for proposals by funding agencies or private companies, reading the literature and thinking of ways to extend or refine previous research, or the translation of basic science discoveries to the clinic or the community. Literature review is always required to identify related research, to define the knowledge gap, to avoid redundancy when the answer is already clear, and to set the research within a proper conceptual and theoretical context based on what is already known. The next step is to generate a researchable question from the general idea. This stage of conceptualization should generate testable hypotheses and delineate the exposure–outcome relationship to be studied in a defined patient population, whether it be a study of prognosis, diagnosis, or treatment. Thus operationalization of the proposed study requires characterization of the specific disease to be studied, establishment of the input variable or exposure (test, risk factor, or intervention) to be associated with an output or clinical outcome. The latter may be the gold standard in a diagnostic test, the clinical event in a cohort study evaluating risk, or the primary clinical outcome in a randomized trial of an intervention. Thus, the broad initial idea is translated into a feasible research project. Narrowing down the area of research is necessary to formulate an answerable question, in which the target population of the study is determined along with a meaningful effect measure—the prespecified study outcome.

In framing researchable questions, it is crucial to define the Patients, Interventions, Controls, and Outcomes (PICO) of relevance. The study question should define the patients (P) to be studied (e.g., prevalent or incident), through clearly defined eligibility criteria. These criteria should specify the problem, the comorbid conditions to include (because the answer(s) to the research question may vary by the condition, e.g., diabetes, cardiovascular disease); and those not to include (because for them the question may be of less interest or hardly answerable, e.g., those with short expected survival). Secondly, the type of exposure (intervention or prognostic factor or test; I) is defined, and its specifics (e.g., what does the exposure actually comprise). Next, the comparison group (C) is defined. Finally, the outcome of interest (O) is declared. Following consideration of the PICO issues the researchable question can then be posed, e.g., "Does a particular statin prevent cardiac events, when compared to conventional therapy, in diabetic patients with stage 3 and 4 chronic kidney disease"?

The operationalization of the study must be consistent with its purpose. If the question is one of *efficacy* (Does it work in the ideal world?), then the measurement tools identified should be very accurate, may be complex and expensive, and may not be necessarily useful in practice. Opposite considerations are involved in *effectiveness* studies (Does it work in the real world?), and trade-offs between rigor and practicality are necessary. Further operational steps in clinical research involve limiting error, whether it be random or systematic error, identifying a representative sample to study, determining a clinically relevant effect to assess, ensuring that the study is feasible, cost-effective, and ethical.

3 Error

The goal of clinical research is to estimate population characteristics (parameters) such as risks by making measurements on samples from the target population. The hope is that the study estimates be as close as possible to the true values in the population (accuracy) with little uncertainty (imprecision) around them (Table 1). However, an error component exists in any study. This is the difference between

Table 1
Precision and accuracy in clinical studies

	Precision	**Accuracy**
Definition	Degree to which a variable has nearly the same value when measured several times	Degree to which a variable actually represents what is supposed to represent
Synonyms	Fineness of a single measurement *Consistency*—agreement of repeated measurements (*reliability*) or repeated sampling data (*reproducibility*)	Closeness of a measurement or estimate to the true value *Validity*—agreement between measured and true values
Value to the study	Increase power to detect effects	Increase validity of conclusions
Threat	Random error (variance)	Systematic error (bias)
Maximization: sampling	Increase sample size	Randomization
Maximization: measurement	Variance reduction	Bias prevention/control
Observer sources	Procedure standardization, staff training	Blinding
Tool sources	Calibration; automatization	Appropriate instrument
Subject sources	Procedure standardization, repetition and averaging key measurements	Blinding
Assessment	Repeated measures (test/retest, inter/intra-observer: correlation, agreement, consistency)	Comparison with a reference standard (gold standard; formal experiments, RCT)

RCT randomized controlled trial

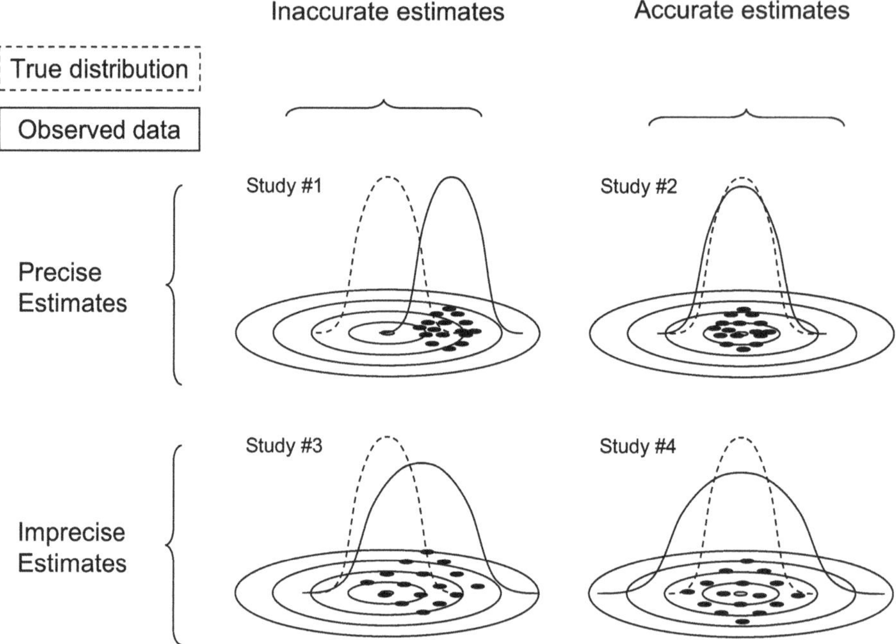

Fig. 1 The effect of the error type on study results. Each panel compares the distribution of a parameter observed in a study (*continuous lines*) and the corresponding true distribution (*dashed lines*). Random error lowers the precision of the estimates increasing the dispersion of the observed values around the average (studies #3 and #4). Systematic error (bias) causes incorrect estimates or "deviations from the truth": the estimated averages correspond to rings distant from the target center (studies #1 and #3) even if results are precise (study #1). With permission Ravani et al., Nephrol Dial Transpl [19]

the value observed in the sample and the true value of the phenomenon of interest in the parent population.

There are two main types of error: random or accidental error, and systematic error (*bias*). Random errors are due to chance and compensate since their average effect is zero. Systematic errors are non-compensating distortions in measurement (Fig. 1). Mistakes caused by carelessness, or human fallibility (e.g., incorrect use of an instrument, error in recording or in calculations), may contribute to both random and systematic error. Both errors arise from many sources and both can be minimized using different strategies. However, their control can be costly and complete elimination may be impossible. Systematic error, as opposed to random error, is not limited by increasing the study size and replicates if the study is repeated.

Confounding is a special error since it is due to chance in experimental designs but it is a bias in non-experimental studies. Confounding occurs when the effect of the exposure is mixed with that of another variable (confounder) related to both exposure and outcome, which does not lie in the causal pathway between them. For example if high serum phosphate levels are found to be associated with higher mortality, it is important to consider the confounding effect of low glomerular filtration rate in the assessment of the relationship between serum phosphate and death [1].

For any given study, the design should aim to limit error. In some cases, pilot studies are helpful in identifying the main potential sources of error (known sources of variability and bias—Table 1) such that the design of the main study can control them [2, 3]. Some errors are specific to some designs and are discussed in a subsequent chapter of this series. Both random and systematic errors can occur during all stages of a study, from conceptualization of the idea to sampling (participant selection) and actual measurements (information collection).

4   Sampling

Once the target population has been defined, the next challenge is to recruit study participants representative of the target population. The sampling process is important, as usually a small fraction of the target population is studied for reasons of cost and feasibility. Errors in the sampling process can affect both the actual estimate and its precision (Table 1, Fig. 2). To reduce sampling errors researchers must set up a proper sampling system and estimate an adequate sample size.

Recruitment of a random sample of the target population is necessary to ensure generalizability of study results. For example if

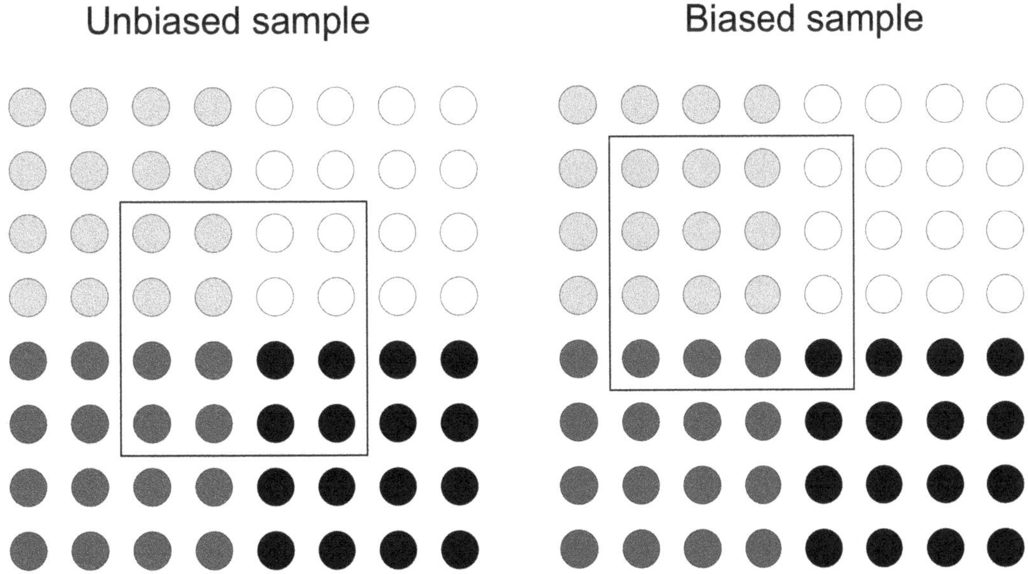

Fig. 2 Sampling bias. An unbiased sample is representative of and has the same characteristics as the population from which it has been drawn. A biased sample is not representative of the target population because its characteristics have different distribution as compared to the original population. With permission Ravani et al., Nephrol Dial Transpl [19]

we wish to estimate the prevalence of Chronic Kidney Disease (CKD) in the general population, the best approach would be to use random sampling, possibly over-sampling some subgroup of particular interest (e.g., members of a racial group) in order to have sufficiently precise estimates for that subgroup [4, 5]. In this instance, a sample of subjects drawn from a nephrology or a diabetic clinic, any hospital department, school, workplace or people walking down the street would not be representative of the general population. The likelihood of CKD may be positively or negatively related to factors associated with receiving care or working in a particular setting. On the other hand, if a study aimed at understanding the characteristics of patients with CKD referred to a nephrologist, a study of consecutive patients referred for CKD would probably provide a reasonably generalizable result.

If the purpose of the study is to estimate a measure of effect due to some intervention, then the sampling problem is not finished. Here the comparability of study groups, other than with regard to the exposure of interest, must be ensured. Indeed to measure the effect of a therapy, we need to contrast the experience of people given the therapy to those not so treated. However, people differ from one another in myriad of ways, some of which might affect the outcome of interest. To avoid such concerns in studies of therapy, random assignment of study participants to therapy is recommended to ensure comparability of study groups in the long run. These must be of sufficient size to reduce the possibility that some measurable or unmeasurable prognostic factors be associated with one or other of the groups (random confounding).

The randomization process consists of three interrelated maneuvers: the generation of random allocation sequences; strategies to promote allocation concealment; and intention-to-treat analysis. *Random sequences* are usually generated by means of computer programs. The use of calendar or treatment days, birth dates, etc. is not appropriate since it does not guarantee unpredictability. *Allocation concealment* is meant to prevent those recruiting trial subjects from the knowledge of upcoming assignment and protect selection biases. Useful ways to implement concealed allocation include the use central randomization, or the use of sequentially numbered sealed opaque envelopes. *Intention-to-treat analysis* consists in keeping all randomized patients in their original assigned groups during analysis regardless of adherence or any protocol deviations. This is necessary to maintain group comparability.

5   Sample Size Estimation

When planning a comparative study two possible random errors (called type I and II errors) are considered. A type I error is made if the results of a study have a statistically significant result when in fact there is no difference between study groups. This risk of false negative results is commonly set at 5 % (equivalent to a significant *P* value of 0.05). A Type II error is made if the results of a study are non-significant when in fact a difference truly exists. This risk of false positive results is usually set at 10 or 20 %. The other factors that determine how large a study should be are the size of the effect to be detected and the expected outcome variability. Different formulae exist to estimate the sample size depending on the type of response variable and the analytical tool used to assess the input–output relationship [6]. In all studies the sample size will depend on the expected variability in the data, effect size (delta), level of significance (alpha error), and study power (1-beta error).

6 Measurement

6.1 Variable Types

As in all sciences, measurement is a central feature of clinical epidemiology. Both input and output variables are measured on the sample according to the chosen definitions. Inputs can be measured once at baseline if their value is fixed (e.g., gender), or more than once if their value can change during the study (such as blood pressure or type of therapy). Outputs can also be measured once (e.g., average blood pressure values after 6 months of treatment) or multiple times (repeated measures of continuous variables such as blood pressure or events such as hospital admissions). The information gained from input and output variables depends on the type of observed data, on whether it be qualitative nominal (unordered categories), qualitative ordinal (ordered categories), quantitative interval (no meaningful zero), or quantitative ratio (zero is meaningful).

In clinical epidemiology the type of outcomes influences study design and determines the analytical tool to be used to study the relationship of interest.

Intermediate variables are often considered *surrogate* outcome candidates and used as an outcome instead of the final endpoint, to reduce the sample size and the study cost (Table 2). Candidate surrogate outcomes are many and include measures of the underlying pathological process (e.g., vascular calcification), or of preclinical disease (e.g., left ventricular hypertrophy). However, well-validated surrogate variables highly predictive of adverse clinical events, such as systolic blood pressure and LDL cholesterol, are very few and only occasionally persuasive (Table 3). Furthermore, although these surrogates may be useful in studies of the general population, their relationship with clinical outcomes is not linear in some conditions making them less useful in those settings [7, 8]. Hard outcomes that are clinically important and easy to define are used to measure disease occurrence as well as to estimate the effects of an exposure.

Table 2
Comparison between final outcome and intermediate (surrogate) response

	Surrogate marker	Hard end-point
Definition	Relatively easily measured variables which predict a rare or distant outcome	The real efficacy measure of a clinical study
Use	May replace the clinical end-point; provide insight into the causal pathway	Response variable of a clinical study (outcome)
Example	Brain natriuretic peptide; left ventricular hypertrophy	Death (from all and specific causes); cardiovascular or other specified events
Advantages	(1) Reduction of study sample size, duration and cost; (2) Assessment of treatments in situations where the use of primary outcomes would be excessively invasive or premature	A change in the final outcome answers the essential questions on the clinical impact of treatment
Disadvantages	1. A change in valid surrogate end-point does not answer the essential questions on the clinical impact of treatment 2. It may lack some of the desired characteristics a primary outcome should have	(1) Large sample size and long duration (cost) of the study; (2) Assessment of treatments may be premature or invasive

Table 3
Validity issues for a surrogate end-point to be tested in an RCT

Surrogate marker validity: *Is the plausible relationship between exposure (E) and the final hard outcome (H) fully explained by the surrogate marker (S)?*	Yes No	E → S → H E → S, E → H, S ↔ H
Desired characteristics of a surrogate		1. Validity/reliability 2. Availability, affordability; suitable for monitoring 3. Dose–response relation predictive of the hard end-point 4. Existence of a cutoff point for normality 5. High sensitivity, specificity, +/− predictive values 6. Changes rapidly/accurately in response to treatment 7. Levels normalize in states of remission

6.2 Measurement Errors

Some systematic and random errors may occur during measurement (Table 1). Of interest to clinical trials are the strategies to reduce performance bias (additional therapeutic interventions preferentially provided to one of the groups) and to limit information and detection bias (ascertainment or measurement bias) by masking (blinding) [9]. Masking is a process whereby people are kept unaware of which interventions have been used throughout the study, including when outcome is being assessed. Patient/clinician blinding is not always practical or feasible, such as in trials comparing surgery with non-surgery, diets, and lifestyles.

Finally, measurement error can occur in the statistical analysis of the data. Important elements to specify in the protocol include: definition of the primary and secondary outcome measure; how missing data will be handled (depending on the nature of the data there are different techniques); subgroup (secondary) analyses of interest; consideration of multiple comparisons and the inflation of the type I error rate as the number of tests increases; the potential confounders to control for; and the possible effect modifiers (interaction). This issue has implication for modeling techniques and is discussed in subsequent chapters.

7 External and Internal Validity

The operational criteria applied in the design influence the external and internal validity of the study (Fig. 3). Both construct validity and external validity relate to generalization. However, *construct validity* involves generalizing from the study to the underlying concept of the study. It reflects how well the variables in the study (and their relationships) represent the phenomena of interest. For example, how well does the level of proteinuria represent the presence of kidney disease? Construct validity becomes important when a complex process, such as care for chronic kidney disease, is being described. Maintaining consistency between the idea or concept of a certain care program and the operational details of its specific components in the study may be challenging.

External validity involves generalizing conclusions from the study context to other people, places, or times. External validity is reduced if study eligibility criteria are strict, or the exposure or intervention is hard to reproduce in practice. The closer the intended sample is to the target population, the more relevant the study is to this wider, but defined, group of people, and the greater is its external validity. The same applies to the chosen intervention, control and outcome including the study context. The *internal validity* of a study depends primarily on the degree to which bias is minimized. Selection, measurement, and confounding biases can all affect the internal validity.

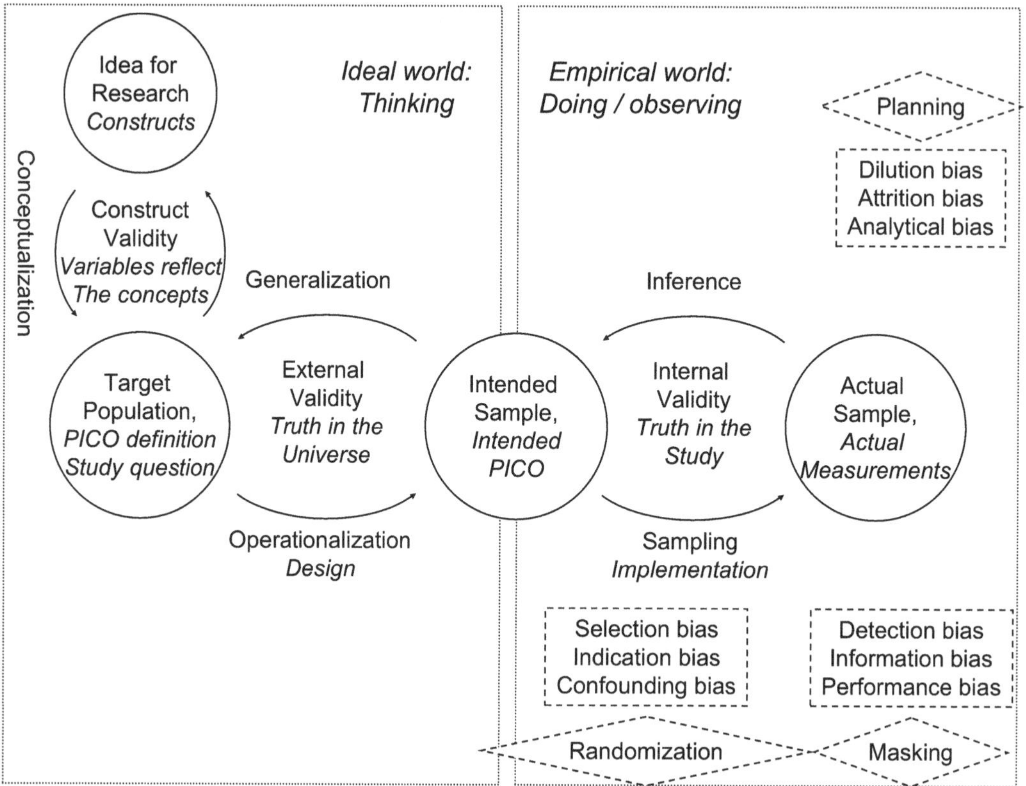

Fig. 3 Structure of study design. The *left panel* represents the design phase of a study, when Patient, Intervention, Control and Outcome (PICO) are defined (conceptualization and operationalization). The *right panel* corresponds to the implementation phase. Different types of bias can occur during sampling, data collection and measurement. The extent to which the results in the study can be considered true and generalizable depends on its internal and external validity. With permission Ravani et al., Nephrol Dial Transpl [19]

In any study there is always a balance between external and internal validity, as it is difficult and costly to maximize both. Designs that have strict inclusion and exclusion criteria tend to maximize internal validity, while compromising external validity. Internal validity is especially important in efficacy trials to understand the maximum likely benefit that might be achieved with an intervention, whereas external validity becomes more important in effectiveness studies. Involvement of multiple sites is an important way to enhance both internal validity (faster recruitment, quality control, and standardized procedures for data collection, management, and analysis) and external validity (generalizability is enhanced because the study involves patients from several regions).

8   Clinical Relevance vs. Statistical Significance

The concepts of clinical relevance and statistical significance are often confused. Clinical relevance refers to the amount of benefit or harm apparently resulting from an exposure or intervention that is sufficient to change clinical practice or health policy. In planning study sample size, the researcher has to determine the minimum level of effect that would have clinical relevance. The level of statistical significance chosen is the probability that the observed results are due to chance alone. This will correspond to the probability of making a type I error, i.e., claiming an effect when in fact there is none. By convention, this probability is usually 0.05 (but can be as low as 0.01). The P value or the limits of the appropriate confidence interval (a 95 % interval is equivalent to a significance level of 0.05 for example) is examined to see if the results of the study might be explained by chance. If $P<0.05$, the null hypothesis of no effect is rejected in favor of the study hypothesis, despite it is still being possible that the observed results are simply due to chance. However, since statistical significance depends on both the magnitude of effect and the sample size, trials with very large sample sizes theoretically can detect statistically significant but very small effects that are of no clinical relevance.

9   Hierarchy of Evidence

Fundamental to evidence-based health care is the concept of "hierarchy of evidence" deriving from different study designs addressing a given research question (Fig. 4). Evidence grading is based on the idea that different designs vary in their susceptibility to bias and, therefore, in their ability to predict the true effectiveness of health care practices. For assessment of interventions, randomized controlled trials (RCTs) or systematic review of good quality RCTs are at the top of the evidence pyramid, followed by longitudinal cohort, case–control, cross-sectional studies and case series at the bottom [10]. However, the choice of the study design depends on the question at hand and the frequency of the disease. Intervention questions ideally are addressed with *experiments* (RCTs) since observational data are prone to unpredictable bias and confounding that only the randomization process will control. Appropriately designed RCTs allow also stronger causal inference for disease mechanisms.

Prognostic and etiologic questions are best addressed with *longitudinal cohort studies* in which exposure is measured first and participants are followed forward in time. At least two (and possibly more) waves of measurements over time are undertaken. Initial assessment of an input–output relationship may derive from *case–control studies* where the direction of the study is reversed.

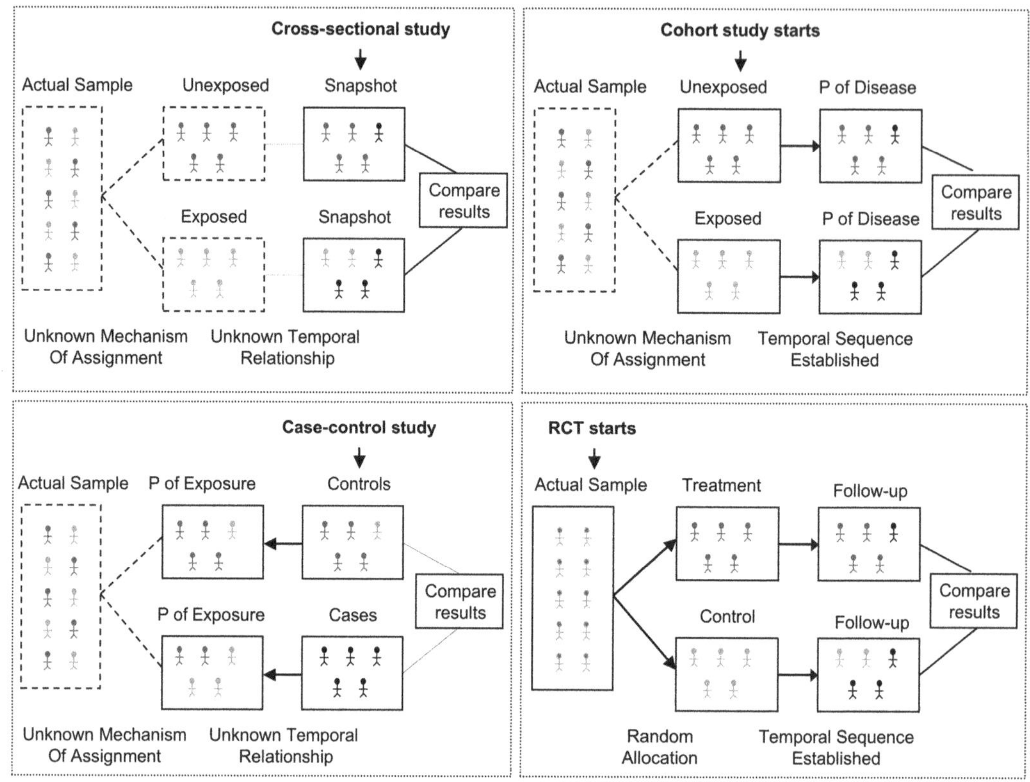

Fig. 4 Examples of study designs. In cross-sectional studies inputs and output are measured simultaneously and their relationship is assessed at a particular point in time. In case–control studies participants are identified based on presence or absence of the disease and the temporal direction of the inquiry is reversed (retrospective). Temporal sequences are better assessed in longitudinal cohort studies where exposure levels are measured first and participants are followed forward in time. The same occurs in randomized controlled trials (RCTs) where the assignment of the exposure is under the control of the researcher. With permission Ravani et al., Nephrol Dial Transpl [20]. *P* Probability (or risk)

Participants are identified by the presence or absence of disease and exposure is assessed retrospectively. *Cross-sectional studies* may be appropriate for an initial evaluation of the accuracy of new diagnostic tests as compared to a gold standard. Further assessments of diagnostic programs are performed with longitudinal studies (observational and experimental). Common biases afflicting observational designs are defined in Chapter 3 and discussed in more detail in Chapter 20.

10   Experimental Designs for Intervention Questions

The RCT design is appropriate for assessment of the clinical effects of drugs, procedures, or care processes, definition of target levels in risk factor modification (e.g., blood pressure, lipid levels, and proteinuria), and assessment of the impact of screening programs. Comparison to a placebo may be appropriate if no current standard therapy exists. When accepted therapies exist (e.g., statins as lipid-lowering agents, ACE-I for chronic kidney disease progression), then the comparison group is an "active" control group that receives usual or recommended therapy.

The most common type of RCT is the two group *parallel-arm* trial (Fig. 4). However, trials can compare any number of groups. In *factorial trials* at least two active therapies (A, B) and potentially their combination (AB) are compared to a control (C). Factorial designs can be efficient since more therapies are simultaneously tested in the same study. However, the efficiency and the appropriate sample size are affected by the impact of multiple testing on both type I and type II error, and whether there is an interaction between the effects of the therapies. In the absence of interaction, the effect of A, for example, can be determined by comparing A+AB to B+C. Interactions where use of A enhances the effectiveness of B, for example, do not reduce the power of the study. However, if there is antagonism between treatments, the sample size can be inadequate.

The *crossover design* is an alternative solution when the outcome is reversible [11]. In this design each participant serves as their own control by receiving each treatment in a randomly specified sequence. A washout period is used between treatments to prevent carryover of the effect of the first treatment to the subsequent periods. The design is efficient in that treatments are compared within individuals, reducing the variation due to subject differences. However, limitations include possible differential carryover (one of the treatments tends to have a longer effect once stopped); period effects (different response of disease to early versus later therapy); and a greater impact of missing data because they compromise within-subjects comparison and therefore variance reduction.

Finally, RCTs may attempt to show that one treatment is not inferior (under a one-sided hypothesis) or equivalent (under a two-sided hypothesis) rather than superior to a comparable intervention. In non-inferiority trials the null hypothesis of inferiority is rejected if the effect of an intervention lies within a certain prespecified non-inferiority margin. In equivalence trials the null hypothesis of non-equivalence is rejected if the effect of an intervention lies within two prespecified margins. These studies are often done when new agents are being added to a class (e.g., another ACE inhibitor), or when a new therapy is already known to be cheaper or safer than an existing standard. In such RCTs the study size is estimated based on a prespecified maximum difference that would still be considered irrelevant. For example, the claim might be made that a new ACE inhibitor is non-inferior to Enalapril, if the mean 24-h blood pressure difference between them was no more than 3 mmHg. Non-inferiority trials have been criticized, as imperfections in study execution, which tend to prevent detection of a difference between treatments, actually work in favor of a conclusion of non-inferiority. Thus, in distinction to the usual superiority trial, poorly done studies may lead to the desired outcome for the study sponsor.

11   Designs for Diagnostic Questions

When assessing a diagnostic test the reference or "gold standard" tests for the suspected target disorders are often either inaccessible to clinicians or avoided for reasons of cost or risk. Therefore, the relationship between more easily measured phenomena (patient history, physical and instrumental examination, and levels of constituents of body fluids and tissues) and the final diagnosis is an important subject of clinical research. Unfortunately, even the most promising diagnostic tests are never completely accurate.

Clinical implications of test results should ideally be assessed in four types of diagnostic studies. Table 4 shows examples from diagnostic studies of troponins in coronary syndromes. As a first step, one might compare test results among those known to have established disease to results from those free of disease. Cross-sectional studies can address this question (Fig. 4). However, since

Table 4

Level of evidence in diagnostic studies using troponin as test (T) and acute myocardial infarction (AMI) as target disorder (D)

Diagnostic question	Direction	Design	Problems	Example	Ref
Do D⁺ patients have different levels of T?	From D back to T	Cross-sectional	Reverse association Sampling bias	Difference in Troponin levels by AMI +/−	
Are patients T⁺ more likely to be D⁺?	From T to D	Cross-sectional	Effectiveness not assessed Sampling bias	Troponin performance in distinguishing AMI +/−	[12]
Does the level of T predict D⁺/⁻?	From T to D	Longitudinal	Missing data Sampling bias	Outcome study in subject at risk for AMI	[12]
Do tested patients have better final outcomes than similar patients who do not?	From T to D	Experiment	Missing data	Outcome (randomized) comparison in subject at risk for AMI	[14]

Positive (+); Negative (−). Missing data are possible in longitudinal or experimental designs: e.g., subjects lost before assessment or with data not interpretable. Strategies should be set up to (1) minimize the likelihood of missing information and (2) plan how subjects with missing information can be treated avoiding their exclusion (e.g., sensitivity analysis, propensity analysis) the direction of interpretation is from diagnosis back to the test, the results do not assess test performance. To examine test performance requires data on whether those with positive test results are more likely to have the disease than those with normal results [12]. When the test variable is not binary (i.e., when it can assume more than two values) it is possible to assess the trade-off between sensitivity and specificity at different test result cutoff points [13]. In these studies it is crucial to ensure independent blind assessment of results of the test being assessed and the gold standard to which it is compared, without the completion of either being contingent on results of the other.

Longitudinal studies are required to assess diagnostic tests aimed at predicting future prognosis or development of established disease [12]. The most stringent evaluation of a diagnostic test is to determine whether those tested have more rapid and accurate diagnosis, and as a result better health outcomes, than those not tested. The RCT design is the proper tool to answer this type of question [14].

12 Maximizing the Validity of Non-experimental Studies

When randomization is not feasible the knowledge of the most important sources of bias is important to increase the validity of any study. This may happen for a variety of reasons: when study participants cannot be assigned to intervention groups by chance either for ethical reasons (e.g., in a study of smoking) or participant willingness (e.g., comparing hemodialysis to peritoneal dialysis); the exposure is fixed (e.g., gender); or the disease is rare and participants cannot be enrolled in a timely manner. When strategies are in place to prevent bias, results of non-experimental studies may approach those of rigorous RCTs.

13 Reporting

Adequate reporting is critical to the proper interpretation and evaluation of any study results. Guidelines for reporting primary (CONSORT, STROBE, and STARD for example) and secondary studies (PRISMA) are in place to help both investigators and consumers of clinical research [15–18]. Scientific reports may not fully reflect how the investigators conducted their studies, but the quality of the scientific report is a reasonable marker for how the overall project was conducted. The interested reader is referred to the above referenced citations for more details of what to look for in reports from prognostic, diagnostic, and intervention studies.

References

1. Chertow GM, Moe SM (2005) Calcification or classification? J Am Soc Nephrol 16:293–295

2. Daugirdas JT, Depner TA, Gotch FA et al (1997) Comparison of methods to predict equilibrated Kt/V in the HEMO Pilot Study. Kidney Int 52:1395–1405

3. Wright JT Jr, Kusek JW, Toto RD et al (1996) Design and baseline characteristics of participants in the African American Study of Kidney Disease and Hypertension (AASK) Pilot Study. Control Clin Trials 17:3S–16S

4. Thorpe LE, Gwynn RC, Mandel-Ricci J et al (2006) Study design and participation rates of the New York City Health and Nutrition Examination Survey. Prev Chronic Dis 3:A94

5. Robbins JM, Vaccarino V, Zhang H, Kasl SV (2000) Excess type 2 diabetes in African-American women and men aged 40-74 and socioeconomic status: evidence from the Third National Health and Nutrition Examination Survey. J Epidemiol Community Health 54:839–845

6. Julious SA (2004) Sample sizes for clinical trials with normal data. Stat Med 23:1921–1986

7. Eknoyan G, Hostetter T, Bakris GL et al (2003) Proteinuria and other markers of chronic kidney disease: a position statement of the national kidney foundation (NKF) and the national institute of diabetes and digestive and kidney diseases (NIDDK). Am J Kidney Dis 42:617–622

8. Manns B, Owen WF Jr, Winkelmayer WC, Devereaux PJ, Tonelli M (2006) Surrogate markers in clinical studies: problems solved or created? Am J Kidney Dis 48:159–166

9. Viera AJ, Bangdiwala SI (2007) Eliminating bias in randomized controlled trials: importance of allocation concealment and masking. Fam Med 39:132–137

10. http://www.cebm.net/levels_of_evidence.asp. Accessed 23 Mar 2007

11. Sibbald B, Roberts C (1998) Understanding controlled trials: crossover trials. BMJ 316:1719

12. Antman EM, Grudzien C, Sacks DB (1995) Evaluation of a rapid bedside assay for detection of serum cardiac troponin T. JAMA 273:1279–1282

13. Sackett DL, Haynes RB, Guyatt GH, Tugwell P (1991) The interpretation of diagnostic data. In: Sackett DL, Haynes RB, Guyatt GH, Tugwell P (eds) Clinical Epidemiology: a basic science for clinical medicine. Little, Brown and Company, Toronto, CA, pp 117–119

14. Alp NJ, Bell JA, Shahi M (2001) A rapid troponin-I-based protocol for assessing acute chest pain. QJM 94:687–694

15. www.equator-network.org. Accessed 4 Apr 2014

16. http://www.consort-statement.org. Accessed 4 Apr 2014

17. http://www.strobe-statement.org. Accessed 4 Apr 2014

18. http://prisma-statement.org. Accessed 4 Apr 2014

19. Ravani P, Parfrey PS, Curtis B, Barrett BJ (2007) Clinical research of kidney diseases I: researchable questions and valid answers. Nephrol Dial Transplant 22:3681–3690

20. Ravani P, Parfrey PS, Dicks E, Barrett BJ (2007) Clinical research of kidney diseases II: problems of research design. Nephrol Dial Transplant 22:2785–2794

Chapter 2

Research Ethics for Clinical Researchers

John D. Harnett and Richard Neuman

Abstract

This chapter describes the history of the development of modern research ethics. The governance of research ethics is discussed and varies according to geographical location. However, the guidelines used for research ethics review are very similar across a wide variety of jurisdictions. The paramount importance of protecting the privacy and confidentiality of research participants is discussed at length. Particular emphasis is placed on the process of informed consent, and step-by-step practical guidelines are described. The issue of research in vulnerable populations is touched upon and guidelines are provided. Practical advice is provided for researchers to guide their interactions with research ethics boards. Issues related to scientific misconduct and research fraud are not dealt with in this paper.

Key words Ethics, Informed consent, Privacy, Confidentiality, Inclusiveness, Protection of human research participants, Vulnerable populations, Risk–benefit assessment, Tri Council Policy Statement (TCPS)

---

1 Research Ethics Development

One of the earliest guides for the ethical conduct of research on humans was provided by Virchow in the Berlin Code of 1900 [1]. The code outlined the requirement for informed consent, excluded participation of minors and those incompetent, and allowed research only under the direction of the institute's medical director. As with most codes for the ethical conduct of research, the Berlin Code arose from the public outcry over unethical research. In this case a "treatment" for syphilis, consisting of serum from "recovering" syphilis patients, was administered to prostitutes without their knowledge or consent resulting in the spread of syphilis among the prostitutes and their clients [1].

The Nuremberg Code (1949; [2]) was conceived by the prosecution as part of the case against physicians conducting "research" under the Nazi regime in Germany after World War II [3]. The Code describes the "legal, ethical and moral" basis on which research could be conducted in humans and served as the basis by which to decide whether research conducted by the

Patrick S. Parfrey and Brendan J. Barrett (eds.), *Clinical Epidemiology: Practice and Methods*, Methods in Molecular Biology, vol. 1281, DOI 10.1007/978-1-4939-2428-8_2, © Springer Science+Business Media New York 2015

defendants met an acceptable public standard. The Nuremberg Code became part of the verdict of the war crimes trial and was later signed by the 51 charter members of the United Nations [3]. An expanded document, the Helsinki Declaration, derived from the Nuremberg Code, but outlining in detail the conduct of acceptable biomedical research was approved by the World Medical Association in 1964 [4].

It should be understood that although the principles and conduct of human research had been to some extent codified, there remained no generalized requirement for mandatory ethical review for research on humans. No systematic process was in place to ensure independent and impartial review to judge whether a research project was ethically sound. It was simply left to the investigator to see that the research was designed and executed in an acceptable manner. However, landmark publications by Pappworth (1965; [5]) and Beecher (1966; [6]) documented numerous studies in the UK and the USA that failed to meet such standards. Standards of consent and protection of vulnerable populations were repeatedly violated in the most egregious manner. Beecher felt that ethical conduct should not be decided by a board or panel, but instead was the responsibility of the investigator. However, public awareness and outrage over the Tuskegee study led to an outcry for action that went beyond the investigator [7]. The Tuskegee study, which started in 1930 and continued until its termination in 1972, employed deception, enticement, and unwarranted medical invasiveness while following the natural course of syphilis in 400 African American males who were consciously denied access to medical treatment. Despite concerns raised within the US Public Health Service, review by the Center for Disease Control in 1969 allowed the study to continue. The unethical conduct in human research documented by Beecher and revealed in the Tuskegee study led to passage of the National Research Act in 1974 [8] which institutionalized mandatory ethical review for all biomedical and behavioral research on humans and set the stage for the Belmont Report [8].

Unlike the previous ethical codes, the Belmont Report (1979; [8]) established a set of ethical principles underpinning the regulatory framework for research on humans. The principles are Respect for Persons, Beneficence, and Justice. Respect for Persons recognizes that humans are autonomous agents and as such must give informed consent to participate in research. Moreover, their privacy must be respected and whatever data is collected from their participation must be held in a confidential manner. Members of vulnerable populations, e.g., children and the institutionalized, require additional measures to ensure their protection. Humans must not be considered the means to an end, i.e., the generation of research results. Beneficence obligates the investigator to design research so as to maximize the benefits and minimize harms. For each study the risks and the benefits must be evaluated and risks must be justified by potential benefits. Justice requires the fair treatment of participants. Those who are likely to share in the potential benefits of the research should equally share in the risks. Vulnerability should not be exploited to provide a pool of research participants, nor should vulnerability exclude a group that might benefit from the research. It is important to appreciate that a particular research design may bring these principles into conflict and that no principle trumps another in the ethical review process.

2   Governance

Ensuring an unbiased evaluation of ethical acceptability requires a governance structure that minimizes real and perceived conflicts of interest by the investigator, the institution, and members of the ethics review committee. Human participants are the means by which research results are generated and as such may be exploited by: (1) the investigator interested in achieving financial gain or career advancement; (2) the institution which may gain status, overhead funding, or a share in patents and other intellectual property arising from the research enterprise; and (3) members of the review body which may have personal or financial interest in the research outcome. Unfortunately, examples of such exploitation at the level of the investigator, institution, and review committee are readily available.

Canadian Research Ethics Boards (Institutional Review Boards, US; Research Ethics Committees, UK) require members with scientific expertise commensurate with the research under review (unscientific research is by definition unethical), expertise in bioethics and relevant law, and representation by the community, the group that is the beneficiary of research in the widest sense. Review committees must follow nationally or internationally accepted regulations or guidelines for the conduct of human research, e.g., Good Clinical Practice [9], Tri-Council Policy Statement (TCPS; Canada; [10]), and Common Rule (US; [11]). As well, institutions must have policies in place to assure independence of the ethical review process. The ethics review body must have written policies and standard operating procedures outlining the detailed operations of the review process and supporting infrastructure and to ensure procedures for research oversight and continuing or ongoing ethical review are in place.

3   Privacy and Confidentiality

Research participates have a right to expect that their privacy will be protected and that data collected will be maintained in a confidential manner by the investigator and study personnel.

Clearly maximum protection is provided when data is collected anonymously, e.g., a survey is completed without disclosing personal information or demographic data that would allow identification of the participant. Collecting identifiable data should be justified in relation to the expected benefits of the study. Once collected the identifier should be coded and only the coded identifier should be stored with the data. The file containing identifiers should be stored in a password protected file or locked file cabinet in a locked room. Access to identifiers should be strictly limited to study personnel on a need to know basis. Retention of identifiable data should be limited in time consistent with institutional policies on research integrity. Long-term retention of such data requires justification. Assurance regarding protection of privacy and confidentiality should be outlined in the consent form or as part of the consent process. Moreover, when confidentiality cannot be maintained, as in a focus group setting, or when privacy is clearly compromised in those cases where facial photographs are published to describe a genetic or medical condition, this must be emphasized in the consent form.

Public concerns with issues of privacy and confidentiality have resulted in extensive legislation guiding the use and dissemination of personal information and in particular the use of personal health information [12]. Investigators and ethics review committees must be aware of this legislation and how it may impact research. Moreover, in many jurisdictions ethics review committees have the authority to grant approval for the use of personal health information in the absence of informed consent when such use can be justified by the nature of the research or the feasibility of obtaining consent is in question or poses additional risks.

4   Composition of a Research Ethics Board

GCP [9] outlines guidelines for the minimum required membership for a research ethics board. It states that the IRB/IEC should consist of a reasonable number of members, who collectively have the qualifications and experience to review and evaluate the science, medical aspects, and ethics of the proposed trial. It is recommended that the IRB/IEC should include:

1. At least five members.

2. At least one member whose primary area of interest is in a nonscientific area.

3. At least one member who is independent of the institution/ trial site.

5   How a Research Ethics Board Functions

As well as being aware of the composition of the REB, applicants should also have some appreciation as to how their local REB functions. Applications are screened by the cochairs and those considered to be of minimal risk are triaged for expedited review by one board member and cochair. If approval is recommended, this is brought to the full REB for ratification only. No further review occurs. If expedited review identifies important ethical issues, then the proposal goes to the full board for review.

In situations in which more than minimal risk is involved, the application goes to the full board for review. One member is assigned the task of detailed review and presentation. The primary reviewer receives the detailed protocol, if available. All members of the board read each application and all applications are discussed at the board meetings which in our institution occur every 2 weeks. Decisions are generally arrived at by consensus, although a vote is taken for the record. Questions are communicated to the researcher. In cases where resolution of the issues proves difficult, the researcher may be invited to present in person to the board. This is generally not required and the majority of applications are approved in a timely fashion. If a proposal is not approved, the researcher has the right of appeal to a duly constituted independent appeals committee.

6   Balancing Risks and Benefits

One of the most important tasks of a research ethics board is deciding if the benefits of a proposed research project outweigh potential risks. In situations where more than minimal risk is involved, more intense scrutiny of the research is required including a scholarly review of the proposed research. In Canada the TCPS defines minimal risk as "If potential subjects can reasonably be expected to regard the probability and magnitude of possible harms implied by participation in the research to be no greater than those encountered by the subject in those aspects of his or her everyday life that relate to the research then the research can be regarded as within the range of minimal risk."

Scholarly review is generally done in the setting of peer review. This poses significant logistical problems for research ethics boards. A true peer review process is time-consuming and could impede timely review and approval of research proposals. There are several approaches to this issue. In large institutions a separate peer review process may be in place. This does delay the timeframe of ethical review. Sometimes funding for the proposal is already secured and comments from a granting agency peer review panel may be available.

More commonly the research ethics board is sufficiently expert and diverse to provide a reasonable assessment of the scientific validity of a research proposal. This review is critically dependent on the quality and clarity of the submission provided by the researcher. Comments on scientific validity are often perceived by researchers as beyond the purview of a research ethics board. However, in situations where more than minimal risk is involved, a research ethics board has the obligation to assess the scientific validity of the proposed research.

A final decision on the risk–benefit ratio of a research proposal involves a review of the quality of the proposal, the likely side effects of the proposed intervention and the potential benefits to participants. Ultimately it is a judgment call of an appropriately constituted research ethics board. In situations where doubt arises, a formal presentation by the researcher to the ethics board may be helpful.

7   Informed Consent

Free and informed consent is a cornerstone of ethical research involving human subjects. It begins with the initial contact and must be sustained until the end of the involvement of the subjects in the research project. Free and informed consent is an iterative process whereby research subjects are informed in understandable terms about the details of the proposed research. While each organization is likely to have their own informed consent template a template developed in Newfoundland and Labrador in Canada [13] provides a practical guide to developing an informed consent document for a clinical trial and addresses the key important questions. This type of approach could easily be modified for other types of research designs.

What is a clinical trial?

This section should address how a clinical trial differs from normal clinical care. It should address the concept of randomization and the possible applicability of the results of the clinical trial to others with a clinical condition similar to the subjects.

Do I have to take part in this clinical trial?

This section needs to stress the voluntary nature of participation in a research project and an assurance of normal clinical care should the subject decide not to participate.

Will this trial help me?

For randomization to be ethical the response here has to be one indicating that benefit is uncertain.

Why is this trial being done?

This section should provide, in lay terms, the rationale for the research question.

What is being tested?

Has the intervention been approved by the appropriate regulatory authorities or is this trial a step towards that approval process. Has the intervention been tested in animals and what, in lay terms was found? Has the intervention been tested in humans? How many were studied and what was shown?

Why am I being asked to take part?

This should include a statement as to how a particular individual was flagged for possible inclusion in the study. This should provide an assurance to the potential participant that their autonomy and privacy has been protected during this process.

Who can take part in this trial?

This should clearly list the inclusion and exclusion criteria in understandable terms and must mirror those criteria outlined in the more detailed protocol.

How long will I be in the trial?

The research participant must be made aware of the overall duration of participation in the study. The amount of time involved in participating in trial activities must be explicitly stated.

How many people will take part in this trial?

Describe whether this is a single-center or multicenter study. If the latter is the case, indicate the number of local and overall participants.

How is this trial being done?

This section should provide a detailed but understandable description of the research methodology. This should include details of randomization and blinding as well as detailed description of what the experimental and control arms entail. Details regarding proposed blood and tissue collection should be described. Clearly describe anything involved in the trial which is not part of standard clinical care.

What about birth control and pregnancy?

Most organizations have standard wording addressing these issues. This should include what is known of the risks of the intervention and what birth control measures (for both the research subject and any sexual partners) are necessary for inclusion in the study. There will often be uncertainty about possible teratogenic effects or effects on breastfeeding babies. In the absence of information it should be assumed that the possibility of such effects exists and individuals should be advised appropriately.

Are there risks to the trial?

Possible adverse effects of the intervention should be listed and grouped according to frequency. Risks of any other procedures being performed as a result of participation in the study must be outlined (e.g., additional radiation exposure as a consequence of imaging procedures that are part of the study and would not be done if normal clinical care applied.) Occasionally certain questions on questionnaires may be distressing or uncomfortable for participants. Subjects should be given the option not to answer such questions. If certain questions have a high likelihood of causing distress, appropriate support services, such as counseling, need to be in place and should be referred to in this section.

Are there other choices?

It must be clearly stated that the subject does not have to participate in the trial and a description of what other treatments are available should be provided. It should also be stated that once enrolled in the trial simultaneous enrollment in another clinical trial is not permissible.

What are my responsibilities?

It is important to point out that research participants should comply with the research protocol, report any changes in health status and provide updated information on the use of other medications.

Can I be taken out of the trial without my consent?

Research participants can be removed from a trial at the discretion of the investigator if he/she feels they are not complying with instructions or if their continued participation is harmful because of side effects or deterioration in their health status. The participant must be informed of the reason for withdrawal from the trial in the event that this happens.

What about new information?

If new information becomes available that may affect the participant's health status or willingness to continue in the study, this must be discussed with the participant.

Will it cost me anything?

Information regarding costs to the participant of being in the trial must be discussed. Reimbursement for expenses may be available and the participant must be made aware of this. If payment of participants is planned, this must be outlined. Payments that constitute an inducement to participate or exposure to excessive risk are not allowed by research ethics boards. Provisions for payment for treatment of or compensation for research related injuries must be addressed in this section of the consent form. If information from the study results in a patented product of commercial value, the participant will not usually receive any financial benefit. This should be made clear to participants.

What about my right to privacy?

Research participants should be assured of privacy and confidentiality. Outside agencies may be privy to private and confidential information for the purposes of audit or licensing. They are expected to observe strict confidentiality when examining the data. The participant must be informed of who will have access to their data. The duration of data storage must be specified. In the case of clinical trials this is generally 25 years after completion of data collection. Details of how the data will be stored and what steps will be taken to ensure secure and confidential storage must be provided. Information on how confidentiality will be assured for any blood or tissue collected must be specifically addressed and will vary depending on the study objectives and the nature of the blood and tissue being stored.

What if I want to quit the study?

Explain the procedure for withdrawal to the participant. Not uncommonly data collected up to the point of withdrawal will be retained and may be used in data analysis to ensure validity of the study. If this is the case, this must be disclosed to the research participant. If the participant has already agreed to blood or tissue storage for future use, he/she must be given the option to withdraw or affirm such an agreement at this point.

What will happen to my sample after the trial is over?

If the sample is to be destroyed, this should be specified. If it is to be used for future research, the sample may be coded to allow future linkage or it may be anonymized in which case future linkage to the participant will not be possible. The participant must be informed and provide consent for either option. If genetic material is to be used for future research, the participant must be informed if the possibility of re-contact is involved and consent to same. The participant may also wish to specify the types of future research that he/she would consent to (e.g., an individual might consent to future use of their DNA for a specific disease and not necessarily for unrestricted use for any research purpose). Studies involving future use of research samples are normally considered sub-studies and require a separate consent form to be signed addressing the issues outlined here.

Declaration of financial interest: If the investigator has a financial interest in conducting the trial, this should be declared. If no financial interest is involved, this should be stated.

What about questions or problems?

If the participant has questions about the trial or has a medical concern, he/she should be provided with contact information for the local principal investigator and study co-coordinator. If a medical concern arises outside normal work hours, details of the process in place to contact help should be provided.

If the participant has questions about their rights or concerns with the way in which the study is being conducted, appropriate contact information should be provided. The contact in this case will vary in different jurisdictions. It will often be through the office of the research ethics board.

The signature page

The signature page should include a statement that the participant has had an ample opportunity to discuss the proposed research, that they understand the proposed research and have had their questions answered satisfactorily. It should indicate that they have been informed of who may access their research records and should indicate that they have the right to withdraw at any time subject to the conditions outlined in the consent form.

The form must be signed by the participant, an independent witness, the principal investigator and the individual who has performed the consent discussion (if not the principal investigator). The signature of the next of kin/legal guardian must be provided for certain types of research (e.g., research involving unemancipated minors and incompetent adults). If the consent form requires translation into another language, the signature of the translator is also required.

8 Inclusiveness in Research

Historically certain groups of individuals have been underrepresented and sometimes deliberately excluded from research. Such groups have included women, the elderly, children and incompetent adults. This list is not exhaustive and the reasons for exclusion of such groups are complex and varied and beyond the scope of this chapter. This issue has been specifically addressed by the Canadian TCPS in Section 5 [13] as follows:

> Where research is designed to survey a number of living research subjects because of their involvement in generic activities (e.g., in many areas of health research, or in some social science research such as studies of child poverty or of access to legal clinics) that are not specific to particular identifiable groups, researchers shall not exclude prospective or actual research subjects on the basis of such attributes as culture, religion, race, mental or physical disability, sexual orientation, ethnicity, sex or age, unless there is a valid reason for doing so.

This statement is based on the principle of distributive justice. Its premise is that it is unethical to exclude individuals from participation in potentially beneficial research. Obviously the protection of these individuals from harm by inclusion in research is equally important. Indeed because some of these groups include potentially vulnerable populations protection from harm and providing fully informed consent does present some unique challenges. For the purposes of this chapter we will confine discussion to two vulnerable groups commonly involved in research: children and incompetent adults.

Often in incompetent adults the incompetence is caused by the disease which requires study. In this case the research cannot be done in a less vulnerable population and the intervention under study may directly benefit participants and others with the same disease. Consent is usually obtained from a proxy in this case, usually the next of kin or legal guardian, who is expected to act in the best interest of the individual participant. When studying incompetent adults it is important to recognize and establish that there are many types of specific competencies. While the individual being studied may not be competent to understand all of the intricacies of the study and the informed consent process they may be perfectly competent to refuse a painful procedure (e.g., needle stick) as part of the study.

Research in adults may not be generalizable to children for a variety of biological, developmental and psychosocial reasons. Quite often the disease being studied is more prevalent in or exclusive to children. Again proxy consent is required for minors with the exception of emancipated minors. However, children beyond a certain age are capable of understanding many of the issues involved and should be involved in the informed consent process and asked to give assent to any proposed research. In certain cases during the course of a study children may reach the age where legal consent is possible. If not incompetent for other reasons, they should then be asked to sign the informed consent document on their own behalf.

9 Practical Tips for Researchers Applying to Research Ethics Boards

- Familiarize yourself with the research ethical guidelines that are used in your jurisdiction.

- Satisfy yourself that the research question is important and the research design is sound.

- Do not cut and paste from the protocol into the ethics application. Summarize the protocol so that it can be easily read by all members of the research ethics board. Remember in most jurisdictions one member of the board is assigned to read the entire protocol and summarize for the other members.

- Identify upfront what you think the ethical issues may be and present these in your application.

- If you have a particular concern, get some advice prior to submission from an appropriate member of the ethics board.

- Ensure that all sections on the form are complete and that the submission is signed.

- If the research requires a consent form, spend time on preparing it at a readable level. Most boards will index this against a certain educational level. Computer programs are available to assess readability level.

- Remember the primary function of the research ethics board is to protect human subjects involved in research. Boards have an ethical obligation to facilitate sound ethical research while fulfilling this function. Interpret any comments or questions from the board with these two concepts in mind.

References

1. http://artandersonmd.com/med_history.pdf
2. https://www.research.buffalo.edu/rsp/irb/forms/Nuremberg_Code.pdf
3. http://www.nccamwatch.org/research/human_guidelines.pdf
4. http://www.wma.net/en/30publications/10policies/b3/index.html
5. Pappworth MH (1967) Human guinea pigs: experimentation on man. Routledge, London
6. Beecher HK (1966) Ethics and clinical research. N Engl J Med 274:1354–1360
7. http://en.wikipedia.org/wiki/Tuskegee_Syphilis_Study
8. http://www.hhs.gov/ohrp/humansubjects/guidance/belmont.html
9. http://www.hc-sc.gc.ca/dhp-mps/prod-pharma/applic-demande/guide-ld/ich/effi-cac/e6-eng.php
10. http://www.pre.ethics.gc.ca/eng/policy-politique/initiatives/tcps2-eptc2/Default/
11. http://www.hhs.gov/ohrp/humansubjects/guidance/45cfr46.html
12. http://www.cihr-irsc.gc.ca/e/documents/et_pbp_nov05_sept2005_e.pdf
13. http://www.hrea.ca/forms.aspx (consent template and consent guidelines)

Chapter 3

Definitions of Bias in Clinical Research

Geoffrey Warden

Abstract

In this chapter a catalog of the various types of bias that can affect the validity of clinical epidemiologic studies is presented. The biases can be grouped into those associated with selection of subjects, misclassification or misinformation, and finally confounding. Definitions are provided for each type of bias listed.

Key words Bias, Definition, Selection, Misclassification, Misinformation, Confounding

1 Introduction

There are three main causes of inaccuracy in clinical epidemiologic research: random variation, confounding, and bias. Of the three causes, bias is the most easily controlled by the investigator and creates systematic errors that distort the measure of a study's true effect when left uncontrolled. Mcitten first classified biases into three broad categories: those that occur during the *selection* and grouping of study participants, the *misclassification* or *misinformation*, and *confounding* [1]. Later, Sackett catalogued 57 biases that can arise in analytical research and listed the likely stages at which bias were likely to occur [2]. Numerous forms of bias have been added to these original lists, making it challenging for investigators to recognize and describe the types of bias they are committing or witnessing. Here, 150 types of bias occurring in clinical and observational epidemiological research have been collected, categorized, and defined with the goal of providing investigators a quick and accessible reference.

First the general terms involving bias have been defined. Secondly, each type of bias has been categorized by the stage of research at which it is most likely to occur, listed alphabetically within each stage, and defined. Table 1 provides reference by stage

Patrick S. Parfrey and Brendan J. Barrett (eds.), *Clinical Epidemiology: Practice and Methods*, Methods in Molecular Biology, vol. 1281, DOI 10.1007/978-1-4939-2428-8_3, © Springer Science+Business Media New York 2015

Table 1
Classification of epidemiological biases by stage of research

General terms (pg 34–35)	
Bias	Non-differential bias
Confounding bias	*Random error*
Differential bias	Selection bias
Design bias	Systematic error
Information bias/misclassification bias	

Literature review and publications (pg 35)	
All's well literature bias	One-sided reference bias
Foreign language exclusion bias	Positive results bias
Hot stuff bias	Rhetoric bias
Literature search bias	

Designing the study and selecting the study sample (pg 35–40)	
Admission rate/Berkson's bias/referral bias	Non-simultaneous comparison bias
Allocation sequence bias	Overdiagnosis bias
Autopsy series bias	Popularity bias
Centripetal bias	Prevalence-incidence bias/Neyman bias
Channeling bias	Previous opinion bias
Consent bias	Procedure selection bias
Diagnostic access bias	Record linkage bias
Diagnostic purity bias	Referral filter bias
Diagnostic vogue bias	Response bias
Ecological fallacy/aggregation bias	Sample size bias
Exclusion bias	Sampling bias
Healthy worker bias/healthy worker effect	Stage bias
Immigrant bias	Self-selection bias
Inclusion control bias	Spectrum bias/case mixed bias
Lead-time bias	Starting time bias
Length bias	Susceptibility bias
Loss to follow-up bias/attrition bias	Survivor treatment selection bias
Membership bias	Solicitation sampling bias
Migration bias	Unacceptable disease bias/faking Good bias
Mimicry bias	Unmasking bias/detection signal bias
Misclassification bias	Volunteer bias
Missing clinical data bias	Will Rogers phenomenon/Will Rogers
Non-contemporaneous control bias	Withdrawal bias/dropout bias
Non-respondent bias	

Executing the intervention (pg 40–41)	
Bogus control bias	Contamination bias
Co-intervention bias	Performance bias/procedure bias
Compliance bias	Proficiency bias

Measuring exposures and outcomes (pg 41–45)	
Apprehension bias	Case definition bias
Attention bias/Hawthorne effect/observer effect	Competing death bias
Confirmation bias	Intraobserver variability bias

(continued)

**Table 1
(continued)**

Context bias	Juxtaposed scale bias
Culture bias	Laboratory data bias
Data capture error/data capture bias	Latency bias
Data entry bias	Obsequiousness bias
Data merging error	Observer bias
Detection bias/surveillance bias	Protopathic bias
Diagnostic suspicion bias	Positive satisfaction bias
Diagnostic review bias	Proxy respondent bias
End-aversion/central tendency bias	Questionnaire bias
End-digit preference bias	Recall bias
Expectation bias	Reporting bias
Exposure suspicion bias	Response fatigue bias
Faking bad bias	Review bias
Family history/family information bias	Scale format bias
Forced choice bias	Sensitive question/social desirability bias
Framing bias	Spatial bias
Hospital discharge bias	Substitution game bias
Incorporation bias	Test review bias
Indication bias	Therapeutic personality bias
Insensitive measure bias	Unacceptability bias
Instrument bias	Underlying cause bias/rumination bias
Interobserver variability bias	Yes-saying bias
Interview setting bias	
Interviewer bias	

Data analysis (pg 45–46)

Anchoring bias/Adjustment bias	Overmatching bias
Data dredging bias	Post-hoc significance bias
Distribution assumption bias	Repeated peeks bias
Enquiry unit bias	Regression to mean bias
Estimator bias	Scale degradation bias
Missing data bias/data completeness bias	Standard population bias
Multiple exposure bias	Treatment analysis bias
Non-random sampling bias	Verification bias/workup bias
Omitted-variable bias	Verification (differential) bias
Outlier handling/tidying-up bias	Verification (partial) bias

Interpretation and publication (pg 47)

Auxiliary hypothesis bias	Magnitude bias
Assumption bias	Mistaken identity bias
Cognitive dissonance bias	Significance bias
Correlation bias	Under-exhaustion bias
Generalization bias	
Interpretation bias	

of biases the investigator may be looking for. Examples have been given when it was thought that definitions did not provide an adequate depiction. Further examples of bias in genetic disease research are provided in Chapter 20.

To create this list of biases, a comprehensive literature search of numerous relevant medical databases (PubMed, EMBASE, The Cochrane Library, Biological Abstracts, Biomedical Reference Collection, CINAHL, Clinical Evidence) was performed using various combinations of the key words "bias," "clinical," "epidemiological," "medical," "error," "systematic error," "research," "outcome measurement," "study design," "confounding," and "methods." Sackett's original list was used to reference biases of analytical research [2]. Rodriguez's review was also used to encompass other forms of bias [3]. Additionally, Porta's "Dictionary of Epidemiology" and Gail's "Encyclopedia of Epidemiologic Methods" were used to shape some definitions [4, 5]. Reference lists of relevant papers were also surveyed to identify additional literature on individual biases. This list of bias may not be complete, but it is an attempt to comprehensively define the majority of biases an investigator will encounter in epidemiologic research.

2   General Terms

Bias: When a systematic error of study design distorts the true effect of the variable under study.

Confounding bias: When a separate variable, with non-intermediate relationship between exposure and outcome, is disproportionally distributed between exposure and control groups and causes a distortion of the true effect of the variable under study. A confounder must be: (1) associated with the exposure in the target population, (2) a causal risk factor for the outcome in the unexposed cohort, (3) and not be an intermediate cause between exposure and outcome.

Differential bias: When a bias unequally affects comparison groups so that the final measurements or outcomes, and the comparison between groups, are both a biased result.

Design bias: When the methodological architecture of a study creates a positive or negative distortion of the study effect.

Information bias/misclassification bias: When a systematic error in the measurement of exposures, outcomes, or covariates, results in information quality discrepancies between comparison groups and distorts the true effect of the variable under study.

Non-differential bias: When a bias affects both comparison groups in an equal manner so that although the final measure is a biased result, the comparison between groups remains unbiased.

Random error: When a study error is due to chance variability and fluctuation of observation and measurement.

Selection bias: When the methods used to select the sample population result in a favoring of a comparison group over another, or neglect a significant proportion of the target population.

Systematic error: When study error is inherent of a system's design and causes repeated inaccuracies of observation and measurement.

3   Biases Associated with Literature Review and Publications

All's well literature bias: When scientific groups publish reports that omit controversial or opposing results.

Foreign language exclusion bias: When foreign language research is less often published or recognized.

Hot stuff bias: When scientific literature is published based on the popularity and excitement around a topic and not the credibility or quality of research.

Literature search bias: When a publication or statement is derived from an incomplete search and review of a topic's literature.

One-sided reference bias: When an investigator or author restricts referenced information to only those publications that support their position.

Positive results bias: When positive results of topic become more frequently published negative results and bias an overall consensus.

Rhetoric bias: When persuasive speech or writing is used to sway a reader's interpretation of data to coincide with the author's interpretation or position.

4   Biases Associated with Study Design and Subject Selection

Admission rate/Berkson's bias/referral bias: When the relationship between exposure and disease is distorted by the selection of study participants from hospitals with inflated admission rates due to the study of the disease at said hospital. Patients in hospitals studying disease will have a higher exposure rate when compared to controls, which may inaccurately define the relationship between the exposure and disease during analysis.

Allocation sequence bias: When the intervention allocation sequence is not concealed to investigators and introduces an intentional or unintentional selection bias.

Autopsy series bias: When disease rates and inferences are derived from a non-random autopsy series sample that does not represent the true population.

Centripetal bias: When incidence and prevalence rates are inflated by the draw of clinician or institution reputation for working with a specific disorder.

Channeling bias: When investigators channel patients who are more likely to have a treatment response to the intervention group rather than the control group.

Consent bias: When a study's sample population does not represent its target population due to systematic differences between consenting and non-consenting patients.

Diagnostic access bias: When the accessibly to diagnostic testing results in the overestimation or underestimation of disease prevalence or incidence rates.

Diagnostic purity bias: When the target population is no longer represented due to the selection of an unrealistic "pure" diagnostic group without the clinical comorbidities seen in the target population.

Diagnostic vogue bias: When a disease receives different diagnostic labels at different points in space or time resulting in the misclassification or exclusion of study participants from the target population.

Ecological fallacy/aggregation bias: When an effect or relationship on an aggregate level is applied to an individual level where it no longer holds true.

Exclusion bias: When eligibility criteria for participant inclusion into a study are applied differently to cases and controls.

Healthy worker bias/healthy worker effect: When the sample population derived from healthy volunteering participants no longer represents the target population. Those who are able to actively participate in a study have shown to be generally healthier and more compliant to study design than those unable or unwilling to participate.

Immigrant bias: When immigrant populations experience different health outcomes than the native population. Immigrants have sometimes been shown to experience better health outcomes. This phenomenon may be due to only those healthy enough to work immigrate to a new population. It may also be due to immigrants returning home when they fall ill and thus shifting the morbidity. Another theory is that an underreporting of disease and inaccessible health care system causes the phenomenon. Regardless of the causality, it is important to ensure that immigrant populations are well represented and equally distributed in study groups.

Inclusion control bias: When the inclusion criteria for controls are associated with the exposure, and a higher than expected rate of disease or outcome in the reference group creates a bias towards the null.

Lead-time bias: When participant survival time is overestimated due to earlier diagnosis of Disease screening can appear to increase survival by providing an earlier diagnosis when compared to no screening. However, earlier diagnosis only creates a greater time interval between diagnosis and death. Without an effective intervention the age of death is often unchanged and only the time interval off known disease diagnosis has increased.

Length bias: When rapidly progressing cases of disease are missed by screening and therefore disproportionately represented when compared to slowly progressing cases of disease. Disease detection is directly proportional to the length of time a disease is in a detectable stage therefore slowly progressing cases are more easily identified by screening.

Loss to follow-up bias/attrition bias: When systematic differences between comparison groups, such as neglectful observation in control groups, cause an uneven loss or withdrawals of participants from one group over another. Those who are lost to follow-up may be more or less likely to develop the outcome of interest and the true relationship between intervention and outcome may be distorted.

Membership bias: When membership in a particular group corresponds with a level of health that is different from others in the target population.

Migration bias: When disease rates are misrepresented due to the migration patterns of those with disease. For example, those with severe seasonal allergies may be more inclined to move away from a rural and country environment and seek refuge in a less pollen rich urban area. This migration could create a surprisingly high prevalence rate of seasonal allergies in an urban setting.

Mimicry bias: When an exposure causes a benign disorder resembling the disease and subsequently becomes suspect of causing the disease. Disease status may be misclassified in their disease status causing investigators to find inaccurate associations between exposure and disease.

Misclassification bias. (Type I) **Non-differential misclassification** is when all classes, groups, or categories of a variable have the same rate of being misclassified for all study participants. (Type II) **Differential misclassification** is when the rate of being misclassified differs between groups of the study.

Missing clinical data bias. When the misclassification of study participants is due to missing or unrecorded clinical data.

Non-contemporaneous control bias. When controls are sampled at a different time period and are no longer comparable to the current sample population due to changes in definitions, exposures, diagnoses, diseases and treatments.

Non-respondent bias. When non-respondents systematically differ from respondents and the sample population is no longer representative of the target population.

Non-simultaneous comparison bias. When exposure/intervention groups are compared to controls or reference standards in a different time and space. Different variables surrounding the time or space when groups are examined may influence the outcomes and cause poor generalizability.

Overdiagnosis bias. When pseudo or subclinical disease, that would not have become apparent before the patient dies of other causes, is diagnosed based on investigator exploration.

Popularity bias. When an interest in a particular disease or therapy causes preferential exposure of patients to observation or procedures.

Prevalence-incidence bias/Neyman bias. When study participants are incorrectly put into the unexposed group due to short or silent evidence of exposure prior to disease.

Previous opinion bias. When a prior diagnostic result affects the subsequent diagnostic process of a patient.

Procedure selection bias. When patients with poor risks are preferentially offered clinical procedures.

Record linkage bias. When those who are not within in a linked database are not represented in the sample population.

Referral filter bias. When an inflated prevalence of rare disease is due to patient referral to a center with a higher level of care.

Response bias. When a study's response rate and participant uptake is not large enough to accurately represent the target population.

Sample size bias. When studies are designed with sample sizes that are too small to ensure that results are not a product of random variability.

Sampling bias: When all members of the target population do not have the same probability of inclusion in the sample population of the study.

Stage bias: When varying methods for determining the stage of disease are used across different geographical areas and time are spuriously used to compare different patient population survival rates.

Self-selection bias: When a proportion of the target population is missed due to the sample population being created from participants deciding whether or not they want to participate in the study.

Spectrum bias/case mixed bias: When the accuracy of a diagnostic test is assessed in a population that differs from the target or clinically relevant population.

Starting time bias: When the inability to use a common starting time for exposure or disease causes the misclassification of exposure or disease status in study participants.

Susceptibility bias: When an exposure causes two separate diseases that precede one another and the treatment of the first disease falsely appears to cause the second disease. Susceptibility bias is a form of confounding.

Survivor treatment selection bias: When an ineffective treatment appears to prolong survival; however, the benefit is due to patients who live longer having more time to select another effective treatment, while those who die earlier are untreated by default.

Solicitation sampling (telephone/e-mail/door-to-door) bias: When a sample population is recruited by a method that is not accessible to a proportion of the target population.

Unacceptable disease or exposure bias/faking good bias: When socially unacceptable diseases or exposures are underreported by participants and investigators and cause misclassification of study participants.

Unmasking bias/detection signal bias: When an otherwise innocent exposure causes a sign or symptom of a disease and precipitates a search for said disease. A well-known example is that menopausal women administered estrogen for hormone replacement therapy experience some associated bleeding which leads to the investigation and potential endometrial cancer detection. When a group of those receiving estrogen is compared to women not receiving estrogen, the diagnosis of subclinical endometrial cancer in the non-estrogen group is delayed and one may interpret that the estrogen caused or lead to a more aggressive form of endometrial cancer.

Volunteer bias: When a sample population does not represent the target population due to volunteer participants exhibiting properties that systematically differ from non-volunteers. This bias is often prevalent in studies that exhibit high participant refusal rates. Studies with refusal rates >20 % should be shown that the volunteering participants do not differ greatly from the refusals.

Will Rogers phenomenon/ Will Rogers bias: When moving a patient from one group to another group raises the average values of both groups. Named after the social commenter, Rogers joked, "When the Okies left Oklahoma and moved to California, they raised the average intelligence in both states." This type of bias occurs when diagnostic ability increases, or disease criteria widens, and previously disease negative patients are classified as disease positive status. Previously subclinical patients were sicker than average healthy individuals; however, they have a better prognosis than the previous disease positive population. Therefore the new inclusion of an early stage disease in the disease positive status group creates a better overall prognosis for both the new positive and negative disease status groups. This phenomenon is most often seen in the new diagnostic tools and criteria of cancer staging as patients move from one stage to another.

Withdrawal bias/ dropout bias: When participants who have withdrawn from a study significantly differ from those who remain. This may cause two different problems with a study. Firstly, an equal withdrawal rate between comparison groups may mean the target population is no longer represented and create clinically irrelevant results; secondly, an unequal withdrawal rate between groups may create an inaccurate comparison from the loss of clinically relevant outcomes in the withdrawals.

5 Biases Associated with Executing the Intervention

Bogus control bias: When the intervention group falsely appears superior due to the reallocation of participants with negative outcomes to the control group.

Co-intervention bias: When the study effect is distorted by comparison groups unequally receiving an additional and unaccounted intervention.

Compliance bias: When non-significant results are due to poor participant adherence to the interventional regime, rather than inadequacy of the intervention.

Contamination bias: When members of the control group inadvertently receive the experimental intervention. For example, if a participant in the placebo-control group were to receive the new medication under study from investigators or another study participant.

Performance bias/procedure bias: When factors within the experimental regime, other than the intervention under study, are systematically employed differently between comparison groups. The maintenance of blinding helps ensure that both groups receive an equal amount of attention, treatment and investigations.

Proficiency bias: When the intervention under study is unequally applied to groups due to differences in resources or the administration of the intervention. This type of bias may occur when there are a number of people administering the intervention at multiple sites. To reduce proficiency bias, it is essential to create clear and efficient methodology for intervention administration.

6 Biases Associated with Measuring Exposures and Outcomes

Apprehension bias: When participant apprehension causes measurements to be altered from their usual levels. A classic example of this phenomenon is known as "White coat syndrome." This common syndrome refers to the elevation patient blood pressure due to the apprehension and nervousness patients feel from a physician's presence. Often a patient's blood pressure will be greatly reduced if they record it themselves at home.

Attention bias/Hawthorne effect/observer effect: When participants alter their natural response or behavior due to investigator observation. Usually people are more likely to give a favorable response or perform better due to their awareness of their involvement in a study and attention received during the study.

Case definition bias: When uncertainty of the exact case definition leads to subjective interpretation by investigators.

Competing death bias: When an exposure is falsely credited with the outcome of death over the causative and competing exposure. This most commonly seen during investigations of disease outcomes in geriatric populations as the increased age and comorbidities create a high competing risk of death.

Confirmation bias: When investigators favor data, outcomes, or results that reaffirm their own hypotheses.

Context bias: When investigators diagnose a participant with disease based on prior knowledge of disease in the population under study, despite test results that are only marginal or suggestive of disease. Examples of context bias often occur in radiology. A radiologist working in Africa is more likely to diagnose tuberculosis than an oncology center radiologist who identifies a cancer from the same abnormality on chest x-ray.

Culture bias: When populations derived from separate cultures experience different outcomes under the same intervention or exposure.

Data capture error/data capture bias: When a recurrent systematic error in the recording of data influences the outcomes and results. Data capture error can result in data collected being equally misrepresentative between groups and create clinically irrelevant results, while data capture bias infers that the data capture errors are favoring or disfavoring the outcomes for one particular group more than the other.

Data entry bias: When the process of converting raw data into a database results in a favorable outcome for either comparison group.

Data merging bias: When the process of merging data results in a favorable outcome for either comparison group.

Detection bias/surveillance bias: When exposure, or knowledge of exposure, influences the diagnosis of disease or detection of an outcome.

Diagnostic suspicion bias: When the intensity or outcome of the diagnostic process is influenced by a prior knowledge of participant exposure status.

Diagnostic review bias: When the interpretation of the reference diagnostic standard is made with knowledge of the results of the diagnostic test under study.

End-aversion/end of scale/central tendency bias: When questionnaire respondents avoid the ends of answer scales in surveys. Most respondents will report more conservatively and answer closer to the middle of a scale.

End-digit preference bias: When observers record terminal digits with increased frequency while converting analog to digital data. A common example is that investigators, nurses, and clinicians prefer to record blood pressures, temperatures, respiratory and heart rates that end in rounded numbers when assessing a patient's vital signs.

Expectation bias: When investigators systematically measure or record observations that concur with their prior expectations.

Exposure suspicion bias: When knowledge of the patient's disease status influences both the intensity and outcome of a search for exposure.

Faking bad bias: When patients try to appear sicker to qualify for supports or study inclusion.

Family history/family information bias: When knowledge of family member exposure or disease status stimulates a search and reveals a new case within the family. This bias causes increased prevalence rates when compared to families without a stimulated search.

Forced choice bias: When study participants are forced to choose predetermined yes or no outcomes without a non-response or undecided option available.

Framing bias: When a participant's response influenced by the wording or framing of a survey question.

Hospital discharge bias: When hospital mortality and morbidity rates are distorted by the health status of patients being transferred between facilities. Some hospitals may discharge patients more frequently or earlier in the disease course and shift the mortality and morbidity to other facilities.

Incorporation bias: When the incorporation of the disease outcome or aspects of diagnostic criteria into the test itself inflate the diagnostic accuracy of a test under study.

Indication bias: When early or preventative treatment in high-risk individuals is falsely credited with causation of disease.

Insensitive measure bias: When outcome measures are incapable of detecting clinically significant changes or differences. Insensitive measure biases often cause a type II error; a statistically significant difference between groups existed however the study was unable to prove the difference.

Instrument bias: When defects in the calibration or maintenance of instruments cause systematic deviations in the measurement of values.

Interobserver Variability bias: When multiple observers produce varying measurements of the same material. Different observers may be more likely to record differing measurements due to occurrences such as "end-digit bias". In order to decrease interobserver variability it is important to have strict measurement criteria that are easy to follow by a number of observers.

Interview setting bias: When the environment in which an interview takes place has an influence on participant response.

Interviewer bias: When an interviewer either subconsciously or consciously gathers selective data during the interview process.

Intraobserver Variability bias: When an observer produces varying measurements on multiple observations of the same material.

Juxtaposed scale bias: When different responses are given to the same item asked on multiple and different self-response scales.

Laboratory data bias: When a systematic error affects all laboratory results. This can be analyzed and confirmed by inter-laboratory comparisons.

Latency bias: When the outcome is measured in a time interval that is too brief for it to occur.

Obsequiousness bias: When participants alter questionnaire responses in the direction they perceive the investigator desires.

Observer bias: When observers have prior knowledge of participant intervention or exposure and are more likely to monitor outcomes or side effects in these participants.

Protopathic bias: When the treatment of early or subclinical disease symptoms erroneously appears to cause the outcome or disease.

Positive satisfaction bias: When participants tend to give positive answers when answering questions in regards to satisfaction.

Proxy respondent bias: When a participant proxy, such as a family member, produces a different response than the study participant would himself or herself.

Questionnaire bias: When survey or questionnaire format influences respondents to answer in a systematic way.

Recall bias: When a systematic error in participant questioning causes differences in the recall of past events or experiences between comparison groups. Recall bias most often occurs in case-control studies when questions about a particular exposure are asked several times to participants with disease but only once to controls.

Reporting bias: When study participants selectively reveal or suppress information to investigators.

Response fatigue bias: When respondents fatigue towards the end of an intervention or survey and become biased to either not finish or respond one-sided manner.

Review bias: When prior knowledge or a lack of blinding influences investigators to make subjective interpretations.

Scale format bias: When response scales are formatted to be an even or odd number of responses. Even scales force the respondent to choose a positive or negative response. Odd scales favor neural responses.

Sensitive question/social desirability bias: When socially sensitive questions elicit socially desirable responses rather than a participant's true belief.

Spatial bias: When spatially differing populations are presented and or represented as a singular entity.

Substitution game bias: When investigators substitute a risk factor that has not been established as causal for an associated outcome.

Test review bias: When the interpretation of a diagnostic test is made with knowledge of the diagnostic reference standard test result of the same material.

Therapeutic personality bias: When an un-blinded investigator's conviction about the efficacy of a treatment influences a patient's perception of the treatment benefit.

Unacceptability bias: When measurements are systematically refused or evaded because they embarrass or invade the privacy of participants.

Underlying cause bias/rumination bias: When cases and controls exhibit differing ability to recall prior exposures due to the time spent by cases ruminating about possible causes of their disease.

Yes-saying bias: When respondents more often agree with a statement than disagree with its opposite statement. Also used to define when survey participants repetitively respond positively without reading the questions after the first few positive responses.

7 Biases Associated with Data Analysis

Anchoring bias/adjustment bias: When an investigator either subconsciously or consciously adjusts the initial reference point so that the result may reach their estimate hypothesis.

Data dredging bias: When investigators review the data for all possible associations without prior hypothesis. This "shotgun approach" to analyses increases the risk of a statistically significant result that has occurred by chance. Type 1 error.

Distribution assumption bias: When the investigator inappropriately applies a statistical test under the incorrect assumption of the data distribution. Many statistical tests require that the data represent a "normal distribution" and should not be applied when this is not the case.

Enquiry unit bias: When the choice of the unit of enquiry affects the analysis, results and impression. For example one could state that 70 % of hospitals do not offer dialysis; however, if the patient becomes the unit of enquiry, the applicable statement could be only 3 % of patients cannot receive dialysis treatment at their hospital.

Estimator bias: When a large difference between an estimator's value and the true value of the parameter occurs. For example, the odds ratio will always overestimate the relative risk.

Missing data bias/handling data/data completeness bias: When data analysis occurs after a systematic loss of data from one of the comparison groups.

Multiple exposure bias: When multiple exposures are responsible for the magnitude of an outcome without being their individual effect being weighted.

Non-random sampling bias: When statistical methods requiring randomly sampled groups are applied to non-random samples.

Omitted-variable bias: When one or more important causal factors are left out of a regression model resulting in an overestimation or underestimation of the other factors effect within the model.

Outlier handling/tidying-up bias: When the exclusion of outliers or unusual results from the analysis cannot be justified on statistical grounds.

Overmatching bias: When comparison groups are matched by non-confounding variables that are only associated with exposure, and not disease.

Post-hoc significance bias: When decision levels of statistical significance are selected during the analysis phase to show positive results.

Repeated peeks bias: When investigators continuously monitor ongoing results and discontinue their study when random variability has shown a temporarily positive result.

Regression to mean bias: When random variability accounts for the majority of a study's significant result and follow-up investigations are found to have less or non-significant results.

Scale degradation bias: When clinical data or outcomes are collapsed into less precise scales which obscure differences between comparison groups.

Standard population bias: When the choice of standard population affects the estimation of standardization rates.

Treatment analysis bias/lack of intention to treat analysis: When study participants are analyzed based on the treatment they received rather than the treatment that they were allocated to during randomization.

Verification bias/workup bias: When the selective referral, workup, or disease verification leads to a biased sample of patients and inflates the accuracy of a diagnostic test under study.

Verification bias: When prior test results are verified by two different reference standards dependent on a positive or negative index test result. The reference standard used for verification of positive results is usually more invasive and therefore not used in patients unlikely to be diagnosed with disease.

8 Biases Associated with Interpretation and Publication

Auxiliary Hypothesis bias: When an ad hoc hypothesis is added to compensate for anomalies not anticipated by the original hypothesis. Often this will be done so that the investigator can state that had experimental conditions been different the original theory would have held true.

Assumption bias: When an audience assumes that the conclusions of a study are valid because they have been published or are presented to them by a speaker, without confirming that statements are accurate and coincide with corresponding data and references.

Cognitive dissonance bias: When an investigator states their belief despite the contradictory evidence of their results.

Correlation bias: When correlation is equated to causation without sufficient evidence. Hill's criteria is often used to show evidence for causation and is defined by nine aspects: (1) the strength of association; (2) the consistency of findings observed; (3) the specificity of a specific site and disease with no other likely explanation; (4) a temporal cause and effect; (5) a biological dose response gradient; (6) a plausible mechanism between cause and effect; (7) coherence of epidemiological and laboratory findings; (8) That effect and condition can be altered by an appropriate experimental regimen; (9) that there has been consideration of alternate explanations:

Generalization bias: When the author or reader inappropriately infer and apply a study's results to different or larger populations for which the results are no longer valid.

Interpretation bias: When the investigator or reader fails to draw the correct interpretations from the data and results achieved.

Magnitude bias: When the selection of the scale of measurement distorts the interpretation of the reader or investigator.

Mistaken identity bias: When strategies directed toward improving the patient's compliance causes the treating investigator to prescribe more vigorously and the effect of increased treatment is misinterpreted as compliance.

Significance bias: When statistical significance is confused with biological or clinical significance and leads to pointless studies and useless conclusions.

Under-exhaustion bias: When the failure to exhaust the hypothesis leads to authoritarian rather than authoritative interpretation.

References

1. Miettinen OS, Cook EF (1981) Confounding: essence and detection. Am J Epidemiol 114:593–603
2. Sackett DL (1979) Bias in analytic research. J Chronic Dis 32:51–68
3. Delgado-Rodríguez M, Llorca J (2004) Bias. J Epidemiol Community Health 58(8):635–641
4. Porta M (1988) A dictionary of epidemiology, 5th edn. Oxford University Press, New York, NY
5. Gail M, Benichou J (2000) Encyclopedia of epidemiologic methods. Wiley, West Sussex

Part II

Longitudinal Studies

Chapter 4

Longitudinal Studies 1: Determination of Risk

Sean W. Murphy

Abstract

Longitudinal or observational study designs are important methodologies to investigate potential associations that may not be amenable to randomized controlled trials. In many cases they may be performed using existing data and are often cost-effective ways of addressing important questions. The major disadvantage of observational studies is the potential for bias. The absence of randomization means that one can never be certain that unknown confounders are present, and specific studies designs have their own inherent forms of bias. Careful study design may minimize bias. Establishing casual association based on observational methods requires due consideration of the quality of the individual study and knowledge of their limitations.

Key words Longitudinal studies, Cohort study, Case–control study, Bias, Risk factors, Sample size estimate

1   Introduction

Randomized, controlled trials (RCTs) are indisputably the gold standard for assessing the effectiveness of therapeutic interventions and provide the strongest evidence of association between a specific factor and an outcome. In this age of evidence-based medicine, "grades of evidence" based on clinical study design universally reserve the highest grade for research that includes at least one RCT. The lowest level of evidence is given to expert opinion and descriptive studies (e.g., case series), and observational studies are considered intermediate levels.

Despite the strengths of an RCT, such a study design is not always feasible or appropriate. It is obvious that human subjects cannot ethically be randomized to exposure to a potentially noxious factor. In some cases, such as surgical versus medical treatments, alternative therapies for the same disease are so different that it is unlikely that patients would be indifferent to their choices to the degree that they will consent to randomization. Sometimes it is not possible to randomize exposure to a risk factor at all. Studies of the genetic contribution to a disease are a good example;

Patrick S. Parfrey and Brendan J. Barrett (eds.), *Clinical Epidemiology: Practice and Methods*, Methods in Molecular Biology, vol. 1281, DOI 10.1007/978-1-4939-2428-8_4, © Springer Science+Business Media New York 2015

subjects either have a family history of the outcome or not, and this cannot be altered. RCTs may not be technically feasible if the outcome is relatively rare or takes a long period of time to become evident. In such instances the sample size will need to be large or the follow-up period long. While it is not true that a RCT will always cost more than an observational study, in many instances a clinical question that requires a very large RCT may be addressed much more cost-effectively with an alternative study design. For these reasons and many others, non-RCT studies make up a large proportion of the published medical literature. Many important clinical questions will never be subjected to an RCT, and clinicians, researchers, and policy-makers must rely on alternative study designs to make decisions.

1.1 Non-randomized Study Designs

As a group, Non-RCT study designs are referred to as non-interventional or observational studies. The investigator does not actually interfere with the study subjects and seeks only to ascertain the presence or absence of either the risk factor or outcome of interest. Some observational designs, particularly cross-sectional studies, are best suited to determining disease prevalence and provide only weak evidence of risk factor and disease association. This focus of this chapter is on observational study designs aimed at providing stronger evidence of causal relationships, including treatment effect. These so-called longitudinal studies include case–control and cohort designs. The strengths and weakness of such designs are discussed, including the biases that may be inherent in each. The interpretation of results and technical issues such as sample size estimation are considered.

2 Cohort Studies

A cohort is a group of subjects, defined at a particular point in time, that shares a common experience. This common factor may be a simple demographic characteristic, such as being born in the same year or place, but it is more frequently a characteristic that is considered a potential risk factor for a given disease or outcome. A cohort is followed forward in time and subjects are evaluated for the occurrence of the outcome of interest.

Cohort studies are frequently employed to answer questions regarding disease prognosis. In this case, the common experience of the cohort is the presence of disease. In its simplest form, patients are enrolled in the study, followed prospectively, and the occurrence of specified symptoms or endpoints, such as death, are recorded. Because comparisons are not being made no control group is required. The data from such a study will be purely descriptive, but provides useful information regarding the natural history of that illness. More commonly researchers will be interested in making some type of comparison. In studies of prognosis, the question may be whether or not a given factor in patients with a disease influences the risk of an outcome such as mortality. In this instance two or more cohorts are assembled—all subjects have the disease of interest, but some have the risk factor under study and others do not. This permits an analysis of the risk attributable to that factor. The risk factor under consideration might be a given disease treatment, and non-randomized trials of therapeutic interventions are in fact cohort studies of prognosis.

Cohort studies are also commonly used to study the association of risk factors and the development of an outcome. In this case the defining characteristic of the cohort is the presence of or exposure to a specified risk factor. A second cohort that does not have the risk factor will serve as the control group. All subjects are followed forward in time and observed for the occurrence of the disease of interest. It is essential that the study and control cohorts are as similar as possible aside from the presence of the risk factor being investigated.

2.1 Types of Cohort Studies

Cohort studies are inherently prospective in that outcomes can only be assessed after exposure to the risk factor. This does not mean that researchers must necessarily begin a cohort study in the present and prospectively collect data. Another approach is to use existing records to define a cohort at some point in the past. Outcomes may then be ascertained, usually from existing records as well, but in some cases subjects or their relatives may be contacted to collect new data. This type of design is referred to as a "historical cohort" and is clearly useful when the outcome takes a long period of time to develop after the exposure. Alternatively, an "ambidirectional" approach may be used, i.e., the cohort may be defined in the past, records used to assess outcomes to the present day, and subjects followed prospectively into the future (Fig. 1).

2.2 Advantages of Cohort Studies

Cohort studies are often an effective way to circumvent many of the problems that make an RCT unfeasible. Potentially harmful risk factors may be ethically studied, as the investigators do not determine the exposure status of individuals at any point. Cohort studies are suitable for studying rare exposures. It is often possible to identify a group of individuals who have been subjected to an uncommon risk factor through occupational exposure or an accident, for instance. The historical cohort design is an excellent approach if there is a long latency period between exposure and outcome.

Cohort studies have an advantage in that multiple risk factors or multiple outcomes can be studied at the same time. This can be easily abused, however, and it is advisable that a single primary outcome be identified, for which the study is appropriately powered, and the remaining secondary outcomes be considered

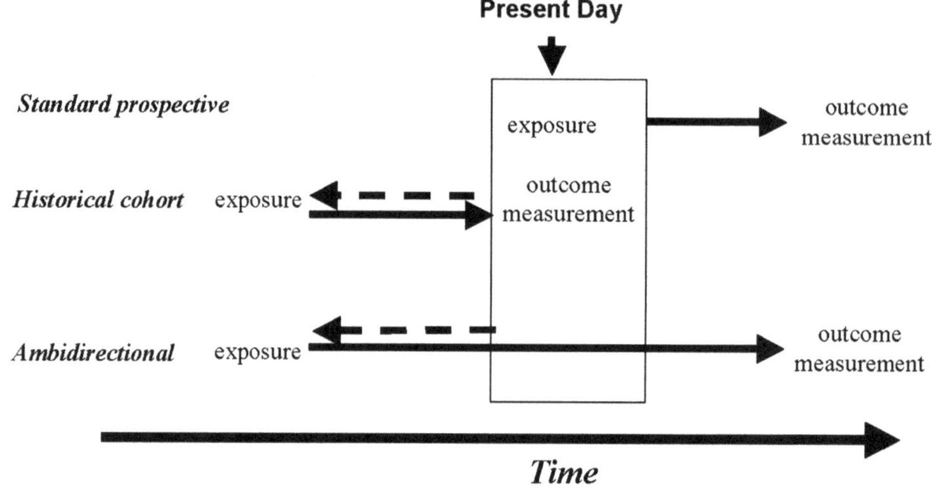

Fig. 1 Types of cohort studies

"hypothesis generating." Depending on the mode of analysis, cohort studies can generate a variety of risk measures, including relative risks (RR), hazard ratios (HR), and survival curves.

In the overall hierarchy of evidence, cohort studies are considered a relatively powerful design to assess the outcome risk associated with a given factor. Unlike a cross-sectional or case–control study, one can usually be certain that the temporal sequence is correct, i.e., exposure precedes outcome. Cohort studies are also less prone to the so-called survivor bias than other observational designs. Disease cases that are instantly or rapidly fatal will be not be sampled in a study that selects cases from a living population. If such patients were included in a cohort study, their deaths would be recorded.

2.3 Disadvantages of Cohort Studies

The cohort design may be used for studying rare diseases or outcomes, but this often necessitates a very large sample size, especially if researchers wish to make comparisons between groups.

2.3.1 Missing Data

A standard, prospective cohort study has the advantage that investigators can establish clear definitions of both the exposure and outcome and then collect all necessary data on subjects as they enroll in the study or meet endpoints. While detailed inclusion criteria and outcome definitions are also required for historical designs, problems may arise when the required data are ambiguous, suspicious, or missing altogether. Differential follow-up between compared groups may be a major problem. Losses to follow-up, whether it is due to study withdrawals, unmeasured outcomes, or unknown reasons are always a concern. This is particularly true when more outcome data is missing in one group than the other, as there is no way to be certain that the factor being studied is not somehow related to this observation.

2.3.2 Ascertainment Bias

The classification of exposed versus unexposed subjects is also critical. One may be confident of exposure status in some cases, e.g., using employment records to determine if an individual worked in a particular factory. For exposures such as smoking or dietary habits, however, reliance upon patient recollection or records not intended to be used for research purposes may lead to misclassification of that subject. In many cohort studies the outcome will also be ascertained through existing records. For objective endpoints such as death there is not likely to be any doubt as the time and certainty of the outcome. Outcomes such as the diagnosis of a specific disease are potentially more problematic. Clinical studies generally require very specific criteria to be fulfilled to diagnose disease outcomes to ensure internal validity. The application of such strict case definitions may not be possible based on past records. The accuracy of administrative databases and hospital discharge records for clinical disease diagnoses varies but may be insufficient for research use.

2.3.3 Contamination

In comparative cohort studies, treatment crossover may occur and is sometimes a substantial source of bias. Subjects initially unexposed to the risk factor of interest may become exposed at a later date. Such "contamination" will tend to reduce the observed effect of the risk factor. If the groups being compared consist of a given treatment versus no treatment or an alternate therapy, it is possible that some controls will start treatment or subjects may switch therapies. It is unlikely that such switches will occur for no reason, and it is possible that subjects not doing well with their current treatment will be the ones changing groups. This will tend to reduce the observed effect and bias the study towards the null hypothesis. Contamination of groups in a cohort study is best dealt with by prevention. This may not be possible, however, and once it has occurred it is not easily addressed in the analysis phase. The conventional approach is to analyze the data in an intention-to-treat fashion, i.e., subjects are analyzed in the group to which they were originally assigned, regardless of what occurred after that point. This method is the only way to eliminate the potential bias that the reason for treatment crossover, or loss to follow-up for that matter, is somehow associated with the outcome [1]. Given that it reduces observed risk, however, some researchers choose to additionally analyze in a "treatment-as-received" manner. A number of statistical methods, including Cox Proportional Hazard modeling and Poisson regression, are suitable for this approach. In the latter technique, rather than allowing a single subject to remain in only one group for analysis, the amount of "person-time" each subjects represents within a study is considered. An individual may therefore contribute person-time to one, two, or more comparison groups depending on whether or not they switched assigned risk factor groups. A major problem, however, is the assignment of outcomes to risk factor groups. Death, for example, can only occur once and is not necessarily attributable to the risk of the group that subject was in at the time that this occurred. Outcome assignment is therefore an arbitrary process and prone to bias in itself. When a treatment-as-received analysis is used, it is in the best interest of the investigator to present both this and the intention-to-treat results. If the results from the two analyses are concordant, there is no issue. When the two techniques five substantially different risk estimates, however, the reasons for the discordance need to be considered.

2.3.4 Selection Bias

Perhaps the largest threat to the internal validity of a cohort studies is selection bias, also called case-mix bias. The major advantage of a randomization is that variables other than the factor being studied, whether they are known to be confounders or not, are balanced between the comparison groups. In a cohort study subjects are assigned to exposure or control groups by themselves, the individuals treating them, or by nature. It is possible, if not probable, that the groups differ in other ways that have an effect of the outcome of interest. In a large cohort study of coffee consumption and coronary heart disease, for example, subjects who drank more coffee were much more likely to smoke, drank more alcohol on average, and were less likely to exercise or use vitamin supplements than subjects consuming lesser amounts [2]. These associated risk factors clearly have an effect on the probability of the outcome, and provide an example of a true confounder—the exposure and disease are not causal, but both are associated with other unmeasured risk factors. When confounders are suspected, they may be quantified and controlled for in the analysis phase. Unfortunately, many confounders will remain unknown to the researchers and will bias the results in an unpredictable manner.

Many variations of selection bias exist. Non-participation is a significant problem if subjects that choose to enroll in a study are not representative of the target population. The resulting risk estimates will not be an accurate reflection of the true exposure–outcome association because of this "response bias." Non-participants have been shown to be older [3], have more illness [3, 4], and less education [4, 5] than subjects who do enroll in clinical studies. Longitudinal genetic epidemiology studies are subject to response bias in often-unpredictable ways. Individuals who perceive themselves at very low risk of a disease, such as those without a family history of a given illness, are less likely to enroll in studies [6]. On the other hand, those that are at very high risk may not participate due to high anxiety regarding the outcome [7]. The subjects who do participate, therefore, may be at more moderate risk but not truly representative of the general population.

2.3.5 Bias by Indication

Bias by indication is another form of selection bias. This occurs when subjects are more likely to be exposed to a factor because they have a second attribute associated with the outcome. Aspirin, for example, may be incorrectly associated with a higher mortality risk if researchers do not account for the fact that individuals with established heart disease are more likely to be prescribed this drug.

2.3.6 Dose-
Targeting Bias

Cohort studies that are intended to compare treatment effect are prone to dose-targeting bias, where subjects who fail to achieve a particular target for treatment have more comorbidity than those who do [8]. It is unlikely that multivariate adjustment for known confounders will compensate for these differences because many of these adverse risk factors will not be known to the investigators.

3 Designing a Cohort Study

Once the researcher has developed a clear, concise question to address, the decision to use a standard prospective or a historical cohort design usually depends on the timelines of the hypothesized exposure–outcome process and the resources available. A historical cohort is only possible when researchers have access to complete records of sufficient quality.

As in a RCT, the investigators should decide on definitions of both the exposure or treatment of interest and the outcome to be measured a priori. It is important that those reading the study have a clear idea of what type of patient was sampled, and whether or not this information can be extrapolated to their own patient population, i.e., to be able to gauge the study's external validity.

3.1 Prevalent Versus Incident Cohorts

Cohort studies that are based on the presence of a fixed characteristic of the subjects, such as the presence of a disease, are performed using a prevalent cohort of subjects, an incident cohort of subjects, or a combination of the two. A prevalent cohort refers to a group of subjects that as of a specified date have that characteristic (e.g., all patients in a center with prostate cancer on January 1st in a specified year). An incident cohort consists of all patients who develop that characteristic within a specified time interval (e.g., all patients who are diagnosed with prostate cancer in a center from January 1st 2013 to December 31st, 2013). A combination of the two, referred to as a period prevalent cohort, may also be used. When a prevalent cohort is used there is a possibility that the onset of the disease or risk factor in one group may be significantly different in the two groups. If the risk of the outcome increases with time the group with the longer duration of exposure or disease will be disadvantaged. This is referred to as "onset bias" [9]. If the risk of the outcome is constant over time this bias may not be a factor, but many outcomes, most notably mortality rates, often increase as the study progresses. This bias may be present in a period prevalent cohort, so an incident cohort design is usually optimal. Unfortunately this option requires more time to accrue subjects and may not be feasible for this reason.

3.2 Data Collection

It is critical that subjects be classified correctly with respect to their exposure and outcome status. In a comparative cohort study, these factors must be measured in precisely the same way in all subjects to minimize the risk of the various forms of information bias. It is not acceptable, for example, to use hospital records to identify outcomes in the exposed group but rely on self-reporting of disease status in controls. Ideally, researchers determining the outcome status should not be aware of the exposure status of individuals so they are not influenced by this knowledge.

3.3 Confounding Variables

Careful study design can help minimize selection bias. Researchers should start by determining all known confounders that may be relevant to their proposed study. A careful review of the literature and consideration of plausible confounding associations may be all that one can do, but this will often result in variables that can be measured and accounted for in the analysis phase.

The anticipated presence of known confounders may be dealt with in a number of ways in the design phase. The investigators may choose to include only subjects that are similar with respect to that factor and exclude those that differ. This process, referred to as restriction, is an effective way to reduce selection bias but comes at a cost—reduced generalizability and a smaller pool of subjects from which to recruit. A second approach is to "match" the exposure groups. Subjects in compared groups are specifically chosen to have the same values for confounding variables, such as age or gender. While effective, matching does not account for unknown confounders and can become quite difficult in larger studies. Alternatively, the researcher may choose to stratify subjects by the confounding factor. Subjects that differ with respect to the confounder may all be included, but they will be analyzed separately. Essentially post-hoc restriction, this approach may improve external validity.

3.4 Selecting a Control Group

The optimal control group for a cohort study will be exactly the same as the study group with the exception of the factor being investigated. Importantly, both groups will have the same baseline risk of developing the outcome prior to the exposure. In all probability this type of control group does not exist, but the researcher must do his or her best to approximate this situation. The control group can be selected from internal or external sources. Internal sources are unexposed subjects from precisely the same time or place as the exposed subjects. For example, one might select workers in a factory who definitely were not exposed to a given chemical to compare to workers in the same factory who were exposed to this potential risk factor. This type of control group is preferred, as one can be fairly confident that these people were similar in many respects. If one could not find enough unexposed controls in that factory, however, researchers might have to select controls from a similar factory elsewhere. Such externally sourced control groups are less likely to be similar to the study patients. The least desirable option would be population-based controls. In this case the risk of the outcome in study subjects is compared to average rates observed in the general population. This is open to many biases, such as the possibility that subjects who work are healthier than those who cannot work (i.e., healthy worker bias).

4   Case–Control Studies

In a cohort study, researchers select subjects who are exposed to a risk factor and observe for occurrence of the outcome. In contrast, researchers performing a case–control study will select subjects with the outcome of interest (cases) and seeks to ascertain whether the exposure of interest has previously occurred (Fig. 2). The probability of exposure in the cases is compared with the probability of exposure in subjects who do not have the outcome (controls) and a risk estimate for that factor can be calculated. Case–control studies are inherently retrospective because knowledge of the outcome will always precede exposure data collection.

Case–control designs are only used to estimate the association of a risk factor with an outcome. Because they are retrospective, these types of studies fall below cohort studies in the hierarchy of medical evidence. It is sometimes not easy to establish the temporal sequence needed to infer a causal relationship. Nevertheless, case–control studies are an efficient and cost-effective method to answer many questions and are thus widely used.

4.1   Nested Case–Control Studies

Nested case–control studies are case–control studies performed on subjects identified during a cohort study. To illustrate this, consider the hypothesis that exposure to a certain trace metal may

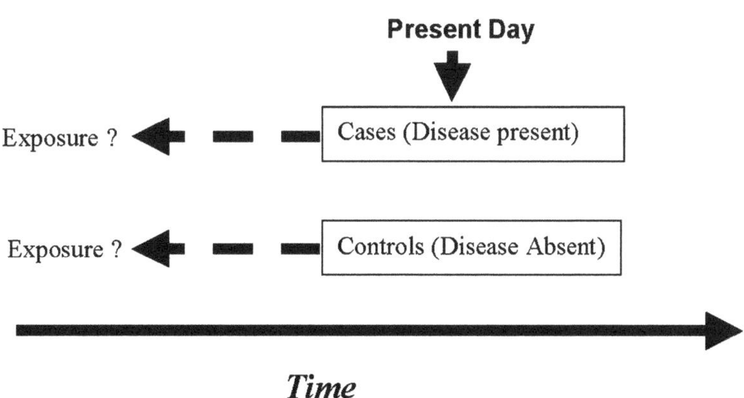

Fig. 2 Design of a case–control study

predispose children to a specific learning disability. To estimate the incidence of this problem, researchers may choose to enroll all school-aged children in a community in a cohort study and periodically test them to detect the disability. While it might be possible to measure blood levels of the metal on all subjects, this would likely be expensive and logistically difficult. Using a nested case–control study, however, the researchers would do the cohort study first and identify the subjects affected by the disability (the cases). They could then randomly choose matched unaffected controls from the remainder of the cohort. Blood levels of the metal may then be collected on the cases and controls and analyzed in a manner similar to a standard case–control study. This approach has the advantage of limiting the need for expensive or difficult risk factor ascertainment.

4.2 Advantages of Case–Control Studies

Case–control designs are often used when the outcome or disease being study is very rare or when there is a long latent period between the exposure and the outcome. A disease with only a few hundred cases identified worldwide, for instance, would require an impossibly large cohort study to identify risk factors. On the other hand, it would be entirely feasible to gather exposure data on the known cases and analyze it from this perspective.

Case–control studies make efficient use of a small number of cases. Additionally, many potential predictor variables can be studied at once. Although a large number of comparisons lead to concerns about statistical validity, this type of study can be hypothesis-generating and quite helpful in planning more focused research.

4.3 Disadvantages of Case–Control Studies

Unlike cohort studies, case–control studies cannot be used to study multiple outcomes. This type of study is not well suited to studying very rare exposures and provides no estimate of disease incidence. The major problems associated with this design, however, are confounding variables and specific types of bias.

4.3.1 Confounding Variables

The issue of confounding variables has been discussed earlier in this chapter. Cases and controls are not randomly assigned and it is highly likely that any confounding variables are not equally distributed in both groups. Most case–control studies will attempt to mitigate the effects of known confounders by matching cases and controls. Appropriate matching has the additional advantage of decreasing the sample size required to find the desired difference between the groups. On the other hand, a variable that is used to match cases and controls can no longer be evaluated for an association with the outcome. "Overmatching," or making the controls too similar to the cases, may result in a situation whereby the controls are no longer representative of the general population. This will result in data that underestimates the true effect of the risk factor. For these reasons it is best to avoid matching for a variable if there is any doubt as to its effect on the outcome

4.3.2 Sampling Bias

Ideally the cases selected for a case–control study should be representative of all patients with that disease. If this is not the case then "sampling bias" may be present. This is not an unusual occurrence. A disease such as hypertension, for example, remains undiagnosed in the majority of people it affects; a case–control study that recruits cases from a hospital setting is not going to be representative of the general hypertensive population. It is often difficult to avoid this form of bias, but the possibility that it exists should be considered when interpreting the results.

4.3.3 Information Bias

Certain types of information bias may be problematic in case–control studies. Because cases are usually more aware of the nature of their disease and potential causes of it compared to the population at large, they are more likely to remember certain exposures in their past. This is known as "recall bias." The effect of this bias may be obviated by ascertaining exposure without relying on the subject's recollections, e.g., by using past medical records. When this is not possible, researchers may try blinding the subjects to the study hypothesis. Careful selection of the control group may help. In a study of the association between family history and all-cause end stage kidney disease, for example, the investigators used the spouses of dialysis patients as controls. These subjects were generally as knowledgeable about kidney disease as their partners and therefore equally likely to report positive family histories if present [10].

A second common form of bias in case–control studies is "diagnostic suspicion bias." This bias relates to the possibility that knowledge of the presence of disease may influence the investigator's interpretation of exposure status. The person recording such data should therefore be blinded as to the outcome status of the subjects if at all possible.

5 Designing a Case–Control Study

Once an appropriate research question is postulated, the investigators should state clear definitions of the outcome or disease of interest and what constitutes exposure to the risk factor(s) to be studied. The target population should be identified and the method for recruiting cases outlined. Potential sampling bias must be considered.

At this stage the investigators should identify potential confounding variables. Restriction and stratification may be useful, but known confounders are most commonly dealt with by matching cases and controls.

5.1 Selecting a Control Group

The selection of controls is a critical step in case–control study design. Subjects that have a higher or lower probability of being exposed to the risk factor of interest based on some other characteristic should not be used. In a study of the association between bladder cancer and smoking, for example, it would not be appropriate to select matched controls from the cardiology ward in the same hospital. Patients admitted with cardiac disease are more likely to have smoked than the general population and an underestimation of the risk is likely to occur. To strengthen the study one might select controls from several populations, such as an inpatient ward, and outpatient clinic and the general population. If the risk estimate relative to the cases is similar across the different control groups the conclusion is more likely to be correct. Finally, if the cases are drawn from a population-based registry it is a common practice to select controls from the general population within that geographic area.

---

6   Power and Sample Size Estimation in Observational Studies

6.1   Statistical Power

Sample size estimation is an important part of the design phase of any study, and observational designs are no different. The sample size requirement is often a major factor in determining feasibility of a study. Obviously, the resources available and population from which to draw recruits must be sufficient for the study to be possible. Less obvious, perhaps, is ability of adequate sample size to ensure that the study is meaningful regardless of whether the result is positive or negative. The probability of a type I error, i.e., finding a difference between groups when one actually does not exist, is expressed by the parameter α. This is typically set at 0.05, and a p-value less than this from statistical tests will be interpreted as indicating a statistically significant difference. The probability of a type II error, on the other hand, is the chance of not finding a difference between groups when one actually does exist. This is expressed by the parameter β, and $1-\beta$ is referred to as the power of a study. It is typically set at 0.8, meaning that there is a 20 % chance of a type II error, or an 80 % chance of reporting a difference if one truly exists. The higher the desired power of the study, the larger the sample size required. A study with too small a sample size will be poorly powered; if such a study does not find a difference between groups, it will be difficult to tell whether there is truly no difference or not. Underpowered studies are uninformative and journal reviewers will generally reject them for this reason alone.

6.2   Factors Determining Required Sample Size

Aside from power and the threshold for statistical significance, several other factors will influence the require sample size. Foremost among these is the minimum difference between the comparison groups that the researcher deems significant. The smaller this difference is, the larger the required sample size will be. Sample size will also be larger given a larger variance of the outcome variable. More "noise" in the outcome will make it more difficult to distinguish any differences.

Sample size calculations are relatively straightforward for RCTs, and most investigators perform them. Unfortunately, sample size or power estimation is often not considered in the design phase of observational studies. Often investigators are limited by the amount of data available, especially in historical studies. Cohort studies are sometimes limited by the total number of exposures, and case–control studies by the total number of cases that can be identified. In these instances power, rather than required sample size, can be calculated and the utility of the study considered from that perspective.

6.3 Calculating Required Sample Size for a Relative Risk or Odds Ratio

The exact approach to sample size estimation depends on the nature of the outcome data and the analyses to be used. The sample size formulas for relative risk (RR) and odds ratio (OR) calculation for two groups are essentially the same the same as one would use for comparing two proportions. In the simplest situation, the sample size will be equal for both groups. This also minimizes the total sample size required. The researcher specifies the desired OR or RR (equivalent to the minimum detectable difference between groups) and the expected proportion of outcomes in the control group; the proportion in the exposed group is calculated as follows:

$$ RR = \frac{p_{exposed}}{p_{unexposed}} = \frac{p_2}{p_1} \quad so \quad p_2 = RR \bullet p_1 $$

$$ OR = \frac{p_{exposed}/(1-p_{exposed})}{p_{unexposed}/(1-p_{unexposed})} = \frac{p_2/(1-p_2)}{p_1/(1-p_1)} \quad so \quad p_2 = \frac{OR \bullet p_1}{1+p_1(OR-1)} $$

With p_1 and p_2 known, the formula for the required sample size in each group is:

$$ n = \left(\frac{Z_\alpha\sqrt{2p_1(1-p_1)} - Z_\beta\sqrt{p_1(1-p_1)+p_2(1-p_2)}}{p_1 - p_2} \right)^2 $$

Z_α is the two-tailed Z value related to the null hypothesis and Z_β is the lower one-tailed Z value related to the alternative hypothesis [11]. These values are obtained from appropriate tables in statistical reference books, but for the common situation where $\alpha = 0.05$ and $\beta = 0.80$, $Z_\alpha = 1.96$ and $Z_\beta = 0.84$.

6.4 Calculating Sample Size for a Log-Rank Test

Studies that produce time-to-event outcome data from two or more groups are generally analyzed using survival methods (discussed later in this chapter). If the Kaplan–Meier method is used, statistical comparisons of groups are made with the log-rank test. The general principles of power and sample size estimation for this method are no different than that discussed above. Again, for maximum simplicity and power one may consider the case where two groups are to be compared with an equal number of subjects in both. One must first estimate the total number of outcomes (d) that must be observed:

$$d = \left(Z_\alpha - Z_{\beta(\text{upper})} \right)^2 \bullet \left(\frac{1 - \psi}{1 - \psi} \right)^2$$

$$\psi = \frac{\ln\left(\text{Survival group 2 at end of study}\right)}{\ln\left(\text{Survival group 1 at end of study}\right)}$$

Z_α is the two-tailed Z value related to the null hypothesis and Z_β is the upper one-tailed Z value of the normal distribution corresponding to $1 - \beta$ [12]. Once this is solved, the sample size (n) for each of the groups is:

$$n = \frac{d}{2 - \left(\text{Survival group 1 at end of study}\right) - \left(\text{Survival group 2 at end of study}\right)}$$

6.5 Calculating Sample Size for a Cox Proportional Hazards Model

Methods have been established to estimate power and sample size for studies to be analyzed using the Cox Proportional Hazards method. The researcher must specify α, subject accrual time, anticipated follow-up interval, and the median time to failure in the group with the smallest risk of the outcome [13]. The minimum hazard ratio (HR) detectable is then used to calculate either the power or the estimated sample size. It is advisable to make use of any of a number of software packages available to perform these relatively complex calculations [14, 15].

7   Analyzing Longitudinal Studies

7.1 Identifying Confounders

Once the data is collected the researcher should analyze information regarding the distribution of potential confounders in the groups. Very often the first table presented in a paper is the baseline characteristics of the study groups. The most common approach to identifying differences is to use simple tests ($\chi 2$ or t-tests) to identify statistically significant differences. The results of such comparisons are highly sensitive to sample size, however. Very large studies may result in statistically significant but clinically unimportant differences, and small studies may not demonstrate significant p-values when differences exist. An alternative approach is to present standardized differences, an indicator that is less affected by study size. The difference between the groups is divided by the pooled standard deviation of the two groups. Standardized differences greater than 0.1 are usually interpreted as indicating a meaningful difference [16].

**7.2 Calculating
an Estimate of Risk**

The desired result of a longitudinal study is most often a quantitative estimate of the risk of developing an outcome given the presence of a specific factor. The method used to generate this estimate depends on three factors—the study design, the nature of the outcome data and the need to control for confounding variables.

In the simplest situation, the outcome data for a cohort study will be the incidence or number of outcomes in each of the compared groups, and for a case–control study the number of exposed individuals in the cases and controls. If confounders are either not known to be present or have been minimized through restriction or matching there is no need to adjust for them though statistical means. The appropriate analysis for a cohort study in this situation is the RR, defined as $\text{Incidence}_{(\text{exposed})}/\text{Incidence}_{(\text{unexposed})}$. This is easily calculated from a 2×2 table (Table 1). A RR greater than 1.0 implies and increased risk, whereas a RR less than 1 is interpreted as demonstrating a lower risk of the outcome if the factor is present. A RR of 0.6, for example, implies a 40 % protective effect, whereas a RR of 1.4 indicated a 40 % increased risk in exposed individuals.

The measure of risk resulting form a case–control study is an OR, the odds of having been exposed in cases relative to controls. The RR cannot be calculated in a case–control study because the researcher determines the number of controls. The OR is generally an accurate approximation of the RR as long as the number of subjects with the outcome is small compared with the number of people without the disease. The calculation of the OR is shown in Table 1.

*7.2.1 Simple Hypothesis
Testing for Risk Estimates*

The most common null hypothesis to be tested for OR or RR is that either parameter is equal to 1, i.e., there is no difference between the compared groups. The traditional approach to direct hypothesis testing is based on confidence intervals (CI). The upper and lower bounds of the CI are calculated based on a specified value of α. This is usually set at 0.5, and the resulting 95 % CI is interpreted as containing the true value of the risk estimate with 95 % confidence. The CI is valuable in itself as a measure of the precision of the estimate. A wide CI indicates low precision.

**Table 1
Calculation of relative risk and odds ratios**

		Disease/ outcome		
		+	**–**	
Risk factor	+	a	b	$\text{Relative Risk}\,(\text{RR}) = \dfrac{\left[\,a\,/\,(a+b)\,\right]}{\left[\,c\,/\,(c+d)\,\right]}$
	–	c	d	$\text{Odd Ratio}\,(\text{OR}) = \dfrac{ad}{bc}$

Table 2
Calculation of 95 % confidence intervals (95 % CI) for relative risks and odds ratios. See Table 1 for parameter definitions

For a Relative Risk:

$$95\% CI = \exp\left(\ln(RR) \pm 1.96 \sqrt{\frac{1-[a\,/\,a+b]}{a} + \frac{1-[c\,/\,c+d]}{c}} \right)$$

For an Odds Ratio:

$$95\% CI = \exp\left(\ln(OR) \pm 1.96 \sqrt{\frac{1}{a} + \frac{1}{b} + \frac{1}{c} + \frac{1}{d}} \right)$$

The calculation of the CI for an OR or RR is complicated by the fact that ratios are not normally distributed. Natural logarithms of the ratios are normally distributed, however, and are thus used in the computation (Table 2). Once the 95 % CI is known, testing the null hypothesis is simple. If the 95 % CI does not include 1.0, it can be concluded that the null hypothesis can be rejected at a significance level of 0.05. An alternate approach to hypothesis testing is to apply χ^2 test to the 2×2 contingency table used to compute the RR or RR [12].

7.2.2 Controlling for Confounders

When confounding variables are present the researcher will normally want to minimize their effect on the risk estimate. Simple RR or OR calculation will not be sufficient. In the analysis phase, the investigator has two methods available to accomplish this—stratification and regression.

Stratification has been discussed earlier in this chapter. In either a cohort or case–control design, study groups are subdivided by values of the confounding variable and analyzed separately. Crude, or unadjusted risk estimates are computed for each stratum. The Mantel–Haenszel technique produces an "adjusted" summary statistic for the combined strata, which are weighted according to their sample size [17, 18]. If the adjusted risk estimate differs from the crude one, confounding is likely present and the adjusted value is the more reliable of the two.

Regression refers to any of a large number of statistical techniques used to describe the relationship between one or more predictor variables and an outcome. It is the ability to simultaneously analyze the impact of multiple variables that makes them valuable for dealing with confounders. The researcher cannot only "adjust" for the confounding variables but can quantify their effect. The appropriate type of regression is primarily determined by the nature of the outcome data. Continuous variable outcomes, such as height or weight, are generally analyzed by multiple linear regression. Although this type of analysis will produce an equation allowing one to predict the impact of a change in the predictor variable on the outcome, linear regression does not produce an estimate of risk. A more common type of outcome data in observational studies is a dichotomous variable, i.e., one that may assume only one of two values. Either the outcome occurred (such as the diagnosis of a disease or death) or it did not. This type of data may be analyzed using logistic regression. Although limited to dichotomous outcomes, logistic regression has the advantage of producing a risk estimate (the risk ratio, interpreted the same way as a RR or OR) and a confidence interval. Multiple predictor variables can be analyzed, adjusting for confounders.

7.3 Analyzing Survival Data

Many cohort studies produce time-to-event or survival outcome data. This type of outcome contains far more information than the simple occurrence of an outcome. Survival data records when an event happened, allowing the researchers to learn much more about the natural history of a disease, for example, and the potential impact of risk factors on how soon an outcome occurs.

Time-to-event data is analyzed by any one of a number of survival techniques. Life table analysis, essentially a table of cumulative survival over time, is not a widely used method because it requires all subjects to reach the specified outcome. If the outcome is death, for example, all subjects must die. It is a descriptive technique that does not allow for comparisons between groups and produces no risk estimate. A more common situation is that not all subjects reach the endpoint by the time the observational study ends. Some subjects may drop out, some may be subject to competing risks, and some will simply not reach the endpoint at the end of the follow-up period. These subjects will be censored, i.e., the data will be incomplete at study end and it will not be known when, or if, they reach the specified outcome. The fact that these subjects had not reached the endpoint up until a specified point is still very informative. A technique that makes use of censored data is the Kaplan–Meier method [19]. This method will generate graphical representations of cumulative survival over time, i.e., survival curves, for one or more groups. Although the overall survival of the different groups may be compared using the Log-Rank test, the Kaplan–Meier method does not produce a risk estimate. Confounders can be analyzed by stratification, but creating many groups quickly becomes cumbersome and difficult to interpret. The commonest multivariate form of survival analysis is based on the Cox-Proportional Hazards Model [20]. This very powerful technique allows researchers to control for the effect of multiple predictor variables and generate "adjusted" survival curves. It generates a risk estimate analogous to the RR, the Hazard Ratio, and corresponding confidence intervals. This technique is widely used in the medical literature. It is discussed in more depth in a later chapter.

7.4 Limitations of Multivariate Techniques

It should be kept in mind that multivariate regression techniques, while extremely useful, still have limitations. Statistical power may be an issue in many studies. In general, the number of predictor variables that may be included in a regression model is a function of the sample size. Using the common rule of thumb that there must be 10 outcomes observed for every variable included in the model, one must have 100 outcomes to analyze the effect of 10 predictor variables. Using too many predictor variables will result in an underpowered analysis incapable of detecting true differences.

It is also important to understand that regression and survival methods all have certain assumptions that must be met to ensure the validity of the results. A detailed discussion of these requirements is beyond the scope of this chapter, but the researcher must understand the assumptions and the methods of assessing them for the analytic technique they are using.

References

1. Gillings D, Koch G (1991) The application of the principle of intention-to-treat to the analysis of clinical trials. Drug Inf J 25:411–424
2. Lopez-Garcia E, van Dam RM, Willett WC, Rimm EB, Manson JE, Stampfer MJ, Rexrode KM, Hu FB (2006) Coffee consumption and coronary heart disease in men and women: a prospective cohort study. Circulation 113: 2045–2053
3. Carter WB, Elward K, Malmgren J, Martin ML, Larson E (1991) Participation of older adults in health programs and research: a critical review of the literature. Gerontologist 31:584–592
4. Benfante R, Reed D, MacLean C, Kagan A (1989) Response bias in the Honolulu Heart Program. Am J Epidemiol 130:1088–1100
5. Evans AM, Love RR, Meyerowitz BE, Leventhal H, Nerenz DR (1985) Factors associated with active participation in a Cancer Prevention Clinic. Prev Med 14:358–371
6. Kash KM, Holland JC, Halper MS, Miller DG (1992) Psychological distress and surveillance behaviors of women with a family history of breast cancer. J Natl Cancer Inst 84:24–30
7. Lerman C, Trock B, Rimer BK, Boyce A, Jepson C, Engstrom PF (1991) Psychological and behavioral implications of abnormal mammograms. Ann Intern Med 114:657–661
8. Parfrey PS (2007) In the literature: on clinical performance measures and outcomes among hemodialysis patients. Am J Kidney Dis 49: 352–355
9. Brookmeyer R, Gail MH (1987) Biases in prevalent cohorts. Biometrics 43:739–749
10. O'Dea DF, Murphy SW, Hefferton D, Parfrey PS (1998) Higher risk for renal failure in first-degree relatives of white patients with end-stage renal disease: a population-based study. Am J Kidney Dis 32:794–801
11. Dawson B, Trapp RG (2004) Basic & clinical biostatistics. McGraw-Hill, Toronto
12. Glantz SA (2005) Primer of biostatistics. McGraw-Hill, Toronto
13. Schoenfeld DA (1983) Sample-size formula for the proportional-hazards regression model. Biometrics 39:499–503
14. Dupont WD, Plummer WD (2004) PS: power and sample size calculation. Available at http://biostat.mc.vanderbilt.edu/twiki/bin/view/Main/PowerSampleSize. Accessed 25 Jun 2014
15. Schoenfeld DA (2001) Find statistical considerations for a study where the outcome is time to failure. Available at http://hedwig.mgh.harvard.edu/sample_size/time_to_event/para_time.html. Accessed 25 Jun 2014
16. Mamdani M, Sykora K, Li P, Normand SL, Streiner DL, Austin PC, Rochon PA, Anderson GM (2005) Reader's guide to critical appraisal of cohort studies: 2. Assessing potential for confounding. BMJ 330: 960–962

17. Mantel N, Haenszel W (1959) Statistical aspects of the analysis of data from retrospective studies of disease. J Natl Cancer Inst 22:719–748

18. Grimes DA, Schulz KF (2002) Bias and causal associations in observational research. Lancet 359:248–252

19. Kaplan EL, Meier P (1958) Nonparametric estimation from incomplete observations. J Am Stat Assoc 53:457–481

20. Cox D (1972) Regression models and life tables (with discussion). J R Stat Soc Series B Stat Methodol 4:187–220

Chapter 5

Longitudinal Studies 2: Modeling Data Using Multivariate Analysis

Pietro Ravani, Brendan J. Barrett, and Patrick S. Parfrey

Abstract

Statistical models are used to study the relationship between exposure and disease while accounting for the potential role of other factors impact upon outcomes. This adjustment is useful to obtain unbiased estimates of true effects or to predict future outcomes. Statistical models include a systematic and an error component. The systematic component explains the variability of the response variable as a function of the predictors and is summarized in the effect estimates (model coefficients). The error element of the model represents the variability in the data unexplained by the model and is used to build measures of precisions around the point estimates (Confidence Intervals).

Key words Statistical models, Regression methods, Multivariable analysis, Effect estimates, Estimate precision, Confounding, Interaction

1 Introduction

Longitudinal data contain information on disease related factors and outcome measures. Clinical researchers use statistical models to test whether an association exists between one of these outcome measures and some exposure, such as a risk factor for disease or an intervention to improve prognosis.

The present chapter provides introductory notes on general principles of statistical modeling. These concepts are useful to understand how regression techniques quantify the effect of the exposure of interest while accounting for other prognostic variables.

2 Principles of Regression and Modeling

2.1 Role of Statistics

The task of statistics in the analysis of epidemiological data is to distinguish between chance findings (random error) and the results that may be replicated upon repetition of the study (systematic component). For example, if a relationship between blood

Patrick S. Parfrey and Brendan J. Barrett (eds.), *Clinical Epidemiology: Practice and Methods*, Methods in Molecular Biology, vol. 1281, DOI 10.1007/978-1-4939-2428-8_5, © Springer Science+Business Media New York 2015

pressure levels and left ventricular mass values exists, the response (left ventricular mass) is expected to change by a certain amount as blood pressure changes. In the Multiethnic Study of Atherosclerosis, a large-scale multicenter application of cardiac magnetic resonance in people without clinical cardiovascular disease, left ventricular mass was found to be on average 9.6 g greater (95 % Confidence Intervals from 8.5 to 10.8) per each standard deviation (21-mmHg) higher systolic blood pressure [1]. A statistical model was used to quantify both the average change in left ventricular mass per unit change in systolic blood pressure (systematic component) and the variability of the observed values unexplained by the model (random error, summarized by the Confidence Intervals).

The estimated effect (left ventricular mass increase) attributed to a factor (greater systolic blood pressure) is considered valid (close to the true left ventricular mass change per blood pressure change) if all sources of sampling and measurement bias have been adequately identified and their consequences successfully prevented and controlled. In fact, statistics only conveys the effect of the chance element in the data but can neither identify nor reduce systematic errors (bias) in the study design. The only bias that can be controlled for during statistical analyses is "measured" confounding. Finally the estimated effect is unbiased if the statistical tool is appropriate for the data. This includes the choice of the correct function and regression technique.

2.2 Concept of Function

Most clinical research can be simplified as an assessment of an exposure–response relationship. The former is also called input (X, independent variable or predictor) and the latter output (Y, dependent variable or outcome). For example, if left ventricular mass is the response variable and the study hypothesis is that its values depend on body mass index, smoking habit, diabetes, and systolic blood pressure [1], then the value of left ventricular mass (y) is said to be a "function of" these four variables (x_1, x_2, x_3, and x_4). Therefore, the term "function" (or equation) implies a link existing between inputs and output.

A function can be thought of as a "machine" transforming some ingredients (inputs) into a final product (output). Technically the ingredients (term or expression on which a function operates) are called the "argument" of that function. Just as any machine produces a specific output and has a typical shape and its own characteristics, similarly any function has its specific response variable and has a typical mathematical form and graphical shape. As in the above example, more than one input variable may take part in the function, or if you prefer, more "ingredients" may be used to make a final product. This is important when studying simultaneously the relative and independent effects of several factors on the same response and during control for confounding.

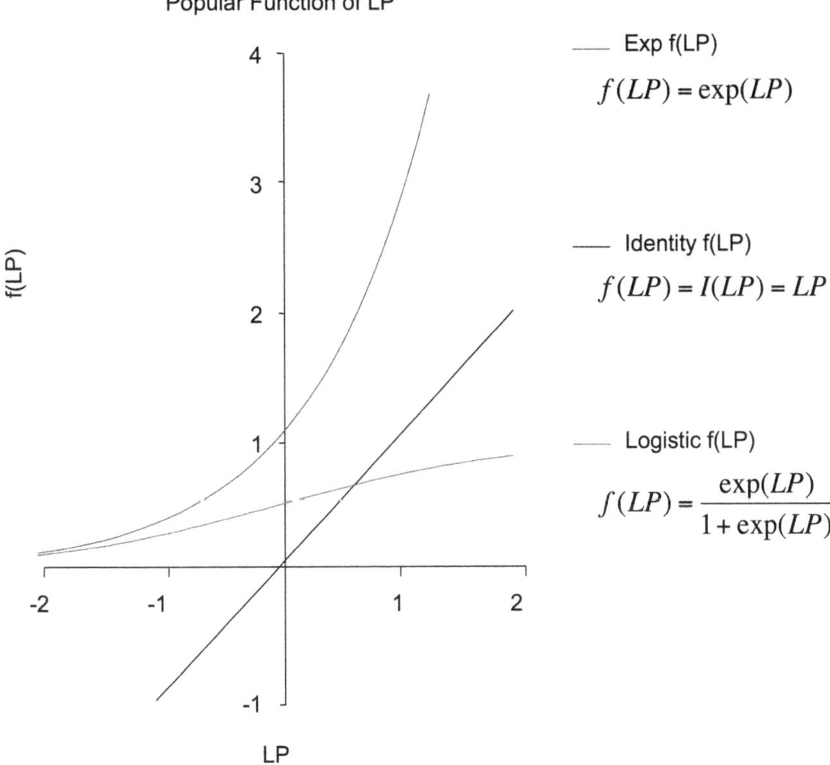

Fig. 1 Example of three common functions of the linear predictor (LP): the identity function does not change the LP (linear model); the exponential function is the exponentiated LP (Poisson model); the logistic function is a sigmoid function of LP (logistic model). Note that different functions have not only different shapes but also different ranges. With permission Ravani et al., Nephrol Dial Transplant [12]

A very important "ingredient" to define is the "linear predictor" (LP), which is the "argument" of the statistical functions that will be discussed in the following chapter. LP contains one or more inputs (the "Xs") combined in linear fashion. Figure 1 shows three important functions of the LP: the identity function, which does not modify its argument and gives LP as output; the exponential function of LP; and the logistic function of LP. The underlying mathematical structure is not important here. However, two aspects should be noted: first, different transformations change the "shape" of the relationship between LP and its function; second despite that the LP can range from $-\infty$ to $+\infty$ (allowing any type of variable to be accommodated into it), its function can be constrained into a range between 0 and 1 (logistic function); can have a lower limit of 0 (exponential function); or can just have the same range as the LP (identity function).

2.3 Regression Methods

2.3.1 Estimation Purpose

Regression strategies are commonly applied in practice. Doctors measure blood pressure several times and take the average in new patients before diagnosing hypertension. Doctors do the same when further checks provide unexpected values. Averages are regarded as more reliable than any single observation. Also in biostatistics the term regression implies the tendency toward an average value. Indeed regression methods are used to quantify the relationship between two measured variables. For example, if there is a linear relationship between age and 5-year mortality, the average change in output (mortality) per unit change in one (age; univariable regression) or more than one input (age and blood pressure; multivariable regression) can be estimated using linear regression. This estimation task is accomplished by assigning specific values to some elements (unknowns) of the specific regression function. These elements are called *parameters* and the values assigned to them by the regression procedure are called *parameter estimates*. For example, in the above example, the linear function of mortality has the following mathematical form: mortality = $LP + \varepsilon = \beta_0 + \beta_{age} \times age + \varepsilon$, where LP is a linear function of the form $\beta_0 + \beta x \times x$ and ε is the variability in the data unexplained by the model. In this simple (univariable) expression there are two "unknowns" to estimate: β_0, representing the intercept of the line describing the linear relationship between the independent variable (age) and the response (mortality); β_x, representing the average change of the response (mortality) per unit change of the independent variable (age).

2.3.2 Meaning of the Model Parameters

The intercept (β_0) is the average value of the response variable "y" (mortality for example) when the independent variable in the model is zero. This makes sense when the independent variable can be zero (for example, when diabetes is coded 0 in nondiabetics and 1 in diabetics). When the independent variable is continuous (age, blood pressure or body weight, for example) the intercept only makes sense if the continuous variables in the model are recoded using the deviates from their means. For example, if the average age in the sample is 50, then the value of age for a 40-year-old subject becomes −10, for a 52-year-old subject is 2, etc. The model of 5-year mortality is the same after this recoding but the intercept of the model now is the value of the response (mortality) when the input (or inputs), such as age or other continuous variables, is (are) zero.

Linear regression allows estimating the terms "β_0," "β_{age}" (as well as more β_s were more inputs modeled), which are the *regression parameters* (or population characteristics). In the above example the most important coefficient is the regression coefficient of age because this coefficient estimates the hypothesized effect of age on mortality. In fact the regression parameters explain how the response variable changes as the predictor(s) change.

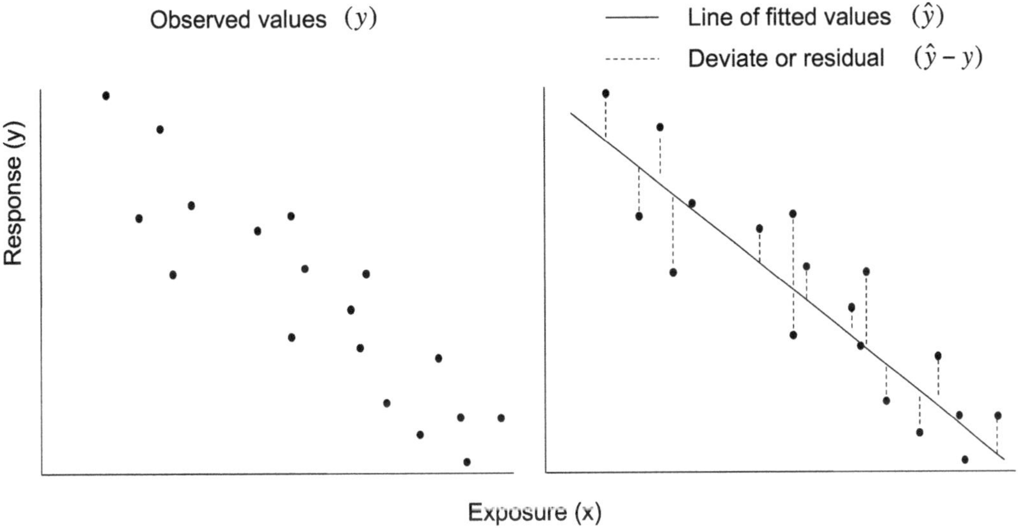

Fig. 2 Ordinary least square method: the regression line drawn through a scatter-plot of two variables is "the best fitting line" of the response. In fact this line is as close to the points as possible providing the "least sum of square" deviates or residuals (*vertical dashed lines*). These discrepancies are the differences between each observation ("y") and the fitted value corresponding to a given exposure value ("ŷ"). With permission Ravani et al., Nephrol Dial Transplant [12]

2.3.3 Estimation Methods

There are different methods to estimate the equation parameters of a regression model. The method commonly used in linear regression, for example, is the *Ordinary Least Square* (OLS) method. In lay words this method chooses the values of the function parameters (β_0, β_{age}) that minimize the distance between the observed values of the response y and their mean per each unit of x (thus minimizing "ε"). Graphically this corresponds to finding a line on the Cartesian axes passing through the observed points and minimizing their distance from the line of the average values (Fig. 2). This line (the LP) is called the line of fitted (expected) values toward which the observed measures are "regressed." Other estimation methods exist for other types of data, the most important of which is *Maximum Likelihood Estimation* (MLE). MLE, as opposed to OLS, works well for both normally (Gaussian) and non-normally distributed responses (for example, Binomial or Poisson). However, both MLE and OLS choose the most likely values of the parameters given the available data, those that minimize the amount of error or difference between what is observed and what is expected. For example, given three independent observations of age equal to 5, 6, 10, the most likely value of the mean parameter is 7, because no other value could minimize the residuals further (give smaller "square" deviates). As another example, given two deaths among four subjects the MLE of the risk parameter is 0.5 because no other values can maximize the MLE function further.

In complex models with several parameters (coefficients) to estimate, the principles of calculus are applied (for all models), as it is very difficult to make even reasonable guesses at the MLE. Importantly, traditional MLE methods (for all models, including those for normally distributed data) are not appropriate if outcome data are correlated because they calculate joint probabilities of all observed outcomes under the assumption that they are independent. For example given (indicated by "|") d failures in n subjects, the likelihood of the observed outcome "π" is the product of each independent event: $\mathrm{MLE}\left(\pi \mid d \,/\, n\right) = \pi \times \left(1 - \pi\right) \times \ldots \times \left(1 - \pi\right) = \pi^{d} \times \left(1 - \pi\right)^{n-d}$. This is the "form" of the ML function of the "risk parameter," which is based on the product of independent probabilities. The most likely parameter estimate (the value of the risk π) after observing two failures in four subjects is 0.5 since no other value of π (given $d=2$ and $n=4$) would make larger the ML function of π (this can be proven in this simple example plugging different values for the unknown "π" given $d=2$ and $n=4$). However, this is valid if each observation is independent (in other words, if measurements are performed on unrelated individuals).

<table><tr><td>

2.3.4 Likelihood and Probability

</td><td>

Likelihood and probability are related functions as the likelihood of the parameters given the data is proportional to the probability of the data given the parameters. However, when making predictions based on solid assumptions (e.g., knowledge of the parameters) we are interested in probabilities of certain outcomes occurring or not occurring given those assumptions (parameters). Conversely, when data have already been observed (the Latin word "datum" means "given") they are fixed. Therefore, outcome prediction is performed estimating the *probability of the data given the parameters*, whereas parameter estimation is performed maximizing *likelihood of the parameters given the observed data*. Examples of probability functions are the Gaussian distribution of a continuous variable (e.g., systolic blood pressure values in a population) given some values of the parameters (e.g., mean and standard deviation); the binomial probability distribution of the number of failures given the parameters π (probability of failure) and n (number of trials); or the Poisson distribution of an event count given the parameter (expected events). For example, assuming known values of k parameters (effects of k independent variables), the probability π of an event d dependent on those k model parameters $\theta = \beta_0, \beta_1, \beta_2, \ldots, \beta k_{-1}, \beta k$ is $\pi(d|\theta)$, which is read "the probability of d given the parameters θ." When the parameters are unknown, the likelihood function of the parameters $\theta = \beta_0, \beta_1, \beta_2, \ldots, \beta k_{-1}, \beta k$ can be written as $L(\theta|d/n)$, which is read "the likelihood of the parameters θ given the observed d/n." The aim of MLE is to find the values of the parameters $\theta = \beta_0, \beta_1, \beta_2, \ldots, \beta k_{-1}, \beta k$ (and, consequently, π or other expected values such as the mean of a quantitative variable) that make the observed data (d/n) most likely.

</td></tr></table>

3   Statistical Models

3.1   Meaning
and Structure

Models are representations of essential structures of objects or real processes. For example, the earth may be approximated to a sphere in astronomical or geographic calculations although it is rather an oblate spheroid being flattened at the poles. Nevertheless depending on the objectives, the inaccuracies deriving from the calculations carried out under the proposition of sphericity may not only be acceptable but also advantageous with respect to precise calculations based on the "real" shape of the planet. The example can be extended to phenomena, such as animal experiments or relationships among different individual characteristics. For example, nephrologists expect that anemia worsens as kidney function decreases. This expectation is based on the idea of a relationship (model) between kidney function and hemoglobin concentration. To study and describe this relationship, epidemiologists may define a statistical model based on a certain model function and regression method. For example, given a reasonably linear relationship, at least within a certain range of kidney function, a linear model may be a good choice to study anemia and kidney function data. Indeed even in the presence of mild deviations from ideal circumstances, the representation of a process by means of a simple model, such as the linear model, helps grasp the intimate nature and the mechanisms of that process. Obviously critical violations of model assumptions would make the model inappropriate. The linear model would be wrong if the relationship was exponential. Similarly the sphere would not be an acceptable model if the earth were a cone. In any case the hope is that a mathematical model can describe the relationship of interest providing a good compromise between appropriateness of the chosen function, simplicity, interpretability of the results, and little amount of residual error (unexplained variation in the data). This error is an important component of statistical models. In fact, biologic phenomena, as opposed to deterministic phenomena of physics or chemistry, do not yield the same results when repeated in the same experimental conditions but are characterized by a considerable amount of unpredictable variability. Therefore, probabilistic rather than deterministic models are applied to biomedical sciences because they include indexes of uncertainty around the population parameters estimated using samples. These indexes allow probability statements about how confident we can be that the estimated values correspond to the truth.

These characteristics of statistical models are reflected in their two major components: the systematic portion or fit and the random or chance element. For example, the fit portion of a linear model is a line and the errors are distributed normally with mean equal to zero (Fig. 3). In other models the fitted portion has

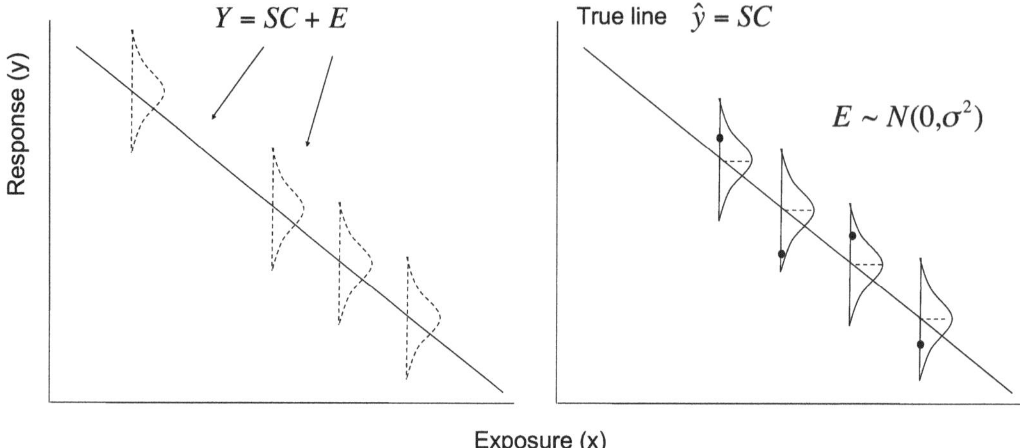

Fig. 3 Components of a statistical model: the statistical model of the response (*Y*) includes a systematic component (SC) corresponding to the regression line (the linear predictor LP in linear regression or some transformation of the LP in other models) and an error term (*E*) characterized by some known distribution (for the linear model the distribution is normal, with mean $= 0$ and constant variance $= \sigma^2$). With permission Ravani et al., Nephrol Dial Transplant [12]

different shapes and the residuals have different distribution. The fit component explains or predicts the output variable whereas the random component is the portion of the output data unexplained by the model. In the previous example of linear regression of mortality the amount of change in mortality per unit change in age is the main "effect" of age. This quantity times age gives the estimated average mortality for that age. For example if the estimated parameters "β_0" and "β_{age}" of the linear model of 5-year mortality are 0.01 (line intercept) and 0.001 (line slope), the expected risk of death of a 60-year-old subject is 7 % in 5 years $(0.01 + 0.001 \times 60)$. However, a 7 % risk of death in 5 years may not correspond to the observed value for the 60-year-old subject in our data. A 60-year-old subject in the current data may even not exist or belong to a category of risk of 0.1 or 0.05. The difference between what has been recorded and the value predicted by the model is the error or residual, and is summarized in the random portion of the model. With biologic phenomena further information can reduce this error, for example refining the precision of the estimate of subject mortality, but even including several inputs into the model the "exact" value of the response (mortality) can never be established. In other words, some amount of variation will remain unexplained after fitting the model to the data.

3.2 Model Choice

3.2.1 General Approach

The most appropriate statistical model to fit the data depends on the type of response variable because this determines the shape of the relationship of interest (fit portion) and the typical distribution of the errors (chance element). Fortunately, the form of most input–output relationships and error distributions are known. This permits orientation in the choice of a model before data are collected. Once the model has been built, its systematic and random components are verified graphically and using formal tests based on residuals in order to ensure that the chosen model fit the data well. These procedures are called assumption verification and model specification check and will not be discussed in this text. However, principles of model choice and checks can be briefly summarized using the linear model as an example. This model is easy to understand because in linear regression the LP is the argument of a function called "identity" (i.e., a function that does not have any effect, like multiplying the argument by 1). In other words, the observed values of the response variable are modeled as "identity" function of the LP, plus an error term (as in the example of 5-year mortality).

3.2.2 Form of the Exposure–Response Relationship

There are three fundamental assumptions to satisfy when using a statistical model: (1) the necessary condition to use a model is that the relationship between the response and the exposure reflect the mathematical form of that model; (2) the difference between what is observed and expected have a distribution compatible with the specific model; and (3) that these residuals be independent. Assumption 1 pertains to the systematic component of the model.

An example of assumption 1 is that to use the linear model there must exist a *linear relationship* between the response variable and the predictors because this is the meaning of the identify function of LP (linear function). In geometry and elementary algebra a linear function is a "first degree polynomial" which eventually has the form of the LP. The coefficients of this function are real constants ("β_0" and "βs") and the inputs "Xs" are real variables. These definitions may seem complex, but all it means is that the effect of each predictor in a linear function results in a constant change in the output for all their values. This function is called linear because it yields graphs that are straight lines. In other models, the response variable is not linearly related to the LP, but the relationship can be exponential or logistic for example. As a result, the input–output relationship has different forms in nonlinear models as compared to the linear model. Yet, independent of the transformation "applied" to the LP, in the most popular statistical models it is still possible to recognize the LP in the right hand side of the model function (Fig. 1). The transformation implies that the change in the response, as the exposure changes, is no longer linear but describable by other curve shapes. Consequently, the change in the form of the relationship (the function) corresponds to a change in the meaning of the coefficients (parameter estimates). These coefficients remain differences in the LP. However, the functional transformation of the LP changed their epidemiological meaning. This is why, for example, differences in the coefficients correspond to odds ratios in logistic

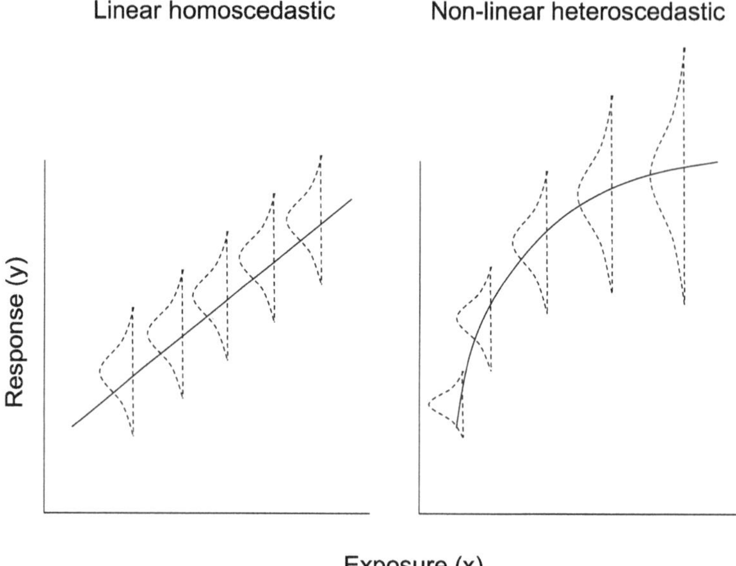

Fig. 4 Linearity and equal variance: in the left panel the response is linearly related to the exposure and has constant variance (homoscedasticity). In the *right plot* two possible important violations are depicted: nonlinearity and unequal variance (heteroscedasticity). With permission Ravani et al., Nephrol Dial Transplant [12]

regression and incidence rate ratios in Poisson regression. Importantly their meaning in the LP remains the same and the linearity of the LP is checked in other models independent of the specific transformation applied to the function argument. This "shape" assumption pertains to the systematic component of all models (Fig. 4).

3.2.3 Random Component

Assumptions 2 and 3, which must be satisfied in order to use a statistical model, pertain to the random component of the model, i.e., the "ε" parameter in linear regression, or more generally the difference between what it is observed and what is expected (residuals). First, the residuals must have some distribution compatible with the specific model. For example, they must be *normally distributed* around the fitted line with *mean equal to zero* and *constant variance* in linear regression; they must follow the *binomial* distribution in logistic regression and the *Poisson* distribution in Poisson regression. For example, in a study of Asymmetric-Di-Methyl-Arginine (ADMA) and levels of kidney function measured as Glomerular Filtration Rate (GFR), the observed GFR of the sample subjects was found to be approximately symmetrically distributed above and below the fitted line of GFR as a function of ADMA, with equal variability along the whole line [2]. This means that the dispersion of the observed GFR values around the fitted line must be symmetrical (error mean = zero) and constant. In other words, the same amount of uncertainty must be observed for all values of ADMA (Fig. 4). Second, the residuals must be *independent* as is true for all models. This is possible only if the observations are independent. This condition is violated if more measures are taken on the same subjects or if there are clusters in the data, i.e., some individuals share some experience or conditions that make them not fully independent. For example, if some subjects share a genetic background or belong to the same families, schools, hospitals, or practices, the experiences within clusters may not be independent and, consequently, the residuals around the fitted values may not be independent. This implies that once some measurements have been made it becomes possible to more accurately "guess" the values of other measurements within the same individual or cluster and the corresponding errors are no longer due to chance alone. This final assumption must be satisfied in the study design and when there is correlation in the data, appropriate statistical techniques are required.

3.2.4 Data Transformation

When the necessary conditions to use a certain model are clearly violated, they can be carefully diagnosed and treated. For instance, often nonlinearity and unstable variance of a continuous response can be at least partially corrected by some mathematical transformations of the output and/or the inputs in order to use the linear model. This can be necessary also for the inputs of other nonlinear models. Urinary protein excretion for example is often log-transformed both when it is treated as output [3] and as an input variable [4]. However, once a transformation has been chosen the interpretation of the model parameters changes accordingly and can become difficult to understand or explain. For these reasons, complex transformations as well as inclusion of power terms in the LP may be useless even if they allow the specific model assumptions to be met. Some reports do not clearly explain the meaning of the parameters (in terms of interpretation of the "change") of some complex models [3–6].

*3.2.5 Meaning
of the Model Assumptions*

The three conditions pertaining to the shape of the relationship, the error distribution and error independence should be imagined in a multidimensional space if the model (as often happens) is multivariable. They have the following meaning. Once the model has been fitted to the data (1) it must be possible to quantify the amount of change of the output per unit change of the input(s), i.e., the parameter estimates are constant and apply over the whole range of the predictors; (2) what remains to be explained around the fit is unknown independent of the input(s) values (3) and is independent of the process of measurements. For more detailed discussion on applied regression the interested reader is referred to specific texts [7].

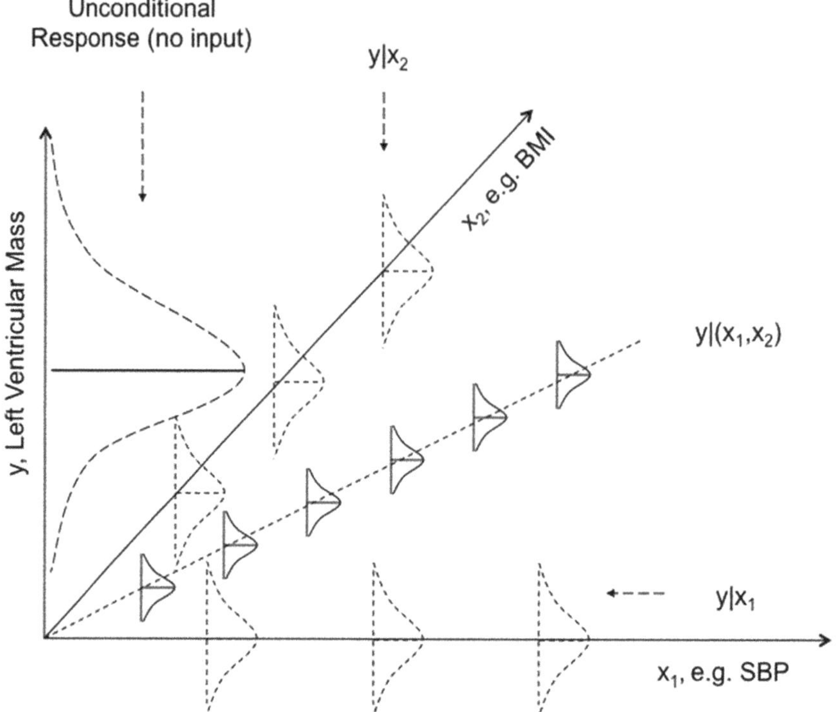

Fig. 5 Information gain and residual variance: the residual variance gets progressively smaller as more informative inputs are introduced into the model as compared to the unconditional response (distribution of the response without any knowledge about exposure). The inputs are systolic blood pressure, SBP (x_1, in mmHg) and body mass index, BMI (x_2, in kg/m^2). With permission Ravani et al., Nephrol Dial Transplant [12]

3.3 Multivariable vs. Univariable Analysis

An important purpose of multiple regression (in all models) is to take into account more effects simultaneously, including confounding and interaction. A graphical approach using the linear model may help understand this meaning of multivariable analysis.

When only the response variable is considered, e.g., the overall mean and standard deviation of left ventricular mass [1], the largest possible variability is observed in the data (Fig. 5, unconditional response). The variability in the output data becomes smaller if the response is studied as a function of one input at a time or, better, two input variables at the same time (conditional distribution of the response). This is accomplished by multiple regression: when more inputs are considered simultaneously the systematic component of the model contains more information about the variability of the response variable and the amount of error or unexplained variability gets smaller. The intercept and standard error of the model without input variables ("null model," i.e., $y = \beta_0 + \varepsilon$) are the parameters of the unconditional distribution of left ventricular mass (mean and standard deviation).

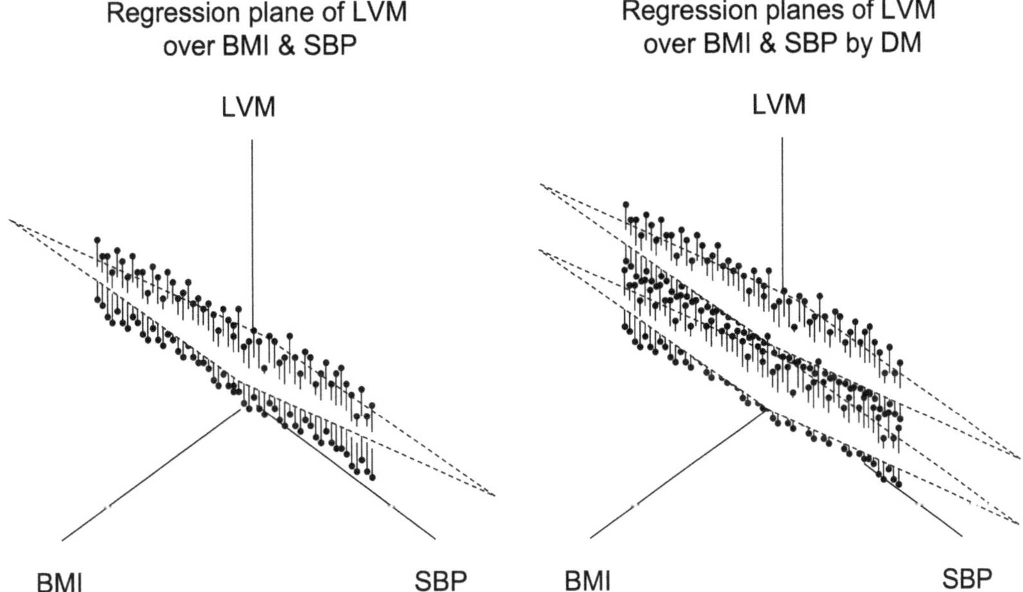

Fig. 6 Three-dimensional representation of the linear model: two quantitative predictors generate a plane in the three-dimensional space (Left Ventricular Mass—LVM over Systolic Blood Pressure—SBP and Body Mass Index—BMI). The number of fitted planes increases with the number of levels of a qualitative input (e.g., Diabetes—DM). With permission Ravani et al., Nephrol Dial Transplant [12]

Figure 6 shows the multidimensional consequences of introducing more inputs. With two quantitative predictors such as systolic blood pressure and body mass index, the fitted values of left ventricular mass lie on a plane in the three-dimensional space, the plane that minimizes the residuals. The addition of a third quantitative variable would create a hyper-plane in the multidimensional space and so on. Of note qualitative inputs, such as diabetes, separate the fitted values on more planes, one per each level of the independent variable. This plane would have S-sigmoid or some other sophisticated shape in case other models are used to fit the data, but the impact of multivariable analysis in the multidimensional space has the same meaning.

4   Confounding and Interaction

4.1   Confounding

A *confounder* is an "extraneous" variable associated with both the outcome and the exposure without lying in the pathway connecting the exposure to the outcome. Conversely, a *marker* is only related to the exposure (indirect relation), whereas an *intermediate variable* explains the outcome. Finally, two inputs are *colinear* when they carry the same or at least similar information (Fig. 7). For example, Heine et al. studied renal resistance indices (a marker of vascular

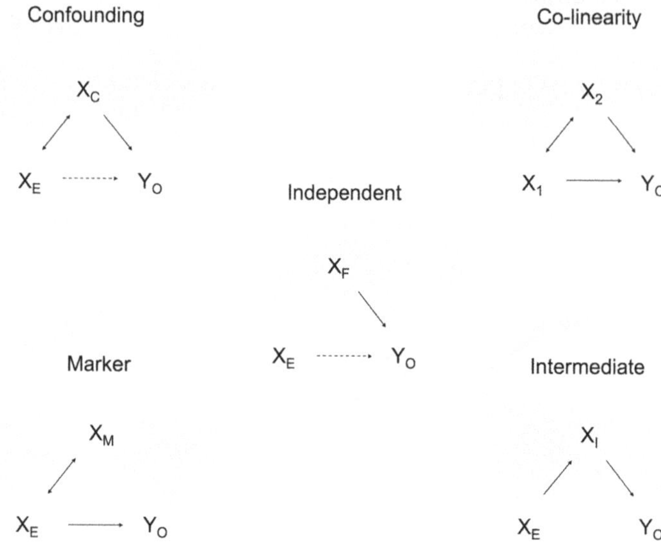

Fig. 7 Possible relationships between input and outcome: a confounding factor (X_C) is an independent variable associated with the response (Y_O) and with the main exposure of interest (X_E) without being in the pathological pathway between exposure and outcome. A marker (X_M) is associated with the exposure only and has no direct relationship with the outcome. Two inputs (X_E and X_F) may also have an independent association with the response: this is the ideal situation as it maximizes the information in the data. Colinearity is a phenomenon whereby two inputs (X_1 and X_2) carry (at least partially) the same information on the response. An intermediate variable (X_I) lies in the pathological path leading to the outcome. With permission Ravani et al., Nephrol Dial Transplant [12]

damage studied with ultrasound examination) in subjects with chronic kidney disease not yet on dialysis [8]. In this study, intima–media thickness of the carotid artery was significantly associated with the response (renal resistance) in baseline models that did not include age. Once age was entered into the model intima–media thickness lost its predictive power. The authors showed that older patients had thicker carotid artery walls. Thus, intima–media thickness may be a confounder, a marker or even an intermediate variable. In the final model of the resistance indices study the introduction of phosphate "lowered" the coefficient of glomerular filtration rate possibly because phosphate increase is one mechanism through which kidney function reduction contributes to higher resistance indices. However, outside an experimental context the nature of these multiple associations can only be hypothesized.

The confounding phenomenon is of particular importance in the analysis of non-experimental data. The way regression analysis removes the association between the confounder and the outcome (the necessary condition for the confounding phenomenon) is straightforward.

Consider the following model including the exposure and the confounding factor: $y = \beta_0 + \beta_E E + \beta_C C + \varepsilon$. The difference between the observed response and the effect of confounding left in the model gives the effect of the exposure: $y - \beta_C C = \beta_0 + \beta_E E + \varepsilon$. The right hand part of the formula is now a simple regression. The same applies to other models estimating odds or incidence rate ratios. This is the epidemiological concept of independence: independent means purified from other effects (including confounding), with this accomplished by going back to simple regression, removing the effect of extraneous variables kept in the model and looking at how the response changes as a function of one input at a time only.

4.2 Interaction in Additive Models

4.2.1 Definition and Examples

A final issue to consider in multiple regression is the existence of an interaction between two inputs. An interaction is a modification of the effect of one input in the presence of the other (and vice versa). For example, Tonelli et al. studied the effect of pravastatin on the progression of chronic kidney disease using data from the CARE trial [9]. They found that inflammation was associated with higher progression rate and pravastatin with significantly slower kidney disease progression only in the presence of inflammation. Inflammation modified the effect of pravastatin (and vice versa).

The interacting variables (called main terms) can be of the same type (qualitative or quantitative) or different type. The interaction effect can be qualitative (antagonism) or quantitative (synergism). For example, in the study of Kohler et al. [5] both body mass index and HbA1C were directly related to the response (albumin/creatinine ratio) when considered separately. However, the coefficient of the interaction had a negative sign indicating that the total change of $\log(ALB/CR)$ in the presence of one unit increase of both inputs $(0.1535 + 0.0386)$ needs to be reduced by that quantity (-0.0036). In linear models interactions involving at least one quantitative variable change the slope of the fitted line since the effects associated with quantitative variables are differences in slope of the line. Interactions involving only qualitative variables change the intercept of the line.

4.2.2 Modeling Confounding and Interaction

Confounding and interaction are two distinct phenomena. Interaction is an effect modification due to the reciprocal strengthening or weakening of two factors, whereas confounding is determined by differential (unequal) distribution of the confounding variable by level of the exposure and its association with the response. All multivariable analyses allow estimation of the exposure effect purified from confounding and interaction. A potential confounding should be kept in the model even if not significant, unless there are reasons not to do so. For example, a likely confounder might be left out if the model is already too complex for the data (there are too many parameters and few observations or event), and the effect of the main exposure does not vary substantially whether the confounder is included or excluded. The amount of acceptable change in the exposure effect in the presence or absence of the confounder in the model can be a matter of debate and the adopted policy should be explained in the reporting. Conversely, the interaction term is kept in the model only if the associated effect is statistically significant (sometimes considering a more generous P value of 0.1 for an interaction model). The formal test for interaction is based on the creation of a product term obtained multiplying the two main terms. For example: inflammation and treatment group [9]; or body mass index and HbA1C [5]. Coding treatment (TRT) 0 for placebo and 1 for pravastatin, and inflammation (INF) 1 if present and 0 if absent, the interaction term (INT) is 1 for active treatment and inflammation and 0 otherwise. If one term is a continuous variable, the interaction term is 0 when the qualitative variable is 0 and equal to the continuous variable when the qualitative variable is 1. If there are two quantitative variables, the interaction term equals their product. Thus, the interaction model in this linear regression is $y = \beta_0 + \beta_{\mathrm{TRT}} T + \beta_{\mathrm{INF}} I + \beta_{\mathrm{INT}} \mathrm{INT} + \varepsilon$ (plus all the other variables in the model). In the absence of a significant effect associated with the interaction term (INT), there is no effect modification (and the interaction term can be left out of the model). This means that the effects of treatment and inflammation are the same across the levels of each other. In the presence of an interaction effect, the effect modification phenomenon must be considered in addition to the main effects. Of note, to be interpretable the interaction must always be tested in the presence of the main terms since any interaction is a difference in differences.

4.2.3 Statistical Meaning of Interaction

The formal test for the presence of interaction (introducing a product term in the model as explained for the linear model) tests whether there is a deviation from the underlying form of that model. For example, if the effect of age and diabetes on some event rate are respectively $\beta_{\mathrm{AGE}} = 0.001$ (rate change per year of age) and $\beta_{\mathrm{DM}} = 0.02$ (rate change in the presence of diabetes) and there is no interaction, then the two fitted lines corresponding to the presence and absence of diabetes are constantly 0.02 rate units apart. The model is called *additive*. Conversely, if there is an interaction effect $\beta_{\mathrm{INT}} = 0.001$ (further rate change per year of age in diabetics), the two lines of the interaction model are not only 0.02 unit of rate apart due to the effect of diabetes but also constantly (proportionally) diverging by a certain amount. This amount is 2 in this example, because $(0.001 \times \mathrm{AGE} + 0.001 \times \mathrm{AGE})/0.001 \times \mathrm{AGE} = 2$. In other words, rates are twice as high in the presence of diabetes at any age category because diabetes modifies the effect of age (and vice versa). This model is called *multiplicative*. More generally, the response ratio is $(\beta_1 + \beta_{\mathrm{INT}})/\beta_1$ when the interaction is between one

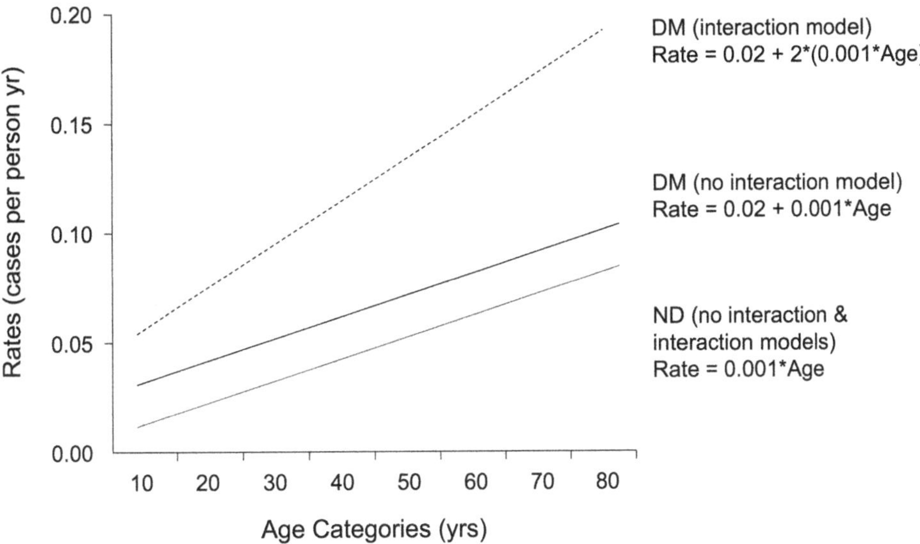

Fig. 8 Interaction parameter as a measure of the departure from the underlying form of a model: the plot shows two models of some event rate as a function of age and diabetes without interaction and with their interaction term. When diabetes is absent (ND, *bottom line*) the event rate is explained by age only in both models. When diabetes is present (DM) the fitted line of the event rate depends on age and diabetes according to the no interaction model (*middle line*) and on age, diabetes, and their product (INT) in the interaction model (*top line*). In the no interaction model the effect of diabetes consists in shifting the event rate by a certain amount quantified by the coefficient of diabetes (change in the intercept of the line). In the interaction model the (*dashed*) fitted line is not only shifted apart for the effect of diabetes but also constantly diverging from the *bottom line* (absence of diabetes). The amount of change in the slope is the effect of the interaction between age and diabetes and is a measure of the departure from the underlying additive form of the model. With permission Ravani et al., Nephrol Dial Transplant [12]

quantitative (x_1) and one qualitative main term with only two values. When both main terms are continuous the response ratio is not constant since $\beta_{INT} \times INT$ varies as the interaction term value varies. However, the coefficient of the interaction term is constant and in all models β_{INT} estimates the amount of departure from the underlying form of the linear model.

Figure 8 shows how the interaction between age and diabetes modifies the slope of the event rate over age. Rate estimates are higher in diabetics by a fixed amount (effect of diabetes) as compared to nondiabetics. This amount (coefficient) remains constant in the no interaction model (rate as a function of age and diabetes, continuous lines). When an interaction is present there is a constant ratio between the two lines resulting in a slope change (because one of the main terms is continuous) in addition to the effect of diabetes (rate as a function of age, diabetes, and their interaction, dashed line and bottom line).

4.2.4 Epidemiological Meaning of the Interaction Coefficient

The coefficient of interaction is always a difference: a difference between differences. In fact considering the example in Fig. 8, there is a rate difference of 0.001 units per year of age; a difference of 0.02 between diabetics and nondiabetics; and a further difference of 0.001 to consider (in addition to 0.021) if a subject is 1 year older and diabetic (total rate difference 0.022 units in a diabetic 1 year older than a nondiabetic). An interaction between two continuous variables would change the slope of the fitted line without affecting the model intercept. For example, if there was an interaction between age (e.g., coefficient 0.001) and systolic blood pressure (e.g., coefficient 0.0001) and the coefficient of interaction was 0.00001, then a subject 1 year older and with 1 mmHg higher systolic blood pressure would have an estimated rate of 0.00111 units (0.00001 + 0.0011) higher.

4.3 Interaction in Multiplicative Models

When the LP is the argument of some non-identity functions, differences in the LP assume different epidemiological meaning. In Cox's, logistic, or Poisson regressions for example, differences in the LP have the meaning of risk ratios. As opposed to linear models in which the combined effect of several factors is the sum of the effects produced by each of the factors, Cox's, logistic, and Poisson regressions are multiplicative models because in these models the joint effect of two or more factors is the product of their effects. For example, if the risk of death associated with diabetes is twice as high as in nondiabetics and is three times as high in men as in women, diabetic men have a risk six times higher than nondiabetic women. However, this multiplicative effect still results from differences in the LP.

A problem with interaction in multiplicative models derives from the definition of interaction as a measure of the departure from the underlying form of the model. This definition meets both statistical and biological interpretation of the interaction phenomenon as an amount of effect unexplained by the main terms. However, when this effect is measured, its statistical and epidemiological interpretation differs, depending on the model scale [10]. This is different from additive models where statistical and epidemiological perspectives coincide: when the input effects are measured as differences, interaction parameters are differences chosen to measure departure from an additive model. In additive models an antagonistic interaction will result in a change lower than expected, i.e., less than additive [5], whereas a synergistic interaction will result in a change greater than expected, i.e., more than additive (Fig. 8). Statistical testing of this departure measures also the biologic phenomenon. When the effects are measured as ratios, interaction parameters are ratios, chosen to measure departures from a multiplicative model. In multiplicative models an antagonistic interaction will result in a change lower than expected (less than multiplicative), whereas a synergistic interaction will result in a change greater than expected (more than multiplicative). Statistical assessment of this departure tests whether there is a departure from

Table 1
Hypothetical cardiac event data expressed as incidence rate ratio (IRR) by level of two risk factors: smoking and hypertension, where there is no interaction on a multiplicative scale but there is on an additive scale

		Hypertension	
		Absent	Present
Smoking	Absent	1 *Ref.*	10 *IRR 10 (1.2, 77.6)*
	Present	5 *IRR 5 (0.5, 42.5)*	50 IRR?

Legend: The 2×2 table shows the number of cardiac events per 1,000 person-years by presence of hypertension and smoking habit. As compared to subjects exposed to neither factor (absence of smoking and hypertension), the event rate in the presence of hypertension only is ten times as high; in the presence of smoking only is five times as high; and in the presence of both exposures is 50 times as high. On a multiplicative scale there is no interaction since there is no departure from the underlying form of a multiplicative risk model (Poisson in this case). In fact, 5 × 10 is exactly 50. Testing the parameter of the product term, the IRR is 1 (95 % CI 0.5, 42.5)
However, risk ratios can be assessed also on an additive scale, where the IRR is 50 (6.9, 359). The two models have the same Log-likelihood (−355.7). The only difference is the "contrast" defining the null hypothesis. In the multiplicative model, the interaction term is a product term assuming the value of 1 for exposed to both and 0 otherwise. The null hypothesis is the absence of deviation from multiplicative risk (and of course it is not rejected). In the additive formulation a factored set of terms is entered into the model with exposed to neither as reference category. The null hypothesis is the absence of difference on an additive scale (departure from additivity). The null hypothesis is rejected because the difference between exposed to both and exposed to neither prove to be larger than the sum of the other two differences, i.e., (50 − 1) − [(10 − 1) + (5 − 1)] = 36. With permission Ravani et al., Nephrol Dial Transplant [12]

multiplicativity and not the existence of a biologic phenomenon. Therefore, from the statistical viewpoint interaction depends on how the effects are measured, although a multiplicative relationship per se is evidence of biologic interaction as the resulting change in the response is greater than the sum of the effects (e.g., if diabetic men have a risk six times as high as nondiabetic women and the relative risk associated with the main effects are 3 and 2, there is no deviation from the multiplicative scale but there is over-additivity). On the other hand, the choice of the model depends on the distribution of the response variable and cannot be dictated by the need to study interaction. However, there are ways to use multiplicative models and still assess the biological meaning of the phenomenon.

Tables 1 and 2 show two different approaches for the analysis of interaction in risk data using multiplicative models. For example, in the Poisson model differences in the coefficients of the LP are interpreted as incidence rate ratios. When the presence of more risk factors is associated with multiplicative risk, there is no deviation from the underlying form of the model and the formal test for interaction is not significant. However, this should be interpreted based on the scale of measurement and biological knowledge. Lack of evidence of deviation from the multiplicative scale implies the existence of over-additivity, which requires a biological explanation. In this case biologic interaction can be assessed using categories of covariate combination with exposed to none as reference.

Table 2
Hypothetical cardiac event data expressed as incidence rate ratio (IRR) by level of two risk factors: smoking and hypertension, where there is antagonism on a multiplicative scale and synergism on an additive scale

		Hypertension	
		Absent	Present
Smoking	Absent	1 *Ref.*	7 *IRR 7 (0.8, 56)*
	Present	3 *IRR 3 (0.3, 28)*	14 IRR?

Legend: The 2×2 table shows the number of cardiac events per 1,000 person-years by presence of hypertension and smoking habit. As compared to subjects exposed to neither factor (absence of smoking and hypertension), the event rate in the presence of hypertension only is seven times as high; in the presence of smoking only is three times as high; and in the presence of both exposures is 14 times as high. If the risk in the interaction cell is less than multiplicative, the estimate of the risk ratio in a multiplicative model is less than 1, giving the misleading impression of a qualitative interaction (antagonism). The formal test for interaction gives an IRR of 0.6 (0.05, 7); using a factored set of terms IRR is 14 (1.8, 106). The additive model support a quantitative interaction because the number of cases in the group exposed to both factors is larger that the sum of the two differences, i.e., $14 - 1 - [(3-1)+(7-1)] = 5$. The two Poisson models have the same Log-likelihood of -166.7. With permission Ravani et al., Nephrol Dial Transplant [12]

This method allows using any regression models to estimate departures from additivity without imposing the multiplicative relation implied by the structure of the chosen function [10].

5   Reporting

The reporting of statistical methods and results in medical literature is often suboptimal. A few tips are summarized in this section. More detailed checklists for reading and reporting statistical analyses are available in textbooks [11].

5.1   Methods

In the methods section there should be a clear statement of the study question, detailed description of study design, how subjects were recruited, how the sample size was estimated to detect the strength of the main association of interest, how all variables (inputs and output) were measured, and how the main biases were prevented or controlled. The main outcome of interest and the main exposure should be clearly defined, since they determine the choice of the regression method and model building strategies.

Number of observations as well as subjects and clusters should be described. This information is important to choose the proper statistical technique to handle correlation in the data.

The statistical model used should be described along with the procedures adopted to verify the underlying assumptions. The type of function used to model the response should be clear, along with the epidemiological meaning of the coefficients, the main exposure and the potential confounders, why and how they appear (or not) in the final model, and why and how possible interactions were taken into account. As different modeling strategies may provide different results using the same data, it is important to describe how the model was built, if any algorithm was followed or if a manual approach was chosen. The regression method to obtain the parameter estimates and to perform hypothesis testing should also be stated. Finally there should be a description of the diagnostics applied, how residuals were studied, how possible violations were excluded, handled or treated (e.g., with transformations), and whether any sensitivity analyses were carried out (running the model excluding some influential observations and checking if the results remained the same). Some models require special checking, e.g., proportionality assumption for the Cox's model and fit tests for logistic and Poisson regression. The description of the statistical package used for analysis should also be provided as estimation algorithms may be different in different packages.

5.2 Results

Since any model has a systematic component and a chance element, both should be reported. The fit component should inform about the relationship between exposure and disease, the strength of the associations (the coefficient estimate), and the effects of other variables (including confounding and interactions). When interactions are included in the model the main terms must also be included.

It is always important to understand the relevance of the effect. Thus, reporting a statistically significant association (a P value) is not enough. Point estimates (parameter estimates) should be reported along with a measure of precision (95 % Confidence Intervals) and the results of statistical testing (exact value of P rather than "<0.05," unless it is <0.001). Often measures of effect, and not measures of disease, are of interest. For example reporting the average blood pressure in group A and B (with their 95 % CI) and the statement of statistically significant difference is not enough: what matters are the estimated difference and the 95 % CI of the difference. Finally, the variability in the response unexplained by the model is important ($1 - R^2$ statistics for linear model, likelihood for MLE methods) as well as the gain obtained from modeling as compared to the unconditional distribution (which can be appreciated from the table of patient characteristics).

The next chapter examines the different multivariable models in more detail.

References

1. Heckbert SR, Post W, Pearson GD, Arnett DK, Gomes AS, Jerosch-Herold M, Hundley WG, Lima JA, Bluemke DA (2006) Traditional cardiovascular risk factors in relation to left ventricular mass, volume, and systolic function by cardiac magnetic resonance imaging: the multiethnic study of atherosclerosis. J Am Coll Cardiol 48:2285–92

2. Ravani P, Tripepi G, Malberti F, Testa S, Mallamaci F, Zoccali C (2005) Asymmetrical dimethylarginine predicts progression to dialysis and death in patients with chronic kidney

disease: a competing risks modeling approach. J Am Soc Nephrol 16:2449–2455

3. Palatini P, Mormino P, Dorigatti F, Santonastaso M, Mos L, De Toni R, Winnicki M, Dal Follo M, Biasion T, Garavelli G, Pessina AC, HARVEST Study Group (2006) Glomerular hyperfiltration predicts the development of microalbuminuria in stage 1 hypertension: the HARVEST. Kidney Int 70: 578–84

4. Malik AR, Sultan S, Turner ST, Kullo IJ (2007) Urinary albumin excretion is associated with impaired flow- and nitroglycerin-mediated brachial artery dilatation in hypertensive adults. J Hum Hypertens 21:231–8

5. Kohler KA, McClellan WM, Ziemer DC, Kleinbaum DG, Boring JR (2000) Risk factors for microalbuminuria in black Americans with newly diagnosed type 2 diabetes. Am J Kidney Dis 36:903–13

6. Verhave JC, Hillege HL, Burgerhof JG, Navis G, de Zeeuw D, de Jong PE (2003) PREVEND study group: cardiovascular risk factors are differently associated with urinary albumin excretion in men and women. J Am Soc Nephrol 14:1330–5

7. Glantz SA, Slinker BK (2001) A primer of applied regression and analysis of variance, 2nd edn. McGraw-Hill, New York

8. Heine GH, Reichart B, Ulrich C, Kohler H, Girndt M (2007) Do ultrasound renal resistance indices reflect systemic rather than renal vascular damage in chronic kidney disease? Nephrol Dial Transplant 22:163–70

9. Tonelli M, Sacks F, Pfeffer M, Jhangri GS, Curhan G (2005) Biomarkers of inflammation and progression of chronic kidney disease. Kidney Int 68:237–45

10. Rothman KJ (2002) Measuring interaction. In: Epidemiology: an introduction. Oxford University Press, New York, pp 168–180

11. Altman DG, Machin D, Bryant TN, Gardner MJ (eds) (2000) Statistics with confidence, 2nd edn. BMJ Books, London

12. Ravani P, Parfrey P, Gadag V, Malberti F, Barrett B (2007) Clinical research of kidney diseases III: principles of regression and modelling. Nephrol Dial Transplant 22(12):3422–30

Chapter 6

Longitudinal Studies 3: Data Modeling Using Standard Regression Models and Extensions

Pietro Ravani, Brendan J. Barrett, and Patrick S. Parfrey

Abstract

In longitudinal studies the relationship between exposure and disease can be measured once or multiple times while participants are monitored over time. Traditional regression techniques are used to model outcome data when each epidemiological unit is observed once. These models include generalized linear models for quantitative continuous, discrete, or qualitative outcome responses, and models for time-to-event data. When data come from the same subjects or group of subjects, observations are not independent and the underlying correlation needs to be addressed in the analysis. In these circumstances extended models are necessary to handle complexities related to clustered data, and repeated measurements of time-varying predictors and/or outcomes.

Key words Generalized linear models, Survival analysis, Repeated measures, Multiple failure times

---

1 Introduction

Longitudinal studies vary enormously in their size and complexity, and this has implications for data analysis. Open cohort studies are of relatively long duration and several patients can leave or join the cohort during follow-up. Closed cohort studies are usually shorter, and fewer participants leave the study during follow-up for reasons unrelated to the outcome of interest.

At one extreme a large population of subjects may be studied over years. For example, Go et al. studied the relationship between reduced kidney function and the occurrence of hospital admissions, cardiovascular events, and death from all causes among 1,120,295 adult members of the Kaiser Permanente Renal Registry [1]. Both levels of kidney function (exposure) and hospital admissions and cardiovascular events (repeatable diseases) were measured multiple times during follow-up. The existence of the hypothesized association between exposure and outcome was tested taking into account these *multiple measurements*.

Patrick S. Parfrey and Brendan J. Barrett (eds.), *Clinical Epidemiology: Practice and Methods*, Methods in Molecular Biology, vol. 1281, DOI 10.1007/978-1-4939-2428-8_6, © Springer Science+Business Media New York 2015

At the other extreme, some longitudinal studies follow up relatively small groups for a few days or weeks. For example Merten et al. compared the effect of sodium chloride and bicarbonate in reducing the occurrence of contrast-induced nephropathy defined as an increase of 25 % or more in serum creatinine within 2 days of contrast [2]. They studied 119 subjects with stable serum creatinine levels of at least 1.1 mg/dL (≥97.2 μmol/L) in a randomized trial. The existence of the hypothesized effect of bicarbonate (exposure–intervention) and reduced risk of contrast nephropathy (disease–outcome) was tested comparing outcome *measured at study end* by treatment group.

These examples introduce an important feature of longitudinal studies: the relationship between exposure and disease can be measured once or multiple times while participants are monitored over time. When data come from the same subjects or group of subjects the underlying correlation need to be addressed in the analysis.

The present chapter provides introductory notes on traditional tools used to model outcome data when each epidemiological unit is observed once. These models include generalized linear models and survival models for time-to-event data. Extensions of these models are necessary to handle complexities related to clustered data, and repeated measurements of time-varying predictors and/or outcomes.

2 Generalized Linear Models

Generalized linear models are "parametric" models because they estimate population characteristics (parameters) based on distributional assumptions. These assumptions specify the shape of the input–output relationship and the distribution of the residuals guiding the choice of the model to study the data (see previous chapter).

The family of generalized linear models is large, but all its members have the following attributes:

1. A specific random component defining the conditional distribution of the response variable (Gaussian or normal for the linear model; binomial for logistic regression; Poisson for Poisson regression, for example).

2. A linear function of the regressors (inputs), or linear predictor (LP), on which the expected (fitted) value of the response $\hat{y}$ of y depends.

3. An "invertible" link function $g(\hat{y}) = \mathrm{LP}$, which transforms the LP into the expectations of the response ($\hat{y}$).

The first attribute pertains to the random portion of the models; the LP and the link function to the systematic component. The LP, introduced in the previous chapter, has the form

Table 1
Some standard link functions and their inverses

Link	$LP = g(\hat{y})$	$\hat{y} = g^{-1}(LP)$	Y range	$\mathrm{Var}(y\,|\,LP)$	Distribution	Model
Identity	$\hat{y}$	LP	$-\infty, +\infty$	$\sum (y-\hat{y})^2 / (n-1)$	Gaussian	Linear
Logit	$\log_e\left[\hat{y}/\left(1-\hat{y}\right)\right]$	$1/\left(1+e^{-LP}\right)$	$(0, 1, 2, \dots, n)/n$	$\hat{y}(1-\hat{y})$	Binomial	Logistic
Log	$\log_e \hat{y}$	e^{LP}	$0, 1, 2, \dots$	$\hat{y}$	Poisson	Poisson

LP is the linear predictor; g represents an invertible link function; $\hat{y}$ is the expected value of the response; y is the observed value of the response; $\mathrm{Var}(y\,|\,LP)$ is the variance of the response given the predictors. An invertible link function is a function linking $\hat{y}$ and LP allowing going back from LP to $\hat{y}$ using its inverse

$LP = \beta_0 + \beta_1 x_1 + \beta_2 x_2 + \cdots + \beta_k x_k$. Each independent variable "xs" (from 1 to "k") may be quantitative or qualitative inputs, their transformations, polynomial terms, contrast generated from factors, and so on. The inputs or regressors can assume different values, whereas the regression coefficients "βs" (from 0 to "k") are constant. In generalized linear models LP is the "argument" of the specific function of that model. The standard link functions, the inverses and the conditional error distributions of the three most popular generalized linear models (linear, logistic, and Poisson) are shown in Table 1. For example, linear models have an *identity link function* and *normally distributed errors*. This means that the observed values of the response (e.g., left ventricular mass index) are modeled as a function of LP (including for example blood pressure and body mass index) and what remains to be explained after the model is fitted to the data (the error component) is normally distributed with mean zero and some non-zero variance. It is possible to go in the opposite direction (using the inverse) from the fitted values (expected averages) and make predictions about future observations taking into account the residuals. In logistic regression a *logit* function links the binary data (e.g., presence of left ventricular hypertrophy) to the LP (with one or more inputs), the inverse function is the *logistic* function that allows estimating probabilities of future outcomes from the LP, and the distribution of the conditional response is *binomial*. In Poisson regression the *natural log* links the expected counts (e.g., death rate or hospitalization) to the LP, its inverse is the *exponential* that allows estimating future incidence rates based on the LP, and the conditional distribution of the response follows the *Poisson distribution*.

The technical explanation of these attributes is complex and beyond the scope of the present chapter. Also the Gaussian, Binomial and Poisson distributions will not be described. However, the important aspect to understand here is that each model has a specific underlying function, which is invertible, and a specific distribution of the "unexplained" variability of the response and, consequently, a specific distribution of the conditional response given the inputs. The type of function has implications on the meaning of the parameters estimated by the model. The distribution of the residual is important to check if the model fits the data well, i.e., to exclude the existence of different links between input and output disregarded by the model.

2.1 General Linear Model for Quantitative Responses

2.1.1 Structure of the Linear Model

Linear regression is appropriate to model quantitative response variables. For example, in a cohort study of chronic kidney disease progression and patient survival, glomerular filtration rate (GFR) was inversely related to asymmetrical dimethylarginine (ADMA) at baseline, being on average 0.17 ml/min per 1.73 m^2 lower per 0.1 µmol/L of ADMA [3]. This inverse relationship suggests that one variable tends to change in the opposite direction of the other, although only 48 % of the change in GFR was explained by the systematic component of the multivariable model (R^2 statistics).

The systematic component of general linear models (LP) includes the model intercept ("β_0") and the estimated effects (e.g., change in GFR) associated with the predictor (e.g., ADMA) and other input variables in the model ("β_k"). The random component is represented by the residuals or differences between the observed response values and their expectations and is summarized by an unexplained variability of GFR as high as 52 % in the ADMA study [3]. Examples of different prediction ability of the same set of covariates used for five cardiac outcomes are described in the Multiethnic Study of Atherosclerosis. In this study the R^2 statistics decreased from almost 60 % for the model of left ventricular mass to less than 20 % for the model of left ventricular ejection fraction [4]. However, the most important use of the R^2 statistics is to compare so called "nested models." These models have the same response and fit the same data (the same set of observations). The best model (i.e., predictors to include, confounding and interaction terms as well as possible transformations to consider) is selected considering the best fit in terms of improvement of the R^2 statistics (reduction of the residual variance).

Linear models can include one or more inputs. For example, t test and one-way ANOVA are special cases of univariable linear models where the input has respectively two and more than two possible levels. The characteristics of the general linear model are summarized in Table 2.

2.1.2 Meaning of the Coefficients in Linear Regression

The regression coefficients of the linear model estimate the average change in the output per unit change in each input. Therefore, they are "differences" in the average response by level or unit of exposure (Table 2). For example, Heine et al. studied renal resistance indices in subjects with chronic kidney disease not yet on dialysis [5]. Among the independent predictors included in the final model of resistance indices there were age, glomerular filtration rate and

Table 2
Characteristics and conditions of validity of the general linear model

Meaning of "β_k"	The regression coefficients of the linear model are differences corresponding to average changes in "y" *(output)* per unit change in "x_k" (*input* "k")
Gauss-Markov assumptions	1. *Linearity:* The shape of the systematic component (LP) must be reasonably linear; mathematically LP is a sum of input(s) raised to the first power, each multiplied by its parameter. This means that it must be possible to quantify the amount of linear change of the output per unit change of the input(s) since the parameter estimates are constant and apply over the whole range of the predictors 2. *Normality:* Residuals are normally distributed around the fitted line with mean = zero and constant variance (homoscedasticity). This means that what remains to be explained around the fit is similarly unknown across all input(s) values 3. *Independency:* The residuals must be independent; this is possible only if the observations are independent. This means that what remains to be explained around the fit is unknown independent of the process of measurement
Purposes of the linear model	1. To predict the value of an output for given input(s) based on estimates obtained from a sample 2. To adjust the effects of an input variable on a quantitative output variable for the effects of other extraneous variables (confounders) 3. To assess whether the effect of an input is unaffected or changes by level of another input variable (interaction)

diabetes, for example. The first coefficient estimated in the model is the model intercept, $b_0 = 50.8$ (95 % Confidence Intervals 42.6–59.1; $P<0.001$). This parameter is the value of the output when everything else is "zero." For example when diabetes is coded "0" (diabetes absent) and "1" (diabetes present) and nothing else is in the model, the intercept estimates the average output value in those without diabetes. However, when quantitative variables (age for example) are in the model this quantity per se has meaning when averages values of those inputs are considered (see previous chapter). The P value is the probability of falsely rejecting the null hypothesis that the coefficient is zero (tested by means of a t-test, for example). The coefficient associated with diabetes (5.59, 95 % CI 2.1, 9) means that diabetics have on average 5.5 higher values of the response. Resistance indices tend to be higher in older subjects (0.18 per year of age) and lower in those with more preserved glomerular filtration rate (−0.07 per ml/min).

2.1.3 Model Check

General linear models are considered the paradigm of all statistical models used in epidemiological research but they cannot be used in all circumstances. Graphical and formal statistical tests must be performed to check if the assumptions of the linear model are reasonably met. More details can be found in specific textbooks [6].

2.2 Logistic Model for Qualitative Responses

When the response variable is a binary outcome that is either present or absent (sometimes termed "success" and "failure"), then an appropriate analysis is often binary logistic regression. The outcome might be the presence of a disease in a survey or the occurrence of an event in a prevention study, such as contrast nephropathy [2]. Researchers are interested in identifying factors associated with the event. However, since it is not possible to predict whether an event will occur or not with certainty, what researchers do is seeking for factors associated with the *probability* (or risk) that an event happens.

2.2.1 Structure of the Logistic Model

Since the logistic function may seem quite complex the characteristics of logistic regression may be more easily introduced by showing why linear regression cannot be used to model probabilities. Consider a sample of 100 subjects on whom the following variables have been measured: age (in years) and coronary heart disease (present or absent) [7]. Researchers may want to study disease status (y) as a function of age (x). Plotting disease status over age in years (Fig. 1, left plot) makes all observation fall on one of two possible values representing the absence of the disease ($y=0$) or the presence of the disease ($y=1$). This plot shows the binary nature of the response and suggests a possible association, as younger individuals tend to fall on the bottom line of no disease. However, the large variability of y at all ages (i.e., subjects with the same age with

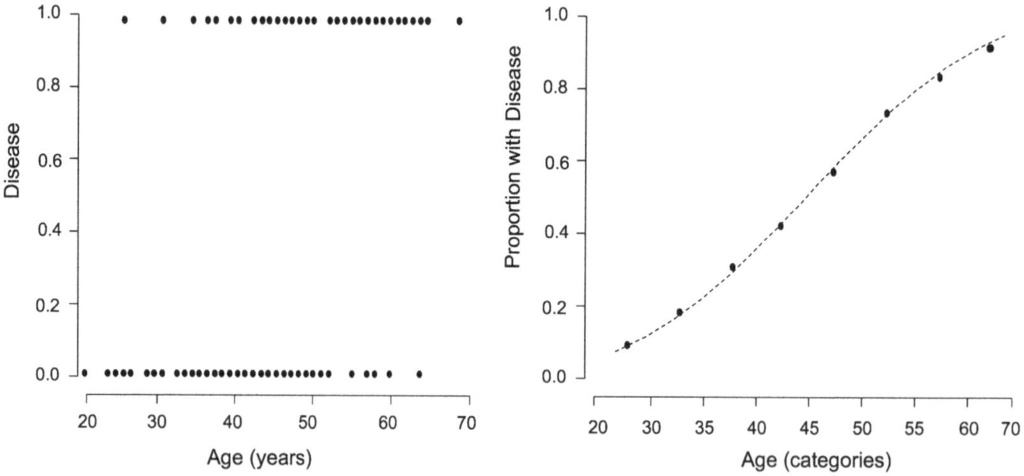

Fig. 1 Study of the presence or absence of a disease as a function of age: The *first scatter-plot* uses the original measurements on 100 study subjects (*left*). The values of the response lie on two lines indicating presence ($y=1$) or absence ($y=0$) of the disease. However, subjects tend to be younger when $y=0$ (older when $y=1$). Since within the age values subjects may be on either line (high variability) the possible relationship cannot be easily appreciated. The *second curve* represents the proportion of subjects with the disease over age category mid-points (*right*). The relationship between the two variables is more clearly appreciated, but the curve is sigmoid rather than straight. With permission from Ravani et al. [39]

and without disease) does not allow appreciation of the relationship. Some variability can be removed categorizing the input and plotting the mean output variable (proportion) value for each input level (Fig. 1, right plot). The relationship becomes appreciable, but the form of the ideal line passing through the points differs from what might have been obtained if the response was quantitative first, the shape of the line is sigmoid rather straight; second, there is no information about the errors. The logistic model rather than the linear model is appropriate for this type of relationship (see previous chapter). In fact in linear regression the conditional response may take any value as LP ranges from $+\infty$ and $-\infty$. Conversely, with dichotomous data the conditional mean (probability) must be ≥ 0 and ≤ 1. The right plot of Fig. 1 shows that this mean approaches 0 and 1 "gradually." In other words, the S-shaped curve implies that the change in the expected value of the response per unit change in the predictor(s) becomes progressively smaller as the response gets closer to 0 or 1. This is what the logistic function does: transform a continuous variable with a range between $+\infty$ and $-\infty$ (LP) into a response ranging from 0 to 1 (probability). Everything else already introduced about the LP (concepts of linearity and meaning of the coefficients) is true also for logistic regression, although the epidemiological meaning of the parameters (coefficients of the LP) changes because of the specific function of the logistic model. The argument (LP) of the logistic function is an "index" combining the contributions of several risk factors, and the logistic function of LP represents the individual risk of the disease for a given value of LP.

Another important difference with linear regression is the distribution of the errors. In linear models the observed values of the response (given the values of the individual inputs) are modeled as function of the LP and the error term is in the model ($y \mid X = LP + \varepsilon$). In logistic regression (logit$[y \mid X] = LP$) the observed values of the dependent variable (y failures in n trials) are not in the equation, but their expectations are linked to the model by the binomial distribution. Of course the values of the population parameter (probability) are unknown. The estimated or fitted values are used instead in the modeling process using Maximum Likelihood Estimation (see previous chapter). The remaining general principles of regression analysis are the same as in linear regression. Therefore, when the response is dichotomous:

1. The conditional mean of the regression equation must be bounded between zero and one (and this is satisfied by the logistic formulation of LP).

2. The binomial and not the normal distribution describes the distribution of the errors.

3. The principles of analysis using linear regression also guide logistic regression.

Table 3
Example of simple logistic regression and meaning of the coefficients

	Failure	Success		
Exposed (E: $x=1$)	30	20		a	b
Unexposed (U: $x=0$)	10	40		c	d
	40	60		
Pre-test odds of failure =	$(a+c)/(b+d)$ =	40/60 =	0.666	
Post-test odds among E =	a/b =	30/20 =	1.500	
Post-test odds among U =	c/d =	10/40 =	0.250	
Odds ratio =	$(a\times d)/(c\times b)$ =	1.5/0.25 =	6.000	

Before considering the predictor (x), the (null) model is $\text{Logit}(\pi_i) = \ln\left[\pi_i/(1-\pi_i)\right]$ which is $\text{Logit}(\pi_i) = \beta_0 = \ln(40/60) = -0.405$. This gives the unconditional probability estimate $\pi_i = \exp(\beta_0)/\left[1+\exp(\beta_0)\right] = 0.4$, or overall risk. However, the conditional probability changes when x is considered. The (full) logistic model is $\text{Logit}(\pi_i \mid x_i) = \beta_0^* + \beta_x x_i$, where $\beta_0^* = -1.386$ represents the log-odds among unexposed, and $\beta_x = 1.791$ is the log-odds ratio (OR). In fact, when $x=0$, the odds are $\exp(-1.386) = 0.25$; when $x=1$ the odds are $\exp(-1.386+1.791) = 1.5$. Therefore, β_x represents the difference of the log-odds between exposed and unexposed, or log-OR. The exponentiated "β_x" gives the OR of exposed vs. unexposed

2.2.2 Meaning of the Coefficients in Logistic Regression

The geometrical meaning of the intercept and the other coefficients of the LP in logistic regression are similar to those of linear regression: they define the position (value of risk corresponding to 0.5) and shape (how much the risk changes as the input values change) of the logistic function. However, differences in the argument of a logistic function have a specific epidemiological meaning since they are related to the odds ratio. This can be best shown using an example. Let us consider a study of a disease such as myocardial infarction and an exposure such as hypertension defined as present or absent. From the 2 by 2 table shown in Table 3 it can be seen that before studying the association between exposure and disease the only available data is that there are 40 failure events among 100 individuals (risk 0.4). Running a "null model" corresponds to ignoring the information related to the exposure: the intercept of the null model informs about the overall risk just as the intercept of a null linear model informs about the overall mean of the continuous response in the sample. The "logit" of the unconditional probability (log-odds) is the intercept of the null model since there is no input in the LP. The "exponentiated" intercept is the pre-test odds for disease. Using the logistic function (inverse) it is possible to estimate the overall risk. However, it may be hypothesized that the risk varies by level of exposure. This can be tested including the predictor in the model. The (full) model has a new intercept. This new intercept carries both the previous knowledge (pre-test odds) and the knowledge gained from considering the exposure "x" (likelihood ratio of being unexposed).

Of course, the logistic model now also contains the coefficient of the input, which has the meaning of the log-odds ratio. In fact when the exposure is present the LP (logit of probability or log-odds) is the sum of β_0 and β_x. When the exposure is absent LP contains only β_0. The difference in these two log-odds, once exponentiated, is simply the odds ratio (OR) of exposed versus unexposed, in the example $\exp(1.8) = 6$. When inputs are categorical or continuous the associated coefficient is the effect per unit change of the variable. For example, if the coefficient is 0.3, the OR associated with each level increase of input (category or unit of exposure) is $\exp(0.3) = 1.35$, which means that each level change in the predictor is associated with a 35 % higher odds for disease (as compared to the previous level). If the coefficient has a negative sign, the predictor is associated with reduced odds for disease. For example, if the coefficient of serum albumin in g/L is -0.2, the OR is 0.81, i.e., there is a 19 % reduction in the odds for the event per each g/L increase in serum albumin. If more inputs are in the model (including confounding and interaction terms), each odds ratio is adjusted for the effect of all the other independent variables in the model. This is clear from the little algebra shown above, as they will appear in both LP terms of the specific difference in question. Of course due to the exponential form of the model the individual odds change on a multiplicative scale as the values of the covariate change. For example, if the OR for a disease associated with male gender is two and the OR for the same disease is three in smokers, the OR for a male subject who smokes as compared to a non-smoking woman will be six. In linear model effects are additive instead because of the identity function linking the response to the LP. However, it is important to remember that the risk index (LP) changes linearly as the covariate levels change and that it is possible to interpret risk change (including the case of interaction) on an additive scale even using multiplicative models (see previous chapter).

Using the full model the background risk can be estimated from the odds among unexposed $[R = O \,/\, (1+O)]$. However, risk estimation from a logistic model only makes sense in longitudinal studies. If subjects were selected based on disease (case control design) the likelihood of exposure is assessed "retrospectively" and the estimate of any risk including the basal risk is biased. The same applies to relative risk (or ratios of estimated risks). For this reason in non-longitudinal designs logistic regression is used to estimate odds ratios only rather than risk and risk ratios.

2.2.3 Model Check and Other Issues

There are a number of ways to check if the model fails to describe the data well. Some of these are based on the same principles as those applied to linear regression because the log-odds for the response must be linearly related to the predictors. Graphical assessment of the residuals is important to assess linearity and study outliers.

In logistic regression (as well as in Poisson and in Cox's regressions) the model likelihood has the same meaning as the R^2 statistic in linear models: the higher the value the better the fit (usually the log-likelihoods of nested models are compared although it is possible to estimate a pseudo—R^2 also for nonlinear models).

Specific to logistic regression are the goodness-of-fit test and the maximum number of parameters that can be simultaneously estimated. The goodness-of-fit test compares the observed probabilities with ones predicted by the model using a chi-squared test. Evidence of lack of fit causes over-dispersion (extra-binomial variation), which means that the standard errors of the model may not be valid. This may arise because some important covariate has been omitted or because outcome data are correlated (e.g., repeated binary outcome in the same subject).

The maximum number of model parameters is another important issue in logistic regression. Hosmer and Lemeshow indicate that a minimum of ten events (the lowest between successes and failures) per parameter is necessary to avoid biased variance estimation [8]. A detailed discussion of logistic regression including special topics and model extensions can be found in specific texts [9].

2.3 Poisson Model for Counts

Poisson regression is used when the risk of an event for an individual is constant and small but the number of individuals is large, and thus the total number of events is considerable. The outcome variable in Poisson regression is a count of independent events over a period of time at risk, such as the number of deaths over years of follow-up. This count is a discrete quantitative variable. The principal covariate in the model is the time at risk, which is recorded for each observation (exposure time). While logistic regression models probabilities, Poisson regression models rates (λ = count of event/ the number of times event could have occurred).

Rates and Rate Ratios: The risk of an event is the expected number of events occurring in a group of people during a specified period of time. Risks are probabilities, dimensionless and with possible values ranging from 0 to 1, and can be estimated in short studies where subject follow-up is approximately complete. Longer studies estimate incidence rates instead of risks because when the study duration is long not all subjects are observed for the same amount of time (e.g., one may be observed for 10 years, another for 20 years, and so on). Rates have the same numerator as risks but person-time of observation as their denominator (e.g., one person observed for 10 years and another for 20 years would contribute for a total of 30 person-years of follow-up or 30 persons per unit time, i.e., 30 person-years). Therefore, rates treat one unit of time as equivalent to another, regardless of whether these time units come from the same subject or different individuals. Furthermore, incidence rates have the dimension of 1/time and range from 0 to $+\infty$. Rates can exceed 1 (100 %)

because they do not measure the proportion of the population that experience disease but the ratio of the number of events to the time at risk for disease. Since the denominator is measured in time units, the numerical value of the incidence rate depends on the chosen time unit. For example, if eight cases occur in 36 subjects observed for 1 month, then the rate is 0.22 cases per person-month or 2.66 cases per person-year, but the two expressions measure the same rate. Finally, if the underlying risk is constant and small (e.g., less than 0.2) it can be estimated as the product of the rate estimate and the observation time. For example, if 1,000 subjects are followed for 10 years and experience a mortality rate of 0.01 per person-year ($0.01\ \text{year}^{-1}$), the risk can be estimated as 0.01×10 or 0.1 over 10 years (each individual has a probability of 10 % to die in 10 years). However, this calculation neglects the shrinking of the population as deaths occur over time, as the same mortality rate applies to a steadily smaller population at risk (exponential decay). The risk approximation of the incidence rate does not work well for high risk or very long time duration. Fortunately, risks of interest to epidemiologists are usually small and epidemiological studies not too long. For these reasons rate estimates approximate true risks reasonably well. For the same reasons, incidence rate (IR) ratios are interpretable as risk (R) ratios since $R_1/R_0 = (\text{IR}_1 \times \text{time})/(\text{IR}_0 \times \text{time}) = \text{IR}_1/\text{IR}_0$. An example will clarify why this is important to Poisson regression. Suppose that "d" independent events are observed during "n" person-years, where d is small as compared to n (note: person-years not persons). For example, in the Framingham Heart Study dataset there are 4,699 individuals and 104,461 person-years of follow-up [10]. The observed incidence of coronary events is $\lambda_1 = d_1\ /\ n_1 = 823\ /\ 42{,}688 = 0.019279\,\text{year}^{-1}$ or 19.27 per 1,000 person-years in men (1) and $\lambda_0 = d_0\ /\ n_0 = 650\ /\ 61{,}773 = 0.010522\,\text{year}^{-1}$ or 10.52 per 1,000 person-years in women (0). The incidence rate ratio of men vs. women is $\text{IRR} = \lambda_1\ /\ \lambda_0 = 1.832$. Poisson regression is used to estimate the IRR associated with "one unit change" of the predictor.

2.3.1 Structure of the Poisson Model

Rates represent the number of events d expected to occur in n person-time (risk over time). The link function in Poisson regression is a simple log transform whose inverse is the exponential function. The Poisson model is $\log(\lambda\,|\,X) = \log(d\,/\,n\,|\,X) = \text{LP}$ in terms of rates or $\log(d\,|\,X) = \log(n) + \text{LP}$ in terms of counts. Using the inverse the expected number of events is $d\,|\,X = \exp\{\log(n) + \text{LP}\}$. Since the risk is assumed to rise directly with n, the coefficient for $\log(n)$ is fixed at one and is known as model offset. The important aspect to note here is that as for logistic regression, the expected rather than the observed counts are modeled. The Poisson distribution links the observed counts to their expectations. Assuming that a Poisson process underlies the event of interest, Poisson regression finds ML estimates of the β parameters.

Let us imagine that ten subjects are observed during a 1-year study divided in one-month bands (unit of n); that the exposure times for the ten subjects (n) are: 1, 2, 3, 4, 5, 6, 7, 8, 9, 10 bands; and that three people die during the study period. Thus, $d = 3$ in 55 1-month bands, each of 0.0833 years duration (1/12). The event rate is $3/(55 \times 0.0833) = 0.655$ per year or, in terms of count, 655 deaths per 1,000 person-years. If the data had been updated every day, then the length of the band would have been 1 day and there would have been $55 \times (365.25/12) = 1,674$ bands (units of n) of 0.002737 year duration. However, the rate would have been the same, i.e., $3/(1,674 \times 0.002737) = 0.655$. Thus, assuming all events occur at the end of the band (which is often a strong assumption), the estimates are not affected by the precision of the measurement. However, time-to-event data are more often modeled rather than rates when individual data and more precise time measurements are available.

From the above example, rates can be viewed as probabilities over time. In fact $\lambda = d/n$, where n represents the number of bands times their duration h and λ can also be expressed as the expected event count per some multiple of unit time (e.g., 0.05 years^{-1} = 5 per 100 person-years). Poisson showed that the binomial distribution of the number of failures d converges to the Poisson distribution of the event count λ as n increases provided that the expected number of failures $\pi n = d$ is constant. In fact when n is large ($\pi = d/n$ is small) then $n\pi$ (expected number of failure events) approaches λ (expected event count). This can be shown also in terms of likelihood function of λ. In fact MLE is also the regression method of Poisson regression. Further details can be found in specific textbooks [10, 11].

2.3.2 Meaning of the Coefficients in Poisson Regression

In the Framingham example of 1,473 deaths in 104,461 patient-years the overall event rate was 0.01410096 per person-year. Therefore, the yearly probability of death per person was 0.0141 (expected count 141 per 10,000 person-years), indicating that the event measured in a large sample occurs with a small probability. This expected rate per person per unit time is the exponentiated coefficient of the null model $\log(\lambda) = LP = \beta_0$. To estimate the effect of gender on mortality the covariate x_i indicating male ($i = 1$) or female gender ($i = 0$) is introduced into the model. The other pieces of information needed for this model are ni, the group exposure time; di, the number of deaths per group; and the true group probability of death πi. The model will estimate the relative risk of death $RR = \pi_1 / \pi_0$ from the estimated π_1 and π_0 as explained in Table 4.

Table 4
Simple Poisson Regression using the Framingham data [10]

Covariate (gender)	Failures	Exposure time (Pt-year)	Rate per unit time (λ)
Male (x_1)	$d_1 = 823$	$n_1 = 42,688$	$\lambda_1 = d_1/n_1 = 0.01927$
Female (x_0)	$d_0 = 650$	$n_0 = 61,773$	$\lambda_0 = d_0/n_0 = 0.01052$

Derivation of the Poisson model: Since π is relatively small λi approximates πi. Then the expected number of deaths is $E(d_1 \mid x_1) = n_1 \pi_1$ in males and $E(d_0 \mid x_0) = n_0 \pi_0$ in females. Since the relative risk is $RR = \pi_1 / \pi_0$ then $\log[E(d_1 \mid x_1)] = \log[\pi_1] + \log[n_1]$ and $\log[E(d_1 \mid x_1)] = \log[n_1] + \log[RR] + \log[\pi_0]$. Renaming $\log[RR]$ with "β" and $\log(\pi_0)$ with "α" we have the Poisson model: $\log[E(d_1 \mid x_1)] = \log[n_1] + \alpha + \beta$ and in more general form: $\log[E(d_i \mid x_i)] = \log[n_i] + \alpha + x_i\beta$. Therefore, the meaning of the coefficient β is $\beta = \log[RR] = \log[\pi_1] - \log[\pi_0]$ and RR is estimated as $\exp(\beta)$

2.3.3 Model Check

There are a number of ways to check if the model fails to describe the data well based on graphical assessment of the residuals and formal tests. The goodness-of-fit test is important also for Poisson regression. Evidence of lack of fit causes over-dispersion (extra-Poisson variation), which means that the standard errors of the model may not be valid. This may arise because some important covariate has been omitted or because outcome data are correlated. The model likelihood has the same meaning as in logistic regression. Further details can be found in specific textbooks [10, 11].

3   Models for Time-to-Event Data

3.1 Survival Data

In many clinical studies, the main outcome under assessment is the time to an event of interest. This time is called survival time, although it may be applied to the time "survived" from complete remission to disease relapse or progression as equally as to the time from diagnosis to death. For appropriate outcome measurement and analysis in survival studies it is especially important to define precisely the event and when the period of observation starts and finishes. For example, in studies of survival post-myocardial infarction, time is recorded from a starting point or "time zero" (the date of diagnosis of myocardial infarction), and the observation continues for each subject until either a recurrent fatal or nonfatal event occurs, the study ends, or further observation becomes impossible.

3.2 Key Requirements for Survival Analysis

A critical aspect of survival analysis arises largely from the fact that some individuals have not had the event of interest at the end of the follow-up and their true time to event remains unknown. This phenomenon is called censoring and it may arise as follows: (a) a patient has not (yet) experienced the outcome event by the study close date; (b) a patient is lost to follow-up during the study period (e.g., due to transfer to another center or for consent withdrawal); (c) a patient experiences another (competing) event that makes further follow-up impossible (e.g., heart transplantation, a new health problem, or even a car accident). Censored observations are those who survived at least as long as they remained in the study but for whom the survival times are not known exactly. Such right-censored survival times underestimate the true (but unknown) time to event. Although some data can be censored in other ways, most survival data are right-censored. If the event occurred in all individuals, other methods of analysis would be applicable. However, the presence of censoring and the distribution of the failure times make survival analysis necessary to study time to event data [12, 13].

The analytical tool used to study survival data assumes that if censoring occurs it occurs randomly and is unrelated to the reason for failure (uninformative or independent censoring principle). In practical terms, this means that censoring must carry no prognostic information about the subsequent survival experience. Note that the assumption would be violated if, just prior to failure, subjects are highly likely to leave the study or if the dropout rate between groups is differential. Other key requirements for a valid survival study are a follow-up duration based on the disease severity and thus sufficient to provide enough power to the study (sufficient to capture enough events); homogeneous cohort effect on survival (similar survival probabilities for subjects recruited early and late in the study); and independence of the failure times (absence of correlation in the data) since estimates of the β parameters are found by ML methods.

3.3 Functions of Time-to-Event Data

Survival data are generally described and modeled in terms of three related functions, namely, the survivor, the hazard, and the cumulative hazard functions. They are different functions of the LP meant to summarize the information on the outcome components described above (time zero, end date, and censor status) in one response variable (Table 5). The *survival probability* (cumulative survival probability or survivor function) is the probability (from 1 at $t=0$ to 0 as time goes to infinity) that an individual survives from "time zero" up to a specified future time t (observation end). Survival probabilities at different times provide essential summary information from time to event data. For example, a survivor function of 0.85 at 30 months informs that 85 % of the subjects (observed from $t=0$) are still event free at 2.5 years (risk of 0.15 at 2.5 years). The *hazard* is the instantaneous probability that an individual who is under observation at time t has an event at that time. So it is a rate rather than a probability, or a probability over a time interval, though very small. Put another way, it gives the instantaneous potential for the event to occur, given that the

Table 5
Functions used to model survival data

Function	Symbol	Reading	Definition	Range
$S f$	$S(t)$	S at t	Cumulative S probability at t	$[0,1]$
$H f$	$\lambda(t)$	H at t	Conditional H rate at t	$[0,\infty]$
$\mathrm{CH} f$	$H(t)$	CH at t	Cumulative H at t	$[0,\infty]$

S survival, t any point in time "t," f function, H hazard, CH cumulative hazard

subject has survived up to that instant (conditional rate). As opposed to the survival probability, which is dimensionless, the hazard has units of 1/time. Also, in contrast to the survivor function, which can only decrease over time, the hazard function can increase, decrease, remain constant or vary with different shapes. For example, at 2.5 years an individual may have a hazard of 0.003 (e.g., events per person-months), but later on this might be higher or lower. This hazard is like a speed, with the risk of failure over time instead of distance covered over time, and may assume different values over time (from 0 to+∞) independent of the average value calculated in an interval. There is a clearly defined relationship between survival and hazard functions, given by calculus formulae incorporated into most statistical packages and each can be determined automatically from the other.

However, unlike the survival function, estimation of the hazard is not simple. Another quantity, the *cumulative hazard*, is calculated instead as an intermediary measure for estimating the hazard. The cumulative hazard at t is the integral of the hazard (or the area under the hazard function between times 0 and t) and is also mathematically related to the other two functions. To understand the concept it is useful to go back to the speed example. If a person faced a hazard rate of death of 0.1 events per hour (a speed of 0.1 mph), then the cumulative hazard is such that were that rate to continue for 2 days (the speed constantly at 0.1 mph) we would expect 4.8 failures to occur (4.8 miles traveled) in 2 days. Since an integral is indeed just a sum, a cumulative hazard is not unlike the total number of times the subject "would fail" over the interval period (cumulative force of mortality).

To compare hazards, survival functions or times across groups, there are different approaches more or less free from specific distributional assumptions (Table 6). Furthermore, some parametric models have an accelerated failure time metric (log-time metric), i.e., the estimated coefficients (the covariate effects) are interpretable as log-time ratios and some have both the proportional hazard and the log-time interpretation. The two interpretations are different. The proportional hazard metric focuses on the actual risk

Table 6
Forms of survival analyses

Form	Parameters	Example	Metrics	Interpretation	Exp(β)
Non parametric	None	Kaplan–Meier	NA	Survival probabilities can be compared across covariates levels	NA
Semi-parametric	Effects	Cox's model	PH	How the risk changes by covariate values	HR
Parametric	Effects and $\lambda(t)$	Gamma Log-normal	AFT	How t changes by covariate values	TR
		Exponential Weibull	PH/AFT	Both PH and AFT	HR or TR

Exp(β), is the number e to the power of β, the estimated value of the coefficient, *NA* not applicable, *PH* proportional hazards, *HR* hazard ratio; gamma, log-normal, exponential, and Weibull are the names of some parametric regression models, *AFT* accelerated failure time, *TR* time ratio

process (the hazard function) that causes failure and how the risk changes with the value of the covariates in the model. The accelerated failure time metric gives a more prominent role to time in the analysis (how the survival time changes with the value of the covariates in the model).

Poisson regression can also be used to study survival times, when individual information on exposure time and event occurrence is available. However, Poisson regression models rates, which are assumed to be low and constant (with variance equal to the mean). When rates are not constant other approaches can be used. For this reason Poisson regression is usually applied to model event counts over a specified time interval (events per person-year) using aggregated data and can be a good way to simplify complex survival models [12, 13].

3.4 The Cox's Model

The Cox's model is by far the most commonly used procedure in current practice [14]. It is a semi-parametric model since it formulates the analysis of survival data where no parametric form of the hazard function (output) is specified and yet the effects of the covariates (inputs) are parameterized (i.e., modeled based on assumptions) to alter the baseline hazard function (the hazard for which all covariates are equal to zero). The Cox's model makes estimation possible assuming that the covariates multiplicatively shift the baseline hazard (Fig. 2).

Besides the ease of coefficient interpretation, freedom from distributional assumption is the greatest advantage of Cox's regression. The cost is a loss of efficiency (precision) since the parameters (coefficients) are estimated comparing subjects at the times when failures happen to occur whereas parametric models maximize the use of the information in the data.

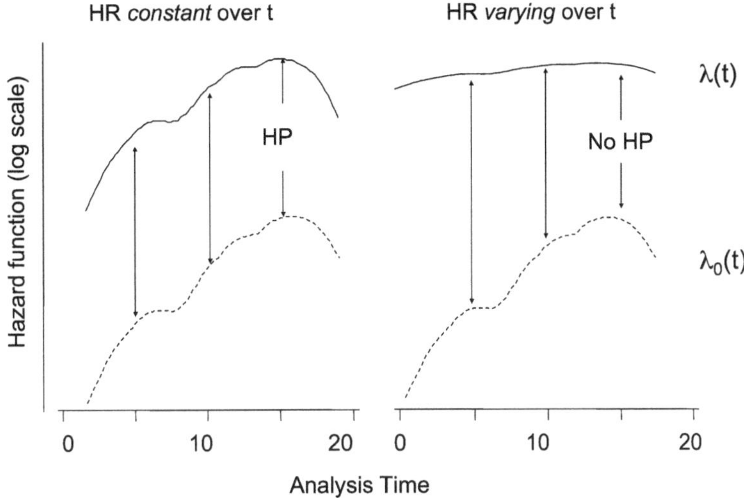

Fig. 2 Hazards proportionality: The *curve* on the *left* shows proportionality of the hazard ratio (HR) over time (e.g., the effect of the covariates is constant); the *right* curve shows a HR varying over time. According to the Cox's model, the hazard at t "$\lambda(t)$" (*continuous line*) is a function of the baseline hazard "$\lambda_0(t)$" (*dotted line*) times the hazard ratio "exp(β)." It can be seen graphically that under the hazard proportionality (HP) assumption (*left curve*) the distance between the two hazards is constant over time, this distance corresponding to "exp(β)" (HR after log transform). This is why estimation is made assuming that the covariates *multiplicatively* shift the baseline hazard function (on the exponential scale). The proportionality assumption can be verified based on these concepts. With permission from Ravani et al. [39]

3.4.1 Structure of the Proportional Hazards Model

The individual hazard at time t is $\lambda\left(t\mid X\right)=\lambda_0\left(t\right)\mathrm{e}^{\mathrm{LP}}$, which means that the hazard experienced at any time during follow-up depends on a basal hazard and the exponentiated LP. No form of the baseline hazard is specified, but there can be groups with different baseline hazard (λ_0). For example if the effect on survival of some categories (gender, age levels for example) is not of interest, a stratification variable can be used to specify the model $\lambda_k\left(t\mid X\right)=\lambda_{k0}\left(t\right)\mathrm{e}^{\mathrm{LP}}$, with "$k$" indicating the stratum. Note that "LP" remains the same. The model, however, allows the basal risk to vary. Since in Cox's regression the intercept β_0 is in the λ_0 rather than in the LP, the stratified Cox's model can be thought of as a multiple regression with intercept varying by stratum. In both cases the difference in the LP between two groups of subjects (e.g., men and women) in terms of hazard (e.g., cardiovascular event), does not involve time and it is constant (Fig. 2). In fact, the ratio $\lambda_k\left(t\mid X^{*}\right)/\lambda_k\left(t\mid X\right)$, where * indicates male gender, is $\lambda k_0(t)\exp(\mathrm{LP}^{*})/\lambda k_0(t)\exp(\mathrm{LP})$ which taking the logs is simply the difference LP*–LP. Since this difference does not involve time, it remains constant and constant difference on a log scale implies proportionality on the natural scale. This is the main assumption of the Cox's model.

*3.4.2 Meaning
of the Coefficients
in Cox's Regression*

As seen from previous models, differences in logs imply taking the exponential to interpret the meaning of the coefficients. The exponentiated coefficient represents the ratio of the hazards or hazard ratio between two levels or unit of exposure, $\exp(\beta) = \text{HR}$.

Hazards ratios estimate the true risk ratios as the ratio of the instantaneous probabilities of event (instantaneous event rates). In fact, as previously discussed with rates, HR is an instantaneous RR, the limiting value for the RR as time approaches zero. As time approaches 0, the risks also approach 0. However, the value of HR is different from zero and approaches that of the true RR. In survival analysis, the incidence rate ratio is the limiting value for the RR as time, over which the risks are taken, approaches 0.

3.4.3 Model Checks

The assumption about linearity of LP, the need to check for leverage and influential observations are similar to that previously discussed. The new important assumption to check is the hazard proportionality. When effects change over time it is possible to modify the formulation of the model to accommodate the problem. Design issues related to independence of the observation are very important as estimation is based on ML. Finally the study protocol must guarantee independent censoring and the other key requirements for a valid survival analysis.

4   Extended Models

Longitudinal studies typically monitor subjects over time and both exposure and outcome variables are often measured more than once in the same subject. Multiple outcome measurements performed at regular intervals on the same subjects (*longitudinal data*) are correlated because their values tend to be closer than values obtained from different individuals. Also cross-sectional measurements repeated in random order in the same individual or the assessments of a paired organ such as the eye (*repeated measures*), or single observations on different members of the same hospital/region or family (*clustered data*) are correlated because different organs of the same subject and different individuals of the same community share biologic experiences, environmental exposures, and genetic background, and therefore are not independent. For this reason traditional regression methods are not appropriate for the analysis of correlated data (see previous chapter).

The term "correlated data" refers to the association between different measurements of the response. The reader is already familiar with other types of correlation in the studied variables, such as the association between exposure and disease (which is the relationship of interest to the study), or multiple associations involving both inputs and output (determining phenomena such as confounding or multi-collinearity). Correlated outcome data arise whenever the unit of observation differs from the epidemiological unit of the study and their analysis can be challenging. However, correlated data are opportunities rather than problems if appropriately analyzed using methods developed to account for the within cluster correlation. In fact, the analysis of correlated data can help decrease the unexplained variability in the response, which is the ultimate goal of any regression analysis.

Although criteria for model choice are the same as for traditional regression models, the choice of the specific extended technique and the corresponding data layout depend on the study question and design. For both correlated generalized linear and time-to-event data two major analytical approaches are introduced here: random effect modeling and variance corrected methods. Other methods and special cases are mentioned at the end of the chapter.

4.1 Extended Generalized Linear Models

4.1.1 Panel Data Layout

Data sets for the analysis of longitudinal data contain more observations (i.e., records) per subject. In these data layouts there are often multiple measurements of the response, as well as time independent and time dependent inputs if data come from longitudinal designs. Time independent inputs are variables that do not change with time, such as gender, or variables measured at baseline, such as starting body weight or initial blood pressure values. Time dependent (or varying) covariates are input variables whose values are updated during the study, such as blood pressure or hemoglobin in studies of left ventricular mass. Also follow-up or cross-sectional studies may generate correlated data, clustered in centers, families, ethnic groups, etc. Correlated data generated by either longitudinal or non-longitudinal designs are also referred to as "panel data."

Multilevel correlations can also be taken into account. For example, each unit of a paired organ can be assessed several times in the same subject and subjects may be grouped in larger clusters. Such panel data would include variables identifying the level (hierarchy) of correlation.

A didactic data set is available from a famous reliability study of Peak Expiratory Flow Rate [15], measured twice on 17 subjects (Fig. 3). In this simple example there are only two rows (observations) per subject (34 in total), both with the same value of subject "identifier" (from 1 to 17); different values for the variable "occasion" (1 or 2); and different values of the response (L/min). Recorded measurements on the same subject tend to lie on the same side of the overall mean and be closer to each other than those taken on different individuals. In diagnostic studies the degree of correlation is expected to be very high as between individual discrimination is a necessary condition for a diagnostic test. However, even small correlations in outcome studies may induce important bias in the estimation process of both the model coefficients (effects)

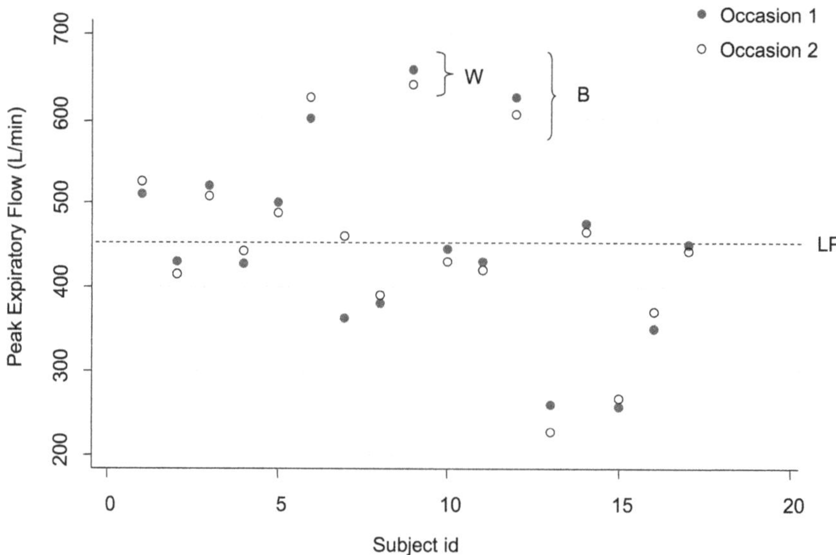

Fig. 3 Between (*B*) vs. within (*W*) subject correlation: Values of Peak Expiratory Flow Rate (L/min) measured in two occasions in the same subject are correlated. In fact they tend to lie on the same side of the overall mean and be closer to each other than those taken on different individuals. *LP* linear predictor (overall mean)

and their standard errors (statistical testing and Confidence Intervals) if not taken into account.

4.1.2 Modeling Random Effects

To understand the philosophy of this approach, it is useful to think of different possible components of the overall variability of the response. Regression methods tend to minimize the residual variance assigning the most likely values to the model coefficients estimating how the response varies as the inputs change. These are called fixed effects associated with *fixed* factors or continuous inputs whose levels of interest are actually measured or measurable. Fixed effects are unknown constant population parameters describing the input–output relationship of interest. Conversely, *random* classification variables are inputs whose levels are "randomly sampled from a population of levels" (e.g., individuals A, B, C; Drs A, B, C; hospitals: A, B, C, and so on). Random effects are unobserved random changes of the response by levels of these random factors. In other words, they are deviations from the relationship described by fixed factors. To distinguish between random and fixed factors, it is useful to answer the following question: "Were the study repeated would the same groups/levels be used again?" If yes (e.g., gender, treatment A vs B, age groups), it implies fixed effects. If not (e.g., centers, regions, subjects), it implies random effects. However, the same variable (e.g., centre) may be treated as a random variable or as a fixed factor, depending on the objective of the study (e.g., to assess a specific centre effect).

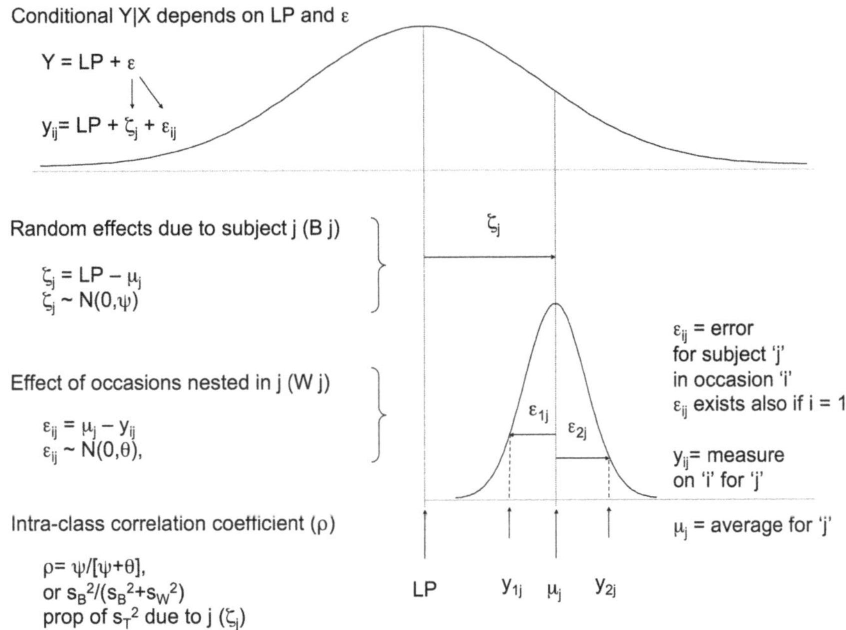

Fig. 4 Variance components: The *top curve* represents the distribution of a hypothetical response variable (such as the Peak Expiratory Flow Rate—Fig. 3). The observed values are equal to the linear predictor (LP) plus an error term (ε). The latter includes two components: the variability due to the effect of subject "*j*" (random effect, ζj equal to the difference between the mean μij of the values yij, measured on *j*, and the LP); and the variability due to measurement on occasion "*i*" (effect of occasion nested in subject, εij equal to the difference between μij and yij). Usually it is assumed that both these components are normally distributed with mean zero and some non-zero variance (here indicated by ψ and θ). The intra-class correlation coefficient ρ is the proportion of the total variance explained by the random effect. With permission from Ravani et al. [40]

Figure 4 shows the main variance components of the data in Fig. 3: the overall variance of the response includes a variability component due to subjects and another component due to measurement. This is true for both the unconditional response without predictors and the conditional response given the inputs. The variability due to subject is thought to be shared within individual but to vary across them. This random effect is assumed to follow a specified distribution (usually normal, with zero mean and some non-zero variance). The variability due to measurement can be estimated when more than one measurement is performed in the same subject, although it exists independent of the number of measurements performed. A random effect model estimates both these variance components. When the variance of the random effect is significantly different from zero, the null hypothesis of absence of correlation is rejected. The ratio between the variance of the random effect and the total variance is called intra-class correlation coefficient and represents the proportion of the total variability in the response due to subjects.

Random effect models are also called mixed effect models as they usually estimate both fixed and random effects. The family of generalized linear models depending on the specified link function includes linear, logistic, and Poisson mixed models, for example. All mixed models require specification of the level of correlation in the data (variance–covariance structure) in addition to the link function. The random effect can affect either or both the intercept and the slope of the curve defining the input–output relationship.

4.1.3 Correcting the Model Variance

Another possible approach to the analysis of correlated data is based on defining the correlation structure in the data and correcting the model variance. For example, in a cross-sectional study where three measurements are made in the same cluster it may be reasonable to assume that any two responses within a cluster have the same correlation. In this case as there is only one correlation parameter ρ the underlying correlation structure is referred to as "exchangeable." Conversely in the "unstructured" correlation structure there are as many ρ parameters as there are paired combinations of n measurements, $n \times (n-1)/2$. In a longitudinal study it may be assumed that the correlation depends on the interval of time between responses, being greater for responses that occur 1 month apart rather than 20 months apart (Fig. 5).

Which structure best describes the relationship between correlations is not always obvious although design issues may help decide. Despite the coefficient estimates are affected by the correct model choice (link function, covariates to include and their possible transformations) and by a sufficiently large number of clusters (e.g., ideally greater than 40 and not less than 20), the choice of the correlation structure is also important because the correlation matrix enters in the estimation process of the variance of the coefficients. Furthermore, the standard model variance estimators are consistent (converge to the true variance value) only if the correlation structure is correctly specified. For this reason a special variance estimator is used to estimate the standard errors of the coefficients when data are correlated. This method corrects the variance incorporating the dependencies in the process of computations by removing one cluster at a time, and providing an honest estimate for correlated data whenever the observations left out at any step are independent of the observations left in. Standard errors are usually larger than the corresponding naïve standard errors, depending on the sign of the correlation in the data (usually positive). Put simply, the variance of the coefficient estimates is corrected for the correlation in the data and the statistical testing is more conservative (the confidence intervals are larger) as compared to a standard procedure applied to the same data as though each observation was independent. This empirical method is called robust because the variance estimation is consistent, even if the chosen correlation structure is incorrect (robust to misspecifications) [16, 17].

	t_1	t_2	t_3	t_4
t_1	1	0	0	0
t_2	0	1	0	0
t_3	0	0	1	0
t_4	0	0	0	1

Independent

	t_1	t_2	t_3	t_4
t_1	1	ρ	ρ	ρ
t_2	ρ	1	ρ	ρ
t_3	ρ	ρ	1	ρ
t_4	ρ	ρ	ρ	1

Exchangeable

	t_1	t_2	t_3	t_4
t_1	1	ρ_{12}	ρ_{13}	ρ_{14}
t_2	ρ_{21}	1	ρ_{23}	ρ_{24}
t_3	ρ_{31}	ρ_{32}	1	ρ_{34}
t_4	ρ_{41}	ρ_{42}	ρ_{43}	1

Unstructured

	t_1	t_2	t_3	t_4
t_1	1	ρ	ρ^2	ρ^3
t_2	ρ	1	ρ	ρ^2
t_3	ρ^2	ρ	1	ρ
t_4	ρ^3	ρ^2	ρ	1

Autoregressive

	t_1	t_2	t_3	t_4
t_1	1	ρ_1	ρ_2	0
t_2	ρ_1	1	ρ_1	ρ_2
t_3	ρ_2	ρ_1	1	ρ_1
t_4	0	ρ_2	ρ_1	1

Stationary m-dependent

	t_1	t_2	t_3	t_4
t_1	1	.3	.1	0
t_2	.3	1	.3	.1
t_3	.1	.3	1	.3
t_4	0	.1	.3	1

Fixed

Fig. 5 Examples of correlation structures: Each panel represents a correlation matrix between any two of four possible measurements in the same cluster (e.g., taken at time 1, 2, 3, 4). Each symmetric matrix has a value of 1 along the main diagonal and some non-1 value off the diagonal. In the absence of correlation (independent errors) the correlation structure is *independent* (identity matrix). The correlation structure is *exchangeable* if there is only one parameter ρ for any pair of measurements; *unstructured* if there are $n \times (n-1)/2$ different parameters ρ; *autoregressive* (AR1) if there is only one ρ parameter raised to a power of the absolute difference between the times of the response; *stationary m-dependent* if the ρ parameter is the same for $k=1, 2, \ldots, m$ occasions apart and zero for more than m occasion apart (here $m=2$); *fixed* if specific values are assigned to the ρ parameters. With permission from Ravani et al. [40]

Generalized Estimating Equations are regression techniques based on specification of the correlation structure, use of an empirical (robust or corrected) variance estimator and freedom from distributional assumption about possible effect of the correlation. Also in this case one of the link functions of the generalized linear family must be specified. In absence of correlation in the data (independent correlation structure) Generalized Estimating Equations coincide with the corresponding Generalized Linear Model. In the presence of correlated data the variance–covariance of the coefficients is estimated based on the working correlation structure, the conditional mean, and a scale parameter to account for the over-dispersion (extra-variability). If the chosen correlation structure is correct there is no need for robust standard errors. The robust method is a nonparametric estimate that does not assume the correlation structure is correct [17, 18]. Another method to estimate the standard errors without making distributional assumption is bootstrapping. In bootstrapping the sample is resampled with replacement a certain (desired) number of times (to approximate what would happen if the population were resampled). Then model coefficients and measures of variance are estimated to obtain a sample of estimates, from which empirical variance and standard errors are obtained.

4.1.4 Model Choice

The choice of the analytical tool for correlated generalized linear data can be guided by different considerations. As opposed to Random Effects Models, Generalized Estimating Equations are based on only one level of clustering, are not designed for inferences about the covariance structure (the working correlation structure is formulated with no distributional assumptions), and do not give predicted values for each cluster. Using random factors involves making extra assumptions, but gives more efficient estimates and allows estimating contributions to variability from different sources.

Generalized Estimating Equations are marginal models as they assume a model holding over all clusters (population average). Therefore, the coefficients represent average change in the response over the entire population for a unit change in the predictor. Random Effects Models are conditional models in that they assume a model specific to each cluster (subject specific). Therefore, the coefficients represent the average change in the response for each cluster given a unit change in the predictor. Although population effects can be derived averaging cluster effects, conditional models are most useful when the objective is to make inferences about individuals rather than the population.

4.2 Extended Survival Models

Correlation in the occurrence and timing of repeated events may occur when individuals experiencing a single event belong to groups or clusters, or where the subject experiences some event more than once due to a recurrent event process [19]. The correlation in the survival times may result from differences in the general tendency to fail across individuals and varying tendency to fail further once the recurrence process has started (Fig. 6). *Heterogeneity* across subjects (*unshared frailty*) may be due to unknown, unmeasured, or unmeasurable effects (different lifestyles, genetic traits, environmental factors, and experiences), which influence the likelihood to succumb to disease. As a result, some individuals are more (and others less) prone to disease, experiencing their first, second, third, etc., recurrent episode more (less) quickly than others. *Event dependence* within a subject emerges when the threshold of further events changes once previous events have occurred (e.g., the baseline risk of thrombosis of the second and third bypass graft is

Heterogeneity: different general tendency to fail across individual (different hazards, $\lambda_{0a} \neq \lambda_{0b} \neq \ldots \neq \lambda_{0i}$)

Event dependence: within cluster *dependence* of the failure times (varying baseline hazard $\lambda_{01} \neq \lambda_{02} \neq \ldots \neq \lambda_{0n}$)

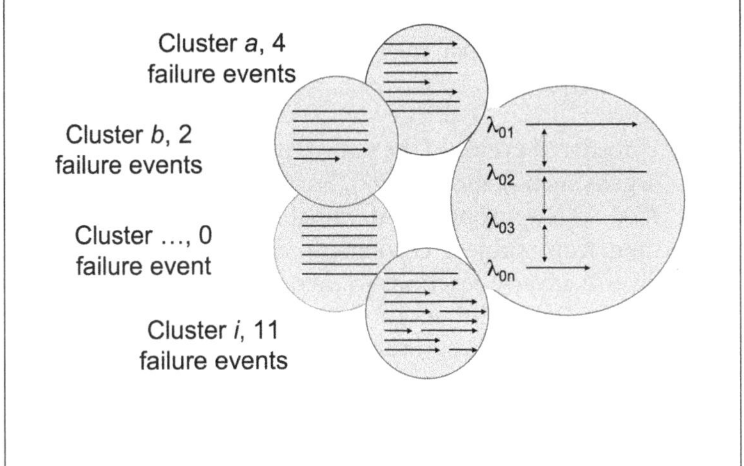

This heterogeneity can be incorporated into the model as **random effect** term $\lambda(t|X) = \lambda_0(t)\,\exp(X\beta + \mathbf{frailty})$

This shift in the baseline hazard can be controlled **stratifying** the model $\lambda(t|X) = \lambda_{0n}(t)\,\exp(X\beta)$

Fig. 6 Sources of correlation within multiple failure-time data. Unknown (or unmeasured) factors can be responsible for heterogeneity across individuals (with consequent different $\lambda_0(t)$, i.e., baseline risk across subjects) and within subject dependence of the failure events ($\lambda_0(t)$ varying within the subject during the recurrent process). With permission from Ravani et al. [40]

progressively higher or lower than that of the first). Further events become more or less likely according to whether the process induces a biological weakening or strengthening of the organism and whether the subject is more or less frail (*shared frailty*). In either case the risk for an event is a function of previous occurrences. Medical research and clinical experience suggest that both individual unshared tendencies and varying shared susceptibility to fail during the recurrent process are likely to be the rule, rather than the exception, in the study of multiple events and that each may enhance the effect of the other [19].

This correlation among events violates the assumption that the timing of events is independent and has two important consequences: the estimates of the coefficients and their standard errors are both biased (wrong) and inefficient (imprecise) in typical repeated events contexts. Variations of the Cox model (and other models), namely, frailty or random effects models and variance-corrected methods, have been proposed to account for the correlation among event times.

<table>
<tr><td valign="top" width="25%">

4.2.1 Risk Sets for Survival Analysis

</td><td valign="top">

Data layouts for survival analysis are more complex as they define the risk set based on the three components of the response variable (time start, time stop, and censor status) and possible distinction of basal risk categories. To define a risk set appropriately, failure events should be first classified according to whether they have a natural order and whether they are recurrences of the same or different event type [19].

</td></tr>
<tr><td valign="top">

Unordered Events

</td><td valign="top">

Unordered events of the same type include lesions studied in paired organs such as the eye [20]. For these data a *Marginal Unstratified Risk Set* is appropriate. Marginal models measure each observation time from subject enrollment. Events of different type include diverse adverse reactions to therapy in an intervention trial, or uremia and mortality in a follow-up study of chronic kidney disease patients [3]. These events are unordered because they occur in random sequence and, in the absence of correlated data and dependent censoring the *Competing Risk Model of Lunn–McNeil* has been suggested for analysis [21]. In this case the likelihood of being censored at time t does not depend on the reason for censoring including failure from a competing risk. The competing risk model is stratified by event type (basal risk allowed to differ) and gives the same results as the combined end point analysis (time to the first event that occurs). The number of observations per subject is a multiple of the number of considered events, all censored and of the same duration if no event occurred or all censored but one if any event occurred. The advantage of the larger data set is that it allows for easy estimation of within-event-type coefficients (stratum specific effects) and the analysis does not taken into account any correlation, as each subject may have at most one event [19]. When there are reasons to believe that the data are correlated, it is possible to analyze multiple events per subject using the *Marginal Model of Wei–Lin–Weissfeld* [22]. As in the previous model all times are measured from the date of patients' enrolment (time zero) but each observation continues in each stratum beyond the first event that occurred. An important characteristic of these failure events is that each can occur only once per subject and that all subjects are at risk for all events (if there are k possible events, each subject will appear k times in the dataset, once for each possible failure). This model may be appropriate when the predictors under investigation are plausibly involved in the pathways leading to more than one event type and, therefore, the censoring mechanism for one event may be informative for the other. For example, plasma levels of asymmetrical di-methyl-arginine (ADMA) have been shown to predict both progression of chronic nephropathies and death in patients with chronic kidney disease [3]. In these situations, the terminating time for observing one event could be correlated with the other (as it happened in that study) and, as a result, the assumption of independent censoring may be violated.

</td></tr>
</table>

Furthermore, considering only time to the first event that occurs reduces the study power. Robust variance is required in this model to account for the occurrence of multiple events in the same subject.

Ordered Events

In end-stage renal disease, catheter infections or dysfunctions, repeated peritonitis or transplant rejection episodes are ordered events in that they may be seen in a study that records the time to first, second, third event, and so on, and the subject is not at risk for further events until a prior one has occurred. Four layout options are available for ordered recurrences.

In the *Counting Process* each subject becomes a multi-event counting process since the total follow-up time of the subject is broken into event defined segments with as many records per individual as there are events plus one if the observation continues after the last event [23]. This model is not stratified, and estimates may be biased if the baseline risk changes during the recurrent event process [19].

In the *Marginal Risk Set* model the layout is identical to the unordered competing risk model [22]. In essence the model is stratified by event number but actually ignores the ordering of events (e.g., a person would be at risk for the fourth infection episode before the first even occurred) and just treats each failure occurrence as a separate process. In agreement with simulation studies the marginal formulation provides a larger estimated effect probably due to the lack of any order implication and the organization of the risk set [19]. However, this model may be useful to model the total time to each of the possible recurrent events, allowing basal risks to differ but with no strict order assumption.

The assumption of the *Conditional Risk Set* model is that each patient is not at risk for a further event until a prior has occurred [24]. Two variations with different time scales and risk sets have been implemented and both stratify the data by event number so that the baseline hazard is allowed to vary with each event. In the conditional risk set model *from entry* (elapsed time) the data is set up as for the counting process (t measured from entry). This variation is useful when modeling the full time course of the recurrent event process. In the conditional risk set model *from previous event* (gap time) the clock is reset at each event (t from previous event with zero time at the beginning of each follow-up segment). This variation is useful to model the gap time between events. Both models are stratified by failure order to track the event number and the structure of the data set reflects this sequence or ordering assumption (conditional risk). However, elapsed time estimation produces the hazard of an event since the study began, while the gap time formulation gives the hazard since the previous event. The choice of gap versus elapsed time depends on the research question at hand. Using gap time presumes there are substantive reasons to believe that the "clock should restart" after each event in order to determine the effect of the covariates on subsequent events. In this case the estimated effects mirror how the covariates affect the risk of failure for each observation (e.g., risk of infection for each catheter). In contrast, elapsed time models assess the effect of the covariates on the risk of failure from the start of the study through the end. In such a case the estimated effects reflect how the covariates affect the risk of failure over the entire course of the recurrent event process (e.g., risk of recurrent infections).

Time Dependent Effects and Time Varying Covariates

Another issue to consider when defining a risk set is related to the values and effects of the input variables. The term *time dependent* is more appropriately used to define the effect associated with an input and the term *time varying* is used for a covariate with updated values over time. For example, an input variable measured at baseline can have different effects during different follow-up periods that can be modeled as a step-function of time. In a follow-up study, baseline values of renal function were associated with increased risk of death only during the first year of observation and not thereafter [3]. These estimated time dependent effects must satisfy the proportionality assumption when using the Cox's model. Conversely a variable measured only once (at baseline) may interact with time and thus have an effect that changes with time, as was found for serum albumin in the HEMO study [25]. By definition, this effect will not satisfy the proportionality assumption. Another possibility is that the risk set contains updated values of a variable. For example, in a study of Urotensin II (a vasoactive substance) in chronic kidney disease patients, end-stage renal disease status (not yet on dialysis vs. already on dialysis) had a different effect on cardiovascular events [26]. This input variable was treated as a time varying covariate as subject could change their status during follow-up. These input-specific effects must also satisfy the proportionality assumption.

4.2.2 Variance Corrected Models

Variations within the family of variance-corrected models are based on different definitions of the risk sets previously described including whether they allow for event-specific baseline hazards using stratification. In these models (Marginal, Counting Process, and Conditional Risk Sets) a robust (cluster) variance estimator is used, as previously described for extended generalized linear models, which incorporates the dependencies in the process of computations.

Variance-corrected models represent one way to deal with the problems produced by heterogeneity across individuals and failure-time dependencies. However, since variance-corrected models do not incorporate any (random) effect into the estimates themselves (the effects are not adjusted for the heterogeneity), these may still remain biased. In other words, although providing corrected confidence intervals around the point estimates, these themselves may still be positively or negatively biased (Fig. 7).

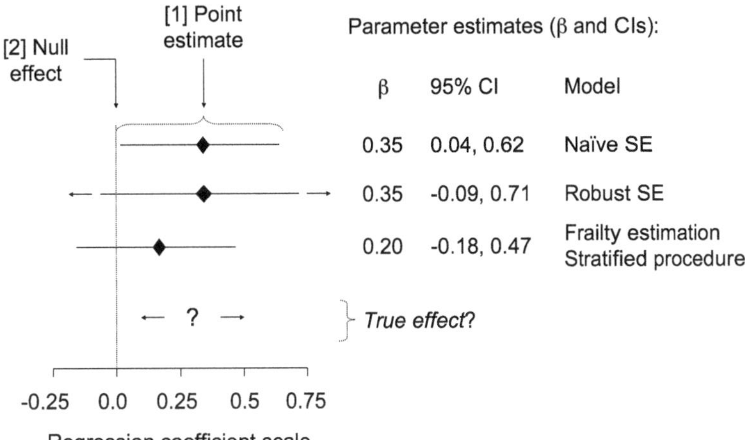

Fig. 7 Plot of the effect (β) of a covariate in the Cox's model (forest plot). In this plot both relevance and precision of the estimated effect can be summarized [1]. Interpretation of the point estimate: the farther its distance from 0 [$\exp(\beta) = HR = 1$] the greater the magnitude (relevance) of the associated effect [2]. Confidence intervals (CIs) and null effect (0 on the β scale; 1 on HR scale): CIs including 0 ($HR = 1$) imply lack of significance due to greater variance relative to the effect (imprecision). Correlation in the data due to recurrent events may affect both chance error (variance) and systematic error (point estimate). Reducing bias (systematic error) makes the point estimate closer to the true value in the population

4.2.3 Frailty Models

In contrast to the variance-corrected models, frailty models do incorporate heterogeneity into the estimated portion of the model by making assumptions about its distribution [27–32]. This latent random effect varies across individuals but it is assumed to be constant over time and shared by a single individual (or all members of a cluster). As a result, under frailty models the event times are assumed to be independent conditional on the patient's underlying frailty and inference can be made in the standard fashion. Standard packages for frailty models estimate the variance of this random effect. When this variance is significantly different from zero, the model supports the hypothesis of a significant heterogeneity in the data based on the shared frailty. Frailty models have been shown to produce unbiased estimates of covariate effects in simulation studies with known variance of the random effect (heterogeneity) and in absence of event dependence [19]. In these situations frailty models have been shown to perform better than variance corrected models. However, the baseline hazard rate for the standard frailty model is assumed to be the same across events (the traditional frailty model has the same risk set as the counting process). This has been viewed as a limitation in presence of event dependence, which is controlled instead by stratified variance-corrected methods, and therefore, these may be preferred in presence of event dependence without heterogeneity. Since repeated events processes are usually characterized by both event dependence and heterogeneity (or it is often unclear which feature of the data mostly underlies the correlation) a stratified frailty model has been proposed with the same risk set as the gap time risk set [28]. This conditional frailty model combines estimation of the unobserved heterogeneity incorporated as random effect with event-based stratification (varying baseline hazards) to control for event dependencies.

4.2.4 Model Choice

The choice of the analytical tool is dictated by the type and order of the failure events and the clinical question to be answered.

For multiple events of different type the marginal model is often the best choice to avoid violation of the uninformative censoring condition. This is true when the model includes factors plausibly involved in the mechanism of more than one event type. Frailty models can be used to specify and account for the sources of correlation in the data [27–32].

For ordered recurrent events of the same type there are more choices, though most often the order condition and the difference in the baseline risks are important issues to be accounted for. The counting process is useful if there is no reason to believe that the baseline risk varies. The marginal risk model may be more appropriate to model repeated hospitalizations (where the reason for hospitalization has no natural order) than repeated bypass graft thrombosis or peritonitis episodes. Conversely, when the clinical course of repeated events supports the conditional assumption, we can either model the entire time course of the disease (from entry) or model the time segments between failures (from previous event). However, variance corrected methods may still provide biased results in presence of heterogeneity since they do not incorporate any random effect in the model.

Heterogeneity and event dependence can be considered components of a latent random effect inducing biased estimates if not taken into account. Both sources of correlation in the data may simultaneously underlie most of the recurrent events processes, although one may prevail over the other. In presence of event dependence without heterogeneity the true variance of the frailty is zero. In these cases stratified variance-corrected methods perform well, whereas the traditional (unstratified) frailty model detects the presence of a random effect that was probably the consequence of event dependence rather than heterogeneity. In presence of heterogeneity without event dependence stratification may not be necessary since the baseline risk should not change by event number. In this case variance corrected models may be inefficient and the unconditional frailty model would perform better. Yet, since repeated events data are very likely to exhibit both sources of correlation, a modeling strategy that is robust to heterogeneity and event dependence may be necessary [28].

4.2.5 Competing Risks

In previous Subheading ("Unordered Events") we introduced two approaches for the analysis of unordered events of different type, including competing events [21, 22]. In these situations the occurrence of one event precludes or alters the risk for other events. If the likelihood that an observation is censored at time t does not depend on the reasons for censoring including failure from a competing risk (non-informative censoring), standard survival analysis methods (Kaplan–Meier and Cox regression) and their extensions [21, 22] can be used in the usual fashion. In the presence of competing risks however, time to competing events and time to censoring may not be independent because the exposure of interest can be associated with one or more competing risks (informative censoring). In these situations an analysis based only on standard methods can lead to misleading conclusions. A more comprehensive analytical approach (including standard methods) will help examine the extent to which the existence of competing risks interferes with the relationship of interest.

The reason the usual survival methods should be applied with caution in the presence of competing risks can be appreciated from the following example. Table 7 shows 12 subjects with kidney disease followed until end-stage kidney disease (ESRD; $N=6$) or death from other causes ($N=6$). Obviously, at 12 months 50 % died and 50 % reached ESRD. However, at 12 months the risk (1 – Kaplan–Meier survival probability; 1 – KM) of ESRD censoring for death is 78 % and the risk for death censoring for ESRD is 100 %. The sum of these two risk estimates is >1. Therefore, in the presence of competing risks, a Kaplan–Meier risk estimate at t can be interpreted as the risk of an event assuming that other types of event do not exist or have not happened at t [33].

The cumulative incidence function (CIF) method has been developed for the analysis of survival data when there are competing risks. According to this approach, the risk for any event is partitioned into the risks for each type of recorded event. Table 7 shows the key difference in the calculation methods. The cumulative risk (1 – KM probability) of ESRD at $t=5$ (censoring for death), for example, is obtained by adding to the 1 – KM estimate at $t=4$ (0.167) the product of the conditional risk for ESRD at $t=5$ ($1-1/8=0.125$) times the *cumulative ESRD-free survival* at $t=4$ (0.833). The CIF at $t=5$ is the sum of the CIF at $t=4$ (0.167) and the product of the conditional risk for ESRD at $t=5$ ($1-1/8=0.125$) times the *cumulative probability of both-event-free survival* at $t=4$ (0.667). The fact that the conditional risk at t is multiplied by a smaller cumulative survival probability at $t=t–1$ explains why the CIF at t is always smaller than the corresponding 1 – KM function when there are competing risks. This calculation method makes sure that the sum of all event-specific CIFs is always ≥0 and ≤1 (first axiom of probability). Figure 8 shows the CIFs and 1–KM probability functions calculated in Table 7.

Table 7
Calculation of the cumulative incidence of events according to the Kaplan–Meier method (KM) and the cumulative incidence function (CIF). Bold emphasis indicates the event of interest in KM analysis

Time	N	Event	Risk of ESRD (R) $R=ESRD/N$	Conditional survival (P) $P=1-R$	Cumulative survival (KM) $KM=P \times KM'$	Complement of Kaplan–Meier (1 − KM) $1-KM=R \times KM' + R'$	Any-event-free survival (KM2) $KM2=KM2' \times (1-(ANY)/N)$	CIF of ESRD $CIF=R \times KM2' +CIF'$
1	12	**ESRD**	0.083	0.917	0.917	0.083	0.917	0.083
2	11	**ESRD**	0.091	0.909	0.833	0.167	0.833	0.167
3	10	DEATH	0.000	1.000	0.833	0.167	0.750	0.167
4	9	DEATH	0.000	1.000	0.833	0.167	0.667	0.167
5	8	**ESRD**	0.125	0.875	0.729	0.271	0.583	0.250
6	7	DEATH	0.000	1.000	0.729	0.271	0.500	0.250
7	6	DEATH	0.000	1.000	0.729	0.271	0.417	0.250
8	5	**ESRD**	0.200	0.800	0.583	0.417	0.333	0.333
9	4	**ESRD**	0.250	0.750	0.438	0.563	0.250	0.417
10	3	DEATH	0.000	1.000	0.438	0.563	0.167	0.417
11	2	**ESRD**	0.500	0.500	0.219	0.781	0.083	0.500
12	1	DEATH	0.000	1.000	0.219	0.781	0.000	0.500

Time	N	Event	Risk of death (R) $R=death/N$	Conditional survival (P) $P=1-R$	Cumulative survival (KM) $KM=P \times KM'$	Complement of Kaplan–Meier (1 − KM) $1-KM=R \times KM' + R'$	Any-event-free survival (KM2) $KM2=KM2' \times (1-(ANY)/N)$	CIF of DEATH $CIF=R \times KM2' +CIF'$
1	12	ESRD	0.000	1.000	1.000	0.000	0.917	0.000
2	11	ESRD	0.000	1.000	1.000	0.000	0.833	0.000
3	10	**DEATH**	0.100	0.900	0.900	0.100	0.750	0.083
4	9	**DEATH**	0.111	0.889	0.800	0.200	0.667	0.167
5	8	ESRD	0.000	1.000	0.800	0.200	0.583	0.167
6	7	**DEATH**	0.143	0.857	0.686	0.314	0.500	0.250
7	6	**DEATH**	0.167	0.833	0.571	0.429	0.417	0.333
8	5	ESRD	0.000	1.000	0.571	0.429	0.333	0.333
9	4	ESRD	0.000	1.000	0.571	0.429	0.250	0.333
10	3	**DEATH**	0.333	0.667	0.381	0.619	0.167	0.417
11	2	ESRD	0.000	1.000	0.381	0.619	0.083	0.417
12	1	**DEATH**	1.000	0.000	0.000	1.000	0.000	0.500

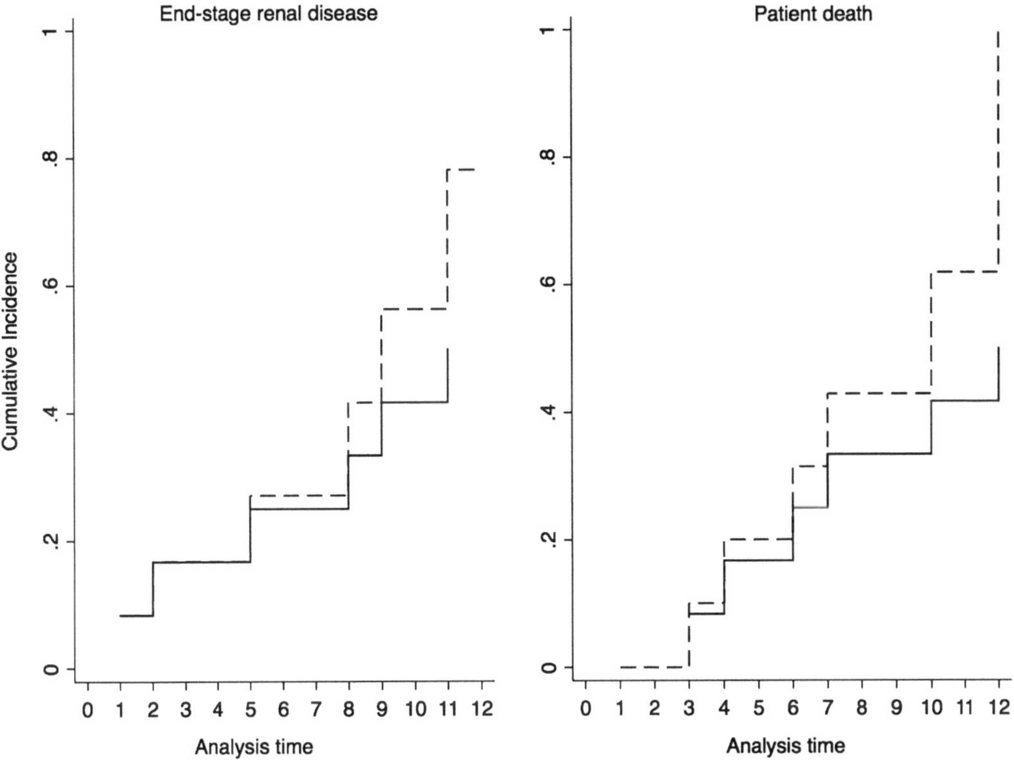

Fig. 8 Cumulative incidence of ESRD (*left*) and death (*right*) according to the Kaplan–Meier method censoring for the competing risk (*dashed line*) and the cumulative incidence function accounting for the competing risk (*solid line*)

While estimating risks ignoring competing risks (e.g., using 1 – KM) is not recommended, because it implies strong assumptions in the presence of competing events, testing covariate effects or making effect estimation using standard procedures (i.e., log-rank test or Cox regression) is useful. Pintilie suggests that survival analysis in the presence of competing risks has two main approaches: testing "pure effects" by ignoring competing risks and incorporating competing risks in the estimation process [33]. Comparing 1 – KM (log-rank) or cause-specific hazards (Cox) gives insight into the biologic mechanism of the disease and is invariant to the size of the competing risks. Censoring for competing events assumes that subjects remain at the same risk following the occurrence of a competing event. This may or may not be true in a given study. Conversely, comparing CIF or sub-hazards does not assume independence between event types as subjects experiencing competing events are counted as they did not have any chance of failing and observed risks or hazard rates are examined [33]. If the non-independent censoring assumption is not violated, then cause-specific and sub-hazards analyses will provide similar results.

The following example illustrates how standard approaches and competing risk methods complement each other in the analysis of time to event when there are competing risks.

Pintilie selected a group of 616 early stage Hodgkin lymphoma patients from a larger Canadian registry cohort [33]. Since all these patients received radiotherapy at a relatively young age (median age 30 years) follow-up is long and late effects of radiation have been recorded, including secondary malignancy and death from other causes unrelated to secondary malignancy. Since the risk of malignancy in general increases as a person grows older and radiation can cause malignancies, the study question is whether older age (age over 30) is associated with increased risk for malignancy secondary to radiotherapy as compared to the younger group (30 years or younger). During follow-up 84 subjects experienced secondary malignancy, 195 patients died from other causes and 337 were alive at the study end date (Fig. 9). Since some patients experienced both secondary malignancy and death the model of Wei, Lin, and Weissfeld [22] would be useful to include multiple (correlated) failure times per subject (Subheading "Unordered Events"). However, since these patients were few, analysis based on the Lunn–McNeil model [21] provided similar results. Both these models are dual event models for cause-specific hazards, as the standard single event Cox model.

Figure 10 clearly shows that older individuals die sooner that younger individuals as expected, irrespective of whether secondary malignancy is treated as competing risk or censored (right plots). Conversely, crude analyses of secondary malignancy differ according to whether death is treated as competing event or is censored. According to the competing risk analysis (top left) age at the time of radiotherapy is not associated with greater incidence of secondary malignancy (Gray test $P=0.56$), while censoring observations for death (bottom left) yields different $1-$ KM functions (log-rank test $P=0.002$). The two approaches convey complementary rather than conflicting information. Competing risk analysis suggests that

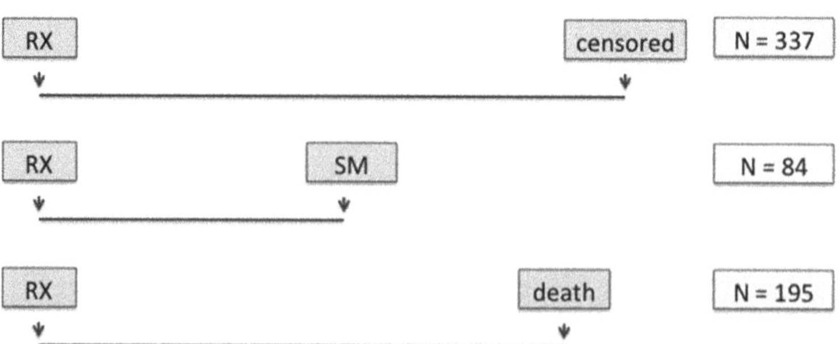

Fig. 9 Events recorded in a cohort of Hodgkin lymphoma patients following radiotherapy

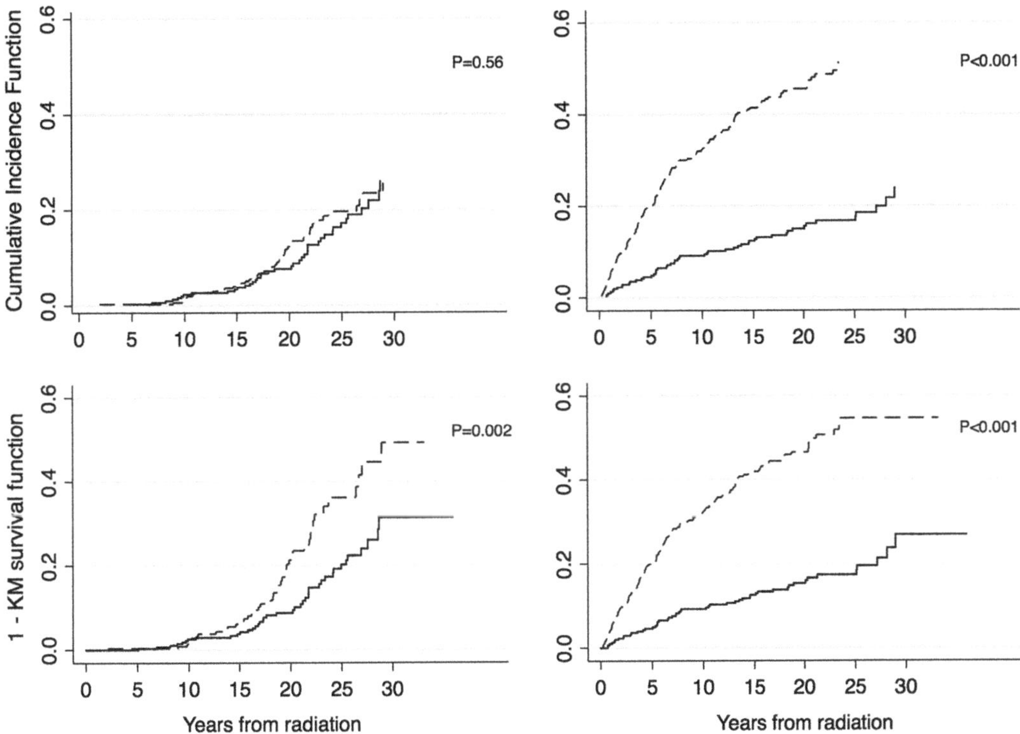

Fig. 10 Cumulative incidence functions (CIF; *top plots*) and 1 – Kaplan–Meier survival functions (1 – KM; *bottom plots*). The event of interest is secondary malignancy (*left plots*) or death (*right plots*). The exposure of interest is age >30 years (dashed lines) vs. 30 years or less (continuous lines)

when death is taken into account secondary malignancy may not have a chance to be observed in the older subjects because these subjects are also more likely to die. However, analysis of cause-specific risks shows that if death did not occur then secondary malignancy also would be more likely in the older subjects (log-rank). Implications may differ according to the purpose of the study and the target stakeholders. From a health policy perspective different preventive measures may not be cost-effective after radiation in older subjects because they are more likely to die than to develop secondary malignancy. However, if they do not die they have higher risk of secondary malignancy, and this finding may inform clinical decision-making in a single patient. Table 8 summarizes the cause-specific hazard ratios (from single event Cox regression models and dual event models) and the sub-hazard ratios (from the Fine and Gray model for competing risk [34] for secondary malignancy and death associated with older age versus younger age at the time of radiation in this Hodgkin lymphoma cohort. Consistent with the data depicted in Fig. 10, the confidence intervals of the sub-hazard ratio for secondary malignancy are not significant at the two-sided significant level of 0.05.

Table 8
Cause-specific and sub-hazard models of time to secondary malignancy and death

MODEL	HR	95 % CI	Outcome	Hazard	Correlation
Cox (single event model)	0.51	0.33, 0.79	Secondary malignancy	Cause-specific	No
Fine and gray (single event model)	0.88	0.58, 1.35	Secondary malignancy	Sub-hazard	No
Cox (single event model)	0.27	0.19, 0.38	Death without secondary malignancy	Cause-specific	No
Fine and gray (single event model)	0.28	0.31, 0.39	Death without secondary malignancy	Sub-hazard	No
Lunn–McNeil (dual event model disregarding events following the first event)	0.51	0.33, 0.79	secondary malignancy	Cause-specific	No
	0.27	0.19, 0.37	Death without secondary malignancy	Cause-specific	No
Wei, Lin, and Weissfeld (dual event model considering all events following the first event)	0.51	0.33, 0.79	secondary malignancy	Cause-specific	Yes
	0.27	0.20, 0.36	Death with or without secondary malignancy	Cause-specific	Yes

In summary, while crude risk estimation in the presence of competing risks requires consideration of the cumulative incidence function, both analysis of cause-specific hazards and analysis of sub-hazards are useful to compare and interpret covariate effects. While cause-specific hazard analysis provides insights into the biologic mechanisms of disease, sub-hazard analysis compares observed risks. In the presence of competing risks the use of both these complementary approaches conveys complementary information and the opportunity to examine the existence of informative censoring and interpretation of its potential consequences.

4.3 Special Topics

Random effect modeling and variance corrected methods are general approaches to model quantitative responses, categorical data, counts, and survival times. The advantage of these methods is that they are natural and very flexible extensions of standard techniques, easily applicable to different circumstances. Special methods exist for specific analytical issues.

Repeated Measures ANOVA is an important model for continuous responses and categorical exposures. The method is based on partitioning between and within subject variance. For example, Dittrich et al. studied residual renal function changes over time in a group of peritoneal dialysis patients receiving contrast media and in a similar control group of unexposed subjects [35]. In this study renal function was assessed repeatedly over time, time was treated as a within subjects factor, and exposure to contrast media as a between subject factor. The effect of the exposure and its interaction with time were studied taken into account intra-subject correlation of the data. However, ANOVA assumes that differences between any two levels of within-subject factor are the same (circular covariance matrix), with constant variance and covariance of any pair of within subject measures (compound symmetry or exchangeable correlation structure). This assumption is rarely met in practice, as adjacent observations tend to be more correlated than distant observations. Sphericity testing and adjustment methods for the underlying F statistics, specific randomized designs, and problems with missing data make this technique a less flexible approach than mixed models.

Multivariate ANOVA (MANOVA) is another approach to repeated measures of continuous data. This model requires that the number of subjects minus the number of between-subjects treatment levels be greater than the number of dependent variables (measurements). MANOVA allows studying the simultaneous change of more outcomes (repeated measures) in response to an exposure. For example, Van Vilsteren et al. showed beneficial effects of an exercise program for dialysis patients on behavioral change, physical fitness, physiological conditions and health-related quality of life [36].

In other longitudinal studies the study objective is the probability of a state change in a population. Markov Chains' models are used for series of system states, where the state change (transition) is studied assuming that a future state is conditionally independent of every prior state given the current state. For example, Weijnen et al. used a Markov chain model to investigate the impact of extended time on peritoneal dialysis using a new dialysis solution, assuming lower cost of the technique as compared to standard hemodialysis and longer durability as compared to peritoneal dialysis with traditional fluid [37]. Different scenarios were forecast over a 10-year period using aggregate data from the End-Stage Renal Registry in the Netherlands.

Time series are other models for longitudinal data. Time series study observations at successive (usually evenly spaced) time intervals to describe, quantify, and test theories on trends, seasonality, cyclic variation, and irregularities. For example, Espinosa et al. used time series analysis to study prevalence trends of Hepatitis C virus infection among hemodialysis patients in the Province of Cordoba, Spain [38].

References

1. Go AS, Chertow GM, Fan D, McCulloch CE, Hsu C (2004) Chronic kidney disease and the risks of death, cardiovascular events, and hospitalization. N Engl J Med 351:1296–1305

2. Merten GJ, Burgess WP, Gray LV, Holleman JH, Roush TS, Kowalchuk GJ, Bersin RM, Van Moore A, Simonton CA 3rd, Rittase RA, Norton HJ, Kennedy TP (2004) Prevention of contrast-induced nephropathy with sodium bicarbonate: a randomized controlled trial. JAMA 291:2328–2334

3. Ravani P, Tripepi G, Malberti F, Testa S, Mallamaci F, Zoccali C (2005) Asymmetrical dimethylarginine predicts progression to dialysis and death in patients with chronic kidney disease: a competing risks modeling approach. J Am Soc Nephrol 16:2449–2455

4. Heckbert SR, Post W, Pearson GD, Arnett DK, Gomes AS, Jerosch-Herold M, Hundley WG, Lima JA, Bluemke DA (2006) Traditional cardiovascular risk factors in relation to left ventricular mass, volume, and systolic function by cardiac magnetic resonance imaging: the Multiethnic Study of Atherosclerosis. J Am Coll Cardiol 48:2285–2292

5. Heine GH, Reichart B, Ulrich C, Kohler H, Girndt M (2007) Do ultrasound renal resistance indices reflect systemic rather than renal vascular damage in chronic kidney disease? Nephrol Dial Transplant 22:163–170

6. Glantz SA, Slinker BK (2001) A primer of applied regression and analysis of variance, 2nd edn. Mc Graw Hill, New York

7. Hosmer DW, Lemeshow LS (2000) Introduction to logistic regression model. In: Applied Logistic Regression, 2nd edn. Wiley, New York, pp 1–30

8. Hosmer DW, Lemeshow LS (2000) Sample size issues when fitting logistic regression. In: Applied Logistic Regression, 2nd edn. Wiley, New York, pp 339–351

9. Hosmer DW, Lemeshow LS (2000) Applied Logistic Regression, 2nd edn. Wiley, New York

10. Dupont WD (2002) Introduction to Poisson regression: inferences on morbidity and mortality rates. In: a simple introduction to the analysis of complex data. Cambridge University Press, p 269–294

11. Kleinbaum DG, Kupper LL, Muller KE, Nizam A (1997) Poisson regression analysis. In: applied regression analysis and multivariable methods. Duxbury Press, p 687–710

12. Hosmer DW, Lemeshow LS (1999) Applied survival analysis, regression modelling of time to event data. Wiley, New York

13. Kleinbaum DG (2005) Survival Analysis, a Self-Learning Text. Springer, New York

14. Cox DR (1972) Regression Models and Life-Tables. J Roy Stat Soc B 34:187–220

15. Bland M, Altman DG (1986) Statistical methods for assessing agreement between two methods of clinical measurements. Lancet 307–310

16. Lin DY, Wei LJ (1989) The robust inference for the Cox proportional hazards model. J Am Stat Assoc 84:1074–1078

17. White H (1982) Maximum likelihood estimation of misspecified models. Econometrica 50:1–25

18. Zeger SL, Liang K-Y (1986) Longitudinal data analysis for discrete and continuous outcomes. Biometrics 42:121–130

19. Therneau TM, Grambisch PM (2000) Multiple events per subject and frailty models. In: modeling survival data: extending the Cox model. Springer-Verlag, New York, p 159–260

20. Lee EW, Wei LJ, Amato D (1992) Cox-type regression analysis for large number of small groups of correlated failure time observations. In: *survival analysis, state of the art*. Netherlands, Kluwer Academic Publishers, p 237–247

21. Lunn M, McNeil D (1995) Applying Cox regression to competing risks. Biometrics 51:524–532

22. Wei LJ, Lin DY, Weissfeld L (1989) Regression analysis of multivariate incomplete failure time data by modeling marginal distributions. J Am Stat Assoc 84:1065–1073

23. Andersen PK, Gill RD (1982) Cox's regression model for counting processes: a large sample study. Anna Statist 10:1100–1120

24. Prentice RL, Williams BJ, Peterson AV (1981) On the regression analysis of multivariate failure time data. Biometrika 68:373–379

25. Eknoyan G, Beck GJ, Cheung AK, Daugirdas JT, Greene T, Kusek JW, Allon M, Bailey J, Delmez JA, Depner TA, Dwyer JT, Levey AS, Levin NW, Milford E, Ornt DB, Rocco MV, Schulman G, Schwab SJ, Teehan BP, Toto R, Hemodialysis (HEMO) Study Group (2002) Effect of dialysis dose and membrane flux in maintenance hemodialysis. N Engl J Med 347:2010–9

26. Ravani P, Tripepi G, Pecchini P, Mallamaci F, Malberti F, Zoccali C (2008) Urotensin II is an inverse predictor of death and fatal cardiovascular events in chronic kidney disease. Kidney Int 73:95–101

27. Huang X, Wolfe RA (2002) A frailty model for informative censoring. Biometrics 58:510–520

28. Box-Steffensmeier JM, De Boef S (2006) Repeated events survival models: the conditional frailty model. Stat Med 25:3518–3533

29. Liu L, Wolfe RA, Huang X (2004) Shared frailty models for recurrent events and a terminal event. Biometrics 60:747–756

30. Mahe C, Chevret S (2001) Analysis of recurrent failure times data: should the baseline hazard be stratified? Stat Med 20:3807–3815

31. Hougaard P (1995) Frailty models for survival data. Lifetime Data Anal 1:255–273

32. Pickles A, Crouchley R (1995) A comparison of frailty models for multivariate survival data. Stat Med 14:1447–1461

33. Pintilie M (2006) Competing risks. Wiley, New York

34. Fine JP, Gray RJ (1999) A proportional hazards model for the sub distribution of a competing risk. J Am Stat Assoc 94:496–509

35. Dittrich E, Puttinger H, Schillinger M, Lang I, Stefenelli T, Horl WH, Vychytil A (2006) Effect of radio contrast media on residual renal function in peritoneal dialysis patients—a prospective study. Nephrol Dial Transplant 21:1334–1339

36. van Vilsteren MC, de Greef MH, Huisman RM (2005) The effects of a low-to-moderate intensity pre-conditioning exercise programme linked with exercise counselling for sedentary haemodialysis patients in The Netherlands: results of a randomized clinical trial. Nephrol Dial Transplant 20:141–146

37. Weijnen TJ, van Hamersvelt HW, Just PM, Struijk DG, Tjandra YI, ter Wee PM, de Charro FT (2003) Economic impact of extended time on peritoneal dialysis as a result of using polyglucose: the application of a Markov chain model to forecast changes in the development of the ESRD programme over time. Nephrol Dial Transplant 18:390–396

38. Espinosa M, Martn-Malo A, Ojeda R, Santamara R, Soriano S, Aguera M, Aljama P (2004) Marked reduction in the prevalence of hepatitis C virus infection in hemodialysis patients: causes and consequences. Am J Kidney Dis 43:685–689

39. Ravani P, Parfrey P, Murphy S, Gadag V, Barrett B (2008) Clinical Research of Kidney Disease IV: standard regression models. Nephrol Dial Transplant 23:475–482

40. Ravani P, Parfrey P, Gadag V, Malberti F, Barrett B (2008) Clinical Research of Kidney Disease V: extended analytical models. Nephrol Dial Transplant 23:1484–1492

Chapter 7

Longitudinal Studies 4: Matching Strategies to Evaluate Risk

Matthew T. James

Abstract

Matching is a strategy that can be used to control for confounding at the design stage of observational studies that examine exposure–outcome relationships. In case–control studies, matching can be used to generate subsamples of case and control units that are similar with respect to one or more confounders. In cohort studies, matching can balance confounder(s) so that they are the same in exposed and unexposed groups. Matching methods have been extended to include multivariable approaches, the most common being propensity score matching in observation studies of interventions. This chapter describes the major principles of matching applied to case–control, cohort, and propensity score studies. Matched study designs provide several advantages for controlling confounding in observational studies; however, they remain vulnerable to residual confounding and can even introduce bias when implemented incorrectly.

Key words Matching, Case–control study, Cohort study, Confounding, Selection bias, Efficiency, Overmatching, Propensity score matching

1 Introduction

In epidemiologic studies, matching refers to the process of selecting a reference group that has one or more similar factors to an index group. Matching is most often employed at the level of individuals. In case–control studies, index cases (members of the group with an outcome of interest) are matched with reference controls (members of the group without the outcome of interest). Matching may also be used in cohort studies, where index subjects in an exposed group are matched with one or more unexposed participants. Matching may also be performed at the level of groups of subjects, a process known as frequency matching [1]. Frequency matching involves selection of a group of reference subjects matched on factors equivalent to the group of index subjects. Whether or not matching is of cases with controls, exposed with unexposed, or individual versus frequency, the process of matching seeks to create groups that are identical or reasonably similar in distribution based

Patrick S. Parfrey and Brendan J. Barrett (eds.), *Clinical Epidemiology: Practice and Methods*, Methods in Molecular Biology, vol. 1281, DOI 10.1007/978-1-4939-2428-8_7, © Springer Science+Business Media New York 2015

on one or more factors that potentially confound the relationship between an exposure and outcome.

Matching can be considered a form of a stratified sampling design, where the distribution of reference and index subjects across strata that are defined by the matching factor, are forced to follow a specific distribution. In case–control studies, when controls are matched to cases, the distribution of cases specifies the distribution. In cohort studies, where the unexposed are matched to the exposed, it is the distribution of the exposed that determines the distribution. Matching is a common strategy in observational studies designed to determine risk, and represents the most common form of stratified sampling in epidemiologic research.

Matching is often described as a strategy to reduce confounding in observational studies. This is true in cohort studies where matching alters the distribution of the matching factors in the study population from which all cases arise, such that the distributions of these factors are made to be similar in exposed and unexposed members of the cohort. Matching of unexposed to exposed thus serves to prevent any association between exposure and the matching factor and thereby controls for confounding in cohort studies. In contrast, although matching in case–control studies increases the efficiency of confounding control, failure to account for the matching factors in later stages of a case–control study can introduce bias. As explained further in this chapter, if matching factor(s) in a case–control study are confounders, it is important to account for the matching factor or factors in the analysis stage in order to avoid introducing selection bias.

2   Matching in Case–Control Studies

The purpose of matching in case–control studies is to select a control group that will provide an estimate of the distribution of an exposure of interest in the source population (Fig. 1a). Matching selects controls that, with respect to the matching factor, are identical or similar to the identified cases.

2.1   Potential for Selection Bias in Matched Case–Control Studies

In case–control studies, when the controls are matched with cases on a factor that is also associated with an exposure, the frequency of that exposure is forced to be similar to that of the cases. Thus if a matching factor is perfectly correlated with an exposure of interest, the distribution of this exposure in controls will be forced to be identical to that of the cases, and no association will be detected between the outcome and exposure (i.e., the result will be an odds ratio of 1.0). Regardless of whether the exposure is positively or negatively correlated with the matching factor, any association between the exposure and matching factor will result in an exposure distribution among controls that is biased towards a similar distribution to that of cases.

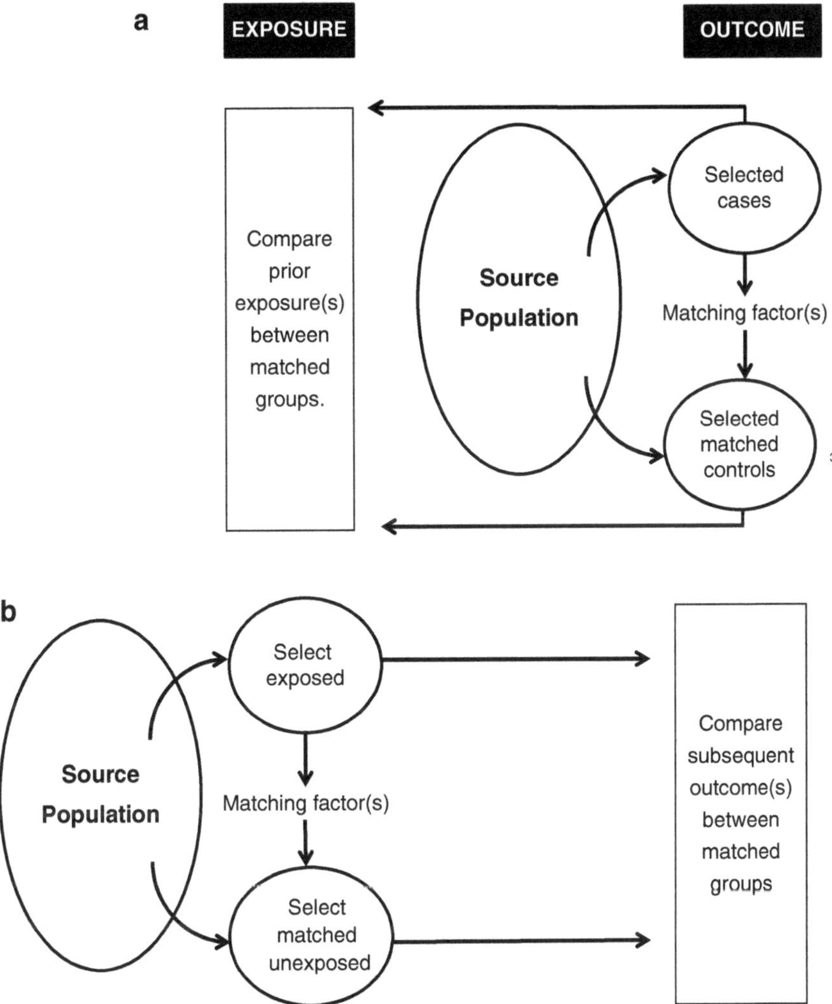

Fig. 1 Use of matching in case–control (**a**) and cohort (**b**) studies. (**a**) Cases (who experienced an outcome) are drawn from a source population, and controls who did not experience the outcome are selected from the source population on the basis of similar matching factor(s). Prior exposures are compared between cases and controls in the matched sample. (**b**) Exposed subjects are drawn from a source population, and unexposed subjects are selected from the source population with similar matching factors. Matched exposed and unexposed subjects are followed for subsequent outcomes

This explains how the process of matching in case–control studies can introduce selection bias [2]. If the matching factors are confounders in the source population, the matching process in a case–control study can superimpose a selection bias, in place of the confounding, that will bias results towards the null, regardless of the nature of confounding in the source population. For this reason, although matching is often intended to control for confounding, matching alone does not remove the potential for bias in a case–control study. However, the selection bias introduced through matching in case–control studies can be controlled for by appropriately accounting for the matching factor as a confounder in subsequent steps of analysis. This can be achieved through stratification on the matching factors, or inclusion of the matching factor as an independent variable in subsequent regression modeling. For example, if cases and controls have been matched on sex and age categories, any stratification or regression adjustment for age and sex categories that is as fine, or finer, than the original matching criteria is required to remove the selection bias introduced by matching.

2.2 Advantages of Matching in Case–Control Studies

Although matching in case–control studies does not by itself prevent confounding, one of its main advantages arises from the efficiency gained for the control of confounding [3]. For example, when the distribution of confounders substantially differs from the distribution in the overall source population, there may be, in the absence of matching, some strata with many cases and few controls and others with few cases and many controls. When controls are matched to cases, the ratio of controls to cases becomes constant across the strata of the matching factor. Matching forces the controls to have the same distribution of matching factors across strata as the cases and hence prevents extreme departures from the optimal distribution among controls. Matching thereby often improves study efficiency by minimizing the variance of subsequent estimates from stratified analysis or regression methods. Although matching on a factor that is a confounder will more often lead to an improvement in efficiency compared to unmatched studies, case–control matching on a variable that is not a confounder will usually harm efficiency.

When the process of measuring an exposure or confounder is difficult or expensive, matching can serve the purpose of optimizing the amount of information obtained for each subject included in the study [4]. This becomes particularly relevant when exposures under study include biological samples which are challenging to obtain or expensive to measure. In these cases it is more efficient to optimize the amount of information from each subject than to increase the number of subjects in the study. Matching on a confounding factor can allow for control of confounding in the analysis, while making maximum use of exposure information that is difficult or expensive to obtain.

In some situations matching is necessary to efficiently control for confounding. This may occur with sparse data that occurs with nominal variables with many categories (e.g., sibship, neighborhood, or care provider) [1]. These variables are often characterized by small numbers of potential subjects within each category of the nominal variable. While many subjects may be eligible for the study, subjects in any given category may have low probability of being included in an unmatched sample, and most strata in a stratified analysis may include only one subject, either a case or control, which would supply no information about the effect under study. Matching can ensure that after stratification by the potentially confounding factor, each case has at least one matched control for comparison. Matching on these types of nominal variables is necessary to obtain an unconfounded and reasonably precise estimate of effect.

2.3 Disadvantages of Matching in Case–Control Studies

There are costs that come with matching. When a factor is used for matching, the true relationship between the factor and disease is disrupted, and it is no longer possible to estimate the association of that factor with the outcome. Although it is no longer possible to study the relationship of the exposure to outcome or evaluate its strength as a confounder in such a scenario, it is still possible to evaluate the factor as an effect modifier.

Matching can also increase the expense required in the process of identifying appropriate control subjects with the same distribution of matching factors found among cases [1, 4]. For example, many potential control subjects may need to be examined to identify one with the same set of matching factors as a case. Thus, if efficiency is judged by the amount of effort or cost required to obtain information for each subject included in a study, matching can decrease the efficiency of the study when the effort required to find matched subjects exceeds the effort that would be required to gather information on a large number of unmatched subjects [1].

Overmatching is another potential disadvantage of matching [5]. One form of overmatching refers to matching that reduces statistical efficiency. This can occur when cases and controls are matched on a variable that is not a confounder. In this situation, matching was not necessary to control for confounding, but in order to avoid introducing selection bias, further stratification or regression adjustment becomes necessary in subsequent steps of analysis of the matched sample, resulting in a loss of information. The inefficiency introduced in such a scenario is proportional to the strength of correlation between the matching factor and the exposure. To avoid this form of overmatching, matching is best done on a confounder that is strongly associated with the disease and has some degree of association with exposure.

A second form of overmatching refers to matching on a variable that is an intermediary between exposure and disease. If matching is performed on a factor that is affected by the study exposure, the exposure prevalence among non-cases will be shifted toward that of the cases, thereby biasing the estimate of association toward the null. The bias introduced by this process will not be corrected by subsequent stratification or regression on the matching factor.

3   Matching in Cohort Studies

The purpose of matching in cohort studies is to select an unexposed group that, with respect to matching factor(s), are identical or similar to an exposed group (Fig. 1b). Matching in a cohort study prevents an association between exposure and the matching factor among the study subjects at the start of follow-up, so the matching factor will no longer act as a confounder of the exposure–outcome relationship. Matching is less often performed in cohort studies than in case–control studies due to the expense of trying to identify suitable unexposed subjects in large cohorts. In cohort studies, it is often more efficient to follow an unmatched group of exposed and unexposed subjects, rather than to use resources to identify unexposed subjects with a similar distribution of matching factors to exposed subjects.

Although matching in cohort studies can control for confounding due to the matching factor(s), it does not necessarily eliminate the need for control of the matching factors. This is because matching prevents the associations between an exposure and matching factor among participants at the start of a cohort study, but matching may not control for subsequent effects of associations between exposure and matching factors that occur during later follow-up time [1]. If an exposure and matching factors affect competing risks and loss to follow-up, the original balance produced by matching will not be maintained across the person time available for analysis. In these cases, additional control of matching factors may be necessary to obtain valid estimates, despite the use of matching at cohort entry.

4   Matching Using a Propensity Score

Matching methods have been extended from matching on one or several covariates individually, to multivariate matching. Matching on multiple covariates between exposed and unexposed groups in cohort studies can be challenging because it becomes more difficult to find matches with close or identical distributions of all matching factors, as the number of matching factors increases. Rather than attempting to match on all of the covariates individually, discriminant matching can be used to overcome this problem. Discriminant matching refers to matching on a scalar function of multiple covariates, which can be used to obtain overall balance of all of the covariates between exposed and unexposed groups. Propensity score methods, developed by Rosenbaum and Rubin, use this approach to control for multiple covariates simultaneously [6].

A propensity score is an individual's probability of being subjected to an exposure of interest, conditional on a set of observed covariates [6]. A propensity score thus reduces a collection of

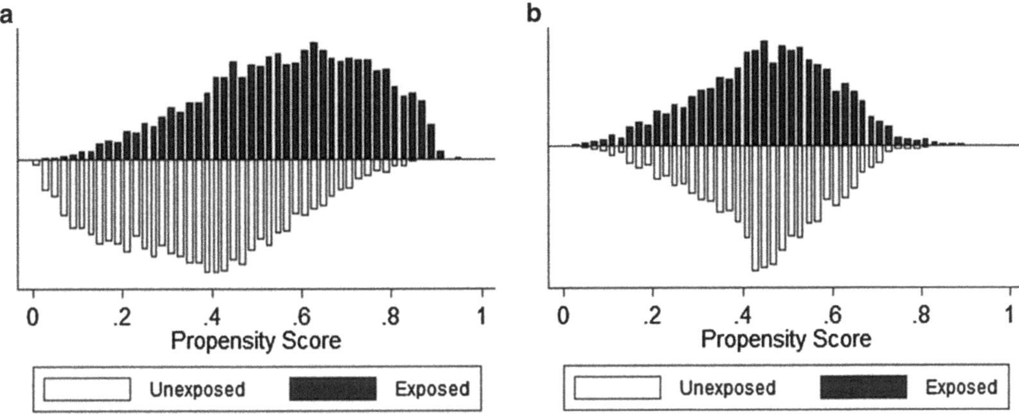

Fig. 2 Overlap of propensity score distributions among exposed and unexposed subjects in the full cohort before matching (**a**) and in the propensity score-matched sample (**b**). In this example, within the full cohort (**a**) a larger proportion of subjects in the unexposed groups had low propensity scores, while a larger proportion of subjects in the exposed group had high propensity score. After matching on the propensity score, the distributions of the propensity scores are similar between the exposed and unexposed groups

multiple covariates into a single scalar score that can subsequently be used for matching. A propensity score can be defined as the probability of being exposed, conditional on a set of measured baseline covariates. An important characteristic of a propensity score arises from the fact that if exposed and unexposed groups have the same distribution of a propensity score, they will also have the same distribution of the observed covariates that were used to generate this propensity score [6]. Thus rather than requiring close or exact matches on all covariates, matching on a propensity score enables the construction of matched sets of exposed and unexposed groups with similar distributions of covariates (Fig. 2). Propensity score matching is thus used to construct matched sets that are balanced on a large number of covariates.

Propensity score matching is often used in cohort studies where the exposure of interest is an intervention or treatment [7]. Such studies of an intervention are vulnerable to confounding due to treatment-selection bias, in which individuals who are selected to receive treatment may have significantly different characteristics than those who are not treated. These preexisting differences between treated and untreated groups need to be controlled to obtain unbiased estimates of the association between treatment and the outcome(s) of interest.

4.1 Advantages of Propensity Score Matching

Matching on a propensity score selects exposed and unexposed groups with a similar distribution of covariates that predict exposure. The result is that the propensity score-matched subsample of exposed and unexposed subjects are "balanced" with respect to their observed covariate distributions, meaning that they are the same in the both groups. This reduces bias due to measured confounders. Furthermore, because the matching process selects unexposed subjects who are most similar to the exposed subjects, the subjects excluded from the matched cohort are those most irrelevant for comparison with exposed individuals [6]. When there are large differences in the covariate distributions between exposed and unexposed groups, standard regression model-based adjustments may be vulnerable to unreasonable extrapolation of model-based assumptions. Matching methods make these differences explicit and avoid sensitivity to untestable model assumptions [8, 9].

When selecting the exposed and unexposed comparison groups by matching on the propensity score, no knowledge about subsequent outcomes of the study is required. Only in subsequent steps of analysis is the relationship between exposure and outcome examined by estimating exposure effects within the matched sample. The separation of these steps may prevent intentional or unintentional bias that might otherwise occur when decisions about exposure and covariate selection occur simultaneously with analysis of their association with outcome [10].

Theoretical and empirical research has demonstrated that propensity score matching methods have advantages to other methods for use of propensity scores, including stratification on a propensity score or covariate adjustment using a propensity score. In prior work, matching on a propensity score was shown to eliminate a greater degree of the systematic differences between exposed and unexposed subjects than did stratification on the propensity score [11, 12]. Also, with propensity score matching, adequate balance of covariates between the exposed and unexposed subjects in the propensity matched sample can be more easily assessed than when using methods of stratification or covariate adjustment using the propensity score. A propensity score-matched study design also facilitates calculation of measures of exposure–outcome relationships such as absolute risk differences or the number needed to treat, analogous to measures of effect reported in randomized trials [8].

4.2 Limitations of Propensity Score-Matched Studies

Although propensity score matching can produce a high degree of balance of covariates between exposed and unexposed groups, it may not achieve balance of variables that were not measured or included in the propensity score. Such unmeasured variables that are not part of the propensity score may remain unbalanced between cohorts, which may result in residual confounding due to these unbalanced variables and lead to biased estimation of exposure–outcome relationships.

Although propensity score methods, including propensity score matching, have been proposed to address confounding by indication in observational studies examining treatment effects and have several theoretical benefits, there is little empirical evidence that they achieve better control of confounding than conventional multivariable regression modeling of exposure–outcome relationships. Although some work has suggested significant differences in treatment effects when estimated using propensity score method versus traditional multivariable regression approaches, the majority of published observational studies have reported similar results using both techniques to adjust for confounding [13–16]. It is not clear whether this is due to inherent properties of propensity score methods, or because studies did not implement propensity score methods properly [12].

5 Steps in Performing a Matched Study

The steps required to perform a propensity score-matched study exemplify how matching can be applied to reduce the effects of confounding in an observational study of an exposure–outcome relationship [8].

5.1 Deriving a Propensity Score

In the first step of a propensity score-matched study, a propensity score is derived for each subject in the cohort. The propensity score is usually estimated using a logistic regression model, in which the exposure of interest is the dependent variable, and several baseline covariates are included as independent variables [17]. When the exposure of interest is a treatment, the propensity score represents the estimated probability, conditional on each subject's covariates, of receiving the treatment.

5.2 Constructing the Propensity Score-Matched Sample

Next, the propensity score-matched sample is constructed. There are several methods for matching a randomly sorted cohort of exposed and unexposed subjects on the basis of a propensity score. In nearest neighbor matching, treated subjects are matched to untreated subject with the closest propensity score. When matching is performed within a specified caliper width, a maximal allowable range in the difference of the propensity score for each pair of exposed and unexposed pairs is specified, and matches are selected only if their difference in propensity score falls within this caliper. Matching using a caliper width of 0.2 of the standard deviation of the logit of the propensity score has been shown to result in good balance [8]. Matching may also be done with or without replacement. In matching with replacement, an unexposed subject remains a possible match for more than one exposed subject, allowing some individuals to be included in multiple matched pair. When matching without replacement, each unexposed and exposed individual is matched only once. Greedy matching approaches match the next unexposed subject to an exposed subject, even if that unexposed subject would have been a better match for a subsequent exposed subject. Conversely, optimal matching algorithms select matches that will minimize the average difference in propensity scores across all possible matches.

5.3 Assessing the Balance of Covariates in the Matched Sample

A comparison of the balance in the baseline covariates between exposed and unexposed subjects in the matched sample is necessary to determine whether the matching process has been successful. Standardized differences are preferred over significance testing because, unlike significance testing (and corresponding p-values) their values will not be influenced by the smaller size of the matched sample compared to the overall cohort [8]. For continuous variables, the degree of imbalance within the matched pairs can be calculated as:

$$d = 100 \times \left| x_{\text{exposed}} - x_{\text{unexposed}} \right| / \sqrt{\left\{ \left(s^2_{\text{exposed}} + s^2_{\text{unexposed}} \right) / 2 \right\}}$$

where x_{exposed} and $x_{\text{unexposed}}$ are the sample means, and s^2_{exposed} and $s^2_{\text{unexposed}}$ are the sample standard deviation of the covariate in the exposed and unexposed groups, respectively.

Similarly, for dichotomous variables, the standardized difference can be calculated as:

$$d = 100 \times \left| P_{\text{exposed}} - P_{\text{unexposed}} \right| / \sqrt{\left\{ \left(P_{\text{exposed}} \left(1 - P_{\text{exposed}} \right) + P_{\text{unexposed}} \left(1 - P_{\text{unexposed}} \right) \right) / 2 \right\}}$$

where P_{exposed} and $P_{\text{unexposed}}$ represent the proportion of exposed and unexposed subjects respectively.

Standardized differences of more than 10 % are generally used as a threshold to suggest imbalance between the groups. The derivation of the propensity score, selection of the matched sample, and assessment of balance between the treated and untreated can be an iterative process, in which earlier steps are modified and repeated until an acceptable balance in is covariates is achieved between the exposed and unexposed groups.

5.4 Estimating the Association Between Exposure and Outcome(s)

In the final step, the association between the exposure and outcome(s) of interest is evaluated within the cohort of matched pairs. Because matched pairs are not independent observations, the subsequent analytical strategy to assess the exposure–outcome relationship should account in the correlation in the matched pairs.

References

1. Rothman KJ, Greenland S (1998) Modern epidemiology, 2nd edn. Lippincott Williams and Wilkins, Philadelphia, PA

2. Siegel DG, Greenhouse SW (1973) Validity in estimating relative risk in case-control studies. J Chronic Dis 26:219–225

3. Greenland S, Morgenstern H (1990) Matching and efficiency in cohort studies. Am J Epidmiol 131:151–159

4. Thomas DC, Greenland S (1983) The relative efficiencies of matched and independent sample designs for case-control studies. J Chronic Dis 36:685–697

5. Walker AM (1982) Efficient assessment of confounder effects in matched cohort studies. Appl Stat 31:293–297

6. Rosenbaum PR, Rubin DB (1983) The central role of the propensity score in observational studies for causal effects. Biometrika 70:41–55

7. Seeger JD, Kurth T, Walker AM (2007) Use of propensity score technique to account for exposure-related covariates: an example and lesson. Med Care 45:S143–S148

8. Austin PC (2007) Propensity-score matching in the cardiovascular surgery literature from 2004 to 2006: a systematic review and suggestions for

improvement. J Thorac Cardiovasc Surg 134: 1128–1135

9. Rubin DB, Thomas N (1996) Matching using estimated propensity scores: relating theory to practice. Biometrics 52:249–264

10. Rubin DB (1979) Using multivariate matched sampling and regression adjustment to control bias in observational studies. J Am Stat Assoc 74:318–328

11. Stukel TA, Fisher ES, Wennberg DE, Alter DA, Gottlieb DJ, Vermeulen MJ (2007) Analysis of observational studies in the presence of treatment selection bias. JAMA 297:278–285

12. Austin PC, Grootendorst P, Anderson GM (2007) A comparison of the ability of different propensity score models to balance measured variables between treated and untreated subjects: a Monte Carlo study. Stat Med 26: 734–753

13. Kurth T, Walker AM, Glynn RJ, Chan KA, Gaziano JM, Berger K, Robins JM (2006) Results of multivariable logistic regression, propensity matching, propensity adjustment, and propensity based weighting under condi-

tions of non-uniform effect. Am J Epidemiol 163:262–270

14. Shah BR, Laupacis A, Hux JE, Austin PC (2005) Propensity score methods gave similar results to traditional regression modeling in observational studies: a systematic review. J Clin Epidemiol 58:550–559

15. Sturmer T, Joshi M, Glynn RJ, Avorn J, Rothman KJ, Schneeweiss S (2006) A review of the application of propensity score methods yielded increasing use, advantages in specific settings, but not substantially different estimates compared with conventional multivariable methods. J Clin Epidemiol 59: 437–447

16. Stukel TA, Fisher ES, Wennberg DE, Alter DA, Gottlieb DJ, Vermeulen MJ (2007) Effects of invasive cardiac management on ami survival using propensity score and instrumental variable methods. JAMA 297(3):278–285

17. Martens EP, Pestman WR, Boer A, Belitser SV, Klungel OH (2008) Systematic differences in treatment effect estimates between propensity score methods and logistic regression. Int J Epidemiol 2008(37):1142–1147

Longitudinal Studies 5: Development of Risk Prediction Models for Patients with Chronic Disease

Navdeep Tangri and Claudio Rigatto

Abstract

Chronic diseases are now the major cause of ill health in both developed and developing countries. Chronic diseases evolve, over decades, from an early reversible phase, to a late stage of irreversible organ damage. Importantly, the trajectory of individual patients with a chronic disease is highly variable. This uncertainty causes substantial stress and difficulty for patients, care providers and health systems. Clinical risk prediction models address this uncertainty by incorporating multiple variables to more precisely estimate the risk of adverse events for an individual patient. In the current chapter, we describe the general approach to developing a risk prediction model. We then illustrate how these methods were applied in the development and validation of the Kidney Failure Risk Equation (KFRE), which accurately predicts the risk of kidney failure in patients with Chronic Kidney Disease Stages 3–5.

Key words Chronic disease, Prognosis, Risk prediction models

1 Introduction

Chronic diseases are now the major cause of ill health in both developed and developing countries. Unlike acute illnesses, chronic diseases evolve over decades, from an early, preclinical, and reversible phase, to a late stage characterized by irreversible organ damage. Importantly, the trajectory of individual patients with a chronic disease is variable and difficult to predict. This prognostic uncertainty causes many difficulties for patients, care providers and health systems. Consider, for example, the specific case of chronic kidney disease.

Chronic kidney disease (CKD) is defined as the presence of persistent reduction in kidney function (i.e., glomerular filtration rate (GFR) <60 mL/min for more than 3 months) or evidence of chronic kidney damage (e.g., proteinuria), and afflicts 10–13 % of adults worldwide [1–5]. The major causes of CKD are hypertension, diabetes, atherosclerotic vascular disease, and certain glomerular diseases (e.g., IgA nephropathy). Even within these

Patrick S. Parfrey and Brendan J. Barrett (eds.), *Clinical Epidemiology: Practice and Methods*, Methods in Molecular Biology, vol. 1281, DOI 10.1007/978-1-4939-2428-8_8, © Springer Science+Business Media New York 2015

categories, however, there is tremendous variation in rates of progression to kidney failure (i.e., needing dialysis) [6–8]: some patients progress rapidly to kidney failure, whereas others remain stable indefinitely with minor reduction in kidney function. In addition, since patients with chronic kidney disease (CKD) often suffer from multiple comorbid conditions, they are at risk of developing competing outcomes, such cardiovascular disease and death. Indeed, many patients will die of cardiovascular disease before their kidney disease progresses to failure. Although the risk of all three adverse events (i.e., kidney failure, cardiovascular disease, death) is high, the risk for each individual event in a given patient is difficult to predict.

This variability is a significant problem for several reasons. For patients, uncertainty hampers psychological adaptation to illness, and degrades quality of life [9–12]. Patients need to know: what will happen to my kidneys? Will I need dialysis? If so, how soon? For health professionals, lack of accurate prognostic estimates makes it difficult to appropriately counsel CKD patients, plan frequency of follow-up, and determine optimal timing for invasive procedures required in preparation for dialysis, such as arteriovenous fistula creation, or referral for preemptive transplantation. From the health systems perspective, CKD care is expensive, and requires specialized resources and frequent visits. These resources should be directed to patients at high risk, and not those at minimal risk of adverse outcomes.

Clinical risk prediction models address this problem by incorporating multiple variables to more precisely estimate the risk of adverse events for an individual patient [13]. Over the last three decades, there has been an increase in the use of risk prediction models with integration into multiple aspects of medical care [14]. In particular, instruments to predict cardiovascular risk have revolutionized the care of patients with cardiovascular disease, and provided novel insights into the prognostic role of individual risk factors and the efficacy of medical interventions [15, 16]. More recently, a robust tool to prognosticate risk of kidney failure has been developed and validated [17].

In the current chapter, we describe the approach to developing a risk prediction model in general terms. We then illustrate how these methods were applied in the development and validation of the Kidney Failure Risk Equation (KFRE), which accurately predicts the risk of kidney failure in patients with CKD Stages 3–5 [17].

2   Methods of Model Development

In order to be clinically useful, a prediction model must be internally valid, show improved reclassification of patients at risk, be externally valid in independent cohorts, and be easily applicable at the bedside.

2.1 Internal Validity: Getting the Basics Right

Internal validity refers to the concept that a prediction model must be derived from the study sample in such a way that the model coefficients accurately reflect the true relationships between the predictor variables and the outcome of interest. Internal validity therefore requires that the prediction model be derived from an appropriately structured and assembled *cohort*. The cohorts chosen for model development (and later validation) are most commonly derived from published prospective cohorts, RCT cohorts, or assembled from administrative databases using specific case definitions. Although a new prospective cohort study could be created for this purpose, such a strategy would offer minimal advantages unless the purpose was to incorporate novel tests or biomarkers into a prediction model; in such cases, suitable stored samples are often not available from an existing cohort, justifying the time and resources required to mount a prospective study. As with any valid prognostic study, the cohort must be structured so that predictor variables of interest are assessed in all patients at a point in time well before the development of the outcome. The proposed predictor variables ideally must have face validity, be clearly defined, and be precisely measurable. To avoid ascertainment bias, the outcome must be defined unambiguously, and assessed equally in all patients by adjudicators blinded to the predictor variable status of patients in the study [13].

Appropriate statistical approaches to model building are also of importance for internal validity. The statistical model chosen should fit the nature of the data. In most cases, if censoring is negligible and the follow-up period clearly defined, logistic regression is used; if censoring is significant or time to event is important, then a survival time approach using a Cox proportional Hazards model is preferred. Other more complex model approaches exist but are beyond the scope of this chapter [18, 19].

To ensure stability of the model coefficients in logistic and Cox regression, an event frequency of at least 10/events per degree of freedom in the model is advised [13]. For example, in a cohort of 1,000 patients where 100 outcomes have been observed, the prediction model should include at most 10 variables. Ratios of less than 10 events per variable can result in over fitting of the data, leading to poor generalizability in other patient cohorts. All these general aspects of study and model specification should be described in the methods to allow assessment of internal validity.

In addition to the general methodological issues enumerated above, which are germane to all studies of prognosis, several metrics specific to prediction model performance have been developed to further assess internal validity.

2.2 Metrics of Predictive Performance

2.2.1 Discrimination

Discrimination measures the ability of a model to accurately assign a higher probability to patients who have the event of interest, versus those who do not. The most commonly used metric of discrimination for logistic and Cox models is the concordance or C-Statistic. The C statistic is defined as the proportion of times the model correctly discriminates between a randomly selected pair of individuals (case and control), and is mathematically equivalent to the area under the receiver operating characteristic curve (AUROC) of the logistic or proportional hazards model. As with the AUROC, a c statistic of 0.50 indicates that the model performs no better than chance; a c statistic of 0.70–0.80 indicates good discrimination; and a c statistic of greater than 0.80 is consistent with excellent discriminatory ability [20].

A necessary step in developing prediction models is comparing the discrimination of two alternative models in order to decide which is better. This has traditionally been done by comparing the difference in c-statistics between the models [20]. However, one of the limitations of using the c statistic for this purpose is that it exhibits asymptotic behavior: as the model c approaches 1, it becomes increasingly difficult to show a meaningful difference in C-statistics despite real improvements in model prediction. An alternative and more sensitive measure of improvement is the integrated discrimination improvement index (IDI) [21, 22]. The IDI measures the difference in discrimination slopes between the two models (i.e., mean predicted probability for those with the outcome vs. those without), and describes this on an absolute and relative scale. As such, the IDI can be an effective method for comparing discrimination between two models where differences in C statistic may be negligible.

2.2.2 *Calibration*

Model calibration refers to how well the model predictions agree with the actual data. For logistic regression models, the Hosmer–Lemeshow chi square statistic is commonly employed for assessing calibration. In this test, patients are ranked into deciles of predicted probability; and the mean probability in each decile is then compared with the actual frequency of outcome among patients in that decile. A chi square test is used to assess whether a significant discrepancy exists between predicted and actual probabilities; a significant chi square statistic is interpreted as evidence that the model calibration is poor [15]. Alternative measures of calibration such as the Brier score which are not dependent on statistically significant differences in each decile have also been studied, but require further testing in the biomedical literature.

Calibration is an important metric for a clinical prediction model, because poorly calibrated models exhibit marked under or over prediction of risk, which is problematic when used for clinical decision making.

2.2.3 *Reclassification*

In clinical medicine, treatments and tests are often prescribed based on the predicted risk category of having an event. When a new prediction model is developed, it is important to consider whether it classifies patients into more appropriate risk strata than the old model. The new model may assign a given patient to the same risk category, a lower risk category, or a higher risk category relative to the old model. If the patient has an event, the new model can be considered successful if it assigns that patient to a *higher* risk stratum, but unsuccessful if it assigns a lower risk. Similarly, for patients who do not have an event, the new model is successful if reclassifies to *lower* risk, and unsuccessful if it reclassifies to a higher risk stratum. This net success or failure is summarized by the Net Reclassification Index. Positive values for NRI indicate correct reclassification and negative values indicate incorrect reclassification. The NRI should be calculated using clinically accepted risk categories, wherever possible [21, 22].

2.2.4 External Validity/Validation	External validity addresses the question of whether the results of the study sample are generalizable to the broader population in which one would like to apply the results. External validity for prediction models can never be assumed, as it is well known that models generated from one set of data (derivation set) usually perform less well in other cohorts. This may be due to a variety of reasons, including true differences in disease or biology between the cohorts, a non-representative derivation or validation cohort, over fitting of the initial models and/or spurious associations between predictors and outcomes in the derivation cohort. Some of these sources or error can be minimized in the derivation phase, by carefully choosing a cohort of patients representative of the clinical condition, and by choosing candidate predictor variables on face value rather than statistical association. Nevertheless, it is critical to perform a validation step by demonstrating that model calibration, discrimination and reclassification remain useful in at least one other, and ideally many other, independent cohorts separated by time, geography or source population. Although typically all the metrics of model performance will be lower in the validation cohort as compared with the original derivation dataset, provided that the drop in performance is not clinically significant, the model can be considered generalizable [13].
2.2.5 Knowledge Translation	The best predictive model is unusable at the bedside unless it can be rapidly and efficiently applied. Most predictive models are derived from complex logistic or proportional hazards models and include multiple coefficients and exponents that cannot be easily permuted using simple arithmetic. This means that the model, once validated, needs to be translated into a clinically useful bedside tool. Until recently, this meant transforming the model into a simpler scoring system, with some inevitable loss of precision, discrimination, and calibration. However, with advent of smartphones, and rapid access to web-based calculators or smartphone apps, the predictive equation can be applied exactly, via a simplified user interface, and without complex calculations. We believe that the integration of prediction models into electronic user interfaces, and particularly into electronic health records and laboratory information systems can greatly enhance knowledge translation [23–26].

3   Practical Application: Development of the Kidney Failure Risk Equation

In the following section, we describe our approach to developing a risk prediction equation for Kidney failure applicable to patients with stage 3–5 chronic kidney disease [17].

3.1 Derivation Cohort Selection

The development cohort was derived from a clinical database, the nephrology clinic electronic health record (EHR) at Sunnybrook Hospital, a part of the University of Toronto Health Network. This database was a prospective registry of patients seen by the nephrology group at Sunnybrook Hospital and included reliable information on predictor variables and outcomes of interest. Patients with CKD stages 3–5 (estimated GFR, <60 mL/min/1.73 m^2) at the time of initial nephrology referral were included and were followed up between April 1, 2001, and December 31, 2008. The outcome of interest, kidney failure requiring dialysis or transplantation, was ascertained by reviewing clinic records and by matching patient ID's with the Toronto Regional Dialysis Registry, a comprehensive registry of all patients receiving dialysis in the Toronto area.

3.2 Selection of Variables

We selected candidate predictor variables on the basis of face validity. The pool of variables explored included age and sex; blood pressure and weight; comorbid conditions, including diabetes, hypertension, and etiology of kidney disease; and laboratory variables from serum and urine collected at the initial nephrology visit. All predictor variables were obtained at baseline from the nephrology clinic EHR in the development data set. Models were developed using Cox proportional hazards regression methods and evaluated using C statistics and integrated discrimination improvement (IDI) for discrimination, calibration plots and Akaike Information Criterion for goodness of fit, and net reclassification improvement (NRI).

3.3 Model Development

We developed a sequential series of models and compared those with more variables (i.e., greater complexity) to simpler ones. We used a combination of clinical guidance and forward selection to determine variable selection. Variables not associated with kidney failure ($P>0.10$) on univariate Cox regression were excluded from further analyses. The 6 models constructed are shown in Table 1. Models 1 through 3 were developed using age and sex, estimated GFR, and albuminuria, successively, and compared with each other. Models 4 through 7 were developed by adding either clinical variables (diabetes and hypertension), physical examination variables (systolic and diastolic blood pressure and weight), laboratory variables of CKD severity (which were associated with the outcome in multivariate forward selection), or all of the above and compared with model 3.

Table 1
Hazard ratios, goodness of fit, and discrimination of prediction models in the derivation cohort[a]

Variable	Models						
	1	2	3	4	5	6	7
Baseline GFR, per 5 mL/min/1.73 m²		0.54	0.57	0.58	0.60	0.61	0.64
Age, per 10 year	0.86	0.75	0.80	0.80	0.79	0.82	0.82
Male sex	1.03[b]	1.46	1.26	1.27	1.34	1.16[b]	1.26
Log spot urine ACR[c]			1.60	1.61	1.55	1.42	1.37
Diabetes				0.86[b]			0.88[b]
Hypertension				1.17[b]			0.89[b]
Systolic BP, per 10 mm Hg					1.15		1.14
Diastolic BP, per 10 mm Hg					1.10		1.15
Body weight, per 10 kg					0.91		0.91
Serum albumin, per 0.5 g/dL						0.84	0.83
Serum phosphate, per 1.0 mg/dL						1.27	1.34
Serum bicarbonate, per 1.0 mEq/L						0.92	0.93
Serum calcium, per mg/dL						0.81	0.82
C statistic[d]	0.56	0.89	0.91	0.91	0.92	0.92	0.92
Akaike Information Criterion[d]	5,553	4,834	4,520	4,521	4,463	4,432	4,378
P value		<0.001	<0.001	0.40	<0.001	<0.001	<0.001

Reproduced with permission from Tangri et al. JAMA 2011; 305:1553–1559 (ref. 17)
ACR albumin-to-creatinine ratio, *BP* blood pressure, *GFR* glomerular filtration rate
[a]Data are presented as hazard ratios unless otherwise specified. Models 2, 3, and 6 columns indicate models based on laboratory data. P values are for comparison of C statistics between successive models, except for models 5, 6, and 7, which are compared with model 3
[b]Hazard ratios with P>0.05; all other hazard ratios are significant (i.e., P<0.05)
[c]Hazard ratio for ACR represents a 1.0 higher ACR on the natural log scale. For the average patient with 20 mg/g of albuminuria, this represents an increase to 55 mg/g
[d]Null values for C statistic and Akaike Information Criterion are 0.50 and 5,569, respectively. Higher values for C statistic and lower values for Akaike Information Criterion indicate better models

3.4 Validation Cohort Selection

The validation cohort was derived from another prospective clinical database, the British Columbia CKD Registry (Patient Registration and Outcome Management Information System), which captures clinical and laboratory data on all patients referred to nephrologists in BC. Patients with CKD stages 3–5 at the time of initial nephrology referral between January 1, 2001, and December 31, 2009, were included. Outcomes such as dialysis, death, and transplantation are all captured in the database, which matches all kidney failure outcomes with provincial and national registries. Note that the use of a separate validation cohort in an entirely different region of Canada and with a different case-mix of patients and practice patterns is a strength and enhances the inference of external validity.

3.5 Results of the Study

The development and validation cohorts included 3,449 patients (386 with kidney failure [11 %]) and 4,942 patients (1,177 with kidney failure [24 %]), respectively.

3.6 Prediction Model Performance in the Development Cohort

The hazard ratios for the variables and statistics for discrimination and goodness of fit for successive models in the development cohort are shown in Table 1. Model 1, including age and sex only, performed poorly (C statistic, 0.561; 95 % confidence interval [CI], 0.529–0.593). The C statistic improved with the inclusion of estimated GFR in model 2 (0.892; 95 % CI, 0.874–0.910; $P<0.001$) and albuminuria in model 3 (0.910; 95 % CI, 0.894–0.926; $P<0.001$), did not improve with the addition of diabetes and hypertension in model 4 (0.909; 95 % CI, 0.893–0.925; $P=0.40$), and did improve with the inclusion of blood pressure and body weight in model 5 (0.915; 95 % CI, 0.899–0.931; $P<0.001$) and laboratory values in model 6 (0.917; 95 % CI, 0.901–0.933; $P<0.001$). Despite a similar C statistic, the AIC was lower (i.e., better fit) for model 6 than for model 5 (4,432 vs. 4,463, respectively). The inclusion of all variables in model 7 improved both the C statistic and the AIC compared with model 3 (0.921 [95 % CI, 0.905–0.937] vs. 0.910 [95 % CI, 0.894–0.926] and 4,378 vs. 4,520, respectively). Given these results, models 1, 4, and 5 were excluded from further evaluation. Models 2, 3, 6, and 7 were then tested in the validation cohort.

3.7 Prediction Model Performance in the Development Cohort

In both cohorts, the C statistic was higher for model 6 compared with models 2 and 3 in the entire population. In the validation cohort, no further improvement was observed with the additional non-laboratory variables (0.835; 95 % CI, 0.819–0.851 vs. 0.841; 95 % CI, 0.825–0.857; $P=0.90$ for model 7 vs. model 6). At all times, both the C statistic and integrated discrimination improvement were greater for model 6 compared with models 2 and 3 ($P<0.001$ for all comparisons). Model 6 was more accurate than model 3 (integrated discrimination improvement, 3.2 %; 95 % CI, 2.4–4.2 %). Figure 1 shows observed vs. predicted probability of kidney failure at 3 years for models 2, 3, and 6 in the validation cohort. The mean absolute difference between the observed and predicted probabilities over quintiles of risk was lower with model 6 compared with models 2 and 3 (1.9 % vs. 2.7 % and 3.1 %, respectively), and the Nam and D'Agostino χ^2 statistic also indicated improved fit with model 6 compared with models 2 and 3 (χ^2 statistic, 19 vs. 37 and 32, respectively).

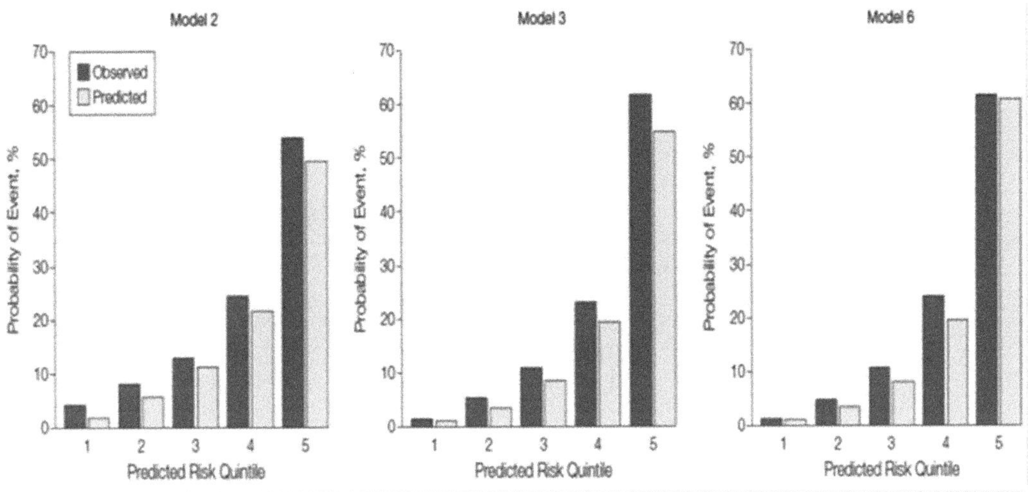

The predicted and observed event probability estimates represent the mean predicted probability from the Cox proportional hazards regression model and the mean observed probability from the population (Kaplan-Meier estimate) divided into quintiles of predicted probability. Predicted risk categories for quintiles 1 through 5 correspond with 0% to 4.3%, 4.4% to 8.1%, 8.2% to 12.9%, 13.0% to 24.5%, and 24.6% to 53.9%, respectively, for model 2; 0% to 1.6%, 1.7% to 5.3%, 5.4% to 11.0%, 11.1% to 23.1%, 23.2% to 61.7%, respectively, for model 3; and 0% to 1.4%, 1.4% to 4.8%, 4.9% to 10.7%, 10.8% to 24.0%, 24.1% to 61.6%, respectively, for model 6. Nam and D'Agostino χ^2 statistic is 37, 32, and 19 for models 2, 3, and 6, respectively.

Fig. 1 Observed vs. predicted risk of kidney failure at 3 years for Models 2, 3, and 6 in the validation cohort. Reproduced with permission from Tangri et al. JAMA 2011; 305:1553–1559 (ref. 17)

3.8 Net Reclassification

As discussed in part 1, the NRI calculates the overall improvement in risk classification as a result of the prediction model. To perform this calculation, it is necessary to have some a priori definition of discrete risk levels for the outcome of interest. Ideally, these risk levels should reflect currently accepted schema that are known to alter clinical decisions (e.g., in cardiovascular disease, many therapeutic decisions are based on the Framingham risk category). As established risk levels for kidney failure do not presently exist, we were obliged to define risk strata according to a "clinical reasonableness" criterion. To enhance the face validity of these thresholds, we asked clinicians what specific levels of risk would likely influence their management decisions for patients with stage 3 and stage 4 disease, respectively. Based on this input, we defined stage-specific CKD risk categories as follows.

1. For CKD stage 3, the risk of kidney failure over *5 years* was classified into the following categories: low (<5 %), medium (5.0–14.9 %), and high (>15.0 %).

2. For CKD stage 4, the risk of kidney failure over *2 years* was classified as: Low (<10 %), medium (10.0–19.9 %), and high (>20.0 %).

Once the risk strata were defined, we then calculated NRI within each CKD stage for Model 6 vs. Model 2, Model 3 vs. Model 2, and Model 6 vs. Model 2 (Table 2). For patients with

Table 2
Net reclassification improvement of the models in the validation cohort

| | No. (%) of participants | | NRI and non-NRI events, |
	NRI events	Non-NRI events	no. (%) [95 % CI]
CKD Stage 3[a]			
Models	$n=248$	$n=2,159$	
3 vs. 2	76 (30.6)	296 (13.7)	372 (44.4) [36.5–52.2]
6 vs. 2	91 (36.7)	296 (13.7)	387 (50.4) [42.7–58.1]
6 vs. 3	21 (8.5)	–11 (–0.5)	10 (8.0) [2.1–13.9]
CKD Stage 4[a]			
Models	$n=400$	$n=1,695$	
3 vs. 2	10 (2.5)	374 (22.1)	384 (24.6) [17.7–31.4]
6 vs. 2	5 (1.3)	432 (25.5)	437 (26.7) [20.1–33.3]
6 vs. 3	–2 (–0.5)	78 (4.6)	76 (4.1) [–0.5 to 8.8]

Reproduced with permission from Tangri et al. JAMA 2011; 305:1553–1559 (ref. 17)
CI confidence interval, *CKD* chronic kidney disease, *NRI* net reclassification improvement
[a]Risk categories for CKD stage 3 are 0–4.9 %, 5.0–14.9 %, and 15.0 % or more over 5 years, and for CKD stage 4 are 0–9.9 %, 10.0–19.9 %, and 20.0 % or more over 2 years

CKD Stage 3 and Stage 4, Model 3 consistently outperformed Model 2 with clinically meaningful improvements in reclassification. Similarly, Model 6 also outperformed Models 2 and 3, albeit with a smaller magnitude in reclassification improvement when compared to Model 3. Together these findings suggested that inclusion of albuminuria (Model 3) is critical for prognostication for kidney failure events, and the additional serum laboratory variables (Model 6) provide an incremental benefit in reclassification.

3.9 Knowledge Translation

Prediction equations are not useful unless they can be readily applied at the bedside to aid clinical decisions. To aid knowledge translation, we provided an online appendix that provided the written risk equation, and an online Excel spreadsheet to calculate the 5 year risk of kidney failure. Furthermore, we partnered with a mobile software developer to include the KFRE in medical calculator applications (QxMD) for use with iOS, Android, and Blackberry based devices. This app was downloaded and accessed >60,000 times in first year of publication.

3.10 Subsequent Validation Steps

Our original analysis comprised a single external validation step, which is really only a minimum requirement for establishing external validity. It is highly desirable to measure the performance of the prediction model in additional populations, as these analyses will provide insight into how reliably the model performs in populations that differ in terms of geography, case mix, and clinical practice. For this reason, our group proceeded to examine the performance of the Kidney Failure Risk Equation in multiple geographically, ethnically, and etiologically diverse CKD cohorts.

In addition to validation studies conducted by other independent investigators [27, 28], we collaborated with investigators from the CKD Prognosis Consortium and performed a validation study of the KFRE (i.e., Models 3 and 6 as described above) in 23 cohorts, spanning 10 countries and 4 continents [29]. This validation study included 562,000 individuals who had 17,000 kidney failure events over a median follow up of 7 years. Across all of our validation cohorts, the original KFRE performed extremely well and achieved discrimination statistics that exceeded the original validation (pooled C Statistic >0.85 for Models 3 and 6 at 5 years). Calibration was also excellent at 2 and 5 years in most cohorts, suggesting that the KFRE could be used globally to facilitate clinical decision making based on absolute risk thresholds at these intervals.

4 Summary

Risk prediction equations are of increasing importance in clinical medicine, particularly in the management of chronic diseases. Risk prediction equations can help patients to better understand their prognosis, health practitioners to more accurately prescribe interventions, and health services organizations to better target populations at risk.

References

1. Chadban SJ, Briganti EM, Kerr PG, Dunstan DW, Welborn TA, Zimmet PZ, Atkins RC (2003) Prevalence of kidney damage in Australian adults: The AusDiab kidney study. J Am Soc Nephrol 14(7 Suppl 2):S131–S138

2. Zhang QL, Rothenbacher D (2008) Prevalence of chronic kidney disease in population-based studies: systematic review. BMC Public Health 8:117

3. Coresh J, Selvin E, Stevens LA, Manzi J, Kusek JW, Eggers P, Van Lente F, Levey AS (2007) Prevalence of chronic kidney disease in the United States. JAMA 298:2038–2047

4. Obrador GT, García-García G, Villa AR, Rubilar X, Olvera N, Ferreira E, Virgen M, Gutiérrez-Padilla JA, Plascencia-Alonso M, Mendoza-García M, Plascencia-Pérez S (2010) Prevalence of chronic kidney disease in the Kidney Early Evaluation Program (KEEP) Mexico and comparison with KEEP US. Kidney Int Suppl 116:S2–S8

5. Shan Y, Zhang Q, Liu Z, Hu X, Liu D (2010) Prevalence and risk factors associated with chronic kidney disease in adults over 40 years: a population study from Central China. Nephrology (Carlton) 15:354–361

6. Levin A, Djurdjev O, Beaulieu M, Er L (2008) Variability and risk factors for kidney disease progression and death following attainment of stage 4 CKD in a referred cohort. Am J Kidney Dis 52:661–671

7. O'Hare AM, Batten A, Burrows NR, Pavkov ME, Taylor L, Gupta I, Todd-Stenberg J, Maynard C, Rodriguez RA, Murtagh FE, Larson EB, Williams DE (2012) Trajectories of kidney function decline in the 2 years before initiation of long-term dialysis. Am J Kidney Dis 59:513–522

8. Li L, Astor BC, Lewis J, Hu B, Appel LJ, Lipkowitz MS, Toto RD, Wang X, Wright JT Jr, Greene TH (2012) Longitudinal progression trajectory of GFR among patients with CKD. Am J Kidney Dis 59:504–512

9. Mishel MH (1981) The measurement of uncertainty in illness. Nurs Res 30:258–263

10. Wineman NM (1990) Adaptation to multiple sclerosis: the role of social support, functional disability, and perceived uncertainty. Nurs Res 39:294–299

11. Livneh H, Antonak R (2005) Psychosocial adaptation to chronic illness and disability: a primer for counselors. J Counseling Dev 83:12–20

12. Schell JO, Patel UD, Steinhauser KE, Ammarell N, Tulsky JA (2012) Discussions of the kidney disease trajectory by elderly patients and nephrologists: a qualitative study. Am J Kidney Dis 59:495–503

13. Clinical SE, Models P (2009) A practical approach to development, validation and updating. Springer, New York

14. Leslie WD, Morin S, Lix LM (2010) A before-and-after study of fracture risk reporting and osteoporosis treatment initiation. Ann Intern Med 153:580–586

15. Dorresteijn JA, Visseren FL, Ridker PM, Wassink AM, Paynter NP, Steyerberg EW, van der Graaf Y, Cook NR (2011) Estimating treatment effects for individual patients based on the results of randomised clinical trials. BMJ 343:d5888

16. Batsis JA, Lopez-Jimenez F (2010) Cardiovascular risk assessment–from individual risk prediction to estimation of global risk and change in risk in the population. BMC Med 8:29

17. Tangri N, Stevens LA, Griffith J, Tighiouart H, Djurdjev O, Naimark D, Levin A, Levey AS (2011) A predictive model for progression of chronic kidney disease to kidney failure. JAMA 305:1553–1559

18. Geddes CC, Fox JG, Allison ME, Boulton-Jones JM, Simpson K (1998) An artificial neural network can select patients at high risk of developing progressive IgA nephropathy more accurately than experienced nephrologists. Nephrol Dial Transplant 13:67–71

19. Tangri N, Ansell D, Naimark D (2008) Predicting technique survival in peritoneal dialysis patients: comparing artificial neural networks and logistic regression. Nephrol Dial Transplant 23:2972–2981

20. Harrell FE Jr, Lee KL, Mark DB (1996) Multivariable prognostic models: issues in developing models, evaluating assumptions and adequacy, and measuring and reducing errors. Stat Med 15:361–387

21. Pencina MJ, D'Agostino RB Sr, D'Agostino RB Jr, Vasan RS (2008) Evaluating the added predictive ability of a new marker: from area under the ROC curve to reclassification and beyond. Stat Med 27:157–172, discussion 207-212

22. Pencina MJ, D'Agostino RB Sr, Steyerberg EW (2011) Extensions of net reclassification improvement calculations to measure usefulness of new biomarkers. Stat Med 30:11–21

23. Bates DW, Ebell M, Gotlieb E, Zapp J, Mullins HC (2003) A proposal for electronic medical records in U.S. primary care. J Am Med Inform Assoc 10:1–10

24. Hillestad R, Bigelow J, Bower A, Girosi F, Meili R, Scoville R, Taylor R (2005) Can electronic medical record systems transform health care? Potential health benefits, savings, and costs. Health Aff (Millwood) 24:1103–1117

25. Maviglia SM, Teich JM, Fiskio J, Bates DW (2001) Using an electronic medical record to identify opportunities to improve compliance with cholesterol guidelines. J Gen Intern Med 16:531–537

26. Muller-Riemenschneider F, Holmberg C, Rieckmann N, Kliems H, Rufer V, Muller-Nordhorn J, Willich SN (2010) Barriers to routine risk-score use for healthy primary care patients: survey and qualitative study. Arch Intern Med 170:719–724

27. Drawz PE, Goswami P, Azem R, Babineau DC, Rahman M (2013) A simple tool to predict end-stage renal disease within 1 year in elderly adults with advanced chronic kidney disease. J Am Geriatr Soc 61:762–768

28. Peeters MJ, van Zuilen AD, van den Brand JA, Bots ML, Blankestijn PJ, Wetzels JF, MASTERPLAN Study Group (2013) Validation of the kidney failure risk equation in European CKD patients. Nephrol Dial Transplant 28:1773–1779

29. Tangri N, Levey AS, Grams M, Coresh J, Astor BC, Collins AJ, Djurdjev O, Elley CR, Hallan SI, Inker L, Kovesdy CP, Kronenberg F, Heerspink H J L, Marks A, Navaneethan SD, Nelson RG, Sarnak MJ, Stengel B, Woodward M, Iseki K. Validation of the Kidney Failure Risk Equation in an International Consortium. Abstract Presented at the Am Soc Nephrol Annual Meeting, November 5—November 10, 2013 Atlanta, GA

Part III

Randomized Controlled Clinical Trials

Chapter 9

Randomized Controlled Trials 1: Design

Bryan M. Curtis, Brendan J. Barrett, and Patrick S. Parfrey

Abstract

Today's clinical practice relies on the application of well-designed clinical research, the gold standard test of an intervention being the randomized controlled trial. Principles of the randomized control trial include emphasis on the principal research question, randomization, blinding; definitions of outcome measures, of inclusion and exclusion criteria, and of comorbid and confounding factors; enrolling an adequate sample size; planning data management and analysis; preventing challenges to trial integrity such as drop-out, drop-in, and bias. The application of pretrial planning is stressed to ensure the proper application of epidemiological principles resulting in clinical studies that are feasible and generalizable. In addition, funding strategies and trial team composition are discussed.

Key words Clinical trial, Randomization, Blinding, Sample size estimate

1 Introduction

The randomized controlled trial (RCT) is the gold standard of clinical research when determining the efficacy of an intervention [1]. Similar to experiments utilizing the scientific control method, it attempts to test a hypothesis about the effect of one variable on another, while keeping all other variables constant. As most epidemiological hypotheses usually relate to populations which are frequently diverse, the role of randomization is to obtain suitably comparable samples for evaluation. Furthermore, pretrial sample size estimation endeavors to ensure that the study will have the ability to detect clinical differences at a statistically significant level. While some clinical research questions may be inherently harder to answer than others (less amenable to the scientific control method), asking the right question coupled with the application of a well-designed trial can yield valuable information for practicing physicians. In addition to the above, the success and applicability of a randomized controlled trial depends on many aspects of research design that will be discussed. Indeed, a poorly designed randomized trial will not generate useful scientific information and

Patrick S. Parfrey and Brendan J. Barrett (eds.), *Clinical Epidemiology: Practice and Methods*, Methods in Molecular Biology, vol. 1281, DOI 10.1007/978-1-4939-2428-8_9, © Springer Science+Business Media New York 2015

a well-designed and executed prospective observational study may be more valuable.

Although the randomized controlled trial is the gold standard test of efficacy in the evidenced-based medicine era, there is emerging concern that the interest of science and society should not prevail over the welfare of individual patients [2, 3]. Ethical Review Boards or Human Investigation Committees composed of medical professionals and nonmedical members attempt to ensure the safety and welfare of the participants in clinical trials. Approval from these bodies is mandatory before undertaking any research involving human subjects. Participants must also enter into the research having freely given informed consent [4, 5].

Other concerns in clinical trials include generalizability, limitations in recognizing small treatment effects, the inability to conduct trials of sufficient duration to mimic treatment of chronic disorders [2] increasing costs, and whether efficacious interventions can be applied effectively in the community.

2   Asking the Question

2.1   Identifying the Problem

Clinical research questions arise from an identified problem in healthcare that requires study to provide evidence for change in clinical practice—specific questions are asked and trials are subsequently designed to obtain answers. Epidemiology provides the scientific foundation for the RCT by identifying risk factors and their distribution in the general population, establishing their role in predicting poor outcomes, as well as quantifying the potential value of treating and preventing the risk in the general population [6]. Furthermore, the RCT also represents the ultimate application of translating basic science research into clinical utility—a process commonly referred to as "bench to bedside." The application of both the epidemiological and basic science research underpins the RCT, the rationale for which is to undertake a safe human experiment, and subsequently apply the premise that observation and interventions in groups can be directly applied to treatment and prevention of disease in individuals [7].

Observational studies remain necessary to plan RCTs, to complement the observations of a randomized controlled trial, to generate hypotheses to be later tested with RCTs, or in some cases to provide answers that cannot be obtained by means of a randomized controlled trial [2]. For example, an RCT would not be appropriate to assess smoking cessation and its impact on preventing lung cancer. RCTs may be impossible in patients with rare diseases or may be logistically difficult when the primary clinical outcome occurs infrequently in large groups. Similarly, RCTs may not be appropriate when dealing with potentially rare but significant adverse effects.

In order to perform a clinical trial, the research question must satisfy a number of requirements: it must be a clinically important one from the perspective of patients, professionals, and society in general; there must be equipoise, meaning uncertainty about the answer to this question; the answer must be generalizable and applicable to a wide enough spectrum of medical practice. A good question will attract funding and help identify potential collaborators who are convinced the question is important. As the RCT is designed specifically to test a hypothesis, the research question must be amenable to the application of an experimental design. It must be logistically feasible as one attempts to keep all other conditions the same while manipulating an aspect of care in the experimental group. As the outcome is measured after a predetermined period, this too must occur within a reasonable time. For example, it would be very difficult to evaluate the effect of an intervention on an outcome if it is very rare or will not occur for 20–30 years.

It is important to know whether the research question has already been answered and how strong the evidence is to support the answer. Extensive literature reviews must be performed using appropriate resources such as Medline or the Cochrane Database to identify related prior work. Demonstration of equipoise is important not only in allocation of scarce research funding but particularly for ethical reasons. Investigators must not deny patients known effective treatment for the sake of new knowledge. For example, it would now be unethical to knowingly treat a hypertensive patient with "placebo only" versus a new drug for prolonged periods to investigate potential benefits. It may, however, be necessary to repeat prior work for confirmation of results or to solidify conclusion through improvements in trial design. Of course, debate exists as to what constitutes good evidence or what determines the strength of evidence. Sometimes a thorough meta-analysis can replace the need for a large RCT. These questions cannot be answered in general and must be considered carefully for each case.

2.2 The Principal Research Question

Once investigators are satisfied that their research question is clinically important, they must outline a specific hypothesis to be tested—referred to as the *alternate hypothesis*. The *null hypothesis*, or the negation of the hypothesis being tested, is then determined. It is the null hypothesis that is tested using statistical methods. Statistical purists believe that one can only reject or fail to reject (versus accept) a null hypothesis. For example, if one wanted to assess the effect of using hydrochlorothiazide versus placebo for treating mild hypertension the alternate hypothesis would be: hydrochlorothiazide is better, on average, than placebo in lowering blood pressure. The null hypothesis would then be: hydrochlorothiazide is not better, on average, than placebo in lowering blood pressure.

3 Trial Design

3.1 Randomization

The goal of randomization is to ensure that participants in different study groups are comparable at baseline. This includes variables that are known, unmeasurable, and unknown. Thus, the only difference between the groups will be the intervention under investigation. In clinical research, there is a mix of demographic and other attributes about which data can be collected during the trial. If these factors are similar in the intervention and control group, we can assume that the objectives of randomization were achieved and that distribution of factors about which the investigators are unaware will not systematically affect results. The probability of a participant's a priori enrollment must be independent of group assignment (i.e., intervention or conventional therapy), ensuring no selection bias. The process is termed "allocation concealment" and prevents participants being enrolled in a trial on the condition they only receive a prespecified intervention [8, 9]. To maximize validity of this process in multicentre trials the randomization and assignment should occur at a central location. This ensures consistency and decreases selection bias. Other options include the use of sequentially numbered, opaque, sealed envelopes or containers, the use of which can be audited.

Simple randomization as described above can be augmented by various means. One such technique is called blocking. This involves the random allocation occurring in blocks in order to keep the sizes of intervention arms similar. For example, if the total sample size is one hundred, participants may be "blocked" into subsets that guarantee an assignment balance after each block is enrolled (e.g., if using blocks of 5, there would be 30 participants in each arm after 60 are enrolled). Another technique is "stratified randomization" and is used when investigators are concerned that one or more baseline factors are extremely important in determining outcome and want to ensure equal representation of this factor in both treatment arms—e.g., diabetics in RCTs of cardiac or chronic kidney disease. When participants are screened they are stratified by whether the factor, like diabetes, is present or not before they are randomized within these strata. "Cluster randomization" involves randomizing entire groups of participants en bloc, for example by hospital or location [10]. This method is particularly useful in the evaluation of nontherapeutic interventions such as education, quality improvement or community based interventions [11].

The principles of randomization discussed above are for two treatment arms with 1:1 representation in each arm. These principles are also applicable to other trial designs where there are three or more treatment arms such as placebo vs. drug A vs. drug B. Additionally, investigators may wish to have more participants in

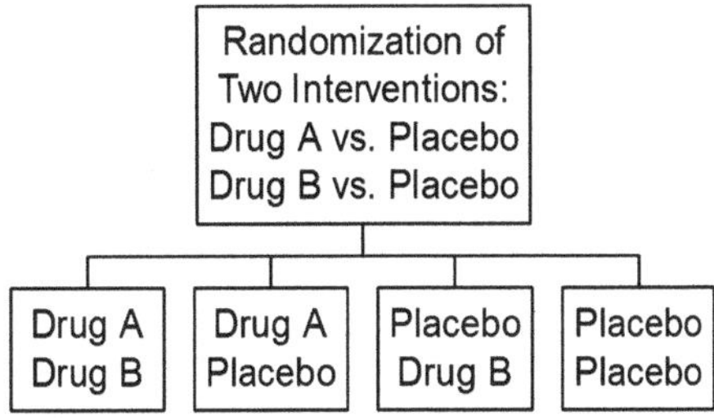

Fig. 1 Possible outcomes in a 2×2 factorial design. Each participant has an equal probability of receiving one of the four intervention combinations

one treatment arm versus the other. For example, 2:1 randomization has two-thirds of the participants randomized to one group and one-third to the other. This technique may be used to ensure adequate participant numbers in a treatment arm to evaluate side effects of a new medication.

A factorial design is one whereby two or more independent interventions are tested simultaneously during the same trial (Fig. 1). The Heart Outcomes Prevention Evaluation (HOPE) trial is one example of factorial design in which patients were randomized to receive either Ramipril, Vitamin E, Ramipril and Vitamin E, or Placebo [12, 13]. Therefore, participants had an equal probability of receiving one of four interventions: (1) Ramipril and Placebo, (2) Placebo and Vitamin E, (3) Ramipril and Vitamin E or (4) Placebo and Placebo. The benefits of this design are reduced costs as compared to testing Ramipril and Vitamin E in two different RCTs, and detecting interactions, such as those between an angiotensin converting enzyme inhibitor (Ramipril) and an antioxidant (Vitamin E). It is possible that an interaction occurs between two interventions such that the effect of the combination is different than the additive effect of both interventions separately—the effect size of one intervention may depend on the presence or quantity of the other intervention.

3.2 Adaptive Trials

Because of concerns that clinical trials are time consuming, expensive and may be prone to failure (failing to demonstrate a clinically important benefit when in fact one exists), newer techniques have been designed to adjust the course of a clinical trial as data accrues [14–16]. These are termed flexible or adaptive trials. They involve changing a newly recruited participant's odds of allocation to different treatment arms based on outcomes already achieved as the trial progresses. Concerns include the ability to maintain equipoise, potential participants delaying enrollment hoping they are more likely to be assigned more effective interventions, and early data signals that may eventually be false [14]. Another alternative is event driven enrollment where the number of participants enrolled (i.e., sample size) is determined by the actual event rate in the RCT, rather than the projected event rate from other studies.

3.3 Crossover

The crossover design is a strategy that may be employed when the outcome is reversible. It involves participants being assigned to one intervention and subsequently getting the competing intervention at a later time, preferably in random order. The advantage is that participants can serve as their own control. It is particularly suited for short-term interventions and outcomes where time related trends are not expected. The design is efficient in that treatments are compared within individuals, reducing the variation or noise due to subject differences. However, loss to follow-up can be particularly problematic when interpreting results. Further limitations include possible differential carryover (one of the treatments tends to have a longer effect once stopped); period effects (different response of disease to early versus later therapy); and a greater impact of missing data because they compromise within subject comparison and therefore variance reduction [17].

3.4 Non-inferiority

Given that there are situations whereby proven effective interventions may exist, placebo-controlled trials may be unethical [18, 19]. Furthermore, as knowledge accumulates, the incremental benefit from interventions may be small, requiring large sample sizes to demonstrate a benefit. Non-inferiority trials (sometimes incorrectly called equivalence) are intended to show that the effect of a new treatment is not worse than that of an active control by more than a specified margin [20]. For example, the claim might be made that a new ACE inhibitor is non-inferior to Enalapril, if the mean 24 h blood pressure of the new ACE inhibitor was not greater than 3 mmHg more than that of Enalopril. One major concern with this type of design is the loss of factors in trial design that ensure conservative interpretation of the outcomes. For example, loss to follow-up will tend to protect against type I error in placebo controlled trials but will bias towards the new treatment in a non-inferiority trial.

3.5 Blinding or Masking

Blinding is a technique utilized to decrease both participant and investigator bias. An "open trial" describes the situation where both the participants and investigators are aware of all treatment assignments and details. A "single-blind" trial is one where the researcher knows the treatment but the participant is unaware. Double-blinding entails both participants and investigators not knowing which treatment arm the participant is enrolled in. This removes bias on the investigators part as it is possible the participant may be treated differently by investigators depending on assignment, even subconsciously so. Double-blinding is sometimes not possible or may be inappropriate, such as with trials of surgical intervention. If double-blinding is not possible, then it is especially important to have objective outcomes and those involved in outcome measurement and adjudication being blind to the intervention received.

3.6 Multicenter

Multicenter trials, although increasing logistical complexity, will allow for greater enrollment opportunities. They also have the advantage of diminished "center effect," making results of the trial more applicable to a wider spectrum of patients. It helps to include academic and nonacademic centers where possible to further decrease case-mix bias, as the spectrum of patients and disease seen at various centers may be different.

3.7 Planned Trial Allocations and Interventions

It is important to precisely outline what the intervention will be and how both the treatment and the control groups will be managed. The goal is to decrease subjectivity in interpreting application of the trial protocol [21]. Other details of dosing, co-therapy, and attainment of therapeutic targets should be clarified as well as contingency plans for side effects. It is important that conventional therapy be applied equally and effectively in both intervention and control groups. This will diminish the chances of extraneous factors, other than interventions being tested, influencing the primary outcome. This may lead to a lower than expected event rate, a common occurrence in well conducted RCTs.

3.8 Inclusion and Exclusion Criteria

Investigators should strive to design trials representative of the relevant clinical practice. Thus, inclusion criteria are important to ensure the study question is answered in a population of subjects similar to that in which the results need to be applied. For logistic reasons participants must be residing in a location amenable to follow up. People who are unable to consent should be excluded. Of course exceptions exist. These may include studies which involve pediatric, dementia, or intensive care patients where third-party consent would be more appropriate. Furthermore, investigators should try to ensure that patients unlikely to benefit from the treatment or prone to side effects from the intervention do not contaminate the study population. For example, in studies of chronic disease it would mean excluding participants with other concomitant diagnoses conferring poor prognosis, such as active cancer. Finally, some people are excluded for general safety or ethical considerations, such as pregnant participants. Clear definitions of inclusion and exclusion criteria are essential.

3.9 Primary and Secondary Outcome Measures

The primary outcome is the most important measure as this provides the answer to the principal research question. Secondary outcome measures may be used to evaluate safety, such as mortality and comorbidities, or additional effects of the intervention. It is important that these measures are specified before the trial is underway and that there are not too many. This prevents post hoc analysis from diminishing the conclusions and interpretation. For example, once a trial is completed and data collected on many outcomes at various follow-up times, it would not be appropriate to analyze all the data points to see which outcome was significantly different.

This is because the more the data are analyzed, the more likely it is to find a statistically significant result just by chance (commit a type I error). This effect of multiple analyses would also limit pre-specified secondary outcomes. Again, clear definitions of primary, secondary, and tertiary outcomes are essential.

3.10 Measuring the Outcome Measures at Follow-Up

Investigators need a relevant, valid, precise, safe, practical, and inexpensive means of judging how a particular treatment affects the outcome of interest [22]. For example, in chronic kidney disease hard end points such as death or dialysis are preferred because of their uniform definition and objectivity. However, it should be remembered that kidney disease progresses at variable rates and the incidence of these advanced end points may be too low in early stage kidney disease. Using surrogate markers, studies may be conducted with smaller sample sizes and over a shorter period. The principal drawback of surrogate markers is their imperfect relationship to hard end points. Nonetheless, for chronic kidney disease for example, it has been suggested to use "intermediate" end points such as both doubling of serum creatinine and reduction in proteinuria by at least 30 % from baseline [22]. Although less accurate, these measures are easy to assess, more practical than more cumbersome measures such as Inulin clearance, and acceptable to some regulators, such as the Food and Drug Administration.

4   Size and Duration of Trial

4.1 Estimating Sample Size

Investigators need to know how many participants are required to enter in an RCT to have a good probability of rejecting the null hypothesis for a clinically meaningful effect of the intervention and to have confidence that the conclusion is true. Because trials test a hypothesis on a subset (sample) of the whole population, it is possible to have results that are skewed due to chance depending on the sample population. A type I error occurs when the results from the sample population permit investigators to reject a null hypothesis which in fact is true. Type II errors occur when investigators fail to reject the null hypothesis when in fact the null hypothesis is false. The risk of committing a type I error is denoted by alpha and the risk of committing a type II error is denoted by beta. It has become convention to accept a 5 % chance of committing a type I error. Failing to reject a true null hypothesis is sometimes called the confidence, equal to one minus alpha (Table 1). The probability of rejecting a false null hypothesis is determined by the power of the RCT. Power is equal to one minus beta, and RCTs are usually designed to have a power of 80–90 %.

An estimate of the likely event rate in the control group, from prior studies or preliminary data, is required to calculate sample size. The clinically relevant effect size due to the intervention is chosen for investigation. When the primary outcome is a continuous

Table 1
Type I and type II errors in a clinical trial

		True state in the population	
		True null hypothesis	False null hypothesis
Trial decision	Reject Null hypothesis	Type I error Probability = alpha	Correct decision Probability = 1—beta (=Power)
	Do not reject Null hypothesis	Correct Decision Probability = 1—alpha	Type II Error Probability = beta

variable the sample size estimation depends on the expected mean and variability (standard deviation) in the control group. A decision is made to use a one-tailed or two-tailed test when comparing the outcomes in the intervention and control groups. Usually a two-tailed test is used because it is possible that the intervention will cause harm as well as benefit.

Computational programs are available to calculate the sample size which take account of type I and type II error, the event rate in the control group, and the effect size to be studied. Sometimes overlooked, but very important, is underestimation of loss to follow-up, and dealing with missing or incomplete data when the trial ends. This must be anticipated beforehand and incorporated into sample size estimation. A practical "rule-of-thumb" is to allow for a minimum of 20 % loss. Finally, the sample size also depends on how the data is to be analyzed, whether by intention-to-treat or by treatment received. Usually the intention-to-treat analysis is the primary analysis.

There are several options available to limit sample size when designing a trial. These include recruitment of subjects at higher risk for an outcome event, thus increasing the event rate, but doing so affects the generalizability of trial results. Another option is to use composite outcomes. Individual components of composites may be uncommon, but together the rate of composite events may be high enough to limit the sample size required. Components of composite outcomes include events that share a likelihood of benefiting from the intervention under study. For example, a trial might seek to determine the effect of a lipid-lowering drug on future myocardial infarction, revascularization, or cardiovascular death. However, the impact of therapy on individual components of the composite may vary, and not all components of the composite are likely to be of equal clinical importance.

4.2 Recruitment Rate

Again, experiences in prior studies, or preliminary data, are required to estimate recruitment rate. It must be stressed that the number of participants willing or able to enroll will be lower than those who are eligible. Reasons such as potential participant's location, enrollment in other trials, unwillingness or inability to consent, simply being overlooked and other physicians hesitant to enter their patients in a particular trial all decrease recruitment rate often to less than 20 % of the eligible population.

4.3 Duration of the Treatment Period

Along with time to recruit an adequate sample, the rate and timing of the primary outcome events may affect the length of the trial. Additionally, the treatment or intervention may not begin when participants are enrolled into the trial. Depending on the protocol there may be run-in periods where participants are monitored for further exclusion to ensure eligibility, or time may be needed for wash-out periods of medications. Similarly, the treatment may end before the trial finishes as time is necessary to follow the participants for long-term outcomes. For example, patients with idiopathic membranous nephropathy and nephrotic syndrome were randomly assigned to receive symptomatic therapy or a treatment with methylprednisolone and chlorambucil for 6 months and clinical outcomes were then determined up to 10 years later [23]. Finally, treatment periods may end when certain outcomes are met, such as transplant, but participants need follow-up for other end points, such as death.

It helps to have a flow diagram (Fig. 2) outlining the streaming of participants through the processes of screening, consent, further

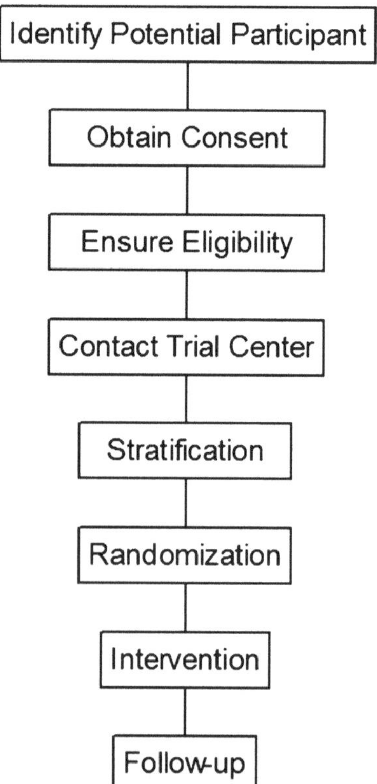

Fig. 2 Example of flow diagram for participants in multicenter randomized controlled trial

assessment of eligibility, contact to trial center, stratification, randomization, and follow-up. This will aid in keeping track of participants in the trial and accounting for them during interpretation and presentation of results.

5 Trial Data

5.1 Data Collection and Management

The database to be analyzed will need to be designed ahead of time and corresponding data collection and collation methods must be accurate but easy-to-use. The data should be collected in a timely fashion. Data entry is becoming more sophisticated with current methods ranging from centralized entry by clerks using the data collection forms to Web-based entry at a remote collection or clinical site. Methods to error check or clean the data must be organized. The final data must be kept secure.

5.2 Details of the Planned Analyses

Appropriate analysis and statistical methods to test the hypothesis depend on the question and must be chosen during the planning phase. Intention to treat analysis is a method where participants are analyzed according to their original group at randomization. This technique attempts to analyze the data in a real world fashion without adjusting for drop-out or drop-in effects. Per protocol analysis, or analysis by treatment received, attempts to analyze the groups according to what the actual treatments were. This way, for example, if a participant drops-out early in the trial, they are excluded from the analysis. Otherwise, the analysis depends on the type of variable, whether repeated measures are used or if "time to event" outcomes are important. The trial design will also affect analysis depending on confounders, stratification, multiple groups or interactions in the case of factorial designs.

5.3 Planned Subgroup Analyses

Subgroup analysis is that done for comparison of groups within the main cohort, for example, diabetics versus nondiabetics in chronic kidney disease. Although not as informative as the whole group analysis because sample sizes may be inadequate, important information may be obtained. It is better to decide upon limited subgroup analysis during trial design than after the data have been collected. The problem in interpreting subgroup analysis is the higher risk of obtaining apparently statistically significant results that have actually arisen due to chance.

5.4 Frequency of Analyses

There may be reasons to analyze a trial while underway. Safety monitoring is probably the most frequent reason. Sometimes during interim analyses the outcomes may be significantly statistically robust (either much better or much worse) than expected such that the continuation of the trial is no longer necessary [24]. In general, statistical stopping rules are used in this circumstance to preserve the originally chosen final alpha by requiring considerably smaller p-values to stop the trial [25]. Another reason for interim analysis is when investigators are uncertain of likely event rates in the control group. Interim analyses that do not address the primary study question do not affect trial type I error rate. Combined event accumulation, or defined intervals or dates, may dictate the precise timing of the interim analysis. An example of a trial halted by the data safety committee is the Beserab erythropoietin trial [26]. That prospective study examined normalizing hematocrit in patients with symptomatic cardiac disease who were undergoing hemodialysis by randomizing participants to receive epoetin to achieve hematocrit of 42 vs. 30 %. The study "was halted when differences in mortality between the groups were recognized as sufficient to make it very unlikely that continuation of the study would reveal a benefit for the normal-hematocrit group and the results were nearing the statistical boundary of a higher mortality rate in the normal-hematocrit group [26]." In addition, the intervention group had a highly significant increased rate of vascular access thrombosis and loss indicating that the intervention group was exposed to harm.

5.5 Economic Issues

Economic issues are a reality when it comes to changing practice patterns and health care policy. It helps if an intervention can be shown to be cost-effective. The methods are reviewed in another chapter. In general, data on resource use is collected prospectively as part of the RCT. Of note, it may be easier to acquire funding from government or hospital sources for the RCT if the outcome is likely to be in their financial interest in the long term.

5.6 Audit Trail

For quality control and scientific integrity, investigators must plan for ongoing record keeping and provide an audit trail. Methods to check for and correct errors should be done concurrently. Similarly, investigators will need to retain records for future access if needed. The length of time for retention is determined by requirements of local or national regulatory agencies, Ethics Review Boards, or Sponsors.

---

6 Challenges to Trial Integrity

One goal of the clinical trial is to estimate the treatment effect, and a well-executed trial should be a model for the real world setting. This section will focus on aspects of trials that will diminish the ability of the trial to detect the true treatment effect.

6.1 Rate of Loss to Follow-Up

Similar to recruitment, where it is not always possible to enroll eligible participants, it is not always possible to keep participants in trials once enrolled. People may "drop-out" because they become disinterested or disenchanted, or they are lost because of relocation, adverse event or death. There are many strategies for preventing this, which depend on the reason participants are lost. Reminders, incentives or regular contact with participants helps keep their interest but this must be done without being too intrusive. Similarly, the trial team must be accessible with efficient and effective measures in place to alleviate concerns participants may have. To deal with relocation or death, it is prudent to have permission from participants to get collateral information from Vital Statistics Bureaus or from relatives.

Another form of "drop-out" has been historically termed non-compliance. In this situation participants are still being followed, yet they are not adhering to the trial intervention. This especially contaminates the active treatment group and may decrease the apparent effectiveness of an intervention. Strategies that have been utilized to reduce this include reinforcement, close monitoring and pill counting.

Similarly, participants in a control arm may inadvertently, or otherwise, receive the experimental treatment. This is termed "drop-in." These phenomena combined act like a crossover design where the investigators are either unaware of its occurrence or may be aware but unable to control it. There is no easy way to deal with this but most investigators will analyze the groups as they were originally assigned (i.e., intention to treat analysis). It is more important to identify areas where this may occur during trial design and try to prevent it. Keeping in mind that some loss is inevitable, the importance of considering these issues when estimating sample size during trial planning is again stressed.

Centers may affect trials in similar ways. They too may "drop-out" and this must be taken into consideration when planning. Prior and ongoing collaboration may decrease this occurrence; however, different center case mix may dictate that some centers will not be able to continue in the trial. For example, they may not have enough potential participants. Otherwise similar strategies to keep participants may be used to keep centers involved.

6.2 Methods for Protecting Against Other Sources of Bias

Standardization of training, methods, and protocol must be undertaken as rigor in these areas decreases variability [27]. Similarly the use of a single central laboratory in multicenter studies can lessen variability in biochemical tests.

7 Funding

The research question must be answerable in a reasonable period of time for practical reasons. Costs will be influenced by the sample size, time to recruit participants, time needed for outcomes to accrue, the intervention, the number of tests and interviews, managing and auditing the trial, and data management and analysis. A budget encompassing all these issues is essential.

7.1 Costs

The majority of today's clinical research is human resource intensive and funding is required for the expertise of research nurses and assistants. Similarly, money is needed to pay for research management, data entry and other staffing necessary for administration of the trial. Employee benefits such as pensions, sick leave, compassionate, maternity/paternity leave, jury duty, and vacation must be factored in to costs. Costs of items such as paper, fax, phone, travel, computers, and other consumables can be significant.

7.2 Licensing

Licensing is required to establish new indications for drugs or techniques. This increases costs for trials as regulations for how these trials are conducted may be very strict, and for safety reasons, monitoring and quality control can be more intense. However, there is usually an increase in industry sponsorship to help alleviate the increased cost.

7.3 Funding Sources

Procuring funding is sometimes the major hurdle in clinical research. Fortunately, it is easier to find money to do topical research. For more expensive trials it may be necessary to obtain shared or leveraged funding from more than one of the following limited sources. Public funding from foundations or institutes such as The National Institutes of Health in the USA is available. These have the benefit of the applications being peer reviewed. Government and Hospital Agencies have funds available for research but they can be tied to quality improvement or research aimed at cost reduction. They may also contribute "in-kind" other than through direct funding by providing clinical space and nursing staff.

It is becoming increasingly difficult to do major clinical research without the aid of the private sector. Issues of data ownership and publication rights must be addressed during the planning phase, as should the relative responsibilities of the applicants and the sponsor. It is usually preferable for the investigator to approach the private funding source with the major planning of the trial already completed.

8 Details of the Trial Team

8.1 Steering Committee

Larger trials may need a steering committee for trial management. The main role is to refine design details, spearhead efforts to secure funding, and work out logistical problems. This may also include protocol organization and interim report writing. The committee may include experts in trial design, economic analysis, data management, along with expertise in the various conditions being studied.

8.2 Trial Manager

Clinical trials require efficient trial management. This ensures finite human and financial resources are utilized efficiently, and in a timely manner. A dedicated trial manager can help improve the success of trial completion [28].

8.3 End-Point Adjudication Committee

An end-point adjudication committee may be utilized to judge clinical end points and is required when there are subjective elements of decision-making or when decisions are complex or error-prone. Criteria for the clinical outcomes have to be prespecified and applicable outside of a trial setting. The committee should include physicians and experts in the respective disease being studied and from specialties related to comorbid end points being assessed. They should not be otherwise involved in the trial and should be blinded with respect to the participants' intervention.

8.4 Data Safety and Monitoring Committee

A data safety and monitoring committee is needed for trials if there is a possibility that the trial could be stopped early [29]. This may be based on interim analysis when sufficient data may exist to provide answer to the principal research question or when unexpected safety concerns emerge. This is especially relevant when outcomes of the trial are clinically important. Another reason would be because of the cost of continuing the trial when interim analysis suggests that continuation of the trial would be futile [30]. This committee, similar to the end-point adjudication committee, should be made up of experts not otherwise involved in the trial and should include specialists from the relevant disciplines and a statistician. The committee may not be provided with group comparisons in some meetings but will meet to consider other issues related to trial quality. They should consider external data that may arise during the trial in considering termination. For example, if an ongoing trial is testing Drug A versus Placebo and another trial is published showing conclusive evidence that Drug A, or withholding Drug A, is harmful then the ongoing trial may be terminated (even before interim analysis). This occurred in The Reduction of Endpoints in NIDDM with the Angiotensin II Antagonist Losartan (RENAAL) trial [31] following publication of the HOPE study [12] after which it was judged unethical to withhold therapy aimed at blockade of the renin–angiotensin system to patients on conventional treatment.

8.5 Participating Centers

If multiple centers are required then each center needs a responsible investigator to coordinate the trial at their center. This may include applying to local ethics boards, coordinating local staff, screening, consenting, enrolling, and following participants. A letter of intent from each center's investigator is usually required to secure funding.

9 Reporting

Accurate reporting of RCTs is necessary for accurate critical appraisal of the validity and applicability of the trial results. All trials should initially be registered in a clinical trials registry, such as clinicaltrials.gov, allowing for transparent public access to information. Registration is required by law in certain countries and can be a requirement for publication in many journals. Trial registries also help to address publication bias, especially in the case of negative or subsequently unpublished trials [32].

The CONSORT (Consolidated Standards of Reporting Trials) Statement, revised in 2010 [33] contains a 25 item checklist and flow diagram. Use of this guidance was associated with improved quality of reporting of RCTs [34]. Twenty-five percent of RCTs involve non-pharmacological treatment, which require more extensive reporting particularly in relationship to the experimental treatment, comparator, care processes, centers and blinding.

References

1. Umscheid CA, Margolis DJ, Grossman CE (2011) Key concepts of clinical trials: a narrative review. Postgrad Med 123:194–204

2. Fuchs FD, Klag MJ, Whelton PK (2000) The classics: a tribute to the fiftieth anniversary of the randomized clinical trial. J Clin Epidemiol 53:335–342

3. Gross CP, Krumholz HM, Van Wye G, Emanuel EJ, Wendler D (2006) Does random treatment assignment cause harm to research participants? PLoS Med 3:e188

4. Robinson EJ, Kerr C, Stevens A, Lilford R, Braunholtz D, Edwards S (2004) Lay conceptions of the ethical and scientific justifications for random allocation in clinical trials. Soc Sci Med 58:811–824

5. Kerr C, Robinson E, Stevens A, Braunholtz D, Edwards S, Lilford R (2004) Randomisation in trials: do potential trial participants understand it and find it acceptable? J Med Ethics 30:80–84

6. Whelton PK (1994) Epidemiology of hypertension. Lancet 344:101–106

7. Whelton PK, Gordis L (2000) Epidemiology of clinical medicine. Epidemiol Rev 22:140–144

8. Schulz KF, Grimes DA (2002) Allocation concealment in randomised trials: defending against deciphering. Lancet 359:614–618

9. Parker MJ, Manan A, Duffett M (2012) Rapid, easy, and cheap randomization: prospective evaluation in a study cohort. Trials 13:90

10. Ivers NM, Halperin IJ, Barnsley J, Grimshaw JM, Shah BR, Tu K, Upshur R, Zwarenstein M (2012) Allocation techniques for balance at baseline in cluster randomized trials: a methodological review. Trials 13:120

11. Weijer C, Grimshaw JM, Taljaard M, Binik A, Boruch R, Brehaut JC, Donner A, Eccles MP, Gallo A, McRae AD, Saginur R, Zwarenstein M (2011) Ethical issues posed by cluster randomized trials in health research. Trials 12:100

12. Yusuf S, Sleight P, Pogue J, Bosch J, Davies R, Dagenais G (2000) Effects of an angiotensin-converting-enzyme inhibitor, ramipril, on cardiovascular events in high-risk patients. The Heart Outcomes Prevention Evaluation Study Investigators. N Engl J Med 342:145–153

13. Yusuf S, Dagenais G, Pogue J, Bosch J, Sleight P (2000) Vitamin E supplementation and cardiovascular events in high-risk patients. The Heart Outcomes Prevention Evaluation Study Investigators. N Engl J Med 342:154–160

14. Scott CT, Baker M (2007) Overhauling clinical trials. Nat Biotechnol 25:287–292

15. Hoare ZS, Whitaker CJ, Whitaker R (2013) Introduction to a generalized method for adaptive randomization in trials. Trials 14:19

16. Brown CH, Ten Have TR, Jo B, Dagne G, Wyman PA, Muthen B, Gibbons RD (2009) Adaptive designs for randomized trials in public health. Annu Rev Public Health 30:1–25

17. Mills EJ, Chan AW, Wu P, Vail A, Guyatt GH, Altman DG (2009) Design, analysis, and presentation of crossover trials. Trials 10:27

18. Avins AL, Cherkin DC, Sherman KJ, Goldberg H, Pressman A (2012) Should we reconsider the routine use of placebo controls in clinical research? Trials 13:44

19. D'Agostino RB Sr, Massaro JM, Sullivan LM (2003) Non-inferiority trials: design concepts and issues—the encounters of academic consultants in statistics. Stat Med 22:169–186

20. Snapinn SM (2000) Noninferiority trials. Curr Control Trials Cardiovasc Med 1:19–21

21. Chan AW, Tetzlaff JM, Gotzsche PC, Altman DG, Mann H, Berlin JA, Dickersin K, Hrobjartsson A, Schulz KF, Parulekar WR, Krleza-Jeric K, Laupacis A, Moher D (2013) SPIRIT 2013 explanation and elaboration: guidance for protocols of clinical trials. BMJ 346:e7586

22. Bakris GL, Whelton P, Weir M, Mimran A, Keane W, Schiffrin E (2000) The future of clinical trials in chronic renal disease: outcome of an NIH/FDA/Physician Specialist Conference. Evaluation of Clinical Trial Endpoints in Chronic Renal Disease Study Group. J Clin Pharmacol 40:815–825

23. Ponticelli C, Zucchelli P, Passerini P, Cesana B, Locatelli F, Pasquali S, Sasdelli M, Redaelli B, Grassi C, Pozzi C, Bizzarri D, Banfi G (1995) A 10-year follow-up of a randomized study with methylprednisolone and chlorambucil in membranous nephropathy. Kidney Int 48:1600–1604

24. Briel M, Lane M, Montori VM, Bassler D, Glasziou P, Malaga G, Akl EA, Ferreira-Gonzalez I, Alonso-Coello P, Urrutia G, Kunz R, Culebro CR, da Silva SA, Flynn DN, Elamin MB, Strahm B, Murad MH, Djulbegovic B, Adhikari NK, Mills EJ, Gwadry-Sridhar F, Kirpalani H, Soares HP, Abu Elnour NO, You JJ, Karanicolas PJ, Bucher HC, Lampropulos JF, Nordmann AJ, Burns KE, Mulla SM, Raatz H, Sood A, Kaur J, Bankhead CR, Mullan RJ, Nerenberg KA, Vandvik PO, Coto-Yglesias F, Schunemann H, Tuche F, Chrispim PP, Cook DJ, Lutz K, Ribic CM, Vale N, Erwin PJ, Perera R, Zhou Q, Heels-Ansdell D, Ramsay T, Walter SD, Guyatt GH (2009) Stopping randomized trials early for benefit: a protocol of the study of trial policy of interim truncation-2 (STOPIT-2). Trials 10:49

25. Whitehead J (2004) Stopping rules for clinical trials. Control Clin Trials 25:69–70, author reply 71-2

26. Besarab A, Bolton WK, Browne JK, Egrie JC, Nissenson AR, Okamoto DM, Schwab SJ, Goodkin DA (1998) The effects of normal as compared with low hematocrit values in patients with cardiac disease who are receiving hemodialysis and epoetin. N Engl J Med 339:584–590

27. Sweetman EA, Doig GS (2011) Failure to report protocol violations in clinical trials: a threat to internal validity? Trials 12:214

28. Farrell B, Kenyon S, Shakur H (2010) Managing clinical trials. Trials 11:78

29. Kasenda B, von Elm EB, You J, Blumle A, Tomonaga Y, Saccilotto R, Amstutz A, Bengough T, Meerpohl J, Stegert M, Tikkinen KA, Neumann I, Carrasco-Labra A, Faulhaber M, Mulla S, Mertz D, Akl EA, Bassler D, Busse JW, Ferreira-Gonzalez I, Lamontagne F, Nordmann A, Rosenthal R, Schandelmaier S, Sun X, Vandvik PO, Johnston BC, Walter MA, Burnand B, Schwenkglenks M, Bucher HC, Guyatt GH, Briel M (2012) Learning from failure–rationale and design for a study about discontinuation of randomized trials (DISCO study). BMC Med Res Methodol 12:131

30. Sully BG, Julious SA, Nicholl J (2014) An investigation of the impact of futility analysis in publicly funded trials. Trials 15:61

31. Brenner BM, Cooper ME, de Zeeuw D, Keane WF, Mitch WE, Parving HH, Remuzzi G, Snapinn SM, Zhang Z, Shahinfar S (2001) Effects of losartan on renal and cardiovascular outcomes in patients with type 2 diabetes and nephropathy. N Engl J Med 345:861–869

32. Scherer RW, Langenberg P, von Elm E (2007) Full publication of results initially presented in abstracts. Cochrane Database Syst Rev MR000005

33. Moher D, Hopewell S, Schulz KF, Montori V, Gotzsche PC, Devereaux PJ, Elbourne D, Egger M, Altman DG (2010) CONSORT 2010 explanation and elaboration: updated guidelines for reporting parallel group randomised trials. BMJ 340:c869

34. Plint AC, Moher D, Morrison A, Schulz K, Altman DG, Hill C, Gaboury I (2006) Does the CONSORT checklist improve the quality of reports of randomised controlled trials? A systematic review. Med J Aust 185:263–267

Chapter 10

Randomized Controlled Trials 2: Analysis

Robert N. Foley

Abstract

When analyzing the results of a trial the primary outcome variable must be kept in clear focus. In the analysis plan consideration must be given to comparing the characteristics of the subjects, taking account of differences in these characteristics, intention to treat analysis, interim analyses and stopping rules, mortality comparisons, composite outcomes, research design including run-in periods, factorial, stratified, and crossover designs, number needed to treat, power issues, multivariate modeling, and hypothesis-generating analyses.

Key words Randomized controlled trials, Analysis, Intention to treat, Research design, Stopping rules, Multivariate modeling

1 Introduction

The objective of this chapter is not to formally explore the mathematics of statistical testing or the pluses and minuses of different statistical software packages. The intent is to focus on selected analytical considerations that may help one to decide whether the evidence in a given randomized trial is valid and useful in real-world clinical practice. For the most part, the chapter discusses issues related to trials with outcomes that are clinically meaningful and that are assumed to lead to permanent changes in health status, where a definitive result would be expected to change clinical practice.

2 What Is the Primary Study Question?

Therapeutic uncertainty is the basis of randomized trials and most trials are designed to answer a single question. When analyzing the results of a trial, the primary hypothesis and the primary outcome variable should be kept in clear focus. The nature of the question should be unambiguous and should immediately suggest major design elements and appropriate methods for statistical analysis. For example, in the primary report of the Diabetes Control and

Patrick S. Parfrey and Brendan J. Barrett (eds.), *Clinical Epidemiology: Practice and Methods*, Methods in Molecular Biology, vol. 1281, DOI 10.1007/978-1-4939-2428-8_10, © Springer Science+Business Media New York 2015

Complications Trial (DCCT) [1], the abstract states the following: "Long-term microvascular and neurologic complications cause major morbidity and mortality in patients with insulin-dependent diabetes mellitus. We examined whether intensive treatment with the goal of maintaining blood glucose concentrations close to the normal range could decrease the frequency and severity of these complications." If one takes the purist approach that there can only be a single primary outcome, this description is ambiguous; for there to be a single primary outcome, the description suggests the possibility that a composite outcome was employed in which the outcome was the first occurrence of any microvascular or neurological complication; equally well, the total number of such complications occurring in a defined period of time is also compatible with the terminology used. Needless to say, the analysis and reporting of these two outcomes are very different. In the first case, time-to-first-event analysis might be employed, whereas a rate-based analysis (allowing multiple events to be counted) might be used in the second scenario. In the introduction to the article, the following statement is made, which helps considerably to clarify the primary intent of the trial: "Two cohorts of patients were studied in order to answer two different, but related, questions: Will intensive therapy prevent the development of diabetic retinopathy in patients with no retinopathy (primary prevention), and will intensive therapy affect the progression of early retinopathy (secondary intervention)? Although retinopathy was the principal study outcome, we also studied renal, neurologic, cardiovascular, and neuropsychological outcomes and the adverse effects of the two treatment regimens." It is clear, then, that two randomized trials were performed in parallel, and retinopathy was the primary study outcome in both. The statement also makes it apparent that the study will most likely use time-to-first-event analysis as the main analytical tool.

In the empirical sciences, hypotheses can never be proven. When reading a trial report, or when deciding an analysis plan, it is often worth spending a little time on a formal enumeration of the null and alternate hypotheses. For example, while the null and alternate hypothesis were not formally reported in the DCCT primary prevention trial study report, the statistical approach makes it clear that these were as follows:

Null hypothesis: retinopathy with intensive treatment = retinopathy with standard treatment

Alternate hypothesis: retinopathy with intensive treatment ≠ retinopathy with standard treatment

Laid out in this fashion, an important analytical issue is immediately addressed. In statistical terms, this is a two-tailed hypothesis. In other words, should intensive treatment truly worsen the primary outcome, this will become apparent in the primary analysis. The principal attraction of a one-tailed design is lower sample size requirements than that of a two-tailed equivalent. Had a one-tailed design been used in the DCCT trial, the null and hypotheses might have been as follows:

Null hypothesis: retinopathy with intensive treatment not better than retinopathy with standard treatment

Alternate hypothesis: retinopathy with intensive treatment better than retinopathy with standard treatment

If, in reality, the experimental treatment proves to be worse than the standard treatment, a one- tailed design will not lead to rejection of the null hypothesis. Ideally, the design and reporting of randomized trials should specify clearly whether one-tailed or two-tailed hypotheses are the basis of the trial. When confronting a one-tailed trial with neutral outcomes, one should immediately ask the question: even though A is not better than B, could B be better than A?

Another situation in which it may be useful to formally write down the null and alternate hypothesis is when an equivalence design is used. With the familiar standard comparative designs typically used in double blind, placebo-controlled trials, the null hypothesis is that no difference between treatments exists, whereas the alternate hypothesis is that a difference exists. In contrast, with equivalence designs, the null hypothesis is that a minimum predefined difference exists between treatments, whereas the alternate hypothesis is that no difference exists.

3   What Are the Characteristics of the Trial Subjects?

It seems intuitively obvious that one should know the maximum amount possible about the subjects included in a given randomized trial. It is difficult to generalize study findings to other populations and to individual patients without detailed descriptions of the study subjects. Secondly, as discussed below, randomization of therapies is rarely perfect with regard to characteristics that increase the chances of developing the study outcome during the trial, quite apart from treatments assigned during the randomization process.

Key pieces of information that are rarely quoted in trial reports are the proportion of potentially eligible subjects available at the study sites, the proportion approached and the proportion of subjects that ultimately enter a trial. Clearly, while adding complexity to the logistics of the trial, all efforts to deliver this information should be made in the planning phase of the trial, as retrospective efforts to obtain these data are often fruitless.

With perfect randomization, known and unknown characteristics are identical in all treatment arms. In practice, even in large trials with careful randomization procedures, the likelihood that one baseline characteristic will be statistically different increases with the number of reported characteristics. It follows that the fewer the number of reported characteristics, the lower the likelihood that any single characteristic will differ between the treatment arms. As discussed above, a strategy of reporting fewer study subject characteristics lowers the generalizability of the study. If one accepts that knowing as much as possible about the study population is inherently better than not, one must accept the possibility of unearthing statistically significant differences between the groups. This situation is not irredeemable, however, as it is easy to adjust for imbalances in baseline characteristics. When appraising a clinical trial, it is critical to inspect whether differences between treatment arms are present. If so, outcome analysis should necessarily adjust for this imbalance. It is equally critical to assess whether important clinical descriptors have been omitted.

4   Intention-to-Treat Analysis

Though perhaps an unfortunate terminology, it is used extensively in the randomized trials literature. Essentially, the philosophy behind the term is that outcome analysis will be based entirely on random treatment assignment. As the latter is completely determined by chance, "analysis by assigned treatment" might be a better description. Essentially, a black box is placed around all information accruing between randomization and assessment of the primary study outcome. One of the main advantages of this approach is the likelihood that unplanned occurrences (like crossovers between treatments, noncompliance, co-interventions) make it less likely that differences between treatments will be seen, so that the intention-to-treat philosophy is conservative in advancing the case of new therapies. In randomized trials designed to determine whether treatments lead to differences in clinical outcomes, intention to treat analysis is the gold standard. All other approaches, including analysis restricted to those who remain throughout on assigned therapy, should be viewed as subsidiary and inadequate in isolation.

5   Interim Analyses

Even in large clinical trials, sample size and event rate projections are often based on guesswork. In addition, new interventions can have unexpected, and sometimes life-threatening, side effects. Equally well, the intervention may lead to more dramatic improvements in the primary outcome than originally expected. It is possible, then, that a difference between treatments could be present much earlier than originally planned in a trial. As a result, interim analyses of the primary outcome are usually planned in latter-day large clinical trials.

While the conceptual basis for the stopping rules used in interim analyses (mainly the problems of dealing with increasing probability of a false-positive result with increasing numbers of primary outcome analyses) are relatively straightforward, confusion still arises, perhaps because of the unfamiliarity of terminology used. For example, the terms "group sequential methods" and "alpha spending functions" are not intuitively helpful to non-statisticians. The first of these terms, "group sequential methods," is used to indicate that the group of patients, and/or endpoints studied at each interim analysis, is likely to have changed, either because new patients have entered the study since the last interim analysis or because new events have accrued. Alpha is the probability level below which a difference between treatments will be accepted, and this is usually set at 0.05. Alpha spending means that, while the alpha level used at each analysis can vary, the overall planned alpha level (or type I error rate) remains constant, typically at 0.05 in most trials.

Several alpha spending methods exist, sharing the common properties that the number of planned interim analyses needs to be specified in advance and that analyses are roughly equally spaced. The Pocock method uses the same critical P-values for all analyses, including the final analysis [2]. For example, in the absence of interim analysis, a two-sided test would generally have a critical value 1.96 for an alpha level of 0.05. With the Pocock method, critical values might be 2.178 with one interim analysis and 2.413 with five interim analyses. Thus, using the Pocock method means that the P-value to reject the hypothesis at the final analysis is considerably lower with greater numbers of interim analyses. The Haybittle–Peto approach uses a very conservative critical value for all interim analyses and then a value close to the usual value of 1.96 at the final analysis [3]. The critical boundary values with the O'Brien–Fleming approach are designed in such a way that the probability of stopping early increases with the amount of information available. For example, with one planned interim analysis, the critical values would be 2.782 at the interim analysis and 1.967 at the final analysis. With five interim analyses, the critical values would very between 4.555 at the first interim analysis and 2.037 at the final analysis [4].

Figure 1 is a schematic example of using the O'Brien and Fleming method in a trial planning four interim and one final analysis. Notable features of this scheme include the fact that the test statistic value and associated P-value for the final comparison are broadly similar to those seen when no interim analysis is planned. In contrast, the absolute magnitude of the test statistic is larger and

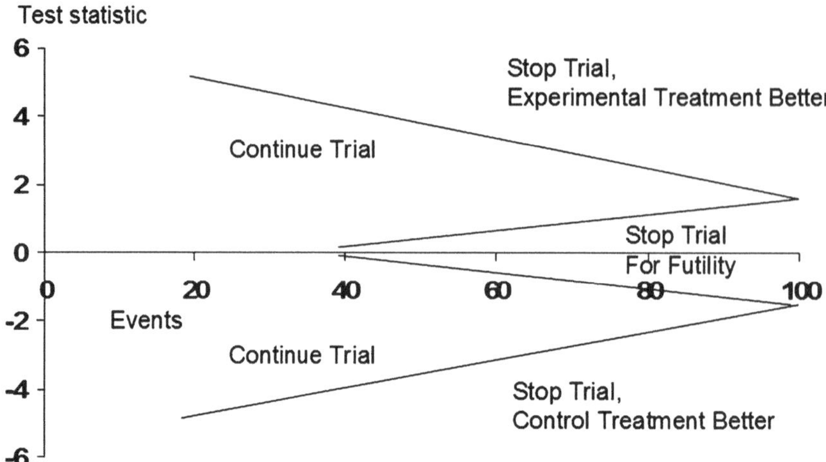

Fig. 1 Hypothetical example of O'Brien and Fleming boundaries in a trial with four planned interim analyses and one final analysis

the boundary *P*-value smaller with ever earlier interim analyses. It is also notable that, while the trial can be stopped for futility, this becomes apparent in later phases of the trial.

None of these stopping rules designs allow for the possibility that an early disadvantage with a given treatment may be more than counterbalanced in the long-term, leading to net benefit. For example, in the secondary prevention arm of the DCCT trial, the intensive treatment group had a higher cumulative incidence of retinopathy in the first 2 years of the trial. By 9 years, however, this initial disadvantage was more than counterbalanced, so that the net effect was a 54 % reduction in the incidence of retinopathy in the intensive treatment group, compared to conventional treatment [1]. It is also worth pointing out that these designs are typically predicated on the primary outcome value only. Typically, major unexpected side effects are not incorporated into stopping rules. Finally, these methods are based entirely on the probability that a difference exists between treatments and do not take the size of this difference into account. With large sample sizes, small absolute differences, can lead to trial termination. Early termination of trials can mean that cost-benefit and cost utility cannot be assessed. In addition, treatment side effects that develop late, such as malignancy, may be difficult to identify.

When reporting trials that were terminated earlier than planned, it should be clear whether the determination was based on preplanned stopping rules, or whether other factors were involved. One high-profile study illustrates the confusion that can result when these matters are not fully clear. In an open-label trial, 1,432 patients with chronic kidney disease and anemia, embarking on erythropoietin therapy, were randomly assigned hemoglobin targets of 113 or 135 g/L, with a primary end-point of time to first occurrence of death or a major cardiovascular event [5]. Four interim analyses were planned using the O'Brien–Fleming alpha-spending boundary method. In the Results section the following statement is made: "The data and safety monitoring board recommended that the study be terminated in May 2005 at the time of the second interim analysis, even though neither the efficacy nor the futility boundaries had been crossed, because the conditional power for demonstrating a benefit for the high-hemoglobin group by the scheduled end of the study was less than 5 % for all plausible values of the true effect for the remaining data." The first part of this statement makes it clear that neither efficacy nor futility boundaries were crossed. In other words, the primary outcome alone cannot have been used as the basis for stopping the trial. The word "because" is therefore inappropriate and the remaining description does not help us to understand why the trial was stopped, as there is no logical connection with the previous information. Unfortunately, when read in isolation, the latter part of the statement sounds very much like the stopping rules were the basis for termination. The situation becomes even more unclear when one learns that the final analysis showed statistically different rates of the primary outcome according to random treatment assignment [5].

6 Mortality Comparisons, Even When Not a Primary Outcome

Most trials examining discrete clinical outcomes use time to event analysis. Typically, every subject in the trial is followed until either the primary outcome or a censoring event occurs. In other words, every subject contributes two variables, time in the study and mode of exit (either with a primary outcome or censored without a primary outcome). Censoring in clinical trials should be examined carefully. To begin with, the term "censoring" is not very intuitive. In practice, this refers to end-of-follow-up events other than the primary study outcome. For example, if primary outcomes are coded 1 and end-of-follow-up events 0, reaching the last day of the study without any clinical event occurring, leaving the study because of a major side effect of the study treatment and loss to follow-up are all treated identically. Similarly, death is a censoring event if it is not included in the primary outcome and it is conceivable that an intervention could improve the primary outcome, while shortening survival. For example, imagine a trial in which every patient had an identical duration of follow. For every hundred patients in the experimental group, 25 exit the study with a primary outcome, 50 die, and 25 exit without a clinical event; the corresponding values in the control group are 50, 25, and 25, respectively. Simple calculation shows that the intervention halves primary outcome rates and doubles death rates. Thus, attention must be paid to the mode of study exit and formal comparison of death rates should be included in studies of clinical outcomes.

Large disparities between the effect of a study treatment on the primary outcome and the effect on mortality can point to unexpected side effects of a study treatment. For example, in the Helsinki Heart Study, 4,081 asymptomatic middle-aged men with dyslipidemia were randomly assigned to gemfibrozil or placebo and cardiac events were the primary outcome. As hypothesized, gemfibrozil reduced the incidence of cardiac events. However, death rates were unaffected by the intervention, which was surprising, as one might have expected that a lower incidence of cardiac events would lead to a lower mortality rate. Ultimately, it was found that gemfibrozil-treated patients had higher rates of violent deaths, including suicide [6]. Thus, it could be argued that a reduction in total mortality is the only dependable evidence that an intervention effects clinical outcomes that should be expected to shorten survival. In practice, this level of evidence usually means very large sample sizes and prolonged follow-up. While this perspective may seem somewhat extreme, failure to consider differential mortality effects can lead to erroneous conclusions about the overall benefit of an intervention.

7 Composite Outcomes

With composite outcomes, it is important to assess whether the components included in the composite are biologically plausible. It is also important to question whether other potentially relevant clinical events have been excluded. While it is seems intuitively obvious that each component of the composite outcome should be analyzed in isolation, many study reports fail to do this.

One study systematically reviewed the use of composite endpoints in clinical trials published in major medical journals between 1997 and 2001. Ultimately 167 original reports were reviewed, involving 300,276 patients where the composite primary outcome included all-cause mortality. 38 % of the trials were neutral for both the primary end point and the mortality component; 36 % reported statistically significant differences for the primary outcome measure, but not for the mortality component; 4 % showed differences in total mortality, but not for the primary composite outcome and finally, 11 % showed differences both in total mortality and in the composite primary outcome [7]. Related to this, while the effect on composite outcomes can be neutral, the intervention may reduce one component of the composite outcome. In this scenario, it must necessarily be the case that intervention increases the risk of at least one of the other components of the composite outcome.

8   Trials with Open-Label Run-In Periods on Active Therapy

Trials with open-label run-in periods require careful analysis and overall conclusions should never forget the run-in phase, even if this was followed by a well-performed placebo-controlled comparison phase. For example, one study examined the effect of carvedilol in 1,094 heart failure patients and found that carvedilol reduced death and hospitalization rates during the placebo-controlled portion of the trial [8]. In the initial open label, run-in phase, eligible patients received 6.25 mg of carvedilol twice daily for 2 weeks and patients tolerating carvedilol were then assigned to receive carvedilol or placebo. The abstract, which is probably the section of a publication with the most relevance to clinicians, failed to report that the seven deaths occurred during the run-in period did not appear in the mortality comparisons, even though they accounted for 24 % of all the deaths in patients who received carvedilol. In addition, 1.4 % of patients were withdrawn prior to randomization because heart failure worsened during the run-in phase. It is probably best, therefore, to avoid this design in general, because it is not reflective of real clinical decision-making, given that the philosophy is predicated on the premise that early effects can be discounted in the assessment of overall benefit. This said, when analyzing data from such a trial, a conservative effect estimate can be generated by assuming that all patients who do not enter the placebo phase are considered to have exited the study because the primary outcome has occurred.

9   Factorial, Stratified, and Crossover Designs

9.1   Factorial Design

It is often advocated that large clinical trials should employ factorial designs, because several interventions can be assessed at one-time. For example, with a typical 2×2 factorial design, subjects are randomized to none, either or both of the treatments A and B. It is possible that the effect of treatment A depends on the presence of treatment B, an example of an interactive effect. Failure to account for this interaction can lead to biased estimates of the effects of treatments A and B. In other words, the primary analysis should jointly included A, B and $A \times B$ as exploratory variables.

9.2   Stratified Design

A similar problem arises when patients are randomized within strata. Stratification is often used in an effort to ensure balance across treatment groups of a dominant characteristic of the study population, often one thought to be highly predictive of the occurrence of the primary outcome variable. It is possible that a study treatment could have differential effects in patients with and without this dominant characteristic. As with factorial designs, it is important to include a treatment-by-stratum term when the effect of the treatment is analyzed in the overall group. In other words, the primary analysis should jointly included treatment, stratum and treatment × stratum as exploratory variables. In addition, even with the risks of multiple comparisons and the likelihood that individual strata may be inadequately powered, it is useful to analyze the effect of the intervention within the individual strata.

9.3 Crossover Trials

In spite of their conceptual simplicity, crossover trials are often analyzed inappropriately in the medical literature. In crossover trials, enrolled subjects are given sequences of treatments and differences in the primary outcome between individual treatments are compared [9]. With this design, the intervention is randomization to a sequence of treatments, for example AB or BA. Because subjects act as their own controls, between-subject variation is eliminated and smaller sample sizes are required to detect a given difference between treatments, in comparison with standard parallel group designs. The principal problem with crossover designs is period-by-treatment interaction, commonly referred to as the carryover effect. Stated briefly, carryover is the persistence of a treatment effect from a single period into a subsequent period of treatment. The possibility of carryover is the reason washout periods are commonly used in crossover trials.

When analyzing crossover trials it is important to pretest the data for carryover effects [10]. In other words, the primary analysis should jointly included treatment, period and treatment × period as exploratory variables. Analysis becomes highly problematic if carryover effects are detected. One approach to dealing with this problem is to treat the study as a standard parallel group trial, confining the analysis to one of the study periods (usually the first periods is chosen). Obviously, the validity of this approach may be threatened by inadequate statistical power, as between subject variability can no longer be assumed to be eliminated, and by the decision to use one of two periods is arbitrary [11]. Another approach, applicable when ≥ 3 treatment periods are used (such as ABB/BAA) is to model the carry over effect and to adjust treatment estimates for this effect [10].

10   Number Needed to Treat

This is defined as the number of cases that have to be treated with an intervention to prevent a single occurrence of the primary study outcome [12]. It is easily computed as the inverse of the absolute risk reduction caused by the treatment and can be very useful in economic analyses, in particular. In analyses based on survival techniques, quoting a number in isolation is meaningless, and an appropriate mode of description might include a measure of the average or median duration of the trial. Similarly, annualizing this measure (as in saying X patients need to be treated per year) may not be accurate, as this approach implicitly assumes that the relative effect of the intervention does not vary with time. Finally, numbers needed to treat are often quoted without associated confidence intervals, which is meaningless from a statistical perspective.

11   Neutral Trials: Power Issues

When trials show no treatment effect, it is important to revisit the issue of sample size and Type II error. In particular, it is worth comparing the projected event rates with the actual event rates observed in the study, especially in the control group. It is also useful to produce numerical estimates of the potential treatment effect the study could have detected with standard power assumptions. As a corollary, it is also very useful to recalculate the sample size needed to detect the originally planned difference between treatments, using the primary outcomes seen in the study.

12   Imbalanced Randomization of Baseline Characteristics and Treatment Comparisons

Earlier in this chapter, the case is made that full and open disclosure of as many characteristics of the study population as possible is vital in assessing the applicability of the study results in other populations and in individual patients. With such an approach, it is to be expected that some baseline characteristics may not be evenly balanced between treatment groups, even with meticulous randomization procedures. If it turns out that these imbalanced characteristics are themselves associated with the primary study outcome, it is imperative that analyses are performed in which adjustment is made for these imbalances.

Because no trials are perfect, it is hard to argue against a policy in which treatment estimates are subjected to a rigorous sensitivity analysis, with regard to adjustment for many potential of covariates.

For example, in the CHOIR study, described above, despite the large sample size, statistically significant differences in two baseline characteristics were observed, namely, more hypertension and more prior coronary artery bypass surgery in the higher hemoglobin target group [5]. Bearing in mind that cardiovascular events were the primary outcome, it is be reasonable to ask "What happens to the treatment effects, when adjustment is made for baseline covariates?" This analysis did not appear in the primary publication. Interestingly, when reported in another forum, with adjustment for baseline characteristics, the P-value for the randomly assigned intervention changed from 0.03 to 0.11 [13]. With a true treatment effect, statistical significance cannot be made to disappear with any adjustment strategy. In essence, therefore, the disparity between the adjusted analysis and the unadjusted analysis is an unequivocal demonstration that the null hypothesis for a true treatment effect cannot be safely rejected.

13   Analysis of Randomized Trials from an Observational Perspective: Assessment of Hypothesized Risk Factors and Surrogates

In some situations, it can be very helpful to combine control groups and intervention groups, and study the outcome associations of the assigned therapy in an observational manner, much like one would do with a prospective cohort study. One ideal situation for this approach is studies where subjects are assigned to target levels of biological variables. For example, in the Hypertension Optimal Trial (H.O.T) 18,790 hypertensive patients were randomly assigned to target diastolic blood pressures ≤ 90, ≤ 85 mmHg or ≤ 80 mmHg, and felodipine was used as primary antihypertensive therapy. In terms of the treatment experiment, the intervention had no effect on cardiovascular event rates. In contrast, when analyzed in a purely observational manner, patients with lower blood pressure levels during the course of the study had lower cardiovascular event rates [14]. The authors of study summarized the findings as showing "the benefits of lowering the diastolic blood pressure down to 82.6 mmHg." While they clearly demonstrated that people with blood pressure levels above this level had higher cardiovascular events, they also showed that an unknown common factor was leading both to high blood pressure and high cardiovascular event rates. In other words, they convincingly showed that the observation between high diastolic blood pressure and cardiovascular disease in the study population was noncausal. Disparities between assigned and observed longitudinal variables in randomized trials strongly suggest the presence an unknown factor causing both the clinical observations and help prove that an epidemiological association is noncausal. This phenomenon might be termed observational–experimental discrepancy.

Randomized trials are the ideal arena for assessing the validity of surrogate markers. For example, imagine the following causal pathway in which A leads to C via the development of B:

$$A \rightarrow B \rightarrow C$$

If this causal pathway is truly valid, the following effects should occur with an intervention that lowers A:

1. The intervention lowers B.

2. The intervention lowers C.

3. When adjustment is made for the development of B, the intervention no longer lowers C.

14 Hypothesis-Generating Analyses

Definition of study subjects, follow-up and assessment of clinical events are often highly detailed in good randomized trials. In addition, high-quality data are often available about outcomes other than the primary study question, and biological samples may be collected sequentially at regular intervals. It may be possible, then, to study many other outcomes with regard to randomly assigned treatment groups. It may be possible to examine the individual components of a composite outcome and even to reexamine the primary outcome many years after the experiment has stopped. Examination of outcomes in segments of time should be possible. In essence, the list of possible comparisons may be impressively long. All these analyses are subject to the problem of multiple comparisons, such that it is a virtual guarantee that an apparently important difference between assigned treatment groups will be found, if one performs enough analyses. While there is nothing intrinsically wrong with examining multiple outcomes in high-quality data sets, these analyses should always be considered as hypothesis generating, at best. Unfortunately, this limitation applies to all non-primary outcome analysis, whether or not these were enumerated in the planning phase of the study.

References

1. The Diabetes Control and Complications Trial Research Group (1993) The effect of intensive treatment of diabetes on the development and progression of long-term complications in insulin-dependent diabetes mellitus. N Engl J Med 329:977–986

2. Pocock SJ (1977) Group sequential methods in the design and analysis of clinical trials. Biometrika 64:191–199

3. Haybittle JL (1971) Repeated assessment of results in clinical trials of cancer treatment. Br J Radiol 44:793–797

4. O'Brien PC, Fleming TR (1979) A multiple testing procedure for clinical trials. Biometrics 35:549–556

5. Singh AK, Szczech L, Tang KL, Barnhart H, Sapp S, Wolfson M, Reddan D, Investigators CHOIR (2006) Correction of anemia with epoetin alfa in chronic kidney disease. N Engl J Med 355:2085–2098

6. Frick MH, Elo O, Haapa K, Heinonen OP, Heinsalmi P, Helo P, Huttunen JK, Kaitaniemi P, Koskinen P, Manninen V et al (1987) Helsinki Heart Study: primary-prevention trial with gemfibrozil in middle-aged men with dyslipidemia. Safety of treatment, changes in risk factors, and incidence of coronary heart disease. N Engl J Med 317:1237–1245

7. Freemantle N, Calvert M, Wood J, Eastaugh J, Griffin C (2003) Composite outcomes in randomized trials: greater precision but with greater uncertainty? JAMA 289:2554–2559

8. Packer M, O'Connor CM, Ghali JK, Pressler ML, Carson PE, Belkin RN, Miller AB, Neuberg GW, Frid D, Wertheimer JH, Cropp AB, DeMets DL (1996) Effect of amlodipine on morbidity and mortality in severe chronic heart failure. Prospective Randomized Amlodipine Survival Evaluation Study Group. N Engl J Med 335:1107–1114

9. Grizzle JE (1965) The two-period change-over design and its use in clinical trials. Biometrics 21:461–480

10. Sibbald B, Roberts C (1998) Understanding controlled trials. Crossover trials. BMJ 316:1719

11. Freeman PR (1989) The performance of the two-stage analysis of two-treatment, two-period crossover trials. Stat Med 8:1421–1432

12. Laupacis A, Sackett DL, Roberts RS (1988) An assessment of clinically useful measures of the consequences of treatment. N Engl J Med 318:1728–1733

13. http://www.clinicaltrials.gov/ct/search;jsessionid=A244B49D3229182015D991D216151230?term=choir&submit=Search Accessed April 2007

14. Hansson L, Zanchetti A, Carruthers SG, Dahlof B, Elmfeldt D, Julius S, Menard J, Rahn KH, Wedel H, Westerling S (1998) Effects of intensive blood-pressure lowering and low-dose aspirin in patients with hypertension: principal results of the Hypertension Optimal Treatment (HOT) randomised trial. HOT Study Group. Lancet 351:1755–1762

Chapter 11

Randomized Controlled Trials 3: Measurement and Analysis of Patient-Reported Outcomes

Michelle M. Richardson, Megan E. Grobert, and Klemens B. Meyer

Abstract

The study of patient-reported outcomes, now common in clinical research, had its origins in social and scientific developments during the latter twentieth century. Patient-reported outcomes comprise functional and health status, health-related quality of life, and quality of life. The terms overlap and are used inconsistently, and these reports of experience should be distinguished from expressions of preference regarding health states. Regulatory standards from the USA and European Union provide some guidance regarding reporting of patient-reported outcomes. The determination that measurement of patient-reported outcomes is important depends in part on the balance between subjective and objective outcomes of the health problem under study. Instrument selection depends to a large extent on practical considerations. A number of instruments can be identified that are frequently used in particular clinical situations. The domain coverage of commonly used generic short forms varies substantially. Individualized measurement of quality of life is possible, but resource intensive. Focus groups are useful, not only for scale development but also to confirm the appropriateness of existing instruments.

Under classical test theory, validity and reliability are the critical characteristics of tests. Under item response theory, validity remains central, but the focus moves from the reliability of scales to the relative levels of traits in individuals and items' relative difficulty. Plans for clinical studies should include an explicit model of the relationship of patient-reported outcomes to other parameters, as well as definition of the magnitude of difference in patient-reported outcomes that will be considered important. It is particularly important to minimize missing patient-reported outcome data; to a limited extent, a variety of statistical techniques can mitigate the consequences of missing data.

Key words Patient-reported outcomes, Health-related quality of life, Quality of life, Functional status, Health status

---

1 History and Definition of Patient-Reported Outcomes

Over the past several decades, it has become common for clinical investigators to use forms and questionnaires to collect observers' reports of human subjects' function and experiences. These instruments measure perception and assessment. Implicitly or explicitly, the investigators hypothesize that such measurement may detect variation in the natural history of disease and treatment effects not

Patrick S. Parfrey and Brendan J. Barrett (eds.), *Clinical Epidemiology: Practice and Methods*, Methods in Molecular Biology, vol. 1281, DOI 10.1007/978-1-4939-2428-8_11, © Springer Science+Business Media New York 2015

described by vital status or by observations recorded in the clinical record. The first instruments designed to assess function were devised in the 1930s and 1940s. These reports of functional status by an observer were not qualitatively different from a detailed account, using a controlled, and hence countable vocabulary, of selected aspects of the medical history. The ensuing nine decades have seen three clinical developments in the measurement of function and experience in clinical investigation: the change in reporting perspective from third person to first person; the broadening of the phenomena of interest from function to quality of life and the subsequent definition of a narrower focus on health-related quality of life; and the merging of the tradition of clinical observation with that of psychometric measurement, which had developed through educational and psychological testing.

The earliest instruments examined aspects of function closely related to impaired physiology, whether related to heart failure and angina (the New York Heart Association classifications), to malignancy and the consequences of its treatment (Karnofsky performance status), or to functional limitations as measured by independence in activities of daily living for aged, chronically ill individuals (e.g., the PULSES Profiles, the ADL Index, the Barthel Index). Development of survey technology by the US military for screening purposes during World War II gave a precedent for directing questions to the individual rather than to clinicians or other observers [1]. Between the 1950s and 1970s, several trends stimulated measurement of quality of life at the societal level. One was the advent of public financing of health care and a second the development of extraordinary, intrusive, and expensive methods of life prolongation. These posed new questions: Was such prolongation desirable at all costs and under all circumstances? (The first indexed reference to "quality of life" in MEDLINE raised questions about dialysis treatment for chronic kidney failure [2].) The third trend contributing to interest in quality of life was the rise of a technocratic approach to public policy, accompanied by statistical argument: Quality of life was a "social indicator," a complement to economic measurement. Interest in it reflected in part ideological rejection of what was seen as materialism and emphasis on quality rather than quantity [3]. Finally, there was an optimistic emphasis on positive health rather than on the absence of disease, first expressed in 1946 in the Constitution of the World Health Organization [4].

In the USA in the 1970s and 1980s, publically funded studies, such as the Health Insurance Experiment and the Medical Outcomes Study, saw the development of health status measurement by scientists trained not primarily as clinicians but in the tradition of psychological and educational testing. They brought mathematical rigor and an emphasis on the theoretical underpinnings of survey construction to measurement of health.

Two traditions of assessment merged: the categorical medical model, and the dimensional psychological and educational model [5]. Beginning in the 1950s, developments in statistics, psychometrics, and the technology of the measurement have fundamentally changed the understanding of patient-reported outcomes, not merely accelerating the process of data acquisition and analysis, but defining new concepts. Computerized adaptive testing use item response theory to adjust the items presented to a respondent on the basis of previous responses. Evolving statistical methods allow comparison of the relative validity of instruments and offer the prospect of being able to "crosswalk" results from one instrument to another, allowing comparison of populations across studies.

The use of questionnaires to elicit reports about all aspects of experience, and the theoretical need to connect the tradition of narrowly focused biological inquiry with broader social concerns led to the formulation of a model in which the individual's physical and mental functioning were at the epicenter of a family of concentric circles; physical aspects of health were measurable as *functional status* and physical and mental aspects as *health status*. Health status was also used to describe the union of these core issues with issues that involved both the individual and his or her immediate social setting: the influence of emotions and physical health on the individual's role functioning, social functioning, and spirituality. The term *health-related quality of life* (HRQOL) is often used to describe aspects of quality of life directly related to health and to distinguish these from aspects of experience more indirectly related to the individual and more dependent on social and political trends. However, the term *quality of life* remains ambiguous shorthand: it refers in some contexts to health related aspects of experience but in others to valuation of those experiences. For example, one university center studying it defines quality of life as "The degree to which a person enjoys the important possibilities of his or her life" [6].

2 Experience and Preference

Patient-reported outcomes are descriptions. These descriptions are measured by instruments that elicit the individual's observation of his or her experience, sometimes experience in the world, sometimes internal experience, sometimes anticipation of future experience. The instruments used to elicit these quantitative descriptions represent a measurement tradition that can be traced back to Fechner's nineteenth century psychophysics. This psychometrically derived description of the individual's experience should be distinguished from the individual's relative valuation of outcomes or states of health. This valuation was classically described as the utility of an outcome to the individual; measures of this valuation are commonly described as preference-based. It is defined by the standard reference gamble described by von Neumann and Morgenstern, in which one chooses between the certainty of an immediate outcome, on one hand, and a gamble between the best and worst possible outcomes, on the other. The utility of the intermediate outcome is defined as being equal to the probability of the best possible outcome at the point of indifference, the point at which one prefers neither the gamble between best and worst outcomes, nor the certainty of the intermediate outcome. For example, imagine that a chronically ill patient faces a choice between continued chronic illness and a treatment that will either return him to perfect health or result in his immediate death. He finds that at a probability of 0.7 of surviving the treatment and returning to perfect health, he is indifferent to the choice. The utility of life in his current state of chronic illness is 0.7. Because of the intuitive difficulty of the standard reference gamble, other approaches to assess the utility of health states have been explored, most successfully, the time trade-off, in which the utility of the intermediate state of health is measured by the number of years of perfect health one would accept in exchange for longer survival in impaired health. Thus, if one is indifferent to a choice between 7 years of perfect health and 10 years of chronic illness, the utility of the state of chronic illness would again be 0.7.

3   Regulatory Standards

Results from reliable patient-reported outcome instruments originating in appropriately designed studies can be used to support claims of therapeutic benefit in medical product labeling. Labeling claims usually relate to patients' signs and symptoms or to an aspect of functioning affected by the disease state. In its Guidance to Industry, the US Food and Drug Administration (FDA) suggests a specific and detailed process by which a patient-reported outcome instrument may be used to prove labeling claims. Four general guidelines require definition of and set standards for [7]:

1. The population enrolled in the clinical trial
2. The clinical trial objectives and design
3. The PRO instrument's conceptual framework
4. The PRO instrument's measurement properties

The European Medicines Agency also provides guidance for quality of life research. In the European Union, efficacy and safety are the basis for drug approval; proving an improvement in quality of life is optional. The European Medicines Agency defines PROs as self-administered, subjective, multidimensional measures and specifies that domains must be "clearly differentiated from the core symptoms of the disease," such as pain. An application submitted claiming global HRQOL improvement must be accompanied by evidence showing robust improvement in all or most of the domains measured. The instrument or questionnaire used must specifically be validated in the condition in question. The observation period must be sufficient to allow distinction of treatment effect on HRQOL from underlying short term fluctuation [8, 9].

4 Instrument Selection

The most fundamental question is whether patient-reported outcomes are important to a study. An affirmative answer to the questions of importance implies that one has a theory or model of the outcomes in question and their relationship to the disease or intervention. A paper from the European Regulatory Issues on Quality of Life Assessment Group suggests that health-related quality of life measurement may be helpful in the following scenarios [8]:

- When one of more HRQOL domain(s) is critical for patients,
- When there is no objective marker of disease activity (e.g., migraine, arthritis),
- When a disease can only be characterized by several possible measures of clinical efficacy (e.g., asthma),
- When a disease is expressed by many symptoms (e.g., irritable bowel syndrome),
- When treatment extends life, possibly at the expense of well-being and HRQOL [...],
- When the new treatment is expected to have a small or non-existent impact on survival [...] but a positive impact on HRQOL [...],
- With highly efficient treatment in severe and handicapping diseases (e.g., rheumatoid arthritis) to ensure that improvement of severity score is accompanied by improvement of HRQOL,
- With not very efficient treatment in less severe diseases (e.g., benign prostatic hypertrophy, urinary incontinence) to ensure that the modest improvement of symptoms is accompanied by improvement of HRQOL,
- In diseases with no symptoms (e.g., hypertension) to ensure that treatment does not alter HRQOL, and
- In equivalence trials, for drugs anticipated to result in a similar disease course, but expected to have HRQOL differences.

If the primary or secondary outcomes of a study are patient-reported, it is important that the investigators make explicit such a conceptual model [10]. In evaluating a specific candidate instrument, the following criteria have been suggested [1]:

1. Will it be used to evaluate a program or to study individuals?
2. What diagnoses, age groups, and levels of disability will be studied?
3. Are short-term or long-term conditions to be studied?
4. How broad and how detailed must the assessment be?
5. Does the instrument reflect an underlying conceptual approach and is that approach consistent with the study?
6. Is scoring clear?
7. Can the instrument detect the changes in question?
8. What evidence exists as to reliability and validity?

In addition to the above questions, the FDA reviews the following characteristics of instruments [7]:

- Concepts being measured
- Number of items
- Conceptual framework of the instrument
- Medical condition for intended use
- Population for intended use
- Data collection method
- Administration mode
- Response options
- Recall period
- Scoring
- Weighting of items or domains
- Format
- Respondent burden
- Translation or cultural adaptation availability

In choosing among instruments, the first question is whether to use a measure of general health-related quality of life alone or to supplement the generic instrument with items regarding experiences particularly relevant to the particular health problem under study. (It would be theoretically possible to ask only questions specific to the instant problem, but it is hard to imagine a situation in which the information elicited by a general instrument would not be important, if only to compare the study population to other populations.) The reason to supplement a generic "core" instrument is that one has reason to believe, on the basis of prior published patient-reported outcome data, clinical experience, or preliminary investigation, that the generic instruments do not elicit important

Table 1
Instruments commonly used in specific clinical settings

Disease	Measures
Coronary heart disease	Minnesota Living with Heart Failure Questionnaire (MLHFQ) Seattle Angina Questionnaire MacNew Heart Disease Health-Related Quality of Life Questionnaire Kansas City Cardiomyopathy Questionnaire (KCCQ)
Geriatrics	Geriatric Depression Scale Life Satisfaction Index
Kidney failure	Kidney Disease Quality of Life—Short Form (KDQOL-SF)
Cancer	EORTC QLQ-C30 Breast Cancer Chemotherapy Questionnaire
Orthopedics/rheumatology	Oswestry Disability Index Fibromyalgia Impact Questionnaire Neck Disability Index Arthritis Impact Measurement Scale (AIMS)
HIV	MOS-HIV MQoL-HIV (Multidimensional Quality of Life Questionnaire for HIV infection)
Diabetes	Diabetes Quality of Life Measure

experiences or adequately detect change. Table 1 shows examples of instruments used in situations in which clinical studies commonly measure health-related quality of life. The empiric literature on whether disease-specific supplements add information to generic instruments is mixed and seems to vary by clinical situation [11]. The content that a "disease-specific" supplement adds to a general measure of health-related quality of life may be quite specific but may also include domains that might be considered of general importance but are not included in all general measures. For example, the SWAL-QOL, which assesses the effects of dysphagia, includes items regarding both the burden of swallowing problems and sleep [12].

Table 2 shows the domains included in seven commonly used short general measures of health-related quality of life. One family of instruments deserves particular note, the series of short forms measuring health status developed in the course of the Medical Outcomes Study. The Short Form-36 Health Survey is probably the most widely used measure of health-related quality of life worldwide. Its translation has been the centerpiece of the International Quality of Life Assessment Project (www.iqola.org). SF-36 domains include physical functioning, role limitations due to physical health, bodily pain, general health perceptions, vitality, social functioning, role limitations

Table 2
Domains included in commonly used short general measures of health-related quality of life

	NHP	COOP	DUKE	EQ-5D	WHOQOL-BREF	SF-36
Pain	√	√	√	√	√	√
Physical functioning	√	√	√	√	√	√
Mental health	√	√	√	√	√	√
General health		√	√	√	√	√
Social functioning	√	√	√		√	√
Sleep	√				√	
Fatigue	√				√	√
Family	√		√			
Work	√		√		√	√
Social support	√	√			√	
Other (recreation, sports, etc.)	√				√	
Intimacy/sexuality	√				√	
Finances					√	

Notes. NHP Nottingham Health Profile, *COOP* Dartmouth COOP Charts, *DUKE* Duke Health Profile, *EQ-5D* EuroQOL EQ-5D Quality of Life Scale, *WHOQOL-BREF* World Health Organization Quality of Life-BREF, *SF-36* Short Form-36 Health Survey

due to emotional problems, and mental health. It yields scale scores for each of these eight health domains and two summary measures of physical and mental health: the Physical Component Summary score (PCS) and Mental Component Summary score (MCS). The SF-6D, a derivative measure, allows assessment of utilities.

In 1996, a second version of the SF-36 was produced, SF-36 v2. Although designed to be comparable to the original form, SF-36 v2 rewords some questions and begins with specific instructions. Several previously dichotomous questions were given more response options to improve fidelity; to streamline the questionnaire, some six-item responses were reduced to five. Formatting was also standardized: all responses are now listed horizontally. The intent was that the SF-36 v2 be more easily used throughout the world. The SF-12, similarly revised in 1996, was developed from the SF-36 as a scannable one-page survey. The SF-12 has 12 items rather than 36, takes about 2 rather than 7 min to complete, and offers results comparable to the SF-36. Numerous studies show PCS and MCS scores calculated from the two instruments to be comparable. The SF-12 is an ideal tool for population-level work. However, the greater reliability of the longer short form makes the SF-36 preferable for interpretation of individual's results, and some investigators argue that even it is too unreliable for this purpose.

In part because of the large number of available surveys, the National Institutes of Health began an initiative called PROMIS® (Patient Reported Outcomes Measurement Information System). This system is intended to be a collection of highly reliable, precise measures of patient-reported health status for physical, mental, and social well-being. PROMIS® is a unique venture in that the measures have been standardized so there are common domains and metrics across conditions, allowing for comparisons across domains and diseases; all metrics for each domain have been rigorously reviewed and tested for reliability and validity; PROMIS items can be administered in a variety of ways, in a different forms; and PROMIS encompasses all people, regardless of literacy, language, physical function, or life course [13].

5 Individualized Measures of Patient Reported Outcomes

The attempt to measure subjective experience, whether health status, health-related quality of life, or broader aspects of experience, arose at least in part as a reaction to the reduction of human experience to economic and clinical measurements. However, some investigators argue that standardized questionnaires are inherently insensitive to the particular issues most important to individuals and the individual should be able to designate the domains important to him or her. McDowell describes this debate as one between nomothetic and ideographic approaches to knowledge [1]. The Schedule for the Evaluation of Individual Quality of Life (SEIQoL) is probably the most widely cited individualized instrument. Because of the complexity and resource requirements of measuring individualized quality of life, such instruments have not been widely used to define clinical trial outcomes [14].

6 Defining the Issues: Focus Groups

The complexity and resource requirements of new instrument development make the use of existing instruments preferable whenever possible. However, even if the intent is to use existing instruments, it is important to confirm their context validity. Focus groups are often recommended but rarely described. Professional facilitators have experience in directing conversation flow and analyzing qualitative results and will also assist in planning focus groups [15–18]. Focus groups should be relatively homogenous, and participants should be strangers to one another; this encourages disclosure and minimizes assumptions in conversation. If sexuality or other sensitive information may be discussed, men and women should be separated. The optimal size is 7–10; too many participants leave some without a chance to talk, and too few create too much pressure to talk. Very few people should be in the room during the conduct of the group itself: only the facilitator, a note taker, and at most one or two members of the research team. Under no circumstances should authority figures, such as clinicians responsible for the care of group members, be present. To protect privacy, it is helpful to use pseudonyms and record only general demographic information. The uses to which transcripts will be put and their eventual disposition should be described explicitly in the process of obtaining informed consent. A focus group meeting should last for 1–2 h and should follow a five- to six-item agenda. Questions should be prepared in advance. Prompts such as posters or handouts may help stimulate discussion. A strong introduction is very important. The facilitator should take a few minutes to explain the purpose of the research and the goals of the group.

7   Characteristics of Scales

There are four kinds of scales: nominal, ordinal, interval, and ratio. A nominal scale simply assigns the subject to a category, for example, yes/no, male/female; the categories have no quantitative relationship. An ordinal scale orders the categories but does not define the magnitude of the interval between categories. An interval scale defines the distance between categories. A ratio scale, by defining a zero point, allows comparison of the magnitude of categories. These distinctions have important implications, and individuals embarking on scale construction, rather than simply mimicking the categories of existing instruments, should consult more detailed discussions [1, 5]. (Clinicians may find it edifying to consider that the traditional medical history is phrased almost exclusively in nominal inquires.)

A major drawback of traditional static surveys is the presence of floor and ceiling effects. These effects limit a scale's ability to discriminate among individuals and to detect change. A scale cannot distinguish between two individuals who give the lowest possible response to every item (floor effect) nor between two who give the highest possible response (ceiling effect). Neither can a scale detect further deterioration in an individual responding at the floor or improvement in an individual responding at the ceiling. The magnitude of floor and ceiling effects obviously depends both on the items' difficulty and the respondents' experience.

Recent advances in survey design have helped minimize the problem of floor and ceiling effects. Computerized adaptive testing (CAT) employs a simple form of artificial intelligence that selects

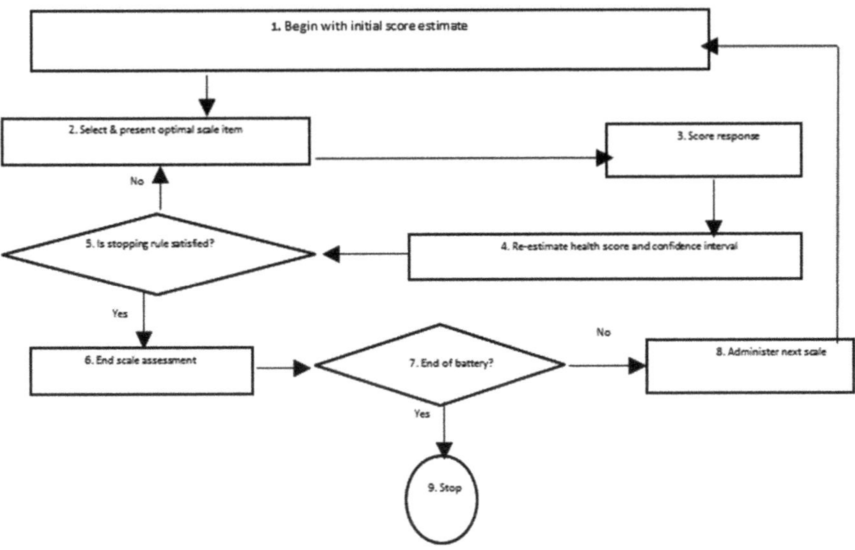

Fig. 1 Logic of computerized adaptive testing

questions tailored to the respondent, shortens or lengthens the instrument to achieve the desired precision, scores everyone on a standard metric so that results can be compared, and displays results instantly [19]. Each administration of an instrument adapts to the level of disease impact the respondent reports in any particular domain or content area. This approach minimizes the number of items required to estimate that impact. Typically, adaptive software first asks a question in the middle of the impact range, and adjusts subsequent items on the basis of the response. With the administration of each item, the score and confidence interval are recalculated (Fig. 1). New items are administered in an iterative fashion until the stopping rule is satisfied. By altering the stopping rule, it becomes possible to match the level of score precision to the specific purpose of measurement for each individual. For example, more precision in scoring will be needed to monitor individual progress than to identify presence of disease impact for an individual respondent.

CAT methodology increases the precision of score estimates, potentially allowing for reliable and valid clinical use in individual patients, eliminates floor and ceiling effects, provides confidence intervals specific to the individual, and allows monitoring of data quality in real time. Although the costs of development and implementation may be considerable, the marginal cost of assessing respondents who are able to use the technology should be considerably less than that associated with other techniques of data collection. If the additional accuracy and precision available from adaptive methods are taken into account, use of the technology may be associated with a very favorable cost-effectiveness ratio.

8 Validity

Validity has been defined as the degree to which an item or an instrument measures the phenomenon of interest in the population of interest. Validity is sometimes described as the extent to which the item or instrument measures what it purports to measure, rather than something else, and is traditionally said to comprise content validity, criterion validity, and construct validity.

Content or face validity describes a conceptual and generally qualitative and intuitive assessment: whether the items capture the experiences that are important and whether they do so accurately. Content validity is most commonly assessed by literature review and conversation, whether unstructured and informal individual conversation or using the techniques of focus groups. The individuals whose opinions are consulted to determine content validity may be professionals accustomed to working with the subjects whose experience is to be measured or representative subjects themselves.

Construct validity is said to be present if responses to a measure exhibit the pattern that might be predicted on the basis of the investigator's theoretical model of the phenomenon of interest. For example, in an opioid-naive population, responses to a pain scale correlate with the dose of narcotic required to treat postoperative pain, and both the pain scale response and the narcotic dose decline day by day following uncomplicated surgery. The pain scale might be said to show construct validity in that population. On the other hand, among the clients of a methadone maintenance program, it might not be so easy to use narcotic doses on the days following surgery to show construct validity of the pain scale.

Criterion validity is a special case of construct validity, examining the correlation between the proposed measure and existing measures, the validity of which have been established or presumed. A scale measuring depression might be validated against the Beck Depression Inventory or the clinical diagnosis of depression by a psychiatrist. References 1–3 explore validity as a theoretical construct in more detail, each from a slightly different perspective, explaining different subtypes of validity that have been described and the mathematical techniques for assessing validity.

9 Reliability

Reliability, the second characteristic defining a scale's performance, describes the consistency of its results. Consider a questionnaire asking women how old they are. If the same women respond to the questionnaire on three consecutive weeks, a reliable instrument will yield approximately the same answer every time (allowing for birthdays). If the subjects give approximately their real ages, the instrument is valid. Reliability does not require validity: An instrument may be highly reliable but also highly biased: the women may all consistently deduct 10 years from their actual ages. Their responses are reliable, in that they do not vary, but not valid. Conversely, however, validity does depend on reliability. If each woman reports a different age on each administration, the instrument clearly is not a valid measurement of age. Formally, reliability is defined by the equation reliability = subject variability/(subject variability + measurement error).

A scale's reliability may be estimated in several ways: the two commonly reported in studies of patient-reported outcomes are test–retest reliability and internal consistency reliability. Test–retest reliability compares the results obtained by administering an instrument to the same subjects on two occasions. Of course, if the subjects' experiences changed between the occasions, any difference observed combines the true change and the error attributed to lack of reliability. If the second occasion occurs too soon, the subjects' responses on the second occasion may be influenced by memories of the first. Empirically, it appears that a reasonable interval is somewhere between 2 and 14 days [5]. Internal consistency reliability is the most common measure of reliability described in contemporary reports of patient-reported outcomes. It represents the logical extension of split-half reliability, which in turn represents a form of equivalent-forms reliability. Equivalent-forms reliability compares the scores of identical subjects or similar groups using two forms of the same instrument. The more highly correlated the scores, the more reliable the instrument. Split-half reliability splits an instrument's questions in half and compares scores from the two halves, presuming that they represent equivalent forms. Internal consistency reliability, most often reported in terms of Cronbach's coefficient α, is equivalent to the average of all possible split-half consistency calculations for an instrument.

Reliability depends on the characteristics of both the instrument and the population. Because subject variability is present in the numerator, the same instrument is more reliable in a population that is heterogeneous with respect to the characteristics being measured than in a more homogeneous population. This is a consideration with respect to the usefulness of an instrument in a population in which it has not previously been used. However, absent information from other comparable measures, the homogeneity of the population and the reliability of the instrument in that population are a matter of conjecture until some data are collected.

Reliability coefficients are correlation coefficients, with a range of 0–1. The scale's reliability determines the width of the confidence interval around a score, and the reliability needed depends on the uncertainty that can be tolerated. In 1978, Nunally suggested a reliability standard of 0.7 for data to be used in group comparisons and 0.9 for data to be used as the basis of evaluating individuals [20]. These standards are often cited, but were arbitrary when proposed and should not be considered absolute. Some of the statistics in which reliability is reported give higher values than others [1]. Finally, by way of comparison, brachial systolic blood pressure, the basis of so many individual treatment decisions in clinical practice, was has been reported to have a reliability coefficient of 0.74 [21].

10 Classical Test Theory and Item Response Theory

Since the middle of the twentieth century, most analyses of tests and survey data followed the principles of classical test theory, which emphasize the characteristics of scales and partitions observed scores into true score and error. Classical test theory describes the characteristics of scales in particular populations; application to new populations requires the empiric measurement of reliability and the establishment of new norms. Further, classical test theory does not distinguish the characteristics of the instrument from the characteristics of the individual whom it measures. A second limitation of classical test theory is that it offers a single reliability estimate for a scale, even though precision is known to vary with the level of a trait. Finally, classical test theory requires long instruments to achieve both precision and breadth [22].

Item response theory, or latent trait theory, is a computationally more intensive approach, which emphasizes the item rather than the scale and allows distinction and definition of the difficulty of a survey or test item and the level of the trait being measured in the individual. Rasch models are closely related and generally considered a subset of item response theory. An important attribute of item response theory is that it allows the ranking of items in difficulty and the development of an item bank, facilitating computerized adaptive testing and making it a key aspect of PROMIS's strategy as it enables the development of more tailored measurement [23, 24]. This technique is widely used in educational testing and is becoming increasingly important in the assessment of patient-reported outcomes in clinical settings [25].

11 Comparing Groups and Assessing Change Over Time

A research plan including study of patient-reported outcomes should include definition of what magnitude of difference is considered clinically important and whether the difference is between groups in a cross-sectional study or in the same group over time. There are at least two approaches. One approach compares the magnitude of observed difference to differences between other defined groups. A conceptually more rigorous, if intuitively less appealing, approach is to calculate an effect size; one calculation indexes the difference by the standard deviation of scores, where a value of 0.2 is considered small, 0.5 is moderate, and 0.8 is large [26–28].

A second and even more important issue in the longitudinal study of patient-reported outcomes is to minimize missing data. Missing items can make entire scale unusable, and missing data can introduce important bias. Response to a questionnaire often requires more involvement by the study participant than giving a blood specimen or undergoing physical or radiologic examination, and it involves interaction between the participant and the study personnel. It is important that everyone involved understand that a response omitted because the participant does not feel like responding, for whatever reason, impairs the interpretability of the entire study. Almost inevitably, however, some patient-reported outcome data will be missing because of patient death or censoring for other reasons. Limiting analysis to those cases on which all observations are available risks important bias. Missing data cannot be ignored if toxicity, worsening of a disease, or the effect of a treatment may be associated with the absence of the data. Such circumstances seem to include many of the very situations in which one would want to measure patient-reported outcomes. A variety of sophisticated statistical methods are available to deal with this problem; in the absence of any clearly correct approach, it may be helpful to perform several analyses to determine whether the conclusions are sensitive to the precise technique used [29, 30].

References

1. McDowell I (2006) Measuring health: a guide to rating scales and questionnaires, 3rd edn. Oxford University Press, New York, NY
2. Elkinton JR (1966) Medicine and the quality of life. Ann Intern Med 64:711–714
3. Noll HH. Social indicators and social reporting: the international experience (Part 1). Canadian Council on Social Development. http://www.gesis.org/fileadmin/upload/institut/wiss_arbeitsbereiche/soz_indikatoren/Publikationen/isscnoll.pdf. Accessed 13 Jan, 2015
4. United Nations (1964) Constitution of the World Health Organization, p 2
5. Streiner DL, Norman GR (2003) Health measurement scales: a practical guide to their development and use. Oxford Medical Publications, 3rd edn. Oxford University Press, New York, NY
6. The Center for Health Promotion, University of Toronto. QOL concepts: the QOL Model. University of Toronto, Canada. Sites.utoronto.ca/qol/qol_model.htm. Accessed 13 Jan, 2015
7. U.S. Food and Drug Administration (2009) Guidance for industry: patient-reported outcome measures: use in medical product development to support labeling claims. U.S. Department of Health and Human Services, Washington, DC
8. European Medicines Agency (2005) Reflection paper on the regulatory guidance for the use of health-related quality of life (HRQL) measures in the evaluation of medicinal products. Committee for Medicinal Products for Human Use (CHMP), London
9. Chassany O et al (2002) Patient-reported outcomes: the example of health-related quality of life. A European guidance document for the improved integration of health-related quality of life assessment in the drug regulation process. Drug Inform J 36:209–238
10. McHorney CA (1999) Health status assessment methods for adults: past accomplishments and future challenges. Annu Rev Public Health 20:309–335
11. Hays RD (2005) Generic versus disease-targeted instruments. In: Fayers PM, Hays RD (eds) Assessing quality of life in clinical trials: methods and practice. Oxford University Press, New York, NY, pp 3–8
12. McHorney CA et al (2002) The SWAL-QOL and SWAL-CARE outcomes tool for

oropharyngeal dysphagia in adults: III. Documentation of reliability and validity. Dysphagia 17(2):97–114

13. PROMIS®: Patient Reported Outcomes Measurement Information System, available at www.nihpromis.org

14. O'Boyle CA, Hoefer S, Ring L (2005) Individualized quality of life. In: Fayers PM, Hayes RD (eds) Assessing quality of life in clinical trials: methods and practice. Oxford University Press, New York, NY, pp 225–242

15. Cote-Arsenault D, Morrison-Beedy D (1999) Practical advice for planning and conducting focus groups. Nurs Res 48(5):280–283

16. International Association of Facilitators (2002) Basic facilitation skills. Freely available 40-page manual on facilitation in general. http://www.iaf-world.org/Libraries/Facilitation_Articles/ASQ-IAF_Facilitation_Primer.sflb.ashx. Accessed 13 Jan 2015

17. Greenbaum TL (2000) Moderating focus groups: a practical guide for group facilitation. Sage Publications, Thousand Oaks, CA

18. Greenbaum TL (2000) On-line summary Sage Publications by Thomas Greenbaum

19. Wainer H, Dorans NJ, Flaugher R et al (2000) Computerized adaptive testing: a primer, 2nd edn. Lawrence Erlbaum Associates, Hillside, NJ

20. Nunnally JC (1978) Psychometric theory, 2nd edn. McGraw-Hill, New York, NY

21. Weatherly BD et al (2006) The reliability of the ankle-brachial index in the Atherosclerosis Risk in Communities (ARIC) study and the NHLBI Family Heart Study (FHS). BMC Cardiovasc Disord 6:7

22. Hays RD, Morales LS, Reise SP (2000) Item response theory and health outcomes measurement in the 21st century. Med Care 38(9, Suppl):II28–II42

23. Reise SP, Waller NG (2009) Item response theory and clinical measurement. Annu Rev Clin Psychol 5:27–48

24. Carle AC et al (2011) Advancing PROMIS's methodology: results of the Third Patient-Reported Outcomes Measurement Information System (PROMIS(®)) Psychometric Summit. Expert Rev Pharmacoecon Outcomes Res 11(6):677–684

25. McHorney CA (2003) Ten recommendations for advancing patient-centered outcomes measurement for older persons. Ann Intern Med 139(5, Pt 2):403–409

26. Guyatt GH et al (2002) Methods to explain the clinical significance of health status measures. Mayo Clin Proc 77(4):371–383

27. Sprangers MA et al (2002) Assessing meaningful change in quality of life over time: a users' guide for clinicians. Mayo Clin Proc 77(6):561–571

28. Osoba D, King M (2005) Meaningful differences. In: Fayers PM, Hays RD (eds) Assessing quality of life in clinical trials: methods and practice. Oxford University Press, New York, NY, pp 243–257

29. Fairclough DL (2002) Design and analysis of quality of life studies in clinical trials: interdisciplinary statistics. Chapman & Hall/CRC, Boca Raton, FL

30. Fairclough DL (2004) Patient reported outcomes as endpoints in medical research. Stat Methods Med Res 13(2):115–138

Other Sources

Streiner DL, Norman GR (2003) Health measurement scales: a practical guide to their development and use, 3rd edn. Oxford University Press, New York, NY, A terse, organized, and elegant introduction to the field with a single authorial voice

Fayers PM, Hayes RD (2005) Assessing quality of life in clinical trials: methods and practice, 2nd edn. Oxford University Press, New York, NY, A collection of essays by well-known investigators

McDowell I (2006) Measuring health: a guide to rating scales and questionnaires, 3rd edn. Oxford University Press, New York, NY, A compendium of over 100 instruments, each accompanied by a critical essay, actual items of the instrument, and a bibliography. It begins with a 35-page essay, "Theoretical and Technical Foundations of Health Measurement." Its areas include physical disability and handicap, social health, psychological well-being, anxiety, depression, mental status testing, pain, general health status and quality of life

Embretson SE, Reise SP (2000) Item response theory for psychologists. L. Erlbaum Associates, Mahwah, NJ

PROQOLID: Patient-Reported Outcomes and Quality of Life Instruments Database, available at www.qolid.org. Online database maintained by MAPI Research Trust, currently cataloging 562 instruments. Basic information is freely available, details for free.

International Quality of Life Assessment Project Links Page, available at www.iqola.org/links.aspx. Links to other patient outcome websites.

Health and Quality of Life Outcomes, available at www.hqlo.com. Freely available online journal.

Centers for Disease Control and Prevention, available at www.cdc.gov/hrqol. Freely available background, concepts and resources.

Chapter 12

Randomized Controlled Trials 4: Biomarkers and Surrogate Outcomes

Claudio Rigatto and Brendan J. Barrett

Abstract

Biomarkers are defined as anatomic, physiologic, biochemical, molecular, or genetic parameters associated with the presence, absence, or severity of a disease process. As such, biomarkers may be useful as prognostic and diagnostic tests. Establishing the utility of a given biomarker as a prognostic or diagnostic test requires the conduct of carefully designed cohort studies in which the biomarker and the outcome of interest are measured independently. The design and analysis of such studies is discussed. Surrogate outcomes in clinical trials consist of events or biomarkers intended to reflect important clinical outcomes. Surrogate outcomes may offer advantages in providing statistically robust estimates of treatment effects with smaller sample sizes. However, to be useful, surrogate outcomes have to be validated to ensure that the effect of therapy on them truly reflects the effect of therapy on the important clinical outcomes of interest.

Key words Biomarkers, Surrogates, Cohort studies, Clinical trials, Statistical methods

1 Introduction

Biomarkers have become very important to medical research and practice in recent years. The search term biomarker is associated with 6,62,548 hits in the PubMed systems as of April 30th, 2014, with 30 % of them being within the past 5 years. Biomarkers are often used to address issues of pathogenesis and as important indicators of prognosis. Furthermore, a role also exists for biomarkers in making a diagnosis and in assessing the efficacy of therapies or interventions. In the latter role, biomarkers are one of a set of possible surrogate outcomes that can be useful in rendering clinical trials feasible or efficient.

2 Definition and Uses of Biomarkers

2.1 Definition

Biomarkers can be defined as anatomic, physiologic, biochemical, molecular, or genetic parameters associated with the presence, absence, or severity of a disease process. Depending on their

Patrick S. Parfrey and Brendan J. Barrett (eds.), *Clinical Epidemiology: Practice and Methods*, Methods in Molecular Biology, vol. 1281, DOI 10.1007/978-1-4939-2428-8_12, © Springer Science+Business Media New York 2015

precise nature, biomarkers are detectable and quantifiable by a variety of methods including physical examination, laboratory assays, and radiological techniques. Often, biomarkers are parameters that are known or hypothesized to be causally involved in mechanisms of disease progression. For example, blood pressure and LDL cholesterol are biomarkers of, and causally linked to, development of atherosclerosis and cardiovascular disease. Evidence of a known or suspected causal link is not strictly necessary, and some biomarkers (e.g., neutrophil gelatinase associated lipocalin (NGAL) in acute renal failure [1], antinuclear antibody (ANA) in lupus, anti neutrophil cytoplasmic antibody (ANCA) in vasculitis) do not have clearly understood pathophysiologic roles. The essential properties of a biomarker are that it be measurable in some way, and that it be associated with the disease of interest.

It is evident from the definition that some clinical signs, such as those observed in the course of a clinical exam (e.g., adenopathy, a rash, crackles on chest auscultation, number of swollen joints), qualify as biomarkers, as do physiologic variables such as blood pressure, even though we are not used to thinking of them as such. Similarly, radiological variables (e.g., tumor size on CT, luminal narrowing on coronary angiography) can also function as biomarkers. Parameters more commonly thought of as biomarkers include proteins such as serum C-reactive protein or troponin T in cardiovascular disease, immunoproteins such as antinuclear antibody in lupus, or genetic biomarkers such as specific gene polymorphisms.

2.2 Conceptual Relationship Between Biomarkers, Risk Factors, and Surrogate Outcomes

These terms overlap significantly in concept and meaning. The term risk factor was coined by epidemiologists over 50 years ago to denote a parameter whose presence or level was associated with a statistically higher probability over time of observing a specific disease in a population. Typically a risk factor was a clinically evident and measurable characteristic, such as age and gender, or behavior, such as smoking or alcohol consumption, but was later extended to include many easily measurable physiological and laboratory parameters (e.g., blood pressure, cholesterol). While the latter quantities would also meet the definition of biomarkers, static, constitutive or irreversible risk factors such as age, gender or race would not. Behaviors can never be considered biomarkers, though they are perfectly legitimate risk factors.

The term biomarker originated in the context of drug discovery for cancer, infections, and cardiovascular disease. Many of these diseases evolve over along periods of time and have imperfect animal analogues, making the process of drug discovery lengthy and difficult. Researchers needed a parameter or metric which might indicate quickly whether an agent possessed promising biological activity directed against disease in vivo in humans. These parameters originally fell into two categories: surrogates of disease progression (e.g., tumor size on X-ray, joint erosions, coronary artery narrowing), or measurement of physiologic, biochemical, or molecular parameters known to be involved in one or more mechanisms of disease development (e.g., cholesterol level, blood pressure level). Implicit in the definition of biomarker, therefore, is the notion of measuring disease activity or progression. Because biomarkers in some way measure mechanisms or intermediate stages in disease evolution, it is not surprising that they are often associated with clinical manifestations of disease, and thus can be considered risk factors in many cases [2].

Surrogates are parameters or measurements that take the place of or stand in for other measurements. In clinical research, one is frequently interested in hard outcomes such as death or the development of some specific disease state (e.g., development of end stage renal disease). Many diseases evolve slowly over time, making it time consuming and costly to study these end points directly. Substitution of a biomarker (e.g., microalbuminuria in diabetic nephropathy) which is measurable sooner can significantly shorten the length of a study and significantly reduce costs. A biomarker used in this way is termed a surrogate outcome. To be useful, the surrogate must be a biomarker possessing very tight association with the development of the disease state in question. Thus, not all biomarkers can be surrogates. Many pitfalls exist, limiting the use or interpretation of a surrogate outcome. These issues are discussed separately below.

2.3 Biomarkers as Indicators of Prognosis

Because biomarkers are by definition associated with disease processes or development, they are potentially useful as markers of prognosis. To be useful prognostically, a biomarker must possess several properties (Table 1). The magnitude of the association must be high, so that the separation in prognosis between biomarker categories is high, and the effect must be independent of other prognostic factors. In addition, the biomarker must improve prediction of outcome beyond clinical variables alone. In statistical terms, this means the biomarker must improve the discrimination (e.g., c-statistic, integrated discrimination improvement (IDI)) and reclassification metrics (net reclassification improvement, vide infra)

Table 1
Characteristics of an ideal prognostic biomarker

Tight association with outcome (e.g., hazard ratio or odds ratio)
Statistically independent
Unconfounded by other prognostic factors
Must improve discrimination and reclassification metrics
Generalizable (e.g., validated in numerous studies and settings)

when added to a multivariate model. Lastly, the prognostic usefulness of biomarker must be shown to be generalizable, which means validating the association in multiple studies and settings. In reality, very few current biomarkers possess these characteristics, which is one reason why biomarkers sometimes add disappointingly little to prognostic or diagnostic certainty [3], despite the common assumption that they are better predictors of disease outcomes than simple clinical data.

2.4 Use in Diagnosis

The discovery of biomarkers capable of replacing the biopsy or other invasive technologies in the diagnosis of many medical ailments is the "holy grail" of biomarker research. The requirements for a useful diagnostic biomarker are if anything more stringent than for a prognostic biomarker. In order to replace a "gold standard" test, such as a biopsy for the diagnosis of cancer, the ideal biomarker must achieve near perfect sensitivity and specificity, with a receiver operating characteristic (ROC) curve that is nearly a perfect square. No biomarker currently fulfills the requirements of an ideal diagnostic test. The diagnostic utility of a particular biomarker, therefore, depends on the strength of the association with disease status and whether the test performance characteristics are better than that of other existing diagnostic markers. The latter are typically measured by parameters calculated from a 2×2 contingency table, such as sensitivity (Sens), specificity (Spec), and positive and negative predictive values (PPV, NPV). In the case of biomarkers with multiple informative levels, an $N \times 2$ table can be created and positive and negative likelihood ratios (LR) calculated for each of the N levels [4].

A direct mathematical relationship exist between the odds ratio (OR) for disease (a measure of strength of association) and test performance characteristics:

$$\mathrm{OR} = [\mathrm{Sens}/(1\text{-}\mathrm{Sens})] \times [\mathrm{Spec}/(1\text{-}\mathrm{Spec})] = [\mathrm{PPV}/(1\text{-}\mathrm{PPV})] \times [\mathrm{NPV}/(1\text{-}\mathrm{NPV})] \quad (1)$$

It is not difficult to see that very high degrees of association (i.e., very high OR) are necessary if a biomarker based test is to yield acceptable performance characteristics. Suppose we desire a test with 95 % sensitivity and specificity. Substituting into Eq. 1, we see that the odds ratio for disease with a positive test (i.e., a test above the threshold) would need to be $(0.95/0.05) \times (0.95/0.05) =$ 361! Relaxing our requirements to 90 % sensitivity and specificity, we would still require an observed odds ratio of $(0.9/0.1) \times (0.9/0.1) = 81$. Suppose instead we would like to use our biomarker test as a screening test for a rare disease, and so require high sensitivity (say, 95 %) but can accept mediocre specificity (say 50 %). The odds ratio for a positive biomarker test would have to be $(0.95/0.05) \times (0.5/0.5) = 19$. Alternatively, suppose we wish the biomarker in question to function as a confirmatory test, and so require a high specificity (99 %) but can accept a low sensitivity (20 %). The OR associated with a biomarker having these performance characteristics would be $(0.2/0.8) \times (0.99/0.01) = 123$! It is evident from these and other examples that a biomarker is unlikely to yield a useful diagnostic test unless it possesses an extremely high association with disease (e.g., $OR \gg 10$).

2.5 Use in Studies of Intervention

Biomarkers may be used in interventional studies as either surrogates (discussed below), or as evidence for an effect on intermediary mechanisms of disease. In the latter case, they can lend an additional mechanistic, causal dimension to a clinical study. For example, consider a randomized clinical trial of cholesterol lowering with placebo vs. low and high dose HMG-CoA reductase inhibitor (i.e., "Statin"). Measurement of the clinical outcome alone can show only whether treatment has clinical efficacy. Simultaneous measurement of serum cholesterol in all groups will allow confirmation of whether the effect is associated with cholesterol lowering, as would be expected based on the known mechanisms of action. Since HMG-CoA inhibitors may have pleiotropic and anti-inflammatory effects, the investigators might wish to address the hypothesis that statin treatment reduces inflammation and that this reduction influences outcome. This could be accomplished by measuring inflammatory markers such as CRP or IL-6 levels during the trial. Thus, integration of biomarker measurements in clinical studies can confirm known mechanisms of action and explore novel and hypothetical mechanisms of disease.

---

3 Validation of Biomarkers

As knowledge of disease mechanisms deepens, new compounds, proteins, and genes are discovered which might prove useful in diagnosing diseases or in prognosticating outcomes. Thus, a common question faced in biomarker research is how to determine the usefulness of a candidate biomarker. Appropriate design of clinical studies, adhering to fundamental epidemiological principles, is a key component of this process. Unless the investigator is experienced in clinical studies of diagnosis and prognosis, collaboration with an epidemiologist and a statistician in the planning stages is highly recommended, because no amount of post hoc statistical manipulation can overcome fatal flaws in study design. Finally, before being widely accepted in clinical use, the observations of one study should be confirmed in another independent set of patients.

3.1 Designing a Study to Assess the Prognostic Value of a Biomarker

Suppose we wish to know if a biomarker x is useful in predicting how long it will take patients at a defined stage of a chronic illness to arrive at a defined disease end point. For example, x could be proteinuria, the disease in question Stage 2 chronic kidney disease, and the defined disease outcome initiation of dialysis. The appropriate study design to address this question is a cohort study.

The fundamental steps in the execution of a cohort study are as follows:

1. *Cohort Assembly:* The investigator must recruit a cohort of patients having the condition in question. Alternatively, a historical cohort may be used, provided (1) adequate stored samples are available for biomarker measurement and (2) the design requirements of a good cohort study are met (vide infra).

2. *Biomarker Assessment:* Levels of the biomarker in question must be assessed at baseline in all patients.

3. *Assessment of other potential prognostic or confounding variables:* Levels of other variables known to be predictive of the outcome must also be assessed at baseline. These measurements will permit multivariate modeling to assess independence and freedom from confounding in the analysis phase, as well as assessment of the incremental predictive value utility (i.e., improvement in net reclassification) of testing for the biomarker.

4. *Unbiased and unambiguous assessment of outcome:* Outcomes must be defined unambiguously and measured in all patients. It is important that the surveillance for outcomes be identical for all patients in the cohort, to avoid the problem of differential surveillance bias. Completeness of follow-up in all patients is also very important, since patients that drop out from a study are systematically different from those that remain and so may bias the results of the study. In cases where the outcome has a subjective component (e.g., extent and severity of joint involvement in rheumatoid arthritis), it is important that the assessor be unaware (blind, masked) to the level of biomarker in order to avoid the possibility of bias. It is important that the outcome be defined completely without reference to and independently of the biomarker being examined. This can be a problem when the biomarker in question is also a criterion for outcome. This scenario is relatively common in the field of rheumatology, where biomarkers of disease activity (e.g., ANA, complement levels, white blood cell count) may also be a component of the outcome definition (e.g., a disease flare in Lupus).

3.2 Analytical Considerations in a Prognostic Biomarker Study

A thorough description of the approach to the analysis and multivariate modeling of cohort studies is the subject of entire textbooks [5], and well beyond scope of this chapter. The single most important principle to be observed is that the plan of analysis should be discussed with a statistician and thoroughly outlined *in the planning stages* of the study, and not after the study is finished! Mathematically disinclined readers can stop here and skip to the section on diagnostic studies. Nevertheless, since a general understanding of the approach to analysis can be helpful in designing a study, we discuss a few broad principles of analysis below.

The objective of the analysis is fourfold: (1) to estimate the strength and statistical significance of the association between biomarker levels and outcome (2) to establish statistical independence of the biomarker in a multivariate model (3) to estimate the degree of confounding with other parameters in the model (4) to establish the degree to which the biomarker improves the predictive power of the prognostic model.

Survival analysis provides the most natural and informative way to analyze cohort data and the effect of biomarker levels on outcome. Survival analysis (also known as time-to-event analysis) very naturally handles the problems of censored data and unequal follow-up times which often can occur in cohort studies. Logistic regression is also commonly used if there is minimal censoring and we are only interested in risk over a defined period of time. Poisson regression and other GLM techniques can also be used although these are less common.

The most common techniques used in survival analysis are Kaplan-Meier (K-M) analysis (bivariate, i.e., one outcome and one predictor variable) and Cox's proportional hazards regression (multivariate, i.e., multiple predictor variables). For a more complete treatment of these techniques, their pitfalls and assumptions, the interested reader is directed to the cited references [6]. The first analytic objective is usually achieved using a bivariate K-M analysis. In this analysis, continuous biomarkers (e.g., serum CRP concentration) are typically stratified into four or more levels (e.g., quartiles), because this involves fewer assumptions about the mathematical nature of the relationship between biomarker levels and outcome. What the analyst is looking for, in addition to statistical significance, is a strong association between biomarker and outcome (e.g., a hazard ratio of at least 10 between highest and lowest quartile/decile). Moreover, a smooth, graded association between biomarker quartile and the hazard ratio for outcome is reassuring and supportive of a causal association.

The second and third objectives are usually achieved by constructing appropriate multivariable models, typically using Cox regression. In this stage, the biomarker is best treated as a continuous variable to maximize power. Log transformation may be required to tame skew. The other prognostic variables included in the models should possess face validity and be known to predict outcome. The statistical independence of the biomarker is usually established by creating a model which includes all variables associated with outcome in the bivariate analysis ($p < 0.1$), and observing whether removal of the biomarker variable from the model results in a significant change in the −2 log-likelihood parameter of the model.

Several metrics of model performance are then calculated and compared between the full multivariate model including the biomarker and the alternative (or base) model which contains all the other important prognostic marker but excludes the biomarker in question. The operative principle here is that to be judged clinically useful, a new biomarker must improve prediction significantly over what is already possible using existing clinical data.

The main metrics of predictive utility are discrimination and reclassification. Discrimination measures the ability of a model to accurately assign a higher probability to patients who have the event of interest, versus those who do not. The most commonly used metrics of discrimination are the concordance or c-statistic and the integrated discrimination improvement (IDI) index [7, 8].

The C statistic is defined as the proportion of times the model correctly discriminates between a randomly selected pair of case and control individuals, and is mathematically equivalent to the area under the receiver operating characteristic curve (AUROC) of the logistic or proportional hazards model. As with the AUROC, a c-statistic of 0.50 indicates that the model performs no better than chance; a c statistic of 0.70–0.80 indicates good discrimination; and a c statistic of greater than 0.80 is consistent with excellent discriminatory ability. Comparing the magnitude and statistical significance of the change in c-statistic between the base and the biomarker model is the traditional metric of biomarker usefulness.

Integrated Discrimination Improvement: A limitation of using the c-statistic for estimating improvement in discrimination is that it exhibits asymptotic behavior: as the model c approaches 1, it becomes increasingly difficult to show a meaningful difference in C-statistics despite real improvements in model prediction. An alternative and more sensitive measure of improvement is the integrated discrimination improvement index (IDI). The IDI measures the difference in discrimination slopes between the two models (i.e., mean predicted probability for those with the outcome vs. those without), and describes this on an absolute and relative scale. As such, the IDI can be an effective method for comparing discrimination between two models where differences in C statistic may be negligible.

Reclassification: In clinical medicine, treatments and tests are often prescribed based on the predicted risk category of having an event. When a new prediction model is developed, it is important to consider whether it classifies patients into more appropriate risk strata than the old model. The new model may assign a given patient to the same risk category, a lower risk category, or a higher risk category relative to the old model. If the patient has an event, the new model can be considered successful if it assigns that patient to a higher risk stratum, but unsuccessful if it erroneously assigns a lower risk. Similarly, for patients who do not have an event, the new model is successful if reclassifies to lower risk, and unsuccessful if it reclassifies to a higher risk stratum. The Net Reclassification Index is essentially the sum of these successes and failures [9]. Positive values for NRI indicate correct net reclassification and negative values indicate incorrect reclassification. The NRI should be calculated using clinically accepted risk categories, wherever possible. For example, the NRI of a model for cardiovascular event prediction might use the Framingham risk categories as the basis for defining successful and unsuccessful reclassification.

3.3 Sample Size Considerations for a Prognostic Biomarker Study

Maximum likelihood based estimation procedures, used in generating coefficients of logistic and Cox regression models, require a minimum of ten outcomes per independent variable included in the multivariate model to ensure model stability [10]. As an example, if the outcome of interest is death, and in addition to the biomarker it is anticipated that six variables (biomarker plus five adjustment variables) will need to be included in the model, then a minimum of $10 \times 6 = 60$ deaths will need to be observed in the cohort. If the mortality of the disease in question is 20 % over 2 years, then 300 patients will need to be observed for 2 years.

Although the above criterion must be satisfied, it does not truly estimate the sample size required to measure a desired improvement in discrimination. Two approaches can be employed

1. *Estimate (guess) the proportion of patients who will experience the outcome in the high biomarker group* vs. *the low biomarker group* (e.g., Biomarker level above the median vs. below the median). This estimate can be based on prior studies, or defined according criteria of clinical significance. For example, if we are interested in a biomarker with high prognostic power, we may only be interested in detecting a relative risk of *at least* 8–10 for mortality in patients with biomarker levels above the median compared with those below the median. If the overall mortality is expected to be 20 %, and the relative risk we are looking for 9, then we would require 18 % mortality in the high biomarker group vs 2 % in the low biomarker group. The sample size can then be calculated using standard formulae for comparing two proportions. In the example cited, the minimum N required will be 111 (assuming two sided $\alpha = 0.05$ and $\beta = 0.2$). In this particular example, applying the first criteria resulted in a higher minimum N than applying the second, but this is not always the case. Nevertheless, to satisfy both criteria, one should select the higher of the two numbers.

2. *Estimate the degree of improvement in the c-statistic.* Although more complex and beyond our scope here, methods exist to calculate sample size for a given anticipated difference in the c-statistic, and references have been provided for the interested reader [7, 11].

In addition, if the cohort is to be prospectively accrued over time, an estimate of the attrition rate must be factored in and the

N increased accordingly. For example, if we anticipate a dropout rate of 10 % over 2 years, and we need 300 patients for the analysis, we would need to enroll 333 patients to ensure 300 patients are followed to the end of the study.

Finally, sample size estimates are the product of multiple assumptions, with the most problematic being the degree discrimination afforded by the biomarker. It is often useful to model sample sizes required for a range of plausible assumptions about effect size.

3.4 Designing a Study to Measure the Diagnostic Usefulness of a Biomarker

A diagnostic study attempts to measure how well a diagnostic test predicts the presence or absence of a specific disease state. For example, a researcher might wish to know whether the presence of cleaved fragments of β2 microglobulin in the urine can correctly distinguish acute rejection of a transplanted kidney from other causes of acute transplant kidney dysfunction (e.g., dehydration, acute tubular necrosis, calcineurin toxicity, viral nephropathy). In all cases, the result of the test (cleavage products present vs absent) is compared to the presence/absence of disease as assessed by a "gold standard" (see below). In order to address this question, the investigator must:

1. *Assemble a diagnostic cohort*: The investigator must enroll a cohort of patients in whom the diagnosis is suspected. In the example cited, patients with transplanted kidneys and evidence of acute kidney dysfunction (e.g., a rise in serum creatinine, oliguria) would be the target population for the hypothetical study.

2. *Define the "gold standard" for diagnosis in all patients*: The term "gold standard" refers to a test or procedure the result of which is considered definitive evidence for the presence or absence of disease. Although conceptually straightforward, identifying an appropriate gold standard can be tricky. In the example cited above, a kidney biopsy might be considered a logical gold standard procedure for identifying rejection in a transplanted kidney. A positive gold standard might therefore be defined as presence of tubulitis, widely accepted as the pathological hallmark of acute rejection. However, tubulitis is a continuum from very mild to severe, raising the question of how much tubulitis needs to be present. In addition, what other criteria might be needed in order to infer that the tubulitis is the main culprit clinically? Suppose there are also prominent viral inclusions or striped fibrosis (thought to represent calcineurin toxicity), what then? Thus, defining the gold standard is not merely a question of choosing a test (or combination of tests!); it is a question of explicitly defining the criteria and procedures employed to judge whether a disease is present or absent. This can be quite a challenge, especially in situations where widely accepted criteria or procedures do not exist.

From a practical viewpoint, the gold standard chosen by the investigator must at minimum be unambiguously defined, and must employ the best techniques/procedures/criteria currently available to define disease status.

3. *Assess biomarker status and disease status independently in all patients in the cohort.* The key concepts here are "all" and "independently". Dropouts (patients who receive one or other test but not both) cannot be included in the analysis and may reduce the power of the study. If the dropouts are a non-random sample (highly likely), their exclusion may bias the data. If outcomes are assessed in only a non-random portion of the cohort (e.g., if pulmonary angiography for gold standard diagnosis of embolism is done only in patients with an elevated d-dimer level), then the assumption of independence is violated, since the assessment of the gold standard will be conditional on the level of the biomarker in question. For the same reasons, assessment of the gold standard should be done without any knowledge of the level of the biomarker, and vice versa, to prevent bias. In practice, this may be achieved by blinding the assessor of the gold standard from any knowledge of biomarker status. These two criteria of completeness and unbiased independence of assessment of both biomarker and disease status are almost impossible to satisfy in administrative datasets, retrospective cohorts (unless stored biological samples are available) and other "found" data, which is why these data sources are in general unsuitable for assessment of diagnostic test performance.

3.5 Analytical Considerations in a Diagnostic Biomarker Study

An in depth discussion of the analytical tools used to characterize test performance is beyond the scope of this chapter (see references). We provide here a broad outline of the analytical approach, highlighting critical aspects of the process.

1. *Dichotomous biomarker.* The simplest case is when the biomarker is dichotomous, i.e., either present or absent. In such instances, a single 2×2 contingency table is created. Patients are classified into four groups according to biomarker and disease status (Fig. 1). Test performance characteristics, with associated 95 % confidence limits, can then be calculated in the usual way. The most helpful statistics are the positive and negative predictive values (PPV, NPV), also known respectively as the true positive and true negative rates (TPR, TNR). To be useful, the test must have a high PPV or NPV, or both.

2. *Continuous biomarker.* The basic approach involves converting the continuous biomarker into a dichotomous variable. This is done by assigning different "thresholds" above which the biomarker is considered a positive test. The individual data are then reclassified as positive or negative for each threshold, and

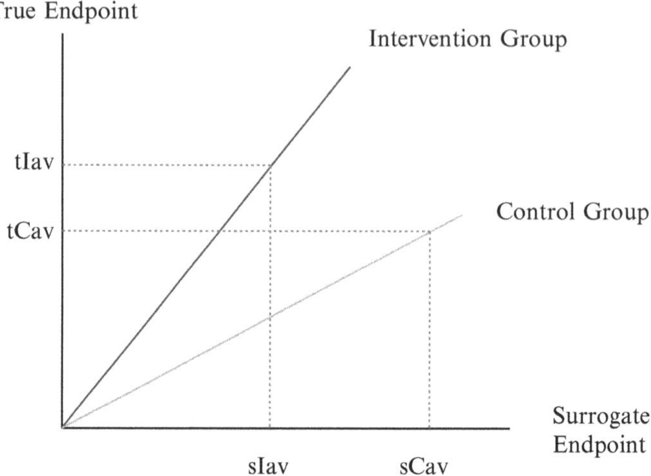

Fig. 1 The *graph* shows the relationship between true clinically important and surrogate end points under treatment with a new intervention (I) and standard control therapy (C). Under both I and C individually there is a perfect correlation between the level of the surrogate and true end points as reflected by the *straight lines*. However, because of the different slopes of the lines, unless the slopes and intercepts were known, it would be possible to reach an incorrect conclusion about the average effect of I and C on true end points (shown as tIav and tCav) from knowledge of their average effects on the surrogate (shown as sIav and sCav)

can be compared to the disease state (present/absent) using the usual 2×2 contingency table. A different contingency table is thus generated for each threshold, from which the sensitivity and specificity associated with each threshold of the biomarker are calculated. A plot of 1-specificity vs. sensitivity for each threshold is then created, forming the ROC curve. Typically, ten or more points (and thus thresholds) reflecting the observed range of the biomarker are necessary to adequately plot the curve. Modern statistical programs automate this process and can generate curves based on hundreds of thresholds. The area under the ROC curve varies between 0.5 (no discrimination, a straight line) and 1.0 (perfect discrimination). An area between 0.8 and 0.9 is generally considered "excellent" test discrimination. The area calculated from separate ROC curves generated from two different biomarkers simultaneously and independently measured in the same population can be formally compared, permitting conclusions about whether one biomarker has statistically better diagnostic performance than another. The optimum threshold for a continuous biomarker is usually defined as the point maximizing both sensitivity and specificity, and corresponds to the point on the ROC curve closest to the point (0,1) on the ROC graph.

3.6 Sample Size Considerations for a Diagnostic Study

Since the area under the ROC curve is a measure of the diagnostic accuracy of the biomarker, a logical approach is to use this statistic as the basis for sample size calculations. A paper by Hanley and McNeil describes an approach using the Wilcoxon statistic and, more importantly, contains useful nomograms and tables that permit direct calculation of sample size needed for (1) estimation of the area under the ROC within a desired range of precision and (2) detection of a statistically significant difference between the ROC areas of two biomarkers [11].

3.7 Establishing Generalizability: Derivation and Validation Sets

A single analysis is never sufficient to establish the validity of a given biomarker. Estimates of association (hazard, odds and rate ratios) and test performance (sensitivities, specificities, etc.) can vary markedly from one study to the next, and can often diminish markedly from early studies to later studies. Early prognostic studies are often small and analyzed intensively, all of which increase the risk of model overfitting and thus observing spuriously inflated associations. Early diagnostic studies often enroll patients exhibiting a discontinuous, bimodal pattern of disease, with patients either having no disease or having severe disease. Biomarkers typically perform better in these bimodal cohorts than in more representative cohorts where a smoother spectrum of disease severity is evident, a phenomenon called "diagnostic spectrum effect (or bias)" [12].

Before being widely accepted in clinical use, the observations of one biomarker study should be objectively confirmed in multiple, independent, clinically relevant populations. At minimum, confirmation in at least one other independent set of patients is required. Since the fundamental purpose of repeating a study is to show the generalizability of the findings of the first study to other similar populations and settings, this final "validation step" is ideally conducted as a completely separate study, in a separate place and at a different time. If the results of such studies are concordant, then there will be reasonably strong evidence of generalizability.

Because conducting two completely independent studies is very costly and often unfeasible, an alternative is to conduct a single study in which patients are randomly grouped into derivation and validation sets. All the model building and statistical testing is conducted in the derivation set (hence the name); the parameters of the same models are then recalculated using data from the validation set, and compared. Because the main purpose of the validation set is to demonstrate that the model parameter estimates (e.g., hazard ratios, odds ratios, specificities, C statistics) are similar to those in the derivation set, and not to retest statistical significance, the validation set can frequently be smaller. Typically, the validation set is half the size of the of the derivation set, but can be larger or smaller depending on need and data availability. The advantage of randomly selecting derivation and validation sets from the same cohort is that the study apparatus does not have to be duplicated. The disadvantage is that random samples from a single cohort are more likely to show congruent results than samples from two completely distinct cohorts, and thus this strategy is a less rigorous test of generalizability.

4 Surrogate Outcomes

Outcome measures or end points are important to all forms of clinical research. For studies of disease prognosis, they usually consist of some identifiable disease state (e.g., development of a cancer, onset of end stage kidney disease, death, or death from some particular cause). Studies of prognosis might seek to describe time from some defined start point (at which point all those studied would be free of the outcome of interest) until either the development of the outcome of interest, or the end of an observation period. Such studies might also assess how well factors measured at the start time, or during the early period of observation predict the outcome of interest. For purely descriptive studies, the frequency of the relevant clinically important outcome does not have to be high to make the study worthwhile. Study sample size, and by extension feasibility, is partly determined by frequency of outcome, but if outcomes are rare, a study of a few hundred cases may still suffice to establish that with reasonable precision. For example, a study of 400 persons where death was observed to occur in 2 % over a 5-year period of observation would be associated with a 95 % confidence interval ranging from about 1–4 % around the estimate. Such a degree of precision might be adequate in many instances.

In situations where the research question relates to the effect of an intervention on outcome, use of "hard" or clinically important end points tends to be most persuasive. Clinically meaningful outcomes are those that reflect how people feel, function or survive. Ultimate outcomes must reflect both the possibility of benefit and harm associated with the choice of intervention. Such outcomes include death rates, disease events and measures of quality of life. For example, in comparing the effect of bare metal stents to drug eluting stents in the therapy of coronary disease, the most important outcomes would include patient survival, rate of subsequent myocardial infarction, and possibly need for future revascularization. Effort and care are also required to determine when an event has occurred. One common strategy is to have blinded adjudication by an end point committee. Demonstrating an effect on such outcomes will tend to be persuasive to clinicians, patients and payers as the meaning of the effect is usually understandable and the events avoided with the more efficacious therapy are themselves meaningful. However, comparative trials often have to be very large to prove superiority of one therapy over another if the rate of events in controls is low and the minimum clinically important difference in outcomes between therapies is small. For example, a 5 % rate of death over 4 years was associated with bare metal stents in a pooled analysis of randomized trials comparing bare metal stents to sirolimus eluting stents [13]. Now, suppose that a 1 % difference in death rates over a 4 year period would be important to identify with statistical significance ($p < 0.05$) in a comparative trial. Such a trial would have to enroll over 9,000 subjects to have a 90 % chance (power) to detect such a difference in death rates. Clearly, a trial of this magnitude would be both costly and difficult to run.

There are several options available to limit sample size when designing a trial. These include recruitment of subjects at higher risk for an outcome event, but doing so affects the generalizability of trial results. Another option is to use composite outcomes. Individual components of composites may be uncommon, but together the rate of composite events may be high enough to limit the sample size required. Components of composite outcomes include events that share a likelihood of benefiting from the intervention under study. For example, a trial might seek to determine the effect of a lipid-lowering drug on future myocardial infarction, revascularization, or cardiovascular death. However, the impact of therapy on individual components of the composite may vary, and not all components of the composite are likely to be of equal clinical importance.

Another commonly employed means to limit trial sample size is to choose an outcome that is measurable in all study participants on a quantitative scale. For example, in studying a new antihypertensive, the initial studies are likely to assess impact on average blood pressure, rather than rates of stroke or kidney failure. In this example, the blood pressure is a surrogate outcome and one would have to rely on data from other sources to judge the likely impact on disease events of the degree of blood pressure lowering observed.

A surrogate outcome is defined as a (bio)marker that is intended to serve as a substitute for a clinically meaningful end point and is expected to predict the effect of a therapeutic intervention. Some examples of surrogate outcomes (and the associated ultimate outcomes) include proteinuria (kidney failure, death, cardiovascular events), LDL cholesterol level (cardiovascular events and death), and left ventricular function (heart failure and death). The advantages associated with using surrogate outcomes as end points in trials of therapy include the smaller sample size as discussed above, as well as the possibility of being able to demonstrate an effect within a shorter time, thus also lowering the cost of the study. As such, early phase trials of an intervention often use surrogates as primary outcome measures. The results of the trials might not be considered definitive enough to drive a change in clinical practice (although they are sometimes marketed in an effort to do so), but the data may be persuasive enough to justify more expensive larger trials with clinically important outcomes. Measurement of surrogates during trials of therapy in which clinically relevant end points make up the primary outcome may be helpful in understanding how a therapy works. Consider a trial comparing a new drug, already known to lower LDL cholesterol level and to have unique effects on inflammation or oxidation pathways, to a statin in terms of cardiovascular event reduction. In such a trial, analyses might seek to determine whether any differential effect of the interventions on inflammatory or oxidation markers was associated with any difference in clinical outcomes. If such an association was found, the new drug might next be tested in other disease states in which inflammation or oxidation were thought to play a role.

Just because a marker is associated with a disease of interest does not necessarily imply that it will be a valid substitute for clinically relevant outcomes in trials of therapy for that condition. For example, low HDL levels are associated with progression of atherosclerotic vascular disease. However, in a trial of torcetrapib, HDL levels were increased but there was no effect on progression of coronary atherosclerosis [14]. A valid surrogate needs to satisfy the following conditions:

- Be predictive of clinically important outcomes

- Predict corresponding changes in clinically important outcomes when itself changed by therapy

- The way therapy affects the surrogate should at least partly explain how therapy affects the clinically relevant outcome

- In the case of a surrogate for drug effects, the dose response should be similar for the surrogate and the clinical effects

It should be noted that a measure may be a valid surrogate for some, but not all clinically important end points. In addition, a surrogate that is valid for the effects of one intervention may not be a valid surrogate for other interventions. For example, both statins and sevelamer lower serum LDL cholesterol. A lower serum LDL cholesterol level may be a valid surrogate for the impact of statins on vascular disease, as reduction in LDL levels in response to statins has been associated with reduced cardiovascular events in numerous trials, and a dose response relationship was also found in trials comparing doses [15]. However, it would not then be correct to assume that sevelamer would have the same impact on cardiovascular events as a statin if given in doses that had a comparable effect on LDL levels. It could well be that the benefit of statins is linked both to how they lower LDL cholesterol as well as to other parallel effects not shared by sevelamer.

To validate a surrogate outcome requires that it be measured during a trial testing the effect of the therapy of interest on clinically relevant outcomes. Demonstrating a simple correlation between the effect of therapy on the surrogate and on the clinical outcome is not sufficient to declare the surrogate valid [16]. This is because, as shown by Baker (Fig. 1), the slope of the relationship between the effect of an experimental therapy E on surrogate and true outcome may differ from that of a control therapy C. Even when a higher level of the surrogate is perfectly linearly associated with a greater frequency of clinical events under either therapy, the difference in slopes can lead to a lower level of the surrogate, but a higher frequency of adverse events with therapy E than therapy C. To avoid this error, Prentice contended that the distribution of true end points given the observed distribution of surrogate end points should not be conditional on treatment group [17]. Graphically this implies that the slope of the lines in Fig. 1 be the same. However, this is overly restrictive, as one only has to know the intercept and slope of the lines to make the correct inference. One can use data from a validation study to estimate the slopes and intercepts. One approach to validating a surrogate relies on hypothesis testing. If in validation trials, the Prentice criterion is met and the slopes and intercepts are similar, then rejection of the null hypothesis for the surrogate will imply rejection of the null hypothesis for the clinical end point. On the other hand, if rejection of the null for the surrogate does not imply rejection of the null for the clinical end point, the surrogate has not been validated. However, this approach is restrictive and does not identify all potentially valid surrogates. An alternative meta-analytic approach uses regression to predict separately the effect of intervention on surrogate and true end points [18]. An advantage of this approach lies in the ability to examine surrogates for harmful as well as beneficial effects of therapy. With this approach, pooled data from several prior intervention studies are analyzed to develop an estimate of the effect of therapy on surrogate and clinical outcomes. These estimates can be validated in a further trial by comparing the predicted to the observed effect of therapy on both surrogate and clinical outcome. The surrogate may be considered valid if the prior estimate and the newly observed effects are sufficiently similar. What constitutes sufficient similarity requires medical judgment as well as consideration of statistics. It should be noted that this whole process is dependent on there being sufficient data from prior trials to develop adequately precise estimates of the effect of therapy on surrogate and clinical outcomes. The decision as to what constitutes adequate validation is also not hard and fast and how surrogates are validated should always be scrutinized before relying heavily on conclusions of future trials using the surrogate as primary end point.

A few caveats need emphasis in relation to surrogate outcomes. Validating a surrogate for one population, intervention or clinical outcome does not imply that the surrogate will be valid for another population, intervention or clinical outcome. A valid surrogate for benefits may not be a valid surrogate for harms associated with an intervention. With these caveats considered, one might question whether there is any real advantage to using surrogates. However, useful surrogates may become accepted if they show a similar relationship to clinical end points under multiple interventions and in different disease states.

References

1. Wagener G, Jan M, Kim M, Mori K, Barasch JM, Sladen RN, Lee HT (2006) Association between increases in urinary neutrophil gelatinase-associated lipocalin and acute renal dysfunction after adult cardiac surgery. Anesthesiology 105:485–491

2. Biomarkers Definitions Working Group (2001) Biomarkers and surrogate endpoints: preferred definitions and conceptual framework. Clin Pharmacol Therap 69:89–95

3. Wang TJ, Gona P, Larson MG, Tofler GH, Levy D, Newton-Cheh C, Jacques PF, Rifai N, Selhub J, Robins SJ, Benjamin EJ, D'Agostino RB, Vasan RS (2006) Multiple biomarkers for the prediction of first major cardiovascular events and death. N Engl J Med 355: 2631–2639

4. Sackett D, Haynes R, Guyatt G, Tugwell P (1991) The interpretation of diagnostic data. In: Sackett DL et al (eds) Clinical epidemiology: a basic science for clinical medicine, 2nd edn. Little, Brown and Company, Toronto, ON

5. Kleinbaum DG (1996) Survival analysis: a self-learning text. Springer, New York, NY

6. Cox DR, Oakes D (1984) Analysis of survival data. Chapman and Hall/CRC, Boca Raton, FL

7. Pencina MJ, D'Agostino RB (2004) Overall C as a measure of discrimination in survival analysis: model specific population value and confidence interval estimation. Stat Med 23: 2109–2123

8. Pencina MJ, D'Agostino RB Sr, D'Agostino RB Jr, Vasan RS (2008) Evaluating the added predictive ability of a new marker: from area under the ROC curve to reclassification and beyond. Stat Med 27:157–172, discussion 207–212

9. Pencina MJ, D'Agostino RB Sr, Steyerberg EW (2011) Extensions of net reclassification improvement calculations to measure usefulness of new biomarkers. Stat Med 30:11–21

10. Peduzzi P, Concato J, Kemper E, Holford TR, Feinstein AR (1996) A simulation of the number of events per variable in logistic regression analysis. Journal of Clinical Epidemiology 99:1373–1379

11. Hanley J, McNeil B (1982) The meaning and use of the area under a receiver operating characteristic (ROC) curve. Radiology 143:29–36

12. Mulherin SA, Miller WC (2002) Spectrum bias or spectrum effect? Subgroup variation in diagnostic test evaluation. Ann Intern Med 137: 598–602

13. Spaulding C, Daemen J, Boersma E, Cutlip DE, Serruys PW (2007) A pooled analysis of data comparing sirolimus-eluting stents with bare-metal stents. N Engl J Med 356:989–997

14. Nissen SE, Tardif JC, Nicholls SJ, Revkin JH, Shear CL, Duggan WT, Ruzyllo W, Bachinsky WB, Lasala GP, Tuzcu EM, ILLUSTRATE Investigators (2007) Effect of torcetrapib on the progression of coronary atherosclerosis. N Engl J Med 356:1304–1316

15. LaRosa JC, Grundy SM, Waters D, Shear C, Barter P, Fruchart JC, Gotto AM, Greten H, Kastelein JJ, Shepherd J, Wenger NK, Treating to New Targets (TNT) Investigators (2005) Intensive lipid lowering with atorvastatin in patients with stable coronary disease. N Engl J Med 352:1425–1435

16. Baker AG, Kramer BS (2003) A perfect correlate does not a surrogate make. BMC Med Res Methodol 3:16–21

17. Prentice RL (1989) Surrogate endpoints in clinical trials: definitions and operational criteria. Stat Med 8:431–440

18. Gail MH, Pfeiffer R, Houwelingen HC, Carroll RJ (2001) On meta-analytic assessment of surrogate outcomes. Biostatistics 3:231–246

Randomized Controlled Trials 5: Determining the Sample Size and Power for Clinical Trials and Cohort Studies

Tom Greene

Abstract

Performing well-powered randomized controlled trials is of fundamental importance in clinical research. The goal of sample size calculations is to assure that statistical power is acceptable while maintaining a small probability of a type I error. This chapter overviews the fundamentals of sample size calculation for standard types of outcomes for two-group studies. It considers (1) the problems of determining the size of the treatment effect that the studies will be designed to detect, (2) the modifications to sample size calculations to account for loss to follow-up and nonadherence, (3) the options when initial calculations indicate that the feasible sample size is insufficient to provide adequate power, and (4) the implication of using multiple primary endpoints. Sample size estimates for longitudinal cohort studies must take account of confounding by baseline factors.

Key words Sample size estimation, Randomized clinical trials, Cohort studies, Type I error, Type II error, Power

1 Introduction

Inferences in clinical research face multiple sources of uncertainty, including bias from uncontrolled confounding, selection bias, errors in generalizing results from a specific study to clinical practice, as well as errors resulting from random variation between the study sample and the population from which the sample was drawn [1]. In contrast to first three of these sources of uncertainty, where quantification of error is usually limited to sensitivity analyses or gross error bounds, uncertainty associated with random variation in the study sample can be quantified with probability theory. Using probability theory, it is possible to derive mathematical relationships between the sample size of the study and probabilities that random sampling error would lead to false positive or false negative conclusions.

Notwithstanding its mathematical precision, the relationship between sample size and the risk of false conclusions depends on

Patrick S. Parfrey and Brendan J. Barrett (eds.), *Clinical Epidemiology: Practice and Methods*, Methods in Molecular Biology, vol. 1281, DOI 10.1007/978-1-4939-2428-8_13, © Springer Science+Business Media New York 2015

characteristics of the study population and of the future conduct of the trial which may not be fully understood when the study is designed [2, 3]. The selection of the sample size also depends on the magnitude of the effect the study should be designed to detect, a complex problem which creates an additional complication for investigators [4, 5]. Finally, because logistical constraints often limit the feasible sample size, control of the risk of false positive and false negative errors often entails consideration of alternative outcomes or alternative study designs which have a greater probability of detecting an effect of the treatment with a smaller sample size. Thus the exercise of sample size calculation encompasses not only the derivation of probabilistic relationships between sample size and the risk of false conclusions, but more fundamentally the elaboration of the assumptions going into the calculations, the determination of the appropriate effect size, and the selection of the primary outcome and study design. This chapter examines each of these elements of sample size calculation. We focus initially on comparisons between treatment and control groups in randomized clinical trials and subsequently extend the discussion to longitudinal cohort studies.

The chapter is organized as follows. Subheading 2 reviews the concept of statistical power within the classical hypothesis testing framework and examines the implications of statistical power for the positive and negative predictive value associated with the findings of a study. Using this framework, we review the fundamental importance of conducting well-powered studies in clinical research. Subheading 3 overviews the fundamentals of sample size calculation for standard types of outcomes for two-group studies. Subheading 4 considers the problem of determining the size of the treatment effect that the study will be designed to detect. Subheading 5 reviews modifications to sample size calculations to account for loss to follow-up and nonadherence. Subheading 6 considers steps which may be taken when the initial sample size calculations indicate that the feasible sample size is insufficient to provide adequate power. This section includes an examination of the use of composite endpoints. Subheading 7 examines the implications of multiple primary endpoints for sample size calculation. Finally, Subheading 8 addresses modifications to sample size calculations for randomized trials which are needed for nonrandomized comparisons in longitudinal cohort studies.

2   The Importance of Statistical Power

2.1   Definition of Statistical Power

Under classical hypothesis testing, the statistical inferences of a randomized clinical trial comparing a treatment to a control group are interpreted as determining whether the trial results provide sufficient evidence to conclude, with low risk of error, that the *null*

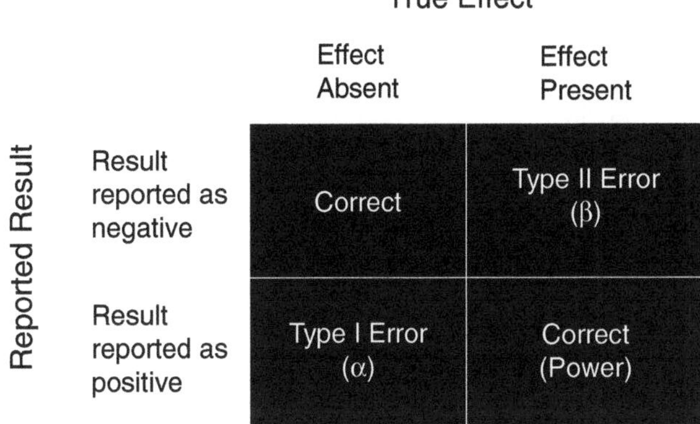

Fig. 1 Classical hypothesis testing. Displayed are the two types of erroneous conclusions under classical hypothesis testing for a comparison of a treatment to a control: type 1 error, which results when the null hypothesis of no effect of the treatment is erroneously rejected, and type II error, which results when a study fails to detect a true effect of the treatment

hypothesis of no difference in outcome between the treatment and control groups should be rejected in favor a *research hypothesis* which corresponds to a clinically or biologically important difference [6]. In this framework, there are two classes of error: A *type 1 error* occurs if the investigators erroneously reject the null hypothesis when the null hypothesis is true, and a *type 2 error* occurs if the investigators fail to reject the null hypothesis when the research hypothesis is true (*see* Fig. 1). The *statistical power* of the trial is defined by subtracting the probability of making a type 2 error from 1 and represents the probability of rejecting the null hypothesis in favor of the research hypothesis when the research hypothesis is true. The goal of sample size calculations is to determine the sample size necessary to assure that statistical power exceeds an acceptable minimum threshold, typically 0.80–0.95, while assuring that the probability of type 1 error is sufficiently small, typically between 0.01 and 0.05. The probabilities of type 1 and type 2 errors are often referred to by the symbols α and β, respectively.

From a mathematical perspective, statistical power is a function which assigns the probability of rejecting the null hypothesis for all possible treatment effects, including the particular treatment effects corresponding to the null and research hypotheses as special cases (*see* Fig. 2). In most cases, the power function equals α when the null hypothesis is true and increases continuously as a smooth curve for nonzero effects until the size of the treatment effect reaches the effect size designated by the research hypothesis, and eventually increases to approximately 1 for arbitrarily large treatment effects. A corollary is that regardless of the sample size, one can define the statistical power to be anywhere between the α-level

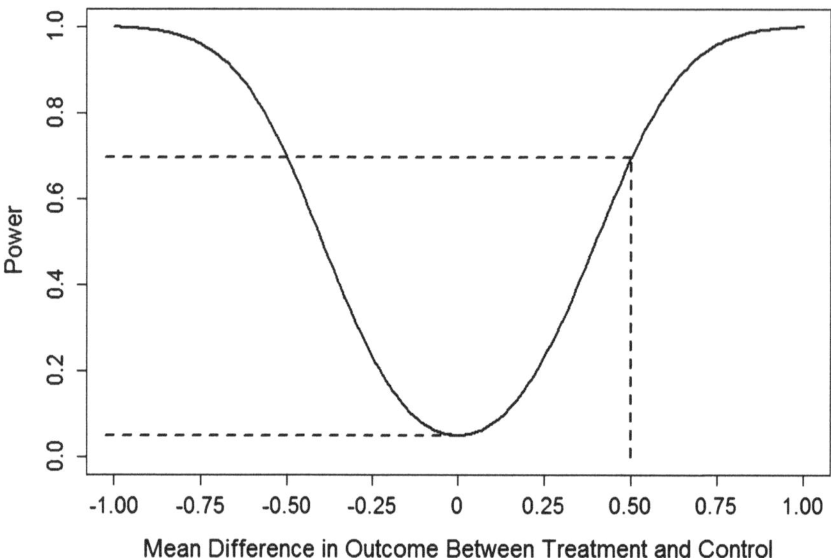

Fig. 2 Power curve for two-sided test. Displayed is the power curve for a two-sided text comparing the mean values of a continuous outcome between treatment and control groups. The *curve* indicates the probability that the null hypothesis is rejected for each possible difference in the outcome means between the two groups. The power is equal to the α-level (0.05 here) when the null hypothesis of no treatment difference is true, and increases to 1 as the differences in mean values increases. In this example, the power is 0.696 for a "moderate" differences in the means equal to one-half of 1 standard deviation in the outcome variable

and 1, depending on what effect size is stipulated for the research hypothesis. This underscores the importance of the appropriate selection of the effect size in sample size calculations.

2.2 Importance of Conducting Well-Powered Studies

There is an extensive body of work spanning both the medical and statistical literatures arguing for the importance of conducting well-powered studies.

Rationale for conducting well-powered studies includes:

(a) *Use of resources.* The conduct of medical research requires expenditure of investigator time and financial resources, which generally come directly or indirectly from funding provided by governments, philanthropic organizations, or profits derived from medical care. Conduct of underpowered studies has been criticized for expending investigator time and funding on studies of low value, thus diverting limited resources from more useful research [7].

(b) *Ethics in relation to study participants.* Multiple studies have shown that individuals often participate in medical research for altruistic motives, to participate in the advance of medical science and help future patients [8–10]. Because underpowered studies may not adequately test the study hypothesis, they have

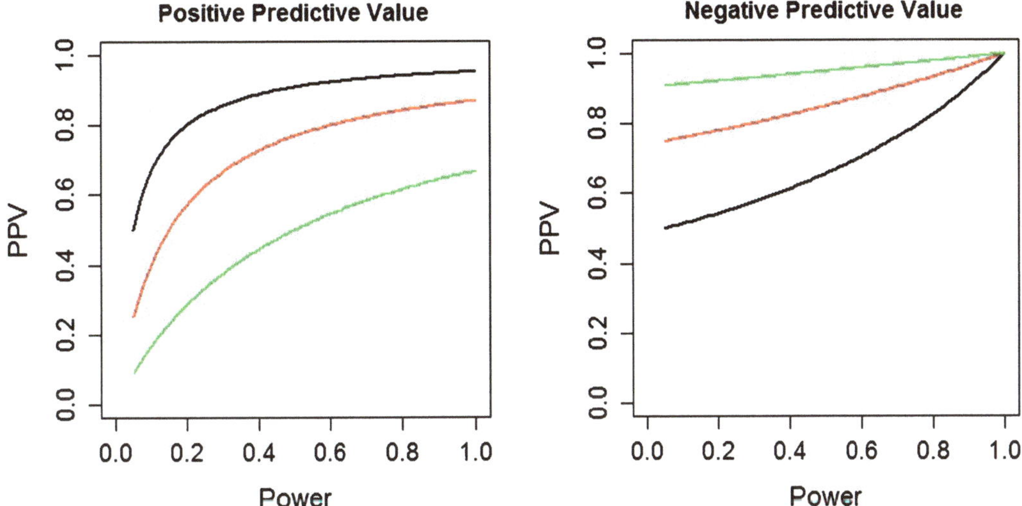

Fig. 3 Positive and negative predictive value and power. Shown are the relationships of positive and negative predictive value to statistical power assuming *R* values of 1 (*black*), 0.333 (*red*), and 0.10 (*green*), respectively. Both positive and negative predictive values are reduced when power is low

been considered of limited scientific value and therefore unethical in their exposure of subjects to the risks and burdens of medical research [10–12] without the benefit of significantly adding to medical knowledge.

(c) *Effects of low power on positive and negative predictive values of study findings.* Recently there has been increased emphasis on the implications of statistical power for the positive and negative predictive values of results published by research programs [13–15]. The risk that a publication by a research program is erroneous is defined either by the probability of a false positive finding given a positive reported result or by the probability of a false negative finding given a negative reported result. These error probabilities can be interpreted as 1 minus the positive and negative predictive values of the study results, respectively. In a simplified model where only the two possible treatment effects corresponding to the null and research hypotheses are considered, the positive and negative predictive values are readily calculated from α and β along with the ratio, usually denoted R, of the proportion of the research program's studies with true research hypotheses versus the proportion of the program's studies with true null hypotheses [13]. Figure 3 displays the positive and negative predictive value as a function of power for $R = 1/16$ and $R = 1$ when $\alpha = 0.05$. Low power leads to substantially reduced positive and negative predictive value at each value of R, implying that both the positive and negative findings reported by the research program may have high risks of error.

Of note, when power is low, the risk that a finding reported as positive is actually a false positive result can be substantially greater than the α-level of 0.05. Positive predictive value is also reduced when R is low, a point we expand on below.

The conduct of underpowered studies may be accompanied by additional shortcomings which can exacerbate the above difficulties. These include:

(d) *Publication bias.* When an underpowered study produces a negative outcome, the precision of the study will typically be insufficient to rule out a clinically important effect that went undetected due to low power, emphasizing the inability of the study design to answer the research question. As a consequence either of this limitation, or a general lack of enthusiasm for negative findings, negative findings from underpowered studies may not be submitted for publication, or, if submitted, they may be less likely to survive the review process. This phenomenon, which has been demonstrated in multiple areas of investigation using meta-analytic techniques [16, 17], can lead to a distorted body of evidence in the medical literature which falsely suggests a beneficial effect of an ineffective treatment or which exaggerates the benefit of a treatment with a small effect.

(e) *Failure to report confidence intervals.* The importance of presenting confidence intervals to indicate the precision of estimated treatment effects has been widely emphasized [18, 19]. In particular, in the absence of a confidence interval, a negative finding may be interpreted incorrectly as demonstrating the absence of an effect when presentation of a confidence interval would show that the results are compatible both with no effect and with a clinically important effect.

(f) *Failure to disclose low power.* Medical journals may be reluctant to publish studies where the power of the primary analysis is reported to be less than 80 %. This often results in a sort of dance, where researchers modify the parameter values, including the targeted treatment effect under the research hypothesis, until the calculated power research is 80 % or higher [20]. In fact, as demonstrated in Fig. 2, regardless of the study's sample size it is almost always possible to achieve any desired statistical power simply by "hypothesizing" a sufficiently large effect. Unfortunately, if the sample size is selected to reflect a hypothesized effect which is not biologically plausible, the consequences are analogous to reducing the ratio R in Fig. 3, leading both to poor positive predictive value and to a low true power. This practice has been viewed as leading to distorted presentations of the evidence to the research community and as misleading trial participants into believing that they are participating in a well-powered study when in fact the study is unable to come to a clear conclusion [12].

2.3 Are Underpowered Studies Ever Justified?

Because there are practical barriers for the conduct of well-powered trials, a number of authors have argued that efforts to prohibit underpowered trials may thwart many investigations, limiting the breadth of medical research [20, 21]. Under this view, underpowered trials may be deemed of value as long as they provide confidence intervals to display the precision of their results and as long as they are published irrespective of whether their results are positive or negative so that they can be subsumed into subsequent meta-analyses in an unbiased fashion. This view is encouraged by progress in registering trials in national data bases, mitigating publication bias [22]. Others have argued that methodological limitations of meta-analyses limit the utility of this approach, and that presentation of confidence intervals, while important, cannot overcome the fact that findings are uninformative if the confidence intervals are so wide as to include both the null hypothesis and clinically important effects [12, 23]. Under the latter view, underpowered studies may be considered ethical only in special cases, such as rare diseases where larger trials are infeasible, or in pilot studies where the primary goals involve feasibility assessments distinct from the determination of the treatment effect on outcomes. An extension of this perspective would hold that well-conducted and properly reported underpowered trials may be acceptable if alternative design and analysis options have been explored and found to be infeasible or inadequate. Recently, efforts have been made to organize prospective meta-analyses of separate studies in which investigators adhere to standardized treatment comparisons and primary outcomes to support a valid meta-analysis of the primary outcome, while allowing variations among participating centers in secondary endpoints and other noncentral aspects of the protocol [24, 25].

3   Basics of Sample Size Calculation

This section illustrates the mechanics of sample size calculation for three types of outcomes: (1) continuous outcomes such as blood pressure or serum lipids levels, (2) binary outcomes such as success or failure, and (3) survival outcomes defined by the time to the occurrence of a clinical event. The statistical literature presenting sample size calculations for different settings is vast, and we will not attempt a complete overview but rather illustrate the main features of sample size calculation with these core examples. Detailed presentations of sample size calculations are given in texts by Chow et al. [26], Cohen [27], and Machin et al. [28].

3.1 Mechanics of Sample Size Calculation

The second column of Table 1 presents standard formulae relating the required sample size in each group of a two-group study for two-sided tests with equal sample sizes per group to the following quantities:

1. The initial multiplying factor 2, which accounts for the fact that the comparison of the outcome between the treatment and control groups involves a comparison of two random quantities.

2. The second term, expressed either as $\left(t_{\alpha/2} + t_{\beta}\right)^2$ or $\left(z_{\alpha/2} + z_{\beta}\right)^2$, determines the effect of the type 1 error α and power $1 - \beta$ on the required sample size. Here $t_{\alpha/2}$ and t_{β} represent quantiles from the t-distribution while $z_{\alpha/2}$ and z_{β} are quantiles from the normal distribution. The type 1 error α is divided by 2 to account for the designation of a two-sided hypothesis test; if a one-sided test is performed, $t_{\alpha/2}$ and $z_{\alpha/2}$ are replaced by t_{α} and z_{α}, respectively. When the sample size is large, $t_{\alpha/2}$ and t_{β} are approximately equal to $z_{\alpha/2}$ and z_{β}, but $t_{\alpha/2}$ and t_{β} are slightly larger than $z_{\alpha/2}$ and z_{β} for small sample sizes to account for the uncertainty in estimating the standard deviation. Typical values of $z_{\alpha/2}$ vary between 1.96 for $\alpha = 0.05$ and 2.58 for $\alpha = 0.01$, and z_{β} varies between 0.84 for 80 % power and 1.28 for 90 % power. It follows that using $\alpha = 0.01$ instead of $\alpha = 0.05$ requires an approximately 49 % larger sample size when power is 80 and a 42 % larger sample size when power is 90 %. Similarly, using 90 % instead of 80 % power requires an approximate 34 % increase in sample size when $\alpha = 0.05$ and a 27 % increase when $\alpha = 0.01$. In general, the clinical trials literature advocates the use of two-sided tests over one-sided tests, in part to acknowledge the possibility of an adverse effect of the treatment and in part to maintain consistency of reporting between different clinical trials [2]. When one-sided tests are performed, it is generally recommend that the significance level be set to one-half the value that would have been used for a two-sided test; this assures that the investigator's decision of whether to use a one- or two-sided test does not change the criteria for concluding a statistically significant effect.

3. The third term, $\dfrac{1}{\delta^2}$, represents the inverse of the square of the hypothesized effect size δ. For continuous outcomes, the effect size is defined as the difference $\mu_{\mathrm{T}} - \mu_{\mathrm{C}}$ in the mean of the outcome between the treatment and control groups under the research hypothesis. Similarly, for binary outcomes, the effect size is defined as the hypothesized difference $\pi_{\mathrm{T}} - \pi_{\mathrm{C}}$ in the proportions between the treatment and control groups. In survival analysis, the effect size is given by the logarithm of the

Table 1
Required sample size for standard two-group comparisons

Setting	Required sample size in each group	Information per patient	Effect size measure	Study population input parameter(s)
Comparison of follow-up means	$2 \times \left(t_{\alpha/2} + t_{\beta}\right)^2 \times \dfrac{1}{\delta^2} \times \sigma^2$	$\dfrac{1}{\sigma^2}$	$\delta = \mu_{\mathrm{T}} - \mu_{\mathrm{C}}$ (hypothesized difference in means)	Outcome SD (σ)
Comparison of mean changes	$2 \times \left(t_{\alpha/2} + t_{\beta}\right)^2 \times \dfrac{1}{\delta^2} \times 2\sigma^2\left(1 - R\right)$	$\dfrac{1}{2\sigma^2\left(1 - R\right)}$	$\delta = \mu_{\mathrm{T}} - \mu_{\mathrm{C}}$ (hypothesized difference in means)	Outcome SD (σ), outcome correlation (R)
Comparison of mean changes, adjusting for baseline values	$2 \times \left(t_{\alpha/2} + t_{\beta}\right)^2 \times \dfrac{1}{\delta^2} \times \sigma^2\left(1 - R^2\right)$	$\dfrac{1}{\sigma^2\left(1 - R^2\right)}$	$\delta = \mu_{\mathrm{T}} - \mu_{\mathrm{C}}$ (hypothesized difference in means)	Outcome SD (σ), outcome correlation (R)
Comparison of mean slopes	$2 \times \left(t_{\alpha/2} + t_{\beta}\right)^2 \times \dfrac{1}{\delta^2} \times \left(\sigma_{\mathrm{B}}^2 + \dfrac{12(P-1)\sigma_{\mathrm{error}}^2}{D^2 P(P+1)}\right)$	$\dfrac{1}{\left(\sigma_{\mathrm{B}}^2 + \dfrac{12(P-1)\sigma_{\mathrm{error}}^2}{D^2 P(P+1)}\right)}$	$\delta = \beta_{\mathrm{T}} - \beta_{\mathrm{C}}$ (hypothesized difference in mean slopes)	Slope SD (σ_{B}), residual SD $(\sigma_{\mathrm{error}})$
Comparison of proportions	$2 \times \left(z_{\alpha/2} + z_{\beta}\right)^2 \times \dfrac{1}{\delta^2} \times \bar{\pi}\left(1 - \bar{\pi}\right)$	$\dfrac{1}{\bar{\pi}\left(1 - \bar{\pi}\right)}$	$\delta = \pi_{\mathrm{T}} - \pi_{\mathrm{C}}$ (hypothesized difference in proportions)	Control group proportion (π_0)
Comparison of event rates (survival analysis)	$2 \times \left(z_{\alpha/2} + z_{\beta}\right)^2 \times \dfrac{1}{\delta^2} \times \left(\dfrac{1}{P_{\mathrm{event}}}\right)$	P_{event}	$\delta = \log(\mathrm{HR})$ (log of hypothesized HR)	Control group event rate

ratio of the hazard rates between the treatment and control groups under the research hypothesis. The fact that the effect size is squared in the expression for the required N has a profound impact on the practice of sample size calculation, as even relatively modest differences in the hypothesized effect size can have a very large effect on the required sample size. For example, suppose that 50 % of subjects are expected to fail in the control group in a study with a binary outcome. Then, hypothesizing that the treatment will lead to a 20 % instead of a 30 % relative reduction in the failure rate would require more than a doubling in the required sample size.

4. The final term, which varies between each type of outcome, represents the variability of the outcome variable for a single patient, and in statistical theory represents the inverse of the amount of information contributed by a single patient to the analysis. Consideration of this variability term accounts for the characteristics of the study population and allows investigators to weigh alternative options for selection of the primary outcome and research design.

For a continuous outcome, the variability of the outcome for a single patient is defined by the square of the standard deviation of the outcome in the study population. In many cases, variability can be reduced (and information per patient increased) by analyzing the change in a continuous variable from baseline, thereby controlling for inter-patient variation at the baseline assessment. For analyses of changes between a baseline and follow-up assessment, the variability per patient is expressed as $2\sigma^2(1-R)$ where R represents the correlation of the outcome between the baseline and follow-up assessments. Thus, if $R = 0.80$, analysis of change from baseline will reduce the variability term, and hence the required sample size, by 60 % relative to an analysis of the outcome without subtracting the baseline level. It is important to note, however, that analysis of changes from baseline leads to increased variability if R is less than 0.50; if $R = 0$, analysis of change scores would double the required sample size compared to analysis of the follow-up outcome variables without consideration of the baseline values. This risk of a loss of power when using change scores can be eliminated by using an analysis of covariance (ANCOVA) model in which the changes from baseline to follow-up are compared between the treatment and control groups after controlling for the baseline levels. The variability term becomes $\sigma^2(1-R^2)$, which is always equal to or smaller than the variability terms both for the analysis of the follow-up value alone and for the analysis of change scores [29]. Compared to analysis of change scores without adjustment for the baseline levels, analysis of covariance provides a 50 %, 37.5 %, 25 %, or 12.5 % lower required sample size if $R = 0$, 0.25, 0.50, or 0.75, respectively.

Outcomes are often measured repeatedly at multiple follow-up times. This provides the investigators with numerous analysis options for contrasting the outcome between the treatment and control group, including, for example, comparisons of the outcome at the final scheduled visit, the average outcome value across all follow-up visits, or comparisons of the mean slope over the baseline and follow-up periods under the assumption of a linear model for change over time. If the follow-up measurements are equally spaced in time, the variability term is given by

$$\left(\sigma_{\mathrm{B}}^2 + \frac{12(P-1)\sigma_{\mathrm{error}}^2}{D^2 P(P+1)} \right)$$ where σ_{B} represents the standard deviation

of the true underlying slopes, $\sigma_{\mathrm{error}}{}^2$ represents the standard deviation of the residuals of the outcome measurements from the underlying linear trajectories, D represents the total duration of follow-up, and P represents the number of measurements. This expression allows investigators to assess the impact of use of different follow-up times and measurement frequencies on the required sample size [30, 31].

For binary outcomes, the variability term is given by $\bar{\pi}(1-\bar{\pi})$, where $\bar{\pi}$ represents the average probability of the outcome across the treatment and control groups under the research hypothesis. For time-to-event analyses, the information per patient is approximated by the proportion of enrolled patients who experience events during the follow-up period of the study. This proportion is determined by the event rate in the study population in conjunction with the durations of the planned enrollment and subsequent follow-up periods of the trial [32].

3.2 Determining Study Population Input Parameters

The practical challenge for calculation of sample size is the determination of the effect size and the study population input parameters listed in the final column of Table 1. We consider these issues during the remainder of this section and the following section.

The ideal approach to estimating the study population input parameters is to perform a systematic review of past research providing summary statistics for similar populations and then pool estimates of the input parameters across these studies. Importantly, it is not necessary to identify studies with interventions similar to the intervention of the proposed study for this exercise. Estimates of standard deviations for continuous outcomes may reasonably consider standard deviation estimates from either treated or control patients in past studies, while estimates of the control group proportion π_{C} or the control group hazard rate should ideally be obtained from populations treated similarly to the control arm of the planned study. It is important to avoid two common methodological errors during this process. First, in order to obtain a smaller required sample size, investigators may be tempted to scan the literature for studies that report favorable standard deviations, outcome proportions, or hazard rates rather than perform an unbiased review. This practice will lead to falsely optimistic estimates of the input parameters compared to those which are observed in the actual study, leading to failure to achieve the desired power. Second, estimates of the population input parameters may be imprecise if obtained from studies with small sample sizes. This issue is especially acute for estimates of variability. For example, with a sample size of 5, the upper endpoints of 75 and 90 % upper one-sided confidence intervals for the standard deviation exceed the reported standard deviation by 44.2 and 93.9 %, respectively, reflecting 2.08 and 3.76-fold differences in the required sample size. With a sample size of 10, the upper endpoints of 75 and 90 % upper one-sided confidence intervals are 23.5 and 46.9 % higher than the reported standard deviation, corresponding to 1.53- and 2.16-fold differences in the required sample size. Due to this uncertainty, it can be advisable to use a 75th or higher upper confidence limit for the standard deviation when small studies are used to obtain the input parameters for sample size calculations or else to formally account for the uncertainty of the estimated standard deviation in the calculation [33]. A third complication arises when considering outcomes defined by adverse events such as mortality. Because the risk of some adverse outcomes is declining over time, event rates from earlier studies may overestimate the risk of the adverse outcome in the control group of the study being designed, leading to underestimation of the required sample size. In addition, patients who enroll in clinical trials often have lower rates of adverse outcomes than observed in the general population; this should be taken into account when applying adverse event rates taken from general population or other observational studies to when designing a clinical trial. In general, if there is uncertainty regarding an input parameter, experience has shown that it is prudent to err on the side of considering less favorable values for the parameter as inputs for sample size calculation.

3.3 Pilot Studies

Some of the above issues can be addressed by performing either external or internal pilot studies. Under this approach, a preliminary sample size target is set based on information from other studies, but the estimated sample size may be adjusted based on estimates of variability or of event rates observed in a pilot study whose entry criteria, outcome measurements, and other protocol elements are formulated to match those of the full-scale trial [3, 34, 35]. The pilot is termed "external" if it is conducted prior to the start of the full-scale trial and the outcome results of the pilot are not included in the analysis of the full-scale trial, and internal if its results are included in the analysis of the full-scale trial. If the results of the internal or external pilot are used only to refine estimates of variability or group event rates, and not estimates of the treatment effect, adjustments to the sample size of the full-scale trial can be implemented with little or no adjustment of the significance level [2].

4 Choosing the Effect Size

Three criteria for choosing the hypothesized effect size have been discussed for sample size calculation: (1) clinical importance, (2) biologic plausibility, and (3) published criteria for "small," "medium," and "large" effects. All three of the criteria involve a certain degree of subjective judgment.

4.1 Minimum Clinically Important Effect

A trial should ideally be designed to detect the "minimum clinically important effect" with high power, thus limiting the risk that an important treatment effect is missed due to a type 2 error. For outcomes defined by clinical events, the minimum clinically important effect size can be assessed by having experts assess the smallest reduction in the event rate felt to justify application of the intervention. This assessment can be aided by computing the number needed to treat, defined as the number of patients who would need to be treated to prevent one event. For binary outcomes, this is $\left(1 / \pi_C - \pi_T \right)$. Judgments of the minimum clinically important effect may also depend on the prevalence of the condition being treated, as the total number of events that could be prevented by an intervention is the ratio of the size of the targeted clinical population and the number needed to treat; for binary outcomes, this is $N_{\text{population}} / \left(\pi_C - \pi_{CT} \right)$. For very large patient populations, even treatments leading to relatively small $\pi_C - \pi_T$ may prevent large numbers of adverse outcomes. The size of the minimum clinically important effect may also be informed by the side effect burden of the treatment, with larger effect sizes needed to warrant application of the treatment for treatments with more severe side effects. For quality of life measures, the minimum clinically important effect has been linked to the minimum clinically important difference, which has been evaluated for many common measures [36]. For biomarker measurements, empirical relationships from previous studies may be used to link differences in the biomarker to differences in clinical outcome, allowing the investigators to identify the difference in the biomarker outcome which is associated with a minimum clinically important difference in the clinical outcome. For example, if a 5 mmHg reduction in blood pressure has been found to be associated with a 15 % relative hazard reduction of adverse cardiovascular in a population, and a 15 % relative hazard reduction is viewed as a clinically important effect, then a 5 mmHg blood pressure reduction may also be interpreted as clinically important for the purpose of power calculations.

4.2 Biologically Plausible Effect

The biologically plausible effect size is assessed primarily by considering the magnitudes of treatment effects observed for similar interventions on similar outcomes in previous studies. Ideally, a meta-analysis may be carried out based on previous studies of treatments in the same class of treatments to provide a provisional estimate of the treatment effect to be tested in a new trial. In many cases, the treatment class under investigation will not have been tested in a previous study; in this situation, investigators may consider the average effect size observed in studies of other treatments having comparable evidence in support of an effect at the time those treatments were evaluated. Two major cautions are warranted when evaluating the range of biologically plausible effect sizes: First, due to publication bias, estimates of treatment effects from early studies in a particular area of investigation may be skewed to overestimate the true treatment effect, particularly if these studies are small. Second, small studies, including internal or external pilot studies, generally do not provide useful estimates of effect size for power calculations. Such studies are not powered to determine the effect of the treatment on outcome; consequently, confidence intervals for the treatment effect from these studies typically include both no effect and very large effects and are consistent with required sample sizes ranging from a small number to positive infinity.

4.3 Standardized Effect Size Conventions

The third approach to determining the effect size is to rely on rules of thumb which have been developed in the literature. The most notable of these are Cohen's "small," "medium," and "large" effect sizes for continuous outcomes, defined in terms of the ratio of the hypothesized mean difference to the standard deviation in the study population. Cohen termed effect sizes standardized in this way as small if they are between 0.2 and 0.3, medium if they are approximately 0.5, and large if they exceed 0.8. While arbitrary, the criteria that studies should usually be powered to detect medium effects have been widely used in the literature [27]. Due to the arbitrariness of this approach, the use of such criteria for sample size calculation is generally recommended for medical studies only when absence of information renders assessment of the minimum clinically important effect and the range of biological plausible effects too difficult [12].

4.4 Noninferiority Trials

The preceding discussion has been framed in the context where the research objective is to determine the superiority of one treatment with respect to a control. In some cases, the research objective is to determine if a new candidate intervention, which may reduce cost or lead to fewer side effects, is at least as effective as an existing standard intervention. The fundamental challenge in noninferiority trials is that it is not possible to demonstrate exact equivalence between interventions. Hence, sample size calculations in noninferiority designs are based on a "noninferiority margin" δ selected, so the treatment effects smaller than δ can be regarded as "clinically equivalent" [37, 38]. In general, the noninferiority margin should be no larger than the minimum clinically important effect.

---

5 Accounting for Loss to Follow-Up and Nonadherence

5.1 Loss to Follow-Up

Documented procedures to minimize loss to follow-up are an essential element of well-designed clinical trials and cohort studies. Even so, it is usually the case that some patients are lost to follow-up prior to the ascertainment of the primary outcome. Hence, for outcomes evaluated at a single follow-up time, it is standard to inflate the sample size of the study design by a factor $1/(1 - P_{loss})$, where P_{loss} is the proportion of patients projected to be lost to follow-up prior to the outcome assessment. For example, if the required sample size is 1,000 patients but 15 % are expected to be lost to follow-up, the target sample size would be set to $1,000/(1 - 0.15) = 1,177$. Adjustment for loss to follow-up is more complex for time-to-event outcomes, as patients who are lost during the follow-up period will contribute partial information to the analysis for the period prior to the time the patient is censored. Hence, standard sample size software for time-to-event analyses requires the user to provide rates of loss to follow-up over the course of the study. Similar considerations apply to longitudinal outcomes such as slopes or the mean value of the outcome throughout the follow-up period [39].

5.2 Nonadherence

Statistical power is also reduced when a subset of patients assigned to the treatment group discontinues the treatment (treatment dropouts) or when a subset of patients assigned to the control group start the treatment (treatment drop-ins). While the occurrence of treatment discontinuation superficially resembles loss to follow-up, the implications of these two processes are fundamentally distinct for the study design and sample size calculation. In accordance with the principle of intention-to-treat, it is essential that all efforts be made to continue to collect outcome information after treatment discontinuation. Since patients who discontinue treatment are likely to have different clinical characteristics than patients who remain on treatment, exclusion of these patients would often lead to important differences in the characteristics of the treatment and control group patients retained in the primary analysis, negating the purpose of the randomized design.

The consequences of treatment drop-ins and dropouts for statistical power are substantial and generally greater than the consequences of comparable rates of loss to follow-up. This can be illustrated most easily for a study comparing a binary outcome between a treatment and control, assuming that the probability of the outcome for treatment dropouts reverts to the outcome

Table 2
Impact of nonadherence on required sample size

Treatment dropout (%)	Treatment drop-in (%)	Overall % nonadherent (%)	Hypothesized biological effect (%)	Hypothesized intent-to-treat effect (%)	Fold increase in required *N* due to nonadherence
10	0	5	10	9	1.25
20	0	10	10	8	1.60
30	0	15	10	7	2.12
40	0	20	10	6	2.92
50	0	25	10	5	4.25
10	10	10	10	8	1.56
20	20	20	10	6	2.78
30	30	30	10	4	6.25
40	40	40	10	2	25.0
50	50	50	10	0	Infinite

Shown are increases in required sample size with varying treatment dropout and drop-in rates for a binary outcome in an RCT with equal allocation to a treatment and control group, where the research hypothesis stipulated an outcome probability of 0.30 under the control and 0.20 under the treatment

probability for patients consistently taking the control and that the outcome probability for treatment drop-ins from the control group assumes the outcome probability for patients consistently taking the treatment. As shown in Table 2, nonadherence in the form of treatment dropouts and drop-ins reduces the treatment effect under the intent-to-treat analysis relative to the biological effect of the treatment with 100 % adherence, which in turn inflates the required sample size. Because of the inverse square relationship between required sample size and the treatment effect, even moderate reductions in the size of the intent-to-treat treatment effect can greatly increase the required sample size; for example, a 20 % treatment dropout rate in conjunction with a 20 % treatment drop-in rate results in a 2.78-fold increase in required sample size. In comparison, a 20 % loss to follow-up in both the treatment and control groups would require a 1.25-fold increase in the required sample size. When considering nonadherence, power calculations are sometimes expressed in terms of the hypothesized biological effect that would hypothetically occur with perfect adherence and sometimes in terms of the intent-to-treat effect after accounting for nonadherence. The ultimate required sample size is the same in either case, as long as the intent-to-treat effect is appropriately discounted to account for the projected effect of nonadherence. We have found that it is useful for investigators to consider both the hypothesized biological effect and the intent-to-treat effect to clarify the implications of nonadherence. Analogous to the loss to follow-up situation, accounting for treatment drop-ins and drop-outs is somewhat more complex in time-to-event analysis, as the expected effect size for patients who dropout or drop-in at a particular follow-up time is usually assumed to match the full biological effect of the treatment until that time. Hence, sample size calculations for time-to-event outcomes also require assumptions regarding the rates of dropouts and drop-ins over successive follow-up intervals [40, 41].

5.3 Pragmatic Trials

Due to the severe effect of nonadherence on power and required sample size, it has historically been a tenet of clinical trial design that efforts should be made to identify and exclude patients at risk for nonadherence prior to randomization and to include adherence promotion efforts after randomization. Recently, there has been increased concern that this approach may compromise the external generalizability of the trial results to clinical practice, and there has been a trend towards the so-called pragmatic trials in which broader patient populations are enrolled irrespective of the risk of nonadherence [42]. Clearly, it is important that realistic projections of nonadherence be incorporated into pragmatic trial designs, with consequent upward adjustments to sample size.

6 Options When the Initial Calculated Sample Size Is Low

As described in Subheading 3, investigators may inflate hypothesized treatment effects to provide the appearance of a well-powered trial when power calculations indicate an infeasible required effect size, with adverse consequences for medical research. Table 3 summarizes more appropriate options when the initial required sample size appears to be infeasible. The first seven settings as well as 8a and 9a represent scenarios in which the primary outcome can be modified to increase statistical information provided per patient, thus reducing the number of patients required to achieve adequate power. For example, if a binary outcome is defined by the occurrence of a normally distributed biomarker value less than a designated threshold, then redefining the primary outcome as the biomarker itself, without dichotomization, typically reduces the required sample size by 30–60 %, depending on the threshold and size of the treatment effect. Basing the treatment group comparison on an average of repeated measurements of the primary outcome can lead to substantial reductions in required sample size if the longitudinal variability within the same patients is substantial compared to the variation of the outcome between patients. For example, if 50 % of the total variance of the outcome is due to within-patient variability, then averaging 2, 3, or 4 repeated measurements would reduce the required sample size by approximately 25, 33, and 37.5 %, respectively.

Table 3
Design options when calculated required sample size is infeasible

Setting	Design option to reduce required sample size
1 Dichotomized continuous outcome	(a) Revert to original continuous outcome
2 Binary clinical endpoint with high probability of occurrence	(a) Perform time-to-event analysis
3 Time-to-event or slope-based analysis	(a) Extend follow-up period
4 Single follow-up assessment of continuous outcome	(a) Employ analysis of covariance (b) Base analysis on multiple follow-up measurements
5 Imprecise outcome	(a) Employ outcome with improved precision
6 Non-normal continuous outcome	(a) Employ transformations to better approximate normality (b) Employ statistical model for non-normal outcome (c) Employ robust statistical methods
7 Highly prognostic covariate available	(a) Employ covariate adjustment or stratified analysis
8 Rare dichotomous endpoint (binary and time-to-event outcomes)	(a) Use composite of 2 or more events (b) Restrict analysis to "enriched" population with higher event rate
9 Small hypothesized effect size	(a) Consider alternative biomarker endpoints more proximate in the causal pathway to the treatment (b) Restrict study subpopulation with larger hypothesized effect size (c) Conduct explanatory trial with intensive adherence promotion
10 Contamination of control group with treatment	(a) Conduct cluster randomized design
11 Treatment effect rapidly attenuates after discontinuation	(a) Employ cross-over design
12 Initial stages of investigation	(a) Revert to pilot study addressing feasibility issues
13 High per-patient cost of protocol	(a) Simplify protocol to focus on primary outcome
14 Multiple treatment arms	(a) Simplify to 2 treatments (b) Organize treatment into factorial design
15 Widespread interest in treatment	(a) Organize or participate in multicenter trial (b) Organize or participate in prospective meta-analysis

Because the information per patient in time-to-event analyses is given by the number of events (Table 1), composite endpoints defined by more than one type of event are often used to reduce the number of patients who must be recruited to observe the required number of events [2, 43]. For example, a study of cardiovascular disease might consider a composite endpoint based on the first occurrence either of death from coronary heart disease or nonfatal myocardial infarction. The savings in required sample size can be substantial; if two types of events are each projected to occur for 5 % of subjects during the planned follow-up period, a composite defined by the first occurrence of either event may reduce the required sample size by nearly 50 %. The use of composite endpoints is most widely recommended when each type of event in the composite reflects the same underlying condition or can be expected to respond to the same underlying mechanism of action of the treatment. The use of composite endpoints is controversial, however, when the different endpoints defining the composite are more disparate. In this case, interpretational difficulties may occur if the treatment effects on different components of the composite go in different directions [44]. Additionally, if there is a substantial possibility that the treatment has no effect on one of the endpoints being considered for inclusion in a composite, then incorporation of that component may reduce the magnitude of the projected treatment effect and thus reduce power in spite of the increase in the total number of events.

The remaining rows of Table 3 represent scenarios in which the study design can be modified to reduce the required sample size. We note that in general, cluster randomization can be expected to increase rather than decrease the required sample size due to correlations of the outcome between subjects belonging to the same cluster [45, 46]. However, an exception to this rule can occur if the effects of a treatment intervention applied to some patients within a given cluster (e.g., hospital, clinic, or physician) are thought likely to spread to subjects in the control group within the same cluster. For example, if the treatment intervention instructs physicians to implement a new checklist to promote smoking cessation, then the physicians may find it difficult to keep themselves from implementing components of the checklist to control subjects as well. Such "contamination" may be prevented by randomization at the cluster level, and if the risk of contamination is high, the increase in effect size may outweigh the effect of correlated outcomes within clusters to reduce the total required sample size.

7 Multiple Outcomes

While the clinical trial literature generally supports the use of a single primary outcome on which to base sample size calculation, there are instances where a clinical trial or cohort study may have more than one primary outcome [47]. For example, multiple distinct research questions may be deemed of equivalent importance, or the investigators may stipulate that a beneficial effect must be demonstrated on more than one outcome to demonstrate an overall benefit to the patient. Sample size calculation for studies with multiple primary outcomes can be complex. While some attempts have been made to develop a single hypothesis test to simultaneously evaluate the effect of a treatment on multiple outcomes [48], the most common approach is to perform separate hypothesis tests for each outcome individually. In this situation, it is necessary to choose the sample size of the study based on the largest of the minimum required sample sizes for each individual outcome. If outcomes have different required sample sizes, this strategy assures that each outcome achieves the desired minimum threshold for power, with even greater power achieved for outcomes requiring smaller sample sizes. Typically, studies including multiple primary outcomes are required to use smaller α-levels for each individual hypothesis test in order to preserve the overall type 1 error of the trial. Such adjustment to the α-level can lead to a substantial increase in sample size if more than 2 or 3 outcomes are included. When power is 90 %, use of 2, 3, or 4 co-primary endpoints increases the required sample size by approximately 18, 29, and 36 %, respectively, if a standard Bonferroni adjustment is used. The increase in required sample size with multiple outcomes can be slightly reduced if estimates exist for the correlations between the different outcomes.

8   Power Calculations for Longitudinal Cohort Studies

The concepts of the preceding sections concerning sample size requirements of randomized clinical trials can also be applied to observational cohort studies estimate the effect of a treatment or exposure on an outcome variable. However, in contrast to randomized clinical trials, where randomization assures that the treatment assignment is approximately unrelated to other baseline factors, in cohort studies the exposure is often associated with multiple confounding factors, which must be controlled for in the study design or data analysis. The range of strategies for controlling confounding is extensive, and a complete review is beyond the scope of this chapter. Here, we consider the most common analytic approach to controlling confounding: covariate adjustment using multiple regression analysis.

For a continuous outcome variable, the formula for the total sample size required for a comparison of the mean level of the outcome between the exposed and unexposed after adjusting for a set of covariates under multiple linear regression is given by the following expression:

$$\frac{1}{2f(1-f)} \times \left(t_{\alpha/2} + t_{\beta}\right)^2 \times \frac{1}{\delta^2} \times \sigma_{\text{resid}}^2 \times \left(\frac{1}{1-R_{\text{rest}}^2}\right)$$

This expression differs from the sample size formula for a two-group comparison of means in a randomized trial in three important respects: (1) in contrast to a randomized trial, where investigators usually allocate equal proportions of subjects to the treatment and control groups, in cohort studies the proportion of exposed reflects the prevalence of the exposure in the study population, and may be anywhere between 0 and 1. The impact of the prevalence of the exposure (denoted f) on the required sample size is indicated by the first term, $\dfrac{1}{2f(1-f)}$, which reduces to the factor 2 in the corresponding formula in Table 1 if 50 % of subjects are exposed, but can be substantially larger than 2 if f is close to 0 or 1; (2) the standard deviation of the outcome is replaced by the adjusted standard deviation that remains after accounting for the covariates included in the model. Typically the adjusted standard deviation is difficult to estimate, so that an estimate of the standard deviation of the outcome without covariate adjustment is often used as a conservative approximation; (3) an additional multiplying factor $\left(\dfrac{1}{1-R_{\text{rest}}^2}\right)$, called the variance inflation factor, is added to sample size formula to indicate the increase in the required sample size that is needed to account for the squared multiple correlation R_{rest}^2 between the exposure and the covariates included in the model. The greater the correlation of the exposure with the covariates, the more difficult it is to separate the effect of the exposure from the covariates, which is reflected in a higher variance inflation factor. The same expression for the variance inflation factor can be used to approximate the effect of inclusion of covariates in analyses of binary or time-to-event outcomes [49–51].

9　Other Issues and Conclusion

This overview has omitted numerous important specialized topics in sample size calculation. These include, but are not limited to, (1) Bayesian sample size calculation, (2) sample size for comparisons of variability, (3) adjustments to sample size to account for the use of stopping rules, (4) sample size calculation in settings with numerous hypothesis tests such as microarray studies, (5) re-estimation of sample size under adaptive designs, and (6) estimation of sample size under complex longitudinal designs. We refer the reader to the text by Chow et al. [26] and references therein for these topics.

Fundamentally, we have stressed the importance of the link between sample size calculation and study design. This linkage highlights the importance of close communication between statisticians and biomedical investigators throughout all stages of the study design process in order to allow for an iterative evaluation required sample size and alternative study design and analysis strategies until a design for an adequately powered study emerges.

References

1. Grimes DA, Schulz KF (2002) Bias and causal associations in observational research. Lancet 359(9302):248–252

2. Friedman LM, Furberg C, DeMets DL (1998) Fundamentals of clinical trials, vol 3. Springer, New York, pp 133–168

3. Birkett MA, Day SJ (1994) Internal pilot studies for estimating sample size. Stat Med 13(23–24):2455–2463

4. Ellis PD (2010) The essential guide to effect sizes: statistical power, meta-analysis, and the interpretation of research results. Cambridge University Press, Cambridge, NY

5. Nakagawa S, Cuthill IC (2007) Effect size, confidence interval and statistical significance: a practical guide for biologists. Biol Rev 82(4):591–605

6. Lehmann EL, Romano JP (2006) Testing statistical hypotheses. Springer, New York

7. Ioannidis J, Greenland S, Hlatky MA, Khoury MJ, Macleod MR, Moher D, Schulz KF, Tibshirani R (2014) Increasing value and reducing waste in research design, conduct, and analysis. Lancet 383(9912):166–175

8. Geller G, Doksum T, Bernhardt BA, Metz SA (1999) Participation in breast cancer susceptibility testing protocols: influence of recruitment source, altruism, and family involvement on women's decisions. Cancer Epidemiol Biomarkers Prev 8(4):377–383

9. Mattson ME, Curb JD, McArdle R (1985) Participation in a clinical trial: the patients' point of view. Control Clin Trials 6(2):156–167

10. Newell D (1978) Type II errors and ethics. BMJ 2(6154):1789

11. Emanuel EJ, Wendler D, Grady C (2000) What makes clinical research ethical? JAMA 283(20):2701–2711

12. Halpern SD, Karlawish JH, Berlin JA (2002) The continuing unethical conduct of underpowered clinical trials. JAMA 288(3):358–362

13. Ioannidis JP (2005) Why most published research findings are false. PLoS Med 2(8):e124

14. Ioannidis JP (2005) Contradicted and initially stronger effects in highly cited clinical research. JAMA 294(2):218–228

15. Wacholder S, Chanock S, Garcia-Closas M, Rothman N (2004) Assessing the probability that a positive report is false: an approach for molecular epidemiology studies. J Natl Cancer Inst 96(6):434–442

16. Easterbrook PJ, Gopalan R, Berlin J, Matthews DR (1991) Publication bias in clinical research. Lancet 337(8746):867–872

17. Dickersin K (1990) The existence of publication bias and risk factors for its occurrence. JAMA 263(10):1385–1389

18. Goodman SN, Berlin JA (1994) The use of predicted confidence intervals when planning experiments and the misuse of power when interpreting results. Ann Intern Med 121(3):200–206

19. Simon R (1986) Confidence intervals for reporting results of clinical trials. Ann Int Med 105(3):429–435

20. Schulz KF, Grimes DA (2005) Sample size calculations in randomised trials: mandatory and mystical. Lancet 365(9467):1348–1353

21. Chalmers TC, Levin H, Sacks HS, Reitman D, Berrier J, Nagalingam R (1987) Meta-analysis of clinical trials as a scientific discipline. I: control of bias and comparison with large co-operative trials. Stat Med 6(3):315–325

22. Horton R, Smith R (1999) Time to register randomised trials: the case is now unanswerable. BMJ 319(7214):865

23. Bailar J 3rd (1997) The promise and problems of meta-analysis. New Engl J Med 337(8):559

24. Ghersi D, Berlin J, Askie L (2011) Chapter 19: prospective meta-analysis. In: Higgins JPT, Green S (eds) Cochrane handbook for systematic reviews of interventions version 5.1.0 (updated March 2011). The Cochrane Collaboration

25. Unit ES (2005) Efficacy and safety of cholesterol-lowering treatment: prospective meta-analysis of data from 90 056 participants in 14 randomised trials of statins. Lancet 366:1267–1278

26. Chow S-C, Wang H, Shao J (2007) Sample size calculations in clinical research. CRC Press, Boca Raton, FL

27. Cohen J (1977) Statistical power analysis for the behavioral sciences (rev.). Lawrence Erlbaum Associates Inc, Hillsdale, NJ

28. Machin D, Campbell MJ, Tan S-B, Tan S-H (2011) Sample size tables for clinical studies. Wiley, New York

29. Borm GF, Fransen J, Lemmens WA (2007) A simple sample size formula for analysis of covariance in randomized clinical trials. J Clin Epidemiol 60(12):1234–1238

30. Schlesselman JJ (1973) Planning a longitudinal study: I. Sample size determination. J Chron Dis 26(9):553–560

31. Schlesselman JJ (1973) Planning a longitudinal study: II. Frequency of measurement and study duration. J Chron Dis 26(9):561–570

32. Fleiss JL, Levin B, Paik MC (2013) Statistical methods for rates and proportions. Wiley, New York

33. Sims M, Elston DA, Harris MP, Wanless S (2007) Incorporating variance uncertainty into a power analysis of monitoring designs. J Agric Biolog Environ Stat 12(2): 236–249

34. Friede T, Kieser M (2006) Sample size recalculation in internal pilot study designs: a review. Biom J 48(4):537–555

35. Wittes J, Brittain E (1990) The role of internal pilot studies in increasing the efficiency of clinical trials. Stat Med 9(1–2):65–72

36. Jaeschke R, Singer J, Guyatt GH (1989) Measurement of health status: ascertaining the minimal clinically important difference. Control Clin Trials 10(4):407–415

37. Fleming TR (2008) Current issues in non-inferiority trials. Stat Med 27(3):317–332

38. Hung H, Wang SJ, O'Neill R (2005) A regulatory perspective on choice of margin and statistical inference issue in non-inferiority trials. Biom J 47(1):28–36

39. Wittes J (2002) Sample size calculations for randomized controlled trials. Epidemiol Rev 24(1):39–53

40. Lakatos E, Lan K (1992) A comparison of sample size methods for the logrank statistic. Stat Med 11(2):179–191

41. Lakatos E (1988) Sample sizes based on the log-rank statistic in complex clinical trials. Biometrics 44:229–241

42. Treweek S, Zwarenstein M (2009) Making trials matter: pragmatic and explanatory trials and the problem of applicability. Trials 10(37):9

43. Cannon CP (1997) Clinical perspectives on the use of composite endpoints. Control Clin Trials 18(6):517–529

44. Freemantle N, Calvert M (2007) Weighing the pros and cons for composite outcomes in clinical trials. J Clin Epid 60(7):658–659

45. Hayes R, Bennett S (1999) Simple sample size calculation for cluster-randomized trials. Int J Epidemiol 28(2):319–326

46. Murray DM, Varnell SP, Blitstein JL (2004) Design and analysis of group-randomized trials: a review of recent methodological developments. Am J Pub Health 94(3):423

47. Pocock SJ (1997) Clinical trials with multiple outcomes: a statistical perspective on their design, analysis, and interpretation. Control Clin Trials 18(6):530–545

48. Tilley BC, Marler J, Geller NL, Lu M, Legler J, Brott T, Lyden P, Grotte J (1996) Use of a global test for multiple outcomes in stroke trials with application to the National Institute of Neurological Disorders and Stroke t-PA Stroke Trial. Stroke 27(11):2136–2142

49. Schoenfeld DA (1983) Sample-size formula for the proportional-hazards regression. Biometrics 39(2):499–503

50. Hsieh FY, Bloch DA, Larsen MD (1998) A simple method of sample size calculation for linear and logistic regression. Stat Med 17(14):1623–1634

51. Hsieh F, Lavori PW (2000) Sample-size calculations for the Cox proportional hazards regression model with nonbinary covariates. Control Clin Trials 21(6):552–560

Chapter 14

Randomized Controlled Trials 6: On Contamination and Estimating the Actual Treatment Effect

Patrick S. Parfrey

Abstract

The intention-to-treat analysis is the gold standard for evaluating efficacy in a randomized controlled trial. However, when non-adherence to randomized treatments is high, the actual treatment effect may be underestimated. The impact of drop-out from the intervention group or drop-in to the control group may be controlled by trial design, increasing the sample size, effective study execution, and a prespecified analytical plan to take contamination into account.

These analyses may include censoring at time of co-interventions associated with stopping treatment, lag censoring which allows an additional period after discontinuation of study treatment to account for residual treatment effects, inverse probability of censoring weights (IPCW), accelerated failure time models, and contamination adjusted intent-to-treat analysis. These methods are particularly useful in assessing the "prescribed efficacy" of the study treatment, which can aid clinical decision-making.

Key words Randomized controlled trials, Non-adherence, Drop-in, Drop-out, Censoring, Inverse probability of censoring weights, Accelerated failure time models

1 Introduction

The intention-to-treat (ITT) analysis is the gold standard for evaluating the efficacy of a study treatment in randomized controlled trials. However, when non-adherence to randomized therapies is high the actual treatment effect may be underestimated. Contamination occurs as a result of a drop-out from the intervention group by patients who prematurely stop taking the study treatment prior to experiencing a primary end point (treatment non-adherence) or of drop-in whereby patients in the placebo group prematurely stop taking placebo and start the commercially available treatment prior to experiencing an end point (treatment crossover) [1]. As both these occurrences lead to the assumption of risk similar to that in the opposite treatment group they diminish the power of the study to observe a treatment effect. The potential impact of contamination needs to be taken into account

Patrick S. Parfrey and Brendan J. Barrett (eds.), *Clinical Epidemiology: Practice and Methods*, Methods in Molecular Biology, vol. 1281, DOI 10.1007/978-1-4939-2428-8_14, © Springer Science+Business Media New York 2015

in the study design, sample size estimate, study execution, and analysis. In particular a prespecified analytic plan to assess the impact of contamination will diminish the bias associated with post hoc data-driven analyses, but also answer the clinically important question: What is the treatment effect size in patients who actually receive the recommended intervention?

2   Controlling the Impact of Contamination

2.1   Trial Design

Planning to limit and quantify treatment contamination is necessary. In particular consideration needs to be given to co-interventions that occur during trial that may induce withdrawal from the treatment. One solution for this is to stop following the patient at time of the co-intervention. However, this action curtails the assessment of the long-term impact of the study intervention on both study outcomes and on safety. The optimal solution is to prespecify in the analytic plan how to take account of co-interventions.

2.2   Sample Size Estimate

The sample size estimate should take account of both drop-in and drop-out rates likely during the trial, with consequent increase in the number to be enrolled. This requires an accurate prediction of the rates of both types of non-adherence which may be difficult. For example, if the trial is of a commercially available treatment the potential for drop-in exists, particularly if clinical practice guidelines identify a clinically important role for the intervention. Even though equipoise exists for the research question being answered in the trial some physicians enrolling patients may feel ethically obligated to follow the clinical practice guideline, even if it is based on inadequate information. The potential for drop-out exists if the trial is for a long duration, particularly if it tests a novel compound in a group of patients with substantial comorbidity. This drop-out rate may be difficult to predict.

2.3   Study Execution

Unanticipated drop-in or drop-out may make a trial uninterpretable. The sponsor of the trial and investigators are blinded to whether a patient has been randomly allocated to the intervention or control group, but careful monitoring is necessary to determine the extent of cessation of investigational product and the prescription of the commercial product. Surveys to assess and optimize adherence, and use of intermediate measures of adherence and effectiveness may limit treatment contamination [1]. Unexpected increase in the rates of treatment non-adherence or prescription of commercial treatment requires immediate intervention in study centers to ensure that the study protocol is being followed and that investigators maintain the belief that equipoise exists regarding the research question. Investment in time by monitors engaging with research nurses and by the study principal investigators communicating with local investigators is likely to enhance the quality of the trial execution, and to determine whether safety issues are the cause of non-adherence. Action on safety is of paramount importance. This will require efficient aggregation of accurate data on all patients enrolled, with subsequent assessment by the independent Data Monitoring Committee, in a timely manner.

2.4 Statistical Plan

The ITT method is comprised of three principles which include: (1) using all randomized patients regardless of whether they have any follow-up data, (2) using randomized treatment assignment regardless of what the patient actually received, and (3) including all follow-up information in the analysis [2]. Based on these principles, prognostic factors of the outcome should be balanced and any differences in outcome that are observed can be attributed to the treatment [3]. However, failure to assess the impact of contamination may mask a beneficial treatment effect.

In the past, treatment contamination was addressed using "as treated" and "per protocol" analyses. With the former technique participants were analyzed entirely on the basis of treatment received and in the latter participants who failed to follow the protocol were dropped from the study. However, these approaches remove the benefits of randomization and result in non-random omission bias, and have appropriately fallen out of favor [1]. However, it is important to obtain the most accurate estimate of efficacy in patients who actually receive the intervention.

Prespecified analyses to assess the impact of contamination on the estimated treatment effect may include censoring at time of co-interventions associated with stopping treatment, lag censoring, inverse probability of censoring weights (IPCW), rank preserving structural failure time model (RPSFTM), and interactive parameter estimation (IPE). Recently contamination adjusted ITT analysis has been proposed [1].

3 Statistical Methods

3.1 Lag Censoring

Lag censoring analysis is a variation of naïve censoring where data are censored at a specific time point (e.g., at the time of non-adherence to study treatment). The lag censoring method allows an additional period after discontinuation of study treatment to account for residual treatment effects. Although lag censoring preserves randomization, and is simple to use and understand, it violates an ITT principle in that it does not include all follow-up information. Furthermore it assumes that stopping study treatment is random between the two treatment groups, but there may be informative bias if non-adherent patients (compared to adherent patients) have different prognostic characteristics predictive of a primary event.

3.2 Inverse Probability of Censoring Weights

With the IPCW method data is censored at time study treatment is discontinued for non-adherent patients, but weighs more heavily on the results from patients who remained on study treatment with similar characteristics [4]. This method models the causal effect of treatment on outcomes, while accounting for time-independent and time-varying confounders [5]. In this context, confounders are variables that are affected by prior exposure to treatment and predict subsequent exposure to study drug and the outcome [6]. A key principle of the IPCW method is to recreate the population that would have been observed had patients remained on assigned study treatment. It does so by censoring data at the time of study treatment discontinuation for non-adherent patients and assigns weights that are proportional to the inverse of the probability of remaining on study drug given each individual patient's characteristics.

To derive the weights, patients' follow-up time until the time of study treatment discontinuation is portioned into several intervals. The probability of remaining on study treatment at the end of each interval adjusted for baseline variables and time-varying confounders is estimated using a pooled logistic regression model. To avoid possible extreme values when taking the inverse of these probabilities, these weights are stabilized by multiplying the probability of remaining on study treatment, conditional only on baseline variables.

The IPCW preserves randomization, takes into account informative censoring, and adjusts for time-dependent confounders, but it is sensitive to the number of non-adherent patients and assumes that there are no unknown confounders. It is computationally difficult to implement since it involves splitting the data into appropriate time intervals, location of the dataset is difficult, and parameter estimates may not be stable, as the model may not converge. Nonetheless, it has been used in many large long-term clinical trials and is accepted by many health care agencies.

3.3 Rank Preserving Structural Failure Time Model

This method is based on an accelerated failure time model, which assumes that exposure to treatment has a multiplicative effect on a patient's survival time. The actual treatment effect can be estimated using a causal model to relate the multiplicative effect and the individuals observed failure time to their counterfactual failure time [7], the time that would have been observed if no treatment was received. In the RPSFTM framework the counterfactual failure time is a pre-randomization variable and is independent of randomization. The treatment effect can be obtained from a grid search over a range of plausible values, until the counterfactual failure times are equally distributed between the treatment groups using a test based method (i.e., log rank) [8].

3.4 Iterative Parameter Estimation

This method is also based on an accelerated failure time model. The principle is that the observed survival time of non-adherent patients can be transformed to the survival time that could have been observed had these patients remained on study treatment, with non-adherent patients assuming the risk of an event of a patient in the opposite treatment arm [9].

IPE models survival time as if drop-in patients never started the commercially available treatment and drop-out patients remained on the study intervention. The survival is contracted for drop-in patients and expanded for drop-out patients. Rather than using a test-based method IPE uses a parametric likelihood estimation method to derive treatment effect. Survival times are transformed through an iterative process until the model converges. IPE preserves randomization and there is no need to model the pattern when patients drop in or drop out. It assumes non-adherence is random, but is prone to informative bias. It requires parametric modelling with the need to specify the correct distribution. It is required to re-censor data when the transformed survival time is beyond the study termination date. Computational methods such as bootstrapping are required to obtain robust confidence intervals.

3.5 Contamination Adjusted ITT

The instrumental variable technique was traditionally used in non-randomized research studies. It used a variable associated with the factor under study but not directly associated with the outcome variable or any potential confounder [1]. The RCT is treated as an instrumental variable with treatment assignment as the "instrument". The effect of treatment assignment on the outcome observed (ITT analysis) is adjusted by the percentage of assigned participants who ultimately receive the treatment (contamination adjusted) [1]. In this way the effect of treatment receipt, rather than treatment recommended, on the risk of the outcome can be obtained. However, this methodology has not been well developed for survival analysis and it is quite complicated to apply.

4 An Example of Analysis of a Trial with Extensive Non-adherence

EVOLVE was a randomized controlled trial in 3,883 patients on hemodialysis with secondary hyperparathyroidism comparing cinacalcet to placebo, during which extensive non-adherence occurred [10, 11]. The data from this trial is used to examine the use of each statistical method.

Cinacalcet (Sensipar®/Mimpara®, Amgen Inc.) is a calcimimetic agent currently approved for the treatment of secondary hyperparathyroidism in patients with chronic kidney disease receiving dialysis. The EVOLVE trial was a global, multicenter, placebo controlled, double-blind, event driven trial ($N = 1,880$) designed to assess the risks and benefits of cinacalcet compared to placebo along with conventional, standard-of-care therapies (including phosphate binders and vitamin D sterols in the majority of patients) on a composite end point consisting of all-cause mortality and major cardiovascular events (myocardial infarction, hospitalization for unstable angina, heart failure, or peripheral vascular event) [11]. Patients were randomized 1:1 to cinacalcet or placebo, stratified by history of diabetes (yes/no) and country. At the time of enrollment, cinacalcet was commercially available in 18 out of the 22 (82 %) countries participating in the study. Although the use of commercial cinacalcet was discouraged, physicians had the option to prescribe commercially available study drug if deemed clinically important.

The original trial duration was anticipated to last 4 years, but due to the lower than expected pooled event rate, the trial was extended to 5.5 years. During the course of the study, a large proportion of patients prematurely withdrew from treatment. Of the 1935 patients randomized to placebo, 1,365 (71 %) discontinued study drug and 1,300 (67 %) of the 1948 patients randomized to cinacalcet also discontinued study drug (Table 1) [10]. Discontinuation for protocol specified reasons was similar in both intervention and placebo groups, but discontinuation for non-protocol specified reasons was higher in the placebo group (Fig. 1). These rates are 2–3 times higher than in other large, long-term cardiovascular outcomes studies of comparable sample size in which study drug discontinuations rates ranged between 20 and 30 % [12]. The time on treatment was approximately half of the total time patients were in follow-up for end points in both treatment groups; the median time on treatment was 17.5 months in the placebo group compared to 21.2 months in the cinacalcet group. In addition, a substantial proportion of patients also received commercially available cinacalcet during the trial (11 % in the group randomized to cinacalcet and 23 % in the group randomized to placebo). Moreover, 14 % of patients randomized to placebo and 7 % of patients randomized to cinacalcet underwent parathyroidectomy, a surgical and more definitive approach to managing hyperparathyroidism. As reported previously [10], 384 (19.8 %) patients randomized to placebo received commercially available cinacalcet prior to the occurrence of a primary event corresponding to an annual rate of 7.4 %. Similarly, 1,207 (62 %) of patients randomized to cinacalcet discontinued study drug prior to the occurrence of a primary event (corresponding to an annual rate of 27.3 %), effectively resulting in crossover between study arms.

For the primary analysis, Kaplan–Meier product limit estimates of event free survival were compared between the two groups using a two-sided, stratified log-rank test. The primary end point did not achieve statistical significance (p-value = 0.112) [10]. The relative hazard for the reduction in the risk of cardiovascular

Table 1
Reasons for discontinuing study drug in EVOLVE [10]

	Cinacalcet (*N*=1,948)	Placebo (*N*=1,935)
Subjects who discontinued study drug (%)	66.7	70.5
Ineligibility determined	0.1	0.3
Consent withdrawn	1.8	2.2
Lost to follow-up	0.6	0.6
Adverse event	15.8	11.8
Protocol-specified reasons	22.1	20.2
Parathyroidectomy	2.4	7.6
Kidney transplant	13.3	11.9
Calcium <7.5 mg/dL or symptoms of hypocalcemia	1.1	0.1
Low PTH	5.2	0.4
Pregnancy	0.0	0.1
Administrative decisions/subject request	20.6	30.7
Hyperparathyroidism	1.9	6.5
Commercial cinacalcet	0.4	1.6
Adverse event	2.3	1.2
Noncompliance	3.5	3.3
Other administrative decision/subject request	12.9	19.7
Commercial cinacalcet	1.2	5.6
Other reasons	5.4	4.5
Missing reason	0.2	0.2
Never received study drug	0.5	0.6

N= Number of randomized patients. Percentages are based on *N*

events or death was 0.93 (95 % confidence intervals (CIs):0.85–1.02) for patients randomized to cinacalcet compared to placebo [10].

Although the ITT analysis is a valid test to compare two treatment policies, it does not provide the best estimate of the actual effect of the study drug when there is considerable non-adherence [1, 3]. No other therapies have effectively reduced the burden of cardiovascular disease or mortality in the hemodialysis population; thus, detailed assessment of the estimated treatment effect in EVOLVE should be particularly relevant to clinical decision-making.

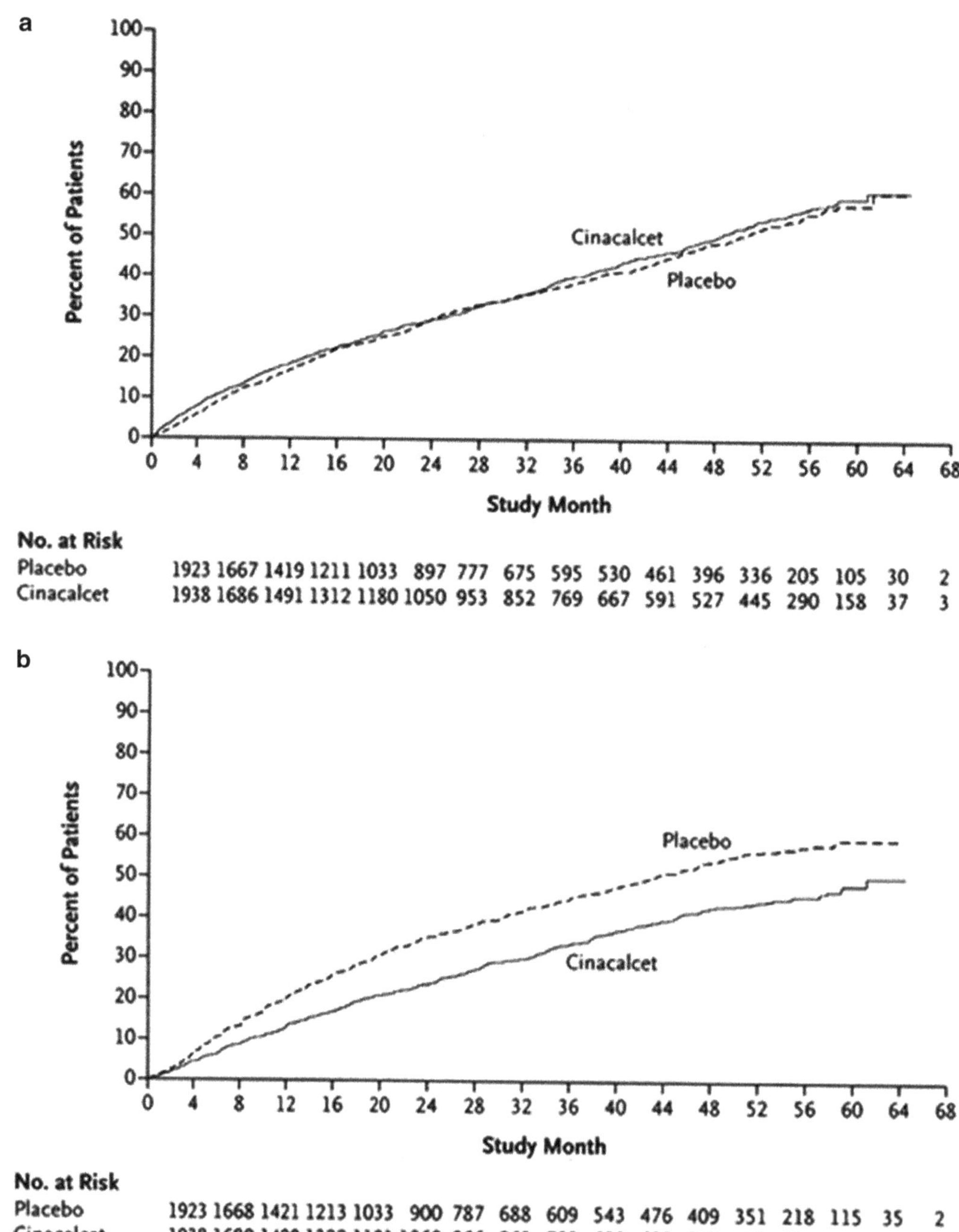

Fig. 1 (**a**) Time to discontinuation of study drug in the EVOLVE trial for protocol-specified reasons [10]. (**b**) Time to discontinuation of study drug for non-protocol specified reasons [10]. From: Effect of cinacalcet on cardiovascular disease in patients undergoing dialysis. The EVOLVE Trial Investigators. N Eng J Med. 367:2488. Copyright 2012 Massachusetts Medical Society. Reprinted with permission

Table 2
Relative Hazard (Cinacalcet vs Placebo) in EVOLVE using different statistical methods [10]

Analysis	HR (95 % CI)
Unadjusted intention-to-treat	0.93 (0.85, 1.02)
Censoring at renal transplant, parathyroidectomy, on commercial cinacalcet[a]	0.84 (0.76, 0.93)
Lag censoring 6 months after drug stop	0.85 (0.76, 0.95)
Inverse probability censoring weight[b]	0.81 (0.70, 0.92)

[a]Co-interventions that reduce serum PTH levels and lead to withdrawal of study cinacalcet
[b]Odds ratio and 95 % confidence intervals (CI) from the final pooled logistic regression model

4.1 Censoring at Time of Co-interventions

As the co-interventions kidney transplantation, parathyroidectomy, and use of commercial cinacalcet reduced parathyroid hormone levels and were associated with cessation of study cinacalcet, Data was censored after each of the co-interventions. For each of these co-interventions the relative hazard for the primary end point was 0.90 (95 % CI = 0.82–0.99; $p < 0.03$) [10]. Censoring at the time of any of these three events yielded a relative hazard of 0.84 (95 % CI = 0.76 = 0.93; $p < 0.001$) (Table 2).

4.2 Lag Censoring

A priori 6 months post-study drug discontinuation was selected as the lag period, as we hypothesized a persistent effect of cinacalcet on the progression of cardiovascular disease related to on treatment parathyroid hormone lowering effects. Study drug discontinuation was defined as the time point at which a subject discontinued study drug permanently for any reported reason or beyond which there was at least 6 months gap in the subject's study drug administration, whichever was earlier. Using this approach, follow-up time and events accrued beyond 6 months following study drug discontinuation were not included in the analysis. Using the lag censoring method, all randomized patients were included and their respective randomized assignments were preserved in the analysis [10]. The relative hazard was 0.85 (95 % CI: 0.76, 0.95) (Table 2).

4.3 Inverse Probability of Censoring Weights

Data were split into time intervals starting from randomization and up until patients had an event, discontinued study drug or completed study, whichever occurred first. The probability of continuing to receive study drug at the end of each time interval was derived using two pooled logistic regression models.

A weight was assigned a weight for each patient based on the inverse of the predicted probability of continuing to receive study drug based on baseline and time-dependent covariates at the end of each interval. To create more stabilized weights, the weight was multiplied by the predicted probability of continuing to receive study drug based only on a baseline covariates. Therefore, heavier weights were assigned to patients who did not drop out but had similar characteristics to those who did. A final cumulative weight for each patient was calculated by multiplying the weights from each time interval. The adjusted treatment effect was estimated using a weighted Cox regression model where data for patients who discontinued study drug were censored at the time of discontinuation. Using the IPCW method, the relative hazard for the primary composite end point was 0.77 (95 % CI 0.66–0.88) [10].

4.4 Interpretation

The sensitivity analyses performed in the EVOLVE trial, that adjust for treatment contamination, suggests that the true effect size in patients who actually received cinacalcet is larger than the effect size in patients recommended for cinacalcet (i.e., randomized to cinacalcet). It seems reasonable to adjust for co-interventions that lower parathyroid levels and induce cessation of the drug. The IPCW method is attractive because it is not prone to informative bias while adjusting for contamination. Although lag censoring is prone to informative bias the hazard ratio is similar to that obtained by censoring at co-interventions or with the IPCW method.

5   Conclusion

While the ITT method remains the gold standard to establish efficacy of a study treatment, additional analyses should be considered to assess the impact of contamination on the treatment effect estimate derived from the ITT analysis. Such analyses are particularly useful in assessing the "prescribed efficacy" of the study treatment, which can aid clinical decision-making.

References

1. Sussman JB, Hayward RA (2010) Using instrumental variables to adjust for treatment contamination in randomized controlled trials. BMJ 340:c2073. doi:10.1136/bmj.c2073

2. Schulz KF, Altman DG, Moher D (2010) CONSORT 2010 Statement: updated guidelines for reporting parallel group randomized trials. BMJ 340:c332

3. Gupta SK (2011) Intention-to-treat concept: a review. Perspect Clin Res 2:109–112

4. Robins JM, Finkelstein DM (2000) Correcting for noncompliance and dependent censoring in an AIDS Clinical Trial with inverse probability of censoring weighted (IPCW) log-rank tests. Biometrics 56:779–788

5. Hernan MA, Brumback B, Robins JM (2000) Marginal structural models to estimate the causal effect of zidovudine on the survival of HIV-positive men. Epidemiology 11:561–570

6. Robins JM, Hernan MA, Brumback B (2000) Marginal structural models and causal

inference in epidemiology. Epidemiology 11:
550–560
7. Morden JP, Lambert PC, Latimer N, Abrams
KR, Wailoo AJ (2011) Assessing methods for
dealing with treatment switching in randomized controlled trials: a simulation study. BMC
Med Res Methodol 11:4
8. Greenland S, Lanes S, Jara M (2008)
Estimating effects from randomized trials with
discontinuations: the need for intent-to-treat
design and G-estimation. Clin Trials 5:5–13
9. Branson M, Whitehead J (2002) Estimating a
treatment effect in survival studies in which
patients switch treatment. Stat Med 21:
2449–2463
10. Chertow GM, Block GA, Correa-Rotter R
et al (2012) Effect of cinacalcet on cardiovascular disease in patients undergoing dialysis.
New Engl J Med 367:2482–2494
11. Chertow GM, Pupim LB, Block GA, Correa-
Rotter R, Drueke TB, Floege J, Goodman
WG, London GM, Mahaffey KW, Moe SM,
Wheeler DC, Albizem M, Olson K, Klassen P,
Parfrey P (2007) Evaluation of cinacalcet therapy to lower cardiovascular events (EVOLVE):
rationale and design overview. Clin J Am Soc
Nephrol 2:898–905
12. Snapinn SM, Jiang Q, Iglewicz B (2004)
Informative noncompliance in endpoint trials.
Curr Control Trials Cardiovasc Med 5:5

Chapter 15

Randomized Controlled Trials 7: Analysis and Interpretation of Quality-of-Life Scores

Robert N. Foley and Patrick S. Parfrey

Abstract

Quality-of-life (QoL) outcomes are important elements of randomized controlled trials. The instruments for measurement of QoL vary but usually multiple comparisons are possible, a concern that can be offset by prespecifying the outcomes of interest. Missing data may threaten the validity of QoL assessments in trials. Therefore familiarity with the strategies used to account for missing data is necessary. Measures that incorporate both survival and QoL are helpful for treatment decisions. The definition of minimal clinically important differences in QoL scores is important and often derived using inadequate methods.

Key words Quality of life, Assessment, Measurement scales, Patient-reported outcome, Missing data, Quality-adjusted survival, Minimal clinically important difference

1 Introduction

Quality-of-life (QoL) outcomes are important elements of most pivotal randomized controlled trials. Even in trials where QoL has secondary importance, some familiarity with the analytical challenges posed by QoL outcomes is important for overall interpretation of trial findings. At their core, QoL outcomes share the same challenges as other measurements that are measured longitudinally in patients in trials. As with studies examining parameters like lipid levels, glycemic control, body mass index or blood pressure, one can anticipate that QoL studies are under constant threat from missing data, and one needs to understand whether the overarching need is to measure time-integrated (or area under curve [AUC]) differences between treatments or to capture differences at a specific point in time. Treatment allocation is intuitively important for patient-reported outcomes like QoL; even where initial treatment allocation is concealed, it is worth pondering how likely long-term concealment may be feasible. While multiplicity of comparisons is not unique to QoL studies, it is often more of a concern, because many QoL studies have multiple instruments, domains,

Patrick S. Parfrey and Brendan J. Barrett (eds.), *Clinical Epidemiology: Practice and Methods*, Methods in Molecular Biology, vol. 1281, DOI 10.1007/978-1-4939-2428-8_15, © Springer Science+Business Media New York 2015

and large numbers of individual items. Some QoL instruments, especially those that capture patient preferences and utilities into single scores, are useful for integrating cost and anticipated survival, allowing direct comparisons across different disease states and treatments. Finally, perhaps the most difficult issue that arises with QoL studies concerns the translation of subjective, patient-reported outcome into objective metrics; although easily applicable, valid estimates are rarely available, the impact of a given QoL difference in a randomized trial would be greatly enhanced if readers knew what constituted a clinically significant increment in QoL for the instrument under consideration.

2   QoL Instruments

In this chapter, we assume that readers have some familiarity with basic statistical techniques, especially regarding longitudinal comparisons of outcomes that are typically interval in nature. This preamble presents some basic steps that an interested, but nonspecialist reader might consider when presented with quality-of-life data in the setting of a large randomized control trial, with major clinical events as the primary outcome. A fundamental principle of patient-reported quality-of-life assessments is that they should come from the patient.

Lack of familiarity with QoL scales and scoring may partly explain a tendency for some health care professionals to consider QoL as lacking in scientific validity and clinical usefulness. Many scales are very simple, and the majority are based on linear templates like rating health status on a line varying from 0 (the worst possible) to 10 (the best possible), or categorical templates with descriptions like "not at all," "a little," "quite a lot," and "very much." When scales contain multiple items, these are usually totaled across all variables, but it is worth checking that this is a feature of the instrument under consideration. In many schemes, the working score is standardized to a range of 0–100, a summary measure that is often called the "scale score." Standardizing scales in this manner can allow readers to discern dominant QoL effects in controlled trials. Where expected scores in the general population are known, scores can be reported in terms of population norms, usually based on age and gender.

Generic instruments, designed to be applicable in a wide range of conditions, have the advantage of allowing comparisons across different health states. In more specific disease states, generic instruments may not be able to capture the health issues of paramount concern to patients with that disease and may not be responsive to disease-specific treatments. This has led to the development of disease-specific questionnaires. Thus, a common approach in large clinical trials is to use both a generic and a disease-specific instrument.

Given that it is the most widely used QoL instrument in clinical trials, all health care professionals should have a familiarity with the Medical Outcomes Study 36-Item Short Form (SF-36) [1]. The SF-36 is measure of general health status, which was developed to fill a gap between much lengthier time-consuming questionnaires and single-item instruments. It was designed to be applicable to all ages, all diseases, and in healthy populations. Capturing information in three main areas (physical, social, and emotional functioning), it can be self-assessed or administered by trained interviewers. It has been validated in a wide variety of health states, demographic subgroups, cultures, and languages. In terms of overall structure, 36 questions addressing eight health concepts produce summary measures for both physical and mental health. Physical health is divided into scales for physical functioning (ten items), role-physical (four items), bodily pain (two items), and general health (five items). Mental health encompasses scales for vitality (four items), social functioning (two items), role-emotional (three items), and mental health (five items). In addition, there is a question about the trajectory of general health, as follows: "Compared to 1 year ago, how would you rate your general health now?" There is also a global question about overall health: "In general, would you say your health is: (excellent, very good, good, fair, poor)?" Regarding time frames, most questions refer to the past 4 weeks, although some relate to the present.

A fundamental qualitative question that needs to be considered is whether the instrument makes intuitive sense in the context of the clinical trial in which it is being used. The main aims of the instrument should be clear, there should be a rational basis for the dimensions of the instrument, and intended usage criteria should be well defined. The procedures used to develop and validate the questionnaire should pass muster. There should be documented information that the instrument is suitable for the target population. Given that missing data is an issue that threatens the validity of many QoL trials, it is useful to have an idea of associated ease of administration and the time required for completion.

2.1 QoL Scoring	As scoring systems for QoL instruments vary widely, a concise, accurate description of the scoring procedure should be easily available. It is important to know whether a global QoL score exists within the instrument and whether multiple scales can be combined to derive a global score for overall QoL. If available, guidelines for clinical interpretation of absolute values and changes in scale scores are very helpful. Many of the more commonly used instruments have multiple scales and it is important to know when and how to group component scales. Some scores have been tested in the general population to produce normative data, usually stratified by age and gender. Thus, scores from these instruments can be reported in terms of expected values from the general population

by a number of different methods, including percentile score, Z-scores, and T-scores. Z-scores are defined as the number of standard deviations from the mean of the reference population; T-scores are quite similar to Z-scores but have a mean of 50 (vs. 0 with Z-scores) and standard deviation of 10 (vs. 1 with Z-scores) in the general population.

3   Analysis of Treatment Effect

Even where QoL is an ancillary outcome in a clinical trial, it is useful to know whether a single variable within a specific time frame was designated as being of principal interest during the planning phase of the trial. As with other outcomes in clinical trials, it is useful to know whether statistical power was considered before the trial and whether the likelihood of dropouts occurring was incorporated in the design. As many QoL instruments have a large number of subsidiary scores and are measured at multiple time points, this approach can mitigate the risk of undue attention, after the fact, on a single test result showing a between-treatment difference at a single time point. Thus, it may be worth checking whether treatment-related P-values are adjusted for multiple comparisons. Given that the intent of randomization is to generate groups with similar clinical and demographic characteristics, it is important to check whether randomization was actually successful. When imbalances are found, it is critical that QoL analyses are presented with and without adjustment for known differences at the time of randomization. For trials showing no differences between treatments, it is very useful to know the statistical power that was actually available when the trial concluded.

Treatment allocation is a critical consideration in trials with QoL outcomes. Even when placebo treatments are used throughout, patients and treatment teams can determine probable treatment in some situations. For example, in a trial where anemic patients are randomly assigned to different hemoglobin targets, it may not be ethical, or feasible, to prevent hemoglobin levels being measured outside of the trial setting, especially when trials are of long duration and patients receive multiple types of specialist clinical care and patients are likely to be hospitalized during the course of the trial. If this situation applies, the likelihood of successful treatment concealment would be expected to decline over time. Although rarely seen in trial reports, it would be very useful in trials predicated on targeted laboratory variables, to know the comparative frequency of nonscheduled, nonconcealed measurements of these laboratory variables.

While several approaches to dealing with missing data are discussed later on, it is important to get a numerical sense of overall compliance and whether this differs between treatment arms. Compliance is calculated as a proportion, with the number of completed QoL questionnaires as numerator, and the number of expected questionnaires as denominator, bearing in mind that QoL forms can only be expected for patients still alive at the time point in question. A related graphical approach is to perform a survival analysis plot of time versus survival without missing the scheduled QoL element.

Most trials measure QoL longitudinally at predetermined, regular intervals. It is rarely feasible, for logistical issues, to perform each QoL assessment at exactly the desired interval, and acceptable time windows are usually employed. While the need for time windows is understandable, readers of trial results need to examine the procedures employed and use their own judgment as to their appropriateness. Ever longer windows can threaten validity, and as elsewhere, it is worth checking whether decisions about window length were planned before the trial began, whether visits occurring outside windows were as likely to be early as late, and whether attendance patterns were the same in all treatment arms of the trial.

While this chapter is not intended to cover statistical techniques in detail, it is worth checking whether the main statistical analysis tool employed is what one would expect for the primary QoL outcome being assessed in the trial. Thus categorical, ordinal, and interval outcomes should use the appropriate type of statistical test, and distributional requirements of the test should be respected. Many trials use an area-under-the curve approach for primary outcomes, and the statistical tools should reflect this. Imbalances of covariates at baseline should prompt the reader to look for analyses that adjust for these imbalances. Decisions to form categories from variables that are intrinsically continuous should have a sound underlying rationale, and decisions made after the fact should be viewed with a degree of skepticism. As journals now have the facility to publish large amounts of additional information as online appendices, word and page limits can hardly justify the lack of availability of comprehensive descriptions of study procedures and results.

4 Missing Data

Missing data commonly threaten the validity of quality-of-life assessment in trials. It is essential to develop a sense of whether the available data are representative of the QoL of the combined group of patients with and without missing data. In the planning phase of trials examining QoL, it is useful to develop a simple system for describing the causes of failure to capture these data elements.

For readers of these trials, tracking the numbers of tests over time and comparisons between treatment arms are essential components of the critical appraisal of these trials. Similarly, where missing data are substantial, a detailed comparison of the baseline characteristics of subjects who do or do not complete all of the scheduled assessments should be available.

Some familiarity with the terminology and strategies used in different missing data scenarios can be useful. It is easy to envisage several situations where the fact of missing data could be informative. For example, subjects may not be able to complete the quality-of-life assessment because of advancing illness or may not appear for testing because symptoms of the illness have abated. Although rarely performed, it is possible to get a numerical estimate of the relationship between failing to complete a QoL assessment and a hard outcome, like death. For example, in a trial where death is the primary outcome and QoL is an ancillary outcome, it would be instructive to treat the time elapsed between baseline and failure to complete a scheduled QoL test as a time-dependent outcome in a statistical model where time to death is the primary outcome.

A simple approach to dealing with missing data is to consider only subjects with complete information. This is a standard technique, often used for outcomes like blood pressure, body mass index, lipid levels, and glycemic control. Unlike these parameters, many widely used QoL instruments have multiple individual items, and it is worth noting what exactly constitutes a missing case. For example, if one of 36 items is missing, it is not possible to use actual data for that scale, and a global score is not available. Scores based on the remaining 35 items are available, however, and may provide useful insights. Whether employed or not, it is worth pointing out that exclusive reliance on complete-case analysis is the equivalent of assuming that missing data are absent completely at random. In practice, it is common practice to add alternative strategies when the totality of missing data exceeds predefined proportions (often 5 % in large trials) or when proportions different by randomized treatment allocation.

Available-case approaches have obvious disadvantages. For example, when many assessments are made, it becomes extremely likely that some, or all, of a single assessment will be missing in most patients. Analyzing available data separately at different time points is an intuitive approach to this problem, although it typically results in different numbers of subjects being available at different time points in the trial. Summary measures, like AUC, or greatest change in QoL are another intuitive, commonly used approach, but deserve scrutiny as it can appear that all patients were compared, even though the extent of missing data is large enough to imperil the conclusions. For example, even if ten postrandomization assessments were planned, only one is required to calculate both an AUC and a largest QoL increment.

A frequently employed approach that attempts to provide a middle ground between complete-case and available-case approach is to substitute missing data with data that are imputed based on an arbitrary set of rules. For example, many investigators elect to carry forward the last available measurement. As with many other facets of randomized trials, it is worth assessing whether the algorithm used for imputation was formulated in the planning phase of the trial. Regardless of whether or not an a priori approach was used, no amount of imputation can eliminate the threat of bias generated by large degrees of missing data. While not often reported, it is often very useful to quantify the total number of complete forms that are missing as well as the number of individual items within the form. A detailed exposition of different imputation techniques is available in large QoL textbooks, but basic dichotomy is the use of existing data from the subject with a missing data element, as opposed to using data from other patients [2].

5   Quality-Adjusted Survival

Changes in survival and QoL may not occur in parallel, and measures that jointly incorporate both elements can be very useful for treatment decisions, both at the level of individual patients and in terms of cost to society as a whole. In most quality-adjusted survival models, health ratings can vary between 0 (the worst imaginable) and 1 (the best imaginable). All of these ratings are patient preferences, but the term "utilities" is usually used when the outcome being assessed is uncertain. Many procedures have been employed to measure these utilities. With visual analog scales, for example, study subjects are asked to rate their current health status on a line bounded by 0 (worst) and 1 (perfect). Standard gamble techniques produce utilities by asking questions like "If there is X percent chance of death in the next year, but you have to take this therapy for the rest of your life, would you take the treatment?", varying X and arriving at a point of indifference. Time trade-off techniques are quite similar, but the point of equipoise is achieved by asking questions like "Would you pick X months in perfect health or 1 year at your current health?" Another variant, Willingness to Pay, asks similar questions that are predicated on the maximum monetary price subjects would be prepared to pay to avoid adverse health states.

Assuming a valid utility measure has been obtained, varying between 0 and 1, quality-adjusted life years are easily calculated. Consider a progressive disease with multiple known states; in the first state, the survival is S_1 years and the utility of that state is U_1, while in the final state, the survival is S_f years and the utility is U_f. The overall number of quality-adjusted life years (QALY) is calculated as: $QALY = U_1 S_1 + U_2 S_2 + \ldots + U_n S_n + \ldots U_f S_f$. When treatment costs are known, the cost-utility per QALY uses cost as numerator and QALY as denominator: Cost-Utility per QALY = Cost/QALY. In intervention trails of control (C) and experimental treatments (E), the cost per QALY gained with the experimental treatment is calculated as: Cost per QALY Gained$_{E \text{ vs. } C}$ = (Cost$_E$ − Cost$_C$)/ (QALY$_E$ − QALY$_C$).

Many variants of the QALY approach can be defined. For example, consider a disease whose treatments have large effects on QoL but are followed by treatment-free periods of good health, and possibly, by a relapse to the original disease state. If the proportions of overall survival spent in each state are known, it is possible to quantify quality-adjusted time without symptoms and toxicity (Q-TWiST). Healthy years equivalents (HYE) are another variant, where study subjects report the number of years in full health they would trade for current health states.

6   Clinical Interpretation and Clinically Important Differences

While many patients struggle with interpreting how meaningful a finite change in blood pressure might be, many health care professionals are quickly able to decide whether such a change is of minimal, moderate, or great importance. Although it is very easy to see that QoL measures could be fundamentally important to patients and changes in QoL have survival implications in many studies, many health care professionals discount real differences in QoL, because they do not understand their clinical meaning. Lack of proof of clinical importance applies equally to many other measures, like changes in blood pressure, body mass index, lipid, or blood glucose levels, not least because proof is difficult to ascertain. It may well be the case that lack of familiarity with QoL scales contributes to the difficulties health professionals have with interpreting clinical importance.

Just like trying to estimate the value of a finite change in blood pressure in randomized trial, determining the clinical significance of a change in a QoL instrument is a challenging proposition. The most obvious approach is to actually ask the patients, as in asking them to rate the importance of the change in overall status, perhaps with a multiple-category Likert scale or with a linear visual analog scale. This approach, often called the anchor-based method, has the critical advantage of actually respecting the core philosophy of quality-of-life assessment by relying on what patients say, as opposed to relying on what health care professionals think [3]. This approach, however, has the disadvantage of requiring another scale to evaluate changes in the scale being evaluated. As this means a formal validation process, it is not surprising that robust anchor-based evaluation of minimal clinically important differences are lacking even for the most frequently used QoL instruments. A more common approach is to evaluate changes in QoL with regard to observed statistical distributions, often called the distribution method. For example, a change in QoL exceeding a specified number of standard deviations is deemed to be the minimal clinically important difference. Many might argue that using something like a standard deviation as a yardstick for assessing a change in QoL is not too different from evaluating a level of statistical significance. Given that a major objective of trying to establish the minimal clinically important difference is to allow separation of clinical significance from statistical significance, using a statistical approach for an essentially clinical question appears to be a logical fallacy.

An interesting example of the challenges of assessing the clinical importance of changes in QoL scores comes from the Trial to Reduce Cardiovascular Events With Aranesp Therapy (TREAT) study [4]. In this study of patients with diabetes, chronic kidney disease, and anemia, 4,038 patients were randomly assigned to darbepoetin alfa, with hemoglobin level of 13 g/dL or placebo, with salvage darbepoetin alfa for levels under 9.0 g/dL. No differences in the primary end points (composites of death or cardiovascular events and death or end-stage renal disease) were seen with the study. The main prespecified patient-reported outcome was the change in patient-reported outcomes at week 25 in the Functional Assessment of Cancer Therapy-Fatigue (FACT-Fatigue) instrument (on which scores range from 0 to 52, with higher scores indicating less fatigue). Among patients with both baseline and week-25 scores, from a baseline score of 30.2 in the group of 1,762 of 2,012 (87.6 %) patients assigned to darbepoetin alfa to a baseline score of 30.4 in the 1,769 of 2,026 (87.3 %) patients assigned to placebo, there was a greater degree of improvement in the mean ($\pm$S.D.) score in the darbepoetin alfa group than in the placebo group (an increase of 4.2 ± 10.5 points vs. 2.8 ± 10.3 points, $P<0.001$ for between-group changes). An increase of three or more points ("considered to be a clinically meaningful improvement") occurred in 963 of 1,762 patients assigned to darbepoetin alfa (54.7 %) and 875 of 1,769 patients assigned to placebo (49.5 %) ($P=0.002$); though the latter comparison was of subsidiary importance in the trial, many interpreted the trial as having shown a statistically significant difference of borderline clinical importance, not least because 19 patients ($100/(54.7-49.5)$) would have to be treated for 1 more patient to achieve a change in FACT-Fatigue score that was clinically meaningful [5].

Given that fatigue is such a debilitating problem in patients with chronic kidney disease and defining clinically important change in FACT-Fatigue score anemia, two questions immediately present themselves: What is the provenance of the ≥3 points change requirement to be considered clinically meaningful? Are data from within the trial available that could allow patients to judge what 1.4-point difference in change scores mean to them? Regarding the first question, the evidence for the three-point requirement for the FACT-Fatigue scale comes from retrospective analyses from a heterogeneous group of studies in patients with cancer, including patients that participated in a nonrandomized validation study of the FACT-An scale; patients from a nonrandomized, observational study of chemotherapy-induced fatigue and patients from a community-based clinical trial of an intervention for anemia in patients with cancer [6]. While the use of the description "anchor" in the study might suggest to an unwary reader that patient input was sought in determining clinically important differences in QoL scales, this was not uniformly the case, as the three anchors consisted of blood test (hemoglobin level), a physician-based assessment of overall functional status (the Karnofsky score), and an evaluation of whether the Fatigue subscale changed in parallel with the overall FACT-An scale within the same patient. It seems hard, then, to conclude, that ≥3 is a valid estimate of the minimally important clinical difference for the FACT-Fatigue scale in patients with anemia, diabetes, and chronic kidney.

Is it safe to conclude that a 1.4 point difference between the two treatment arms should be discarded as clinically meaningless? A subsequent report from the TREAT investigators was instructive in this regard [7]. This study included regression coefficients for FACT-Fatigue scores as a time-integrated outcome, measured at weeks 25, 49, and 97 of the study. In this patient group, each additional year of life was associated with a decline in FACT-Fatigue of 0.073 years. Thus, a treatment difference of 1.4 points would be equivalent to 1.4/0.073 or 19.2 additional years of age. Using a similar approach, the treatment effect in the TREAT trial exceeded the fatigue associations of having recreation activity classed as heavy or medium (vs. none or light), and the presence of overt pulmonary disease or cardiovascular disease (Table 1). In this framework, a change of 1.4 points on the FACT-Fatigue score may not be trivial after all. Thus, observational models of changes in key QoL parameters may be very useful for gauging the clinical importance of treatment effects in randomized trials.

In conclusion measurement of QoL in randomized trials is important, but care must be taken to prespecify outcomes, to develop strategies to account for missing data and to understand the clinical importance of statistically significant changes in QoL.

Table 1
Multivariate repeated measure model for FACT-Fatigue changes at 25, 49, 97 weeks ($N=3,531$) in the TREAT trial darbepoetin therapy in patients with CKD, diabetes, and anemia (7)

FACT-Fatigue change ($n=3,531$)	Model covariates (P)	Estimates (SE)
Randomization to darbepoetin	1.001 (0.402)	0.013
History of cardiovascular disease	−0.990 (0.299)	<0.001
Baseline FACT-Fatigue score (per 1 unit increase)	−0.504 (0.012)	<0.001
Baseline factors		
Race (black versus white)	1.108 (0.382)	0.004
Recreation activity (heavy/medium versus other)	1.066 (0.320)	<0.001
Age (per 1 year increase)	−0.073 (0.016)	<0.001
Pulmonary disease	−1.299 (0.329)	<0.001
Any nonsedentary job activity	0.933 (0.338)	0.006
Baseline diastolic BP (per 1 mmHg increase)	−0.044 (0.015)	0.004
Body mass index (per 1 kg/m^2 increase)	−0.045 (0.021)	0.030
Baseline white blood cells (10^9/L)	−0.191 (0.070)	0.006
Baseline triglycerides (per 10 mg/dL)	−0.070 (0.019)	<0.001
Baseline potassium (mmol/L)	0.535 (0.234)	0.023
Baseline serum ferritin (per 10 µg/L)	0.012 (0.006)	0.036
History of diabetic nephropathy	−0.570 (0.293)	0.052
History of atrial fibrillation	−0.999 (0.480)	0.038
Known duration of diabetes (per 1 month increase)	−0.003 (0.001)	0.013
Postrandomization factors		
Interim stroke	−5.040 (1.300)	<0.001
Number of hospitalizations	−1.007 (0.128)	<0.001
Any hemoglobin <9 g/dL status	−1.100 (0.314)	<0.001

Estimates were from repeated-measure model adjusted for baseline FACT-Fatigue scores, stratification factors, treatment groups, covariates listed in Table 1, and postrandomization factors (i.e., interim heart failure event, number of days transfused, interim myocardial ischemia/infarctions, and development of ESRD). *n* Number of subjects in PRO FACT-Fatigue analysis set. With permission from Lewis E et al. (2011). Darbepoetin alfa impact on health status in diabetes patients with kidney disease: a randomized trial. Clin J Am Soc Nephrol 6:845–855

References

1. McHorney CA, Ware JE Jr, Raczek AE (1993) The MOS 36-Item Short-Form Health Survey (SF-36): II. Psychometric and clinical tests of validity in measuring physical and mental health constructs. Med Care 31:247–263

2. Fayers PM, Machin D (eds) (2007) Quality of life: the assessment, analysis and interpretation of patient-reported outcomes, 2nd edn. Wiley, Chichester, England

3. Hays RD, Woolley JM (2000) The concept of clinically meaningful difference in health related QoL search. How meaningful is it? Pharmacoeconomics 18:419–423

4. Pfeffer MA, Burdmann EA, Chen CY, Cooper ME, de Zeeuw D, Eckardt KU, Feyzi JM, Ivanovich P, Kewalramani R, Levey AS, Lewis EF, McGill JB, McMurray JJ, Parfrey P, Parving HH, Remuzzi G, Singh AK, Solomon SD, Toto R, Investigators TREAT (2009) A trial of darbepoetin alfa in type 2 diabetes and chronic kidney disease. N Engl J Med 361:2019–2032

5. Marsden PA (2009) Treatment of anemia in chronic kidney disease-strategies based on evidence. N Engl J Med 361:2089–2090

6. Cella D, Eton DT, Lai JS, Peterman AH, Merkel DE (2002) Combining anchor and distribution-based methods to derive minimal clinically important differences on the Functional Assessment of Cancer Therapy (FACT) anemia and fatigue scales. J Pain Symptom Manage 24: 547–561

7. Lewis EF, Pfeffer MA, Feng A, Uno H, McMurray JJ, Toto R, Gandra SR, Solomon SD, Moustafa M, Macdougall IC, Locatelli F, Parfrey PS, TREAT Investigators (2011) Darbepoetin alfa impact on health status in diabetes patients with kidney disease: a randomized trial. Clin J Am Soc Nephrol 6:845–855

Chapter 16

Randomized Controlled Trials: Planning, Monitoring, and Execution

Elizabeth Hatfield, Elizabeth Dicks, and Patrick S. Parfrey

Abstract

Large integrated multidisciplinary teams have become recognized as an efficient means by which to drive innovation and discovery in clinical research. This chapter describes how to plan, budget and fund these large studies and execute the studies with well-designed governance and monitoring protocols in place, to efficiently manage the large, often dispersed teams involved. Sources of funding are identified, budget development, justification, reporting, financial governance and accountability are described, in addition to the creation and management of the multidisciplinary team that will implement the research plan.

Key words Clinical research, Randomized controlled trials, Management, Multisite, Multidisciplinary teams, Budgeting, Funding

1 Introduction

Evidence-based research is the primary mechanism utilized to inform health policy, improve health, and strengthen health care through a focused system of translational health research. Successfully funded proposals have four key elements: (1) A clearly stated research question, (2) Strategic alignment of the research question with the mission of the funding agency, (3) A clear description of a well-thought-out experimental design, and (4) A cost effective budget that demonstrates maximum allocative and technical efficiency of the resources required [1, 2].

2 Alignment of the Research Question with Agency Research Themes

One of the key elements of successful proposals is the alignment of research questions with agency funding priorities. In Canada, four national health priorities have emerged and are defined as the four pillars of health research. These include biomedical, clinical, health systems, and population health and are to be investigated using a

Patrick S. Parfrey and Brendan J. Barrett (eds.), *Clinical Epidemiology: Practice and Methods*, Methods in Molecular Biology, vol. 1281, DOI 10.1007/978-1-4939-2428-8_16, © Springer Science+Business Media New York 2015

273

problem based multidisciplinary approach. In addition to the national priorities, local and regional strategic health plans should not be overlooked as they will have their own unique set of priorities in addition to those defined at the national level. These will require information through evidence-based research in areas such as wait times and resource utilization and present opportunities for funded research.

3   Sources of Funding for Clinical Research

Funding sources vary from country to country, but first world countries usually have multiple sources including government, foundations, private industry, and professional organizations, for example in Canada, these include the following:

3.1   Federal

The Canadian Institutes of Health Research (CIHR), the Natural Sciences, Engineering and Research Council of Canada (NSERC)-Collaborative health Research projects (CHRP) Program and Genome Canada fund clinical research. The Canadian Institutes of Health Research is the government of Canada's health research funding agency and reports to Parliament through the Minister of Health. It is comprised of 13 institutions, each with its own scientific director and advisory board. The mandate of CIHR is "to excel, according to internationally accepted standards of scientific excellence, in the creation of new knowledge and its translation into improved health for Canadians, more effective health services and products and a strengthened Canadian health care system" [3]. Across the 13 institutes, CIHR has a research budget of approximately $1 billion per annum and leverages approximately $100 million from partner agencies per annum. These combined sources fund training, salary, equipment, and operating grants. In 2013–2014 approximately 50 % of CIHRs budget was awarded, $465.8M for open operating grants [4], which includes randomized controlled trials. Additionally a number of new signature initiatives were launched including Personalized Medicine, Patient Oriented Research, Community Based Primary HealthCare and the Canadian Epigenetics, Environment and Health Research Consortium [5]. Strategic initiatives launched included the Canadian Longitudinal Study on Aging, the Drug Safety and effectiveness network, and the Strategic Training Initiative in Health Research [3, 6]. By comparison in the United States, the National Institutes of Health invested $30.1 billion in medical research in 2014 [7]. NSERC, reports to Parliament through the Minister of Industry. NSERC has invested over $6 Billion in basic research and university-industry projects in the past decade. It has an annual budget of $1.1 Billion and is the largest funder of science and engineering research in Canada [8]. It has established CHRP program in partnership with CIHR. This program funds interdisciplinary collaborative projects that benefit the health of Canadians through the translation of the research outcomes to health policy. In 2012–2013 NSERC invested $170.4M in Health and Related Life Sciences Technologies [8].

Genome Canada is the principle proteomics and genomics funding center in Canada and has received $700 million from the government of Canada over the last decade for investment in research. Genome Canada's vision is "To harness the transformative power of genomics to deliver benefits to Canadians." Implementation of this vision is achieved by "(1) Connecting ideas and people across public and private sectors to find new uses and applications for genomics; (2) Investing in large-scale science and technology to fuel innovation; and (3) translating discoveries into applications to maximize impact across all sectors" [9]. Genome Canada invests in large-scale multidisciplinary research projects through a system of international peer review. In 2013–2014 it invested $47.6M in support of research projects, $15.7M for S& T Innovation Centres and $4.8M for base funding of the regional Genome Centres [10]. As part of its mandate it must raise 50 % of the funding required for any project from the investment of partners in the public, not-for-profit, and private sectors in Canada and abroad. In addition to research projects, Genome Canada also continues to build national capacity with leading edge technical platforms which facilitate the design and implementation of more efficient genomic and proteomic methodologies.

3.2 Foundations (Public and Private)

Foundations include charitable or not-for-profit agencies. Private foundations are usually funded by one major source, an individual, a family, or a corporation. Public foundations are usually, funded through multiple sources which includes private foundations, individuals, and government agencies [11]. There are many foundations which provide grants for health research and often their funding is directed toward specific research priorities. A search of the web, lists in the United States alone over 60,000 foundations which provide research grants.

3.3 Private Industry

These include pharmaceutical companies and equipment manufacturers primarily. Often these companies will provide unrestricted grants in response to specific requests for funding. In addition, they also provide contractual funding to academic researchers to conduct randomized controlled trials (RCT) as part of multinational networks.

3.4 Professional Organizations

Professional organizations often provide small amounts of funding often between 10,000 and 45,000 that can be used as seed funding to develop a research question and conduct preliminary work.

A number of mechanisms exist to track calls for proposals. Almost all agencies publish calls for proposals on the web and have online searchable databases which list funding opportunities and identify the research themes, relevant procedures, forms, and deadlines for submission of research proposals for funding. Foundations and corporations also publish annual reports and newsletters which include outlines of funded projects. Professional associations provide information on funding opportunities within their organization and also those available through major funding agencies and foundations, via the web, and periodic newsletter. In addition funded peers within a professional organization can be a valuable source of information on potential sources of funding available. A review of professional literature also can help anticipate new research trends that will be funded. Most academic institutions, research hospitals, and other research institutions provide an annual web-based public report of funded projects which list funding sources and research projects. Memorial University of Newfoundland provides such a report annually http://www.mun.ca/research/publications/matters.php.

4   Budget Development and Justification

A well-thought-out budget is a critical component of a successfully funded project and it must demonstrate the most cost-efficient means to investigate the research question. Funding agencies require a carefully detailed budget and justification summarizing costs and describing why each item in the budget is needed to complete the work outlined in the proposal and the time frame over which the item will be required. In addition, the justification must clearly articulate how the calculations were arrived at for each item. All budgeted items should be adjusted for inflation within the limits of the funding agency guidelines. Agencies often provide a budget template together with a list of guidelines for eligible expenses. These may vary by funding program within an agency. In addition to the requirements and procedures of the funding agency, the investigator should also be aware of his or her institutional policies and guidelines when preparing the budget.

4.1   Direct Costs

Budgets have a number of basic elements in common; these include direct costs which include those required to complete the work outlined in the proposal, such as salaries for personnel, consumables, services, equipment, travel, and renovations.

4.1.1   Personnel

In terms of personnel the number and types of personnel and time allocation calculated in full-time equivalents must be identified annually. Salary and Fringe Benefits costs for each type of personnel required are available from the investigators institution human resources division. Where multiple institutions are involved, this becomes more complex but is required as rates differ across institutions. Fringe benefits rate which include group medical, life, and disability insurance may account of between 20 and 25 % of salary costs depending on the type of personnel. It is also important to be aware of the status of professional bargaining agreements, as renewed agreements are often applied retroactively. This should be factored into budget costs for personnel, particularly since personnel costs may represent between 65 and 75 % of total operating budget.

For each person to be hired, or for each type of personnel required, the justification should include in addition to salary costs, the title the person will have on the project, their name, if known, degree(s), the experience, and expertise the individual brings to the project, as well as a description of the responsibilities of the position.

4.1.2 Services

Many projects include a budget item for services, for example costs for services not part of usual clinical care, such as a specific blood panel or EKG stipulated in the protocol. The fee for service is negotiated in writing with the hospital and the mechanism is put in place for billing the project.

4.1.3 Consumables

Consumables may represent 20–25 % of an operating budget and include lab and office consumables required to do the work. Individual expenses for consumables greater than $1,000 should be justified clearly in the budget.

4.1.4 Equipment

Where lab equipment is an allowable expense, each piece of equipment should be justified with a full explanation of what it will be used for and vendor quotes should be supplied, outlining costs, taxes, shipping, and maintenance agreements. The investigator must also take into account whether basic infrastructure equipment is required such as computers and software, desks and chairs, telephones, and identify what is available in existing office equipment. There are often associated institutional guidelines regarding the purchase of equipment with requirements for tendering for single equipment purchases of $10,000 or greater, which may vary by institution.

4.1.5 Travel

Travel is often required for investigators and trainees for dissemination of results to their peers at academic meetings, and also for the provision of research results back to the community of study participants and their families. This kind of travel may include costs for airfare, taxis, and overnight accommodation and per diem rates. In addition patient travel costs incurred to participate in the study should be included where necessary. Institutional guidelines will determine the rates for per diems, allowable taxi rates, gas, or mileage.

Depending on the funding agency, minor renovations budgets are allowable expenses such as improving existing lab space to accommodate required equipment. These kinds of budgets often have maximum budget threshold defined by the agency. Some types of funding programs are designed entirely for space and large infrastructure proposals, such as the Canada Foundation for Innovation Research Hospital fund.

4.2   Indirect Costs

Indirect costs are associated with infrastructure and include overhead for space and equipment provided by the institutions. These costs are often calculated as a percentage of the total direct costs. Indirect costs are negotiated in advance between the institution and funder, and the rates are often standardized.

5   Reporting and Governance

Following notification of grant approval, which usually takes between 3 and 6 months following submission of the full proposal, the investigator will receive a notice of award together with reviewers' comments. This is generally copied to the institution's Office of Research. The notice of award will outline the approved final budget and if reduced from the original request, the investigator will be asked to adjust the budget allocation appropriately and outline whether the reduction will negatively impact on the scope of work proposed. Upon acceptance of the award by the investigator, the funding agency will release the funding to the institution with certain provisions in place which are covered in a memorandum of understanding between the institution and the funding agency. In the case of CIHR these include the following: (1) Prior to release of funding to the investigator, the institution must ensure that the investigator has full ethics approval to conduct the study and that the required infrastructure is in place. (2) The institution must ensure that expenditures allocated to the grant meet eligibility criteria as defined by the funding agency and by the institution. (3) The institution must provide a financial statement of account to the funding agency 1 month after the fiscal year ends or April 30th for each year of the grant. Funding is released in annual allocations as outlined in the budget.

The investigators and team need to familiarize themselves with the budget, be able to identify eligible and non eligible expenses, and understand the reporting and accounting spreadsheet formats utilized to track and report spending activities and the nature of financial accountability.

Generally, the funding agencies provide one additional year to allow utilization of small amounts of surplus funding remaining at the conclusion of the funding period to allow a wind down phase. The investigators may have further reporting responsibilities to the funding agency and this may require the co-submission of scientific progress reports at the end of each fiscal year and upon completion of the project.

For projects supported by multiple sources, reporting and governance regulations may be much more demanding. In the case of Genome Canada, a collaborative research agreement (CRA) is signed between the institutions and the regional Genome centre. The CRA, in addition to outlining those details above, requires that the investigator and institutions provide very detailed financial statements of accounts to Genome Canada on a quarterly basis as well as details for each of the co-funders' budgeted expenses. A detailed explanation of variance is also required for variances of 15 % or greater from the original budget defined for each activity. Scientific reports outlining progress toward milestones are also required on a quarterly basis. Where multiple sites are involved in such a project it is wise to invest in a project manager who can coordinate these activities. Genome Canada funding is released by the regional Genome Centre on a quarterly basis following review of the reports.

6 Management of Clinical Research Projects

6.1 Overview

Interdisciplinary or multidisciplinary studies have emerged as a means to fuel innovation in research and facilitate scientific progress [11–13]. If funded, the research plan has been clearly articulated and the research team is defined. Key to implementing the plan successfully with large teams is the efficient communication of the research objectives and the budget that is meant to support these. This should be communicated to the entire team, including staff, trainees, collaborators, and co-investigators and each member of the team must understand what their individual and collective responsibilities are. The following sections describe how productive teams can be built and managed effectively to ensure the success of the research project.

6.2 Leadership and Organization

Multisite projects, requires an overall team leader, or principal investigator who directs the project and is responsible for the project. This individual is usually someone who has a proven track record of leading these kinds of studies and has enough time to commit to the study. Large multidisciplinary and multisite projects integrate discipline teams each with its own team leader. In addition to the principal investigator (team leader), each individual site requires a co-investigator who directs site operations.

A clearly defined governance framework is invaluable to the seamless implementation and ongoing oversight of a multisite study comprised of the following components:

6.2.1 Executive Steering Committee

Multisite studies require an executive steering committee which is composed of the Principal investigator and co-investigators [14] and they are responsible for management of the project. They oversee the design, execution, and analysis of the study, and report and communicate the study results in conjunction with the study sponsors.

6.2.2 Scientific Advisory Board

A scientific advisory board with relevant areas of expertise is often put in place to consult with the steering committee on overcoming challenges and barriers to achievement of milestones when necessary.

6.2.3 Clinical Endpoint Committee

For randomized controlled trials a Clinical Endpoint Committee is put in place to adjudicate achievement of study endpoints in an unbiased and consistent manner according to prespecified end point criteria outlined in the trial protocol.

6.2.4 Data Safety and Monitoring Committee

Most funding agencies including NIH and CIHR as well as national health regulatory organizations including the FDA and Health Canada, require the inclusion of a Data Safety and Monitoring Committee (DSMC) for interventional studies (e.g., RCTs) and also for some observational studies (OSMC). For RCTs, the DSMC is responsible for monitoring the quality of the data and evaluating the efficacy and safety of the study intervention, and they will make recommendations to the Executive Committee regarding interim analysis and early termination.

6.2.5 Independent Biostatistics Group

For multinational studies, an independent biostatistics group to support the DSMC through independent analysis of safety and efficacy study data is often put in place.

6.2.6 Central Laboratory and Biobanking

Where biospecimens are collected, a central laboratory is required for biospecimen management, analysis, and biobanking as defined for each of these components under the study protocol.

6.2.7 Study Sites

The study sites are responsible for recruitment of participants, and ethical conduct of the study in accordance with the study protocol and all applicable guidelines.

6.2.8 Data Management

For large multisite studies, a data management center is recommended to integrate data collected and ensure consistent application of pre specified ISO data standards across sites, as well as to ensure ongoing data quality and control. The data management center will ensure confidentiality and privacy of the data is maintained as defined by national and provincial/ or state legislation by the provision to the sites of appropriate data collection and transfer protocols to collect and enter the data to the central platform and transfer data collection documents such as abstraction forms to the DMC for quality control and backup.

Data transfer agreements should be put in place as part of the site agreements defining; ownership of the data, standardized data entry protocols including comprehensive data dictionary and protocols for secure transfer of digital and hardcopy data.

6.2.9 Interactive Voice Response System

Randomization of study participants, assignment of investigational product dosing and drug supply management is handled by an automated interactive voice response system.

In addition to this, a study coordinator or project manager is required who will be responsible for establishing and maintaining ongoing communications between the teams and across sites, and who will have responsibility for monitoring and reporting on progress, ensuring adherence of the sites to the study protocol, and achievement of milestones, as well as identifying challenges and barriers for collaboration between principals. Each site as well will require its own site coordinator responsible for implementing site operations and communication of challenges to the study coordinator.

Hiring team members defined by the roles and mix of skills as outlined in the project proposal must be timely. Successful implementation of the research plan requires an effective communication strategy during study startup which must be led by the executive steering committee of the study. Such a communication strategy should include focused team meetings, a shared network where tasks are assigned, and completion of milestones monitored and acknowledged, and communication between team members is encouraged. Microsoft's SharePoint is a good example of collaborative software that allows sharing of data files by team members via secure web access.

Don't discount the importance of support staff. Clinic-based staff such as nurses or attendants may be the first point of contact to help recruit patients or to notify investigators when a participant is admitted to hospital. Take the time to present your study and orientate these groups to the project. Although they are not paid team members, oftentimes a small contribution to an education fund or the donation of a particular book to their unit will enhance collaboration.

A successful and productive team has to have a collective commitment to a common goal inspired by its leadership to overcome challenges. Working together, a team demonstrates a shared leadership role, individual and mutual accountability, a clearly defined objective that the team delivers, a sense of shared commitment and purpose, collective work products, a work environment that encourages opened ended discussion and active problem solving, and measurement of performance through assessment of collective work-products [15].

6.3 Distribution of Funding

Following the disbursement of funding from the funding agency to the lead institution and ethics approval, funding is released to the principal investigator. An account is established for the investigator to which he can apply eligible expenditures outlined in the budget. Where multiple sites are involved, individual site budgets must be negotiated based on economies of scale, during the grant writing phase. The lead institution provides the collaborating institutions with separate inter-institutional agreements or sub-contracts which outline the site budgets, the scope of work, and the reporting required, authorship guidelines, and data transfer clauses Participating institutions' legal, administrative, and risk management offices will review the agreements and make recommendations for changes to the agreements based on institutional requirements if needed. When this has been completed, the institutional signing authorities, the principal investigator, and the site investigators may complete signing on the agreements. When the lead institution receives confirmation of ethics approvals, funding is released to the sites.

6.4 Training and Orientation

During study startup each component leader and staff member should have received a copy of the study binder which includes the study protocol, a copy of ethics approval, a copy of the budget and copies of any other associated documentation, including data abstraction and collection forms, and study questionnaires. The written protocol should be thought of as the Standard Operating Procedures for the study. Any subsequent protocol changes involving study participants must be reviewed and approved by the site research ethics boards prior to their implementation. The revised protocol must then be circulated to the entire team, and a dated revision of the protocol with (ethics approval) archived to a secure site. It is also useful to include a brief statement regarding why the changes were made, particularly, for studies that span several years. The importance of this documentation is that people who were involved in changing the protocol may move and with them, the rationale for the changes. It is important to keep documented track of protocol changes in this manner because the changes made will need to be identified in the methods section as manuscripts are written, and because it is necessary for the orientation of new staff.

6.5 Ethics

As discussed in another chapter, all research involving human investigation requires application to an ethics board for approval. Multiple site involvement is complex, and timelines for submission must be achieved to ensure all sites startup in as timely a manner as possible. A standardized ethics submission should be prepared by the study coordinator and distributed to the sites with the original protocol and any subsequent amendments. In Canada, most ethics boards have similar requirements and if the coordinating center of a multisite project receives approval, in all likelihood the sites will receive approval as well from their own ethics boards. However, this is not always the case, and it is incumbent on each site coordinator to ensure that the specific guidelines for ethics submissions at each site are followed.

The study coordinator and/or project manager is responsible for maintaining copies of all ethics approvals submitted across sites to ensure institutional and funding agency guidelines are met. In addition each site coordinator must maintain copies of their own site ethics submissions as part of routine study documentation.

For RCT's many ethics boards also require registration of the trial on a publicly available clinical trials registry such as ClinicalTrials.gov. Details of the trial including the sponsorship, list of investigators, purpose, population, sample size, outcomes, and publications are listed. The site documentation for the trial is maintained by the trial coordinator over the life of the study.

6.6 Memorandum of Understanding (MOU)

Verbal agreements between study personnel and departments or institutions may be expedient in getting the project started; however, failure to have a written MOU may prove disastrous later as the project evolves. An MOU may help when people change positions (from intellectual and career perspectives) which may put the project at risk. Therefore, to ensure what is negotiated in the early stages of the project continues throughout its life an MOU should be negotiated. The MOU does not need to be a legal contract involving lawyers, but simple documentation between the team and the agreeing party or institution. The MOU will need to describe what has been agreed upon detailing the contribution for both sides and the duration. If monetary stipulations are also agreed upon at the beginning of the study, it is better to have it documented in an agreement. Also, policies concerning authorship should be recorded at the start of the project.

6.7 Execution of the Research Plan

The implementation phase of a study may take time but the steps taken at this phase should enhance the productivity of the group, and assure completion of the project. This phase of the study is also where the team needs to evaluate whether a pilot study is advisable. Although a pilot study entails added work, time, and expense, the information returned may be invaluable. The findings from the pilot study allow the investigator to determine if the protocol, which may look very good on paper, actually works in the real world. The researchers may find that accessing the participants in the manner they had designed may not be viable. The numbers of study participants planned to enroll may not actually be available, or the protocol may be so complex or time consuming that individuals see it as too difficult and decline to participate. If the study involves asking participants to complete a questionnaire(s), the questionnaire(s) should be piloted on a small sample of individuals other than the study participants. For example, if one plans to send a dietary questionnaire to 150 males who are 75 years of age with colon cancer, one could test the questionnaire on 15 men in the same age group without the condition. This will allow one to determine if specific questions can be answered, or answered in the manner stated by the protocol. This small time saving maneuver may lessen the workload on the research team who may subsequently have to re-contact the study participants to fill in the unanswered questions, or it may prevent finding at study conclusion that that vital information is incomplete. Input from participants at the pilot phase will allow the researchers to evaluate and redesign certain pieces of the study, thereby saving time and energy before initiating the main study.

6.8   Public Relations

Once the project is ready to start it is important to introduce it to the eligible population. It may be helpful to have different component leaders prepare presentations to various community groups to let them know about the study and how they might help. Oftentimes, local newspapers will publish a story on research that is being conducted within the community, or the university information officer might present it in their next bulletin. Other avenues that may help disseminate the study could be the local TV channel, or community groups affiliated with the disease of interest. Getting information regarding the project into the community will help educate potential participants even before direct contact has started.

6.9   Networking

If the study involves enrolling individuals for long term follow up, it is extremely important to maintain contact with them. It may be worthwhile to create a newsletter that could be forwarded to each participant every 6 months. These newsletters could highlight a different member of the team and their involvement, or explain the rationale for a particular blood test. As the project evolves and data is analyzed, results should be provided to participants as they deserve this, and it creates with them, a sense of value and pride.

If the study is a one-time project, a newsletter could be sent at the end of the study as it will demonstrate genuine appreciation for their participation.

6.10   Biospecimen Collection

In large multisite studies, the protocol is written to include standard operating procedures for collection, coding, shipment, and storage of biospecimens to a central lab for analysis. This ensures that analysis of samples is standardized and not impacted by variations in analytical protocol between labs. Data from the central lab is transferred to a centralized database for analysis as defined in the protocol.

6.11   Data Collection and Management

Each team or component leader or his designate is responsible for orientation and training of his team in the relevant sections of the protocol. This ensures consistent application and interpretation of the protocol and ensures standardized collection of data.

Ongoing supervision of staff and oversight of data by the investigator or site coordinator is essential to ensure accuracy of the data. Data is best managed using a secure centralized data platform that allows the maintenance and linkage of large collaborative data sets using ISO data standards. Centralization of the data sets in this manner facilitates quality control of the data, as well as the rapid dissemination of preliminary results. The data set should be maintained and analyzed by those individuals on the team specifically trained to handle the data. Tracking of key variables and interim data analysis also enables early identification of problems [16, 17]. However interim analysis of study outcomes must be preplanned and outlined in the protocol.

6.12 Achievement of Milestones

Achievement of milestones within the timeframe specified in the original proposal may be taken into consideration by the funding agencies during interim review. Feasibility of the study may be questioned if it is impossible to recruit the target number of patients into the study across sites within the given time frame. Therefore the importance of timelines and their linkage to achievement of milestones must be clearly communicated to the sites so that they can identify problems at an early phase.

6.13 Reporting

During the course of the study both financial and scientific progress reports are provided to the funding agencies at least on an annual basis. In addition these reports should be provided to the team as they are useful in identifying and developing strategies for resolving problems that crop up from time to time. In addition to the generation of formal reports, it is important for the full team to meet at least once a year in person together with the stakeholders including funders to review progress While it is cost prohibitive for dispersed inter-disciplinary teams to meet regularly in person, it is productive to meet using a combination of tele- and web conferencing where results can be presented and discussed with the team.

It is important at the outset of a study to establish authorship guidelines through the study steering committee and these are often aligned with funding agency and journal guidelines. All abstracts, presentations, manuscripts should be circulated to the steering committee for review and comment before submission.

Dissemination of study outcomes through peer reviewed publication is essential for the ongoing success of the team and greatly enhances opportunities for further funding. A number of published guidelines, widely endorsed by the scientific community are available to help standardize reporting on a number of study designs. Many high impact journals require that manuscripts submitted for publication follow these guidelines. These guidelines include the Consolidated Standards of Reporting Trials (CONSORT) Statement for reporting randomized trials [18]. The CONSORT statement has the endorsement of over 600 journals.

The Strengthening the Reporting of Observational Studies in Epidemiology (STROBE) Statement. The STROBE statement provides guidelines for reporting cohort, case-control, and cross-sectional designs [19]. The Strengthening the Reporting of Genetic Association Studies (STREGA) [20] this statement builds on the STROBE statement and addresses population stratification, genotyping errors, and the Hardy Weinburg equilibrium, and treatment effects in quantitative traits. Reviewers and editors use these guidelines to assess strengths and weaknesses of the manuscripts submitted and it helps to ensure complete reporting on the part of the authors.

References

1. Reif Lehrer L (1995) Getting funded: it takes more than just a good idea. Scientist 9(14):1

2. Gitlin L, Lyons K (2004) Becoming familiar with funding sources. In: Successful grant writing strategies for health and human service professionals. Springer Publishing Company, New York, pp 35–49

3. Canadian Institutes of Health Research. An overview of CIHR. http://www.cihr-irsc.gc.ca/e/7263.html. Accessed 28 Aug 2014

4. CIHR Internal Assessment_Report for the 2011 International Review. http://www.cihr-irsc.gc.ca/e/43812.html. Accessed 28 Aug 2014

5. CIHR Signature Initiatives. http://www.cihr-irsc.gc.ca/e/43567.html. Accessed 2 Sept 2014

6. CIHR Strategic Initiatives. http://www.cihr-irsc.gc.ca/e/12679.html. Accessed 2 Sept 2014

7. NIH About the NIH. http://www.nih.gov/about/budget.htm. Accessed 2 Sept 2014

8. Natural Science and Engineering Council of Canada. http://www.nserc-crsng.gc.ca/NSERC-CRSNG/vision-vision_eng.asp. Accessed 28 Aug 2014

9. Genome Canada. Mandate and objectives. http://www.genomecanada.ca/en/about/news.aspx?i=505. Accessed 28 Aug 2014

10. Genome Canada Annual Report. http://www.genomecanada.ca/medias/PDF/EN/annual_report_2014/index.html. Accessed 2 Sept 2014

11. Pearce C (2003) Managing the multisite team. In: Hawkins J, Haggerty L (eds) Diversity in Health Care Research: Strategies for Multisite, Multidisciplinary, and Multicultural Projects. Springer Publishing Company New York, pp 81–115

12. Horwitz A (2003) Building bridges through collaboration – a pathway for interdisciplinary research. Trends Cell Biol 13(1):2–3

13. Metzger N, Zare R (1999) Interdisciplinary research: from belief to reality. Science 283(5402):642–643

14. Altshuler J, Altshuler D (2004) Organizational challenges in clinical genomic research. Nature 429(6990):478–481

15. Stone KS (1991) Collaboration. In: Mateo MA, Kirchhoff KT (eds) Conducting and using nursing research in the clinical setting. Williams & Wilkins, Baltimore, pp 58–68

16. Katzenbach J, Smith D (1998) The discipline of teams. In: Katzenbach J (ed) The work of teams Harvard Business School Publishing. Boston MA USA, pp 35–49

17. Selby-Harrington M, Donat P, Hibbard H (1993) Guidance for managing a research grant. Nurs Res 41(1):54–58

18. Moher D, Hopewell S, Schulz K, Monton V, Gotzsche P, Devereaux P, Elbourne D, Egger M, Altman D (2010) J Clin Epidemiol 63:1–37

19. von Elm E, Altman D, Egger M, Pocock S, Gotzsche P, Vandenbroucke J (2007) The strengthening of the reporting of observational studies in epidemiology (STROBE) statement: guidelines for reporting observational studies. Lancet 370:1453–1457

20. Little J, Higgins J, Ioannidis J, Moher D, Gagnon F, von Elm E, Khoury M, Cohen B, Davey-Smith G, Grimshaw J, Scheet P, Gwinn M, Williamson R, Zou G, Hutchings K, Johnson C, Tait V, Wiens M, Golding J, van-Duijn C, McLaughlin J, Paterson A, Wells G, Fortier I, Freedman M, Zecevic M, King R, Infante-Rivard C, Stewart A, Birkett N (2009) STrengthening the REporting of Genetic Association Studies (STREGA) – an extension of the STROBE statement. Eur J Clin Invest 39:247–266

Part IV

The Basics for Other Clinical Epidemiology Methods

Chapter 17

Evaluation of Diagnostic Tests

John M. Fardy and Brendan J. Barrett

Abstract

As technology advances, diagnostic tests continue to improve, and each year we are presented with new alternatives to standard procedures. Given the plethora of diagnostic alternatives, diagnostic tests must be evaluated to determine their place in the diagnostic armamentarium. The first step involves determining the accuracy of the test, including the sensitivity and specificity, positive and negative predictive values, likelihood ratios for positive and negative tests, and receiver operating characteristic (ROC) curves. The role of the test in a diagnostic pathway has then to be determined, following which the effect on patient outcome should be examined.

Key words Diagnostic tests, Sensitivity, Specificity, Positive predictive value, Negative predictive value, Likelihood ratio, Receiver operating characteristic curve

1   Introduction

Diagnostic tests are used to increase the likelihood of the presence or absence of illness, to provide prognostic information and, in some situations, to predict a response to treatment. The ability of a diagnostic test to identify a potential underlying disorder depends not only on the characteristics of the test itself, but also on the particular situation in which it is used. The prevalence of the disease in the population and the spectrum of the disease being sought may influence the way a diagnostic test performs. In this chapter the characteristics of diagnostic tests will be examined together with how these characteristics can be used to choose the most useful diagnostic tests.

In order to determine the accuracy of a diagnostic test, an arbiter is necessary to decide whether the test result is correct or not. This is known as the "gold standard" or reference standard. In some instances the "gold standard" is an established test or combination of tests which confirms the diagnosis, while in other cases the "gold standard" requires follow-up over time to confirm or refute the diagnosis. When considering the characteristics of a diagnostic test,

Patrick S. Parfrey and Brendan J. Barrett (eds.), *Clinical Epidemiology: Practice and Methods*, Methods in Molecular Biology, vol. 1281, DOI 10.1007/978-1-4939-2428-8_17, © Springer Science+Business Media New York 2015

one must consider the "gold standard" to which it is compared and determine whether or not it is an appropriate one. The comparison to the "gold standard" should be carried out in a blinded fashion so as to prevent bias in the interpretation of the diagnostic test or the reference standard. Further issues in the design of diagnostic accuracy studies are discussed in a later section.

In the past, assessment of diagnostic tests might have been limited to studies of accuracy, but it is now well recognized that tests form part of a diagnostic pathway. Test results are used to alter the probability of diagnoses in the context of what is already known about the case and the results of other tests that might have been completed at the same time. There is recognition that the results of groups of tests may not be independent. As such, the specific contribution of a particular test needs to be determined. This has recently been discussed by Moons and colleagues, where the information gain from adding a test can be quantified in terms of an increase in the area under the ROC curve (*see* below), net reclassification improvement, or by decision curve analysis [1]. Furthermore following studies of the clinical validity of a test, the clinical utility of the test then needs to be established [2]. There has been much recent literature on the best approach to assessing the clinical utility of tests. Such evaluations may include learning about the full range of effects of tests on patients: psychological, behavioral, and social effects together with the impact of subsequent therapies on longer term health outcomes [3].

2   Diagnostic Test Accuracy Criteria

2.1   Sensitivity and Specificity

The classic parameters used to characterize a diagnostic test are the sensitivity and specificity of the test. The sensitivity of a test refers to its ability to identify persons with the disease. It can be defined as "the proportion of people who truly have a designated disorder who are so identified by the test" [4]. A very sensitive test is one which identifies most people with the disorder in question. A test which is very sensitive is prone to false positive results, i.e., it may incorrectly label people as having the disease when, in fact, they do not have it.

The specificity of a test, on the other hand, refers to its ability to correctly identify the disease in question. It can be defined as "the proportion of people who are truly free of a designated disorder who are so identified by the test" [4]. A very specific test would be unlikely to incorrectly label an individual as having the disorder in question if, in fact, they do not have the disorder. However, a test which is very specific is more prone to false negative results, i.e., it may fail to identify the disease in some persons who actually have it.

Table 1
Assessment of diagnostic tests using 2 × 2 contingency table

		Gold standard		
		Positive	Negative	Total
New test	Positive	True positive a	b False positive	a+b
	Negative	False negative c	d True negative	c+d
	Total	a+c	b+d	

Sensitivity: a/(a+c), Positive predictive value: a/(a+b)
Specificity: d/(b+d), Negative predictive value: d/(c+d)

There is always a trade-off between sensitivity and specificity; as one increases, the other tends to decrease [5]. The higher the cut-off used to say a test is positive, the more specific the test becomes, but this higher specificity comes at a price. As the cut-off is increased, the sensitivity decreases and the test is more likely to miss affected individuals. In some situations, such as screening for a disease, a lower cut-off might be used to create a very sensitive test so as not to miss anyone with the disorder in question. In other situations, when using a test to confirm a diagnosis, a higher cut-off making the test highly specific would be more desirable so as not to incorrectly label anyone with the disorder.

The sensitivity and specificity of a diagnostic test can be calculated using information obtained by comparing the performance of a diagnostic test to a gold standard or reference standard. Typically these results are summarized in a 2 × 2 contingency table as shown in Table 1. Such tables can of course be extended to illustrate the distribution of data at different test cut-offs. Sensitivity and specificity are not directly influenced by disease prevalence, but are affected by the disease severity spectrum. A test that is sensitive for detection of advanced disease may be less sensitive for detection of earlier stages. An example would be the Chest X-Ray for detection of lung cancer.

2.2 Positive and Negative Predictive Values

The sensitivity and specificity of a diagnostic test are useful to describe how well a test performs, but they do not give us much information on the significance of a positive or negative test for an individual patient. This information can be obtained from the positive and negative predictive values of the test. The positive predictive value describes "the proportion of people with a positive test who have the disease" [5]. Similarly, the negative predictive value describes "the proportion of people with a negative test who are free of disease" [5]. These ratios are calculated across the table rather than down the table using the formulae in Table 1. These parameters are more useful to the clinician and the patient as they give the predictive value of a positive and a negative test. A test with a high positive predictive value makes the disease quite likely in a subject with a positive test. A test with a high negative predictive value makes the disease quite unlikely in a subject with a negative test.

Although the positive and negative predictive values of a test are intuitively more useful to the clinician and patient, the predictive values are less stable and are dependent on the prevalence of disease. This makes them less portable from population to population. It also means that positive and negative predictive values derived from a study may not apply to any given patient if that patient's pre-test probability of disease differs from the prevalence of the disease in the study sample.

2.3 Case Study

Let's take a hypothetical new test used to rapidly detect an infectious process usually diagnosed by a culture technique which may take up to a month to provide a result (this is the case for several newer tests for tuberculosis). In a cohort of affected and unaffected subjects in which the prevalence of disease is 50 %, how does the new test compare to the culture technique? The results in Table 2 show a new test with excellent sensitivity and good specificity. This test would be a good screening test and a reasonable confirmatory test. The positive predictive value of 82 % and the negative predictive value of 88 % suggest the new test is quite beneficial to patients and doctors.

However, if the prevalence of the disease is 10 % instead of 50 %, and the sensitivity and specificity are the same, the positive and negative predictive values change as shown in Table 3. Although the negative predictive value has increased from 88 to 98 %, the positive predictive value has dropped to 33 %. This test which was initially a very good predictor of disease when prevalence was 50 %, has much poorer positive predictive value when the disease prevalence drops to 10 %. In fact, with lower disease prevalence, the test produces twice as many false positives as true positives. In general, diagnostic tests will function most efficiently

Table 2

Assessment of a new diagnostic test when prevalence of disease is 50 %

		Gold standard		
		Positive	Negative	Total
New test	Positive	45 (a)	10 (b)	55
	Negative	5 (c)	40 (d)	45
	Total	50	50	100

Prevalence of disease = 50/100 = 50 %

Sensitivity = a/(a+c) = 45/50 = 90 %

Specificity = d/(b+d) = 40/50 = 80 %

Positive predictive value = a/(a+b) = 45/55 = 82 %

Negative predictive value = d/(c+d) = 40/45 = 88 %

Table 3
Assessment of a new diagnostic test when prevalence of disease is 10 %

		Gold Standard		
		Positive	Negative	Total
New Test	Positive	45 (a)	90 (b)	135
	Negative	5 (c)	360 (d)	365
	Total	50	450	500

Prevalence of disease = 50/500 = 10 %
Sensitivity = a/(a+c) = 45/50 = 90 %
Specificity = d/(b+d) = 360/450 = 80 %
Positive Predictive Value = a/(a+b) = 45/135 = 33 %
Negative predictive value = c/(c+d) = 360/365 = 98 %

when the prevalence (or pre-test probability) is between 40 and 60 % and provide much less information at the extremes of pre-test probability [5].

2.4 Likelihood Ratios

The ideal test parameter would be one which has predictive value and is stable with changes in prevalence. The likelihood ratio is such a parameter. A likelihood ratio expresses the relative odds that a given level of a diagnostic test result would be expected in a patient with (as opposed to one without) the target disorder [4]. As with the other parameters, likelihood ratios are calculated from the 2×2 table.

Likelihood ratio for a positive test

$$LR+ = (a \, / \, a+c) \, / \, (b \, / \, b+d) = \text{sensitivity} \, / \, (-1 \, \text{specificity})$$

Likelihood ratio for a negative test

$$LR- = (c \, / \, a+c) \, / \, (d \, / \, b+d) = (-1 \, \text{sensitivity}) \, / \, \text{specificity}$$

Because the likelihood ratios are calculated from the sensitivity and specificity, they are also stable with changes in prevalence of disease. The predictive value of the likelihood ratio calculates the post-test odds of disease from the pre-test odds of disease using the following formula:

$$\text{Post} - \text{test odds} = \text{Pre} - \text{test odds} \times LR+$$

The pre-test odds of disease are similar to the pre-test probability of disease and can be calculated with the following formula:

$$\text{Pre} - \text{test odds} = \text{Pretest probability} \, / \, (-1 \, \text{Pre} - \text{test probability})$$

The pre-test probability of disease is usually estimated from the clinical information or from published reports.

A diagnostic test with likelihood ratios near unity does not have much effect on the post-test probability of disease and therefore is not very useful for decision making. On the other hand, very large LR+ or very small likelihood LR- ratios have a significant impact on the post-test probability of disease. An LR for a positive test of 10 or more means that a positive test is good at ruling in a diagnosis while an LR for a negative test of 0.1 or less means that a negative test is good at ruling out a diagnosis [6]. Likelihood ratios between 5 and 10 if test positive or 0.1–0.2 if test negative lead to moderate changes in the post-test probability while those between 2 and 5 (0.2–0.5) lead to smaller changes.

The use of likelihood ratios to characterize diagnostic tests highlights the importance of the pre-test probability of disease in the performance of a diagnostic test. If the pre-test probability of disease is very high or very low, a diagnostic test will have to be very good to make a significant difference in the post-test probability of disease. Diagnostic tests will perform best when the pre-test probability of disease is about 50 % and generally will perform less well at the extremes of pre-test probability [5]. If the pre-test probability of disease is so high or so low as to rule in or rule out a diagnosis, a diagnostic test is not warranted [6].

2.5 Overall Test Accuracy

These various parameters used to characterize diagnostic tests can help in choosing one test over another, but they do not provide a summary estimate of the accuracy of the test. The receiver operating characteristic (ROC) curve can be used for this purpose. An ROC curve is a plot of test sensitivity (plotted on the y axis) versus its false positive rate ($1 -$ specificity) (plotted on the x axis) [7]. As the cut-off value for a positive test is moved up or down, the sensitivity and specificity of the test change. Figure 1 is an example of an ROC curve for a hypothetical diagnostic test. In this example, raising the cut-off value would lead to high specificity and low sensitivity, with coordinates toward the lower left hand corner of the curve. Lowering the cut-off value for a positive test would lead to a progressive increase in sensitivity and a progressive decrease in specificity moving up along the curve toward the upper right hand corner. The point on the curve closest to the upper left hand corner (which represents 100 % sensitivity and 100 % specificity) would represent the cut-off value which offers the best balance between sensitivity and specificity. This may not always be the best cut-off to choose, depending on the purpose of the test. For a screening test, sensitivity would be favored over specificity, while for a confirmatory test specificity would be favored over sensitivity. In general one needs to consider the clinical impact of false positive and false negative test results and weigh these against each other to determine the most useful cutoff for any given context.

The ROC curve also provides information on the overall accuracy of the diagnostic test. The area under the ROC curve (the area

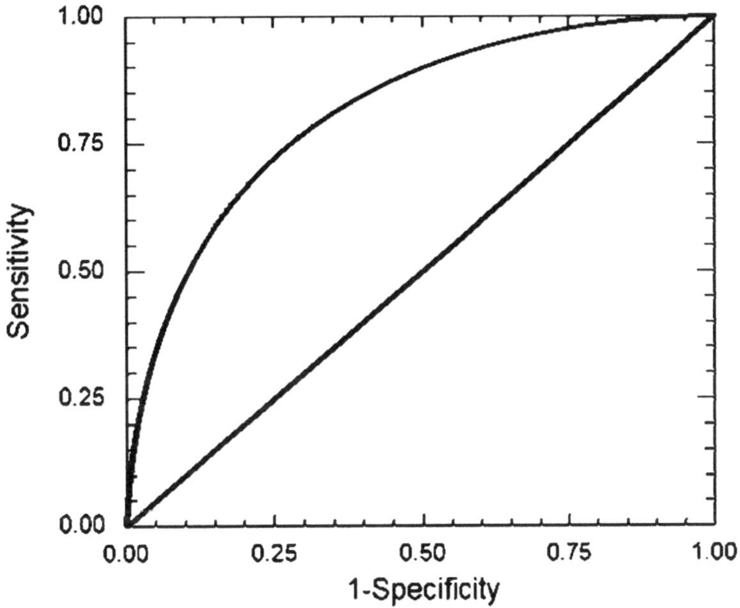

Fig. 1 Receiver operating characteristic (ROC) curve for assessing diagnostic tests

to the right of the curved line in Fig. 1) is a popular measure of the accuracy of a diagnostic test [7]. The ROC curve area can take on values between 0.0 and 1.0, with an area of 1.0 representing a perfectly accurate test. A test with an area of 0.0 is perfectly inaccurate; all patients with the disease have negative results, while all those without the disease have positive results. Such a test would have perfect accuracy if the interpretation of the test were reversed. Therefore, the practical lower bound for the area under the ROC curve is 0.5, which is bounded by the straight line from coordinates 0,0 to 1,1. This line is known as the chance diagonal on an ROC plot [7]. The area under the ROC curve can be used to compare the accuracy of diagnostic tests. It should be noted that in a given study the area under the curve is an estimate with an associated standard error. This can be used to calculate confidence intervals around the estimated area and is also used when the areas under the ROC curves associated with different tests are being compared. Both parametric and nonparametric statistical procedures exist to compare areas under ROC curves, including adjustments for paired samples if the two tests being compared were completed within the same subjects [8, 9].

If the concern is the accuracy of a test, the percentage of patients correctly classified by the test under evaluation can be assessed. In Table 1, accuracy can be calculated as follows:

$$\text{Accuracy} : (a + d) / (a + b + c + d)$$

Unfortunately, the overall accuracy is highly dependent on the prevalence of the disease. Another option for a single indicator of test performance is the diagnostic odds ratio (DOR). This is the ratio of the odds of positivity in the diseased relative to the odds of positivity in the nondiseased [10]. Like the odds ratio in any 2×2 table it is calculated using the following formula:

$$DOR = ad \: / \: bc$$

There is also a close relationship between the DOR and the likelihood ratios:

$$DOR = LR + /LR - (10)$$

The value of the DOR ranges from 0 to infinity with higher values associated with better performance of a diagnostic test. A value of 1 suggests that a test does not discriminate well between those with and without the target disorder, while values lower than 1 suggest improper interpretation of the diagnostic test (more negative tests among the diseased). As with likelihood ratios, the DOR is not dependent on the prevalence of disease, but like sensitivity and specificity is influenced by the disease spectrum in the study population [10]. The DOR can also be useful in meta-analysis of diagnostic studies.

In all of the previous discussion it has been assumed that the reference or "gold" standard will yield a binary outcome of disease presence or absence. However this is not always the case, as for example when echocardiographically determined left ventricular mass as a continuous measure serves as the reference standard when evaluating features of the ECG as a diagnostic test. In that case, a different statistical approach has been proposed for estimating sensitivity, specificity and the ROC curve [11]. An alternate approach using information theoretical concepts also permits consideration of quantitative reference results while explicitly taking into account variation in pre-test probabilities [12].

In addition the reference standard itself may not always be perfect, and in that situation the use of Bayesian Latent Class Models can allow evaluation of novel tests [13–15]. Recently a Web-based application has been developed to allow the less statistically accomplished researcher to complete the required analyses via a user-friendly interface [16].

3   Design of Diagnostic Accuracy Studies

Given the various tools available, how would one set out to evaluate a new diagnostic test? The criteria have been discussed in standard textbooks of clinical epidemiology and are outlined below [4, 5]. These criteria center around a blinded evaluation of the new test versus a "gold standard" in an appropriate population. The reproducibility and the interpretation of the test should be standardized and the test procedure should be well described. Finally, the clinical utility should be documented.

The importance of a blinded evaluation of the diagnostic test versus the reference standard is paramount in the evaluation of a new diagnostic test. Knowledge of the results of either the diagnostic test or the reference standard could lead to bias when interpreting the results of the other. Lack of a blinded comparison would invalidate the results of the study.

The population chosen for study is also a critical factor in the assessment of a diagnostic test. Test performance will vary with disease prevalence and with disease severity, such that diagnostic test performance often varies across population subgroups [17]. The sample population chosen for evaluation of the diagnostic test should be similar to the population for which the test is intended, in terms of both the prevalence and severity of the disease. The comparison group should be comprised of individuals from that group, those suspected of having the target disorder but not actually having the disease as opposed to "normal" individuals. In essence, the test should be evaluated under the same conditions that it will be used. Assessing test accuracy in samples selected to include cases with obvious or severe disease as well as healthy controls will tend to overestimate the accuracy of the test under routine conditions.

In studies of the accuracy of diagnostic tests, it is important that all members of the sample population undergo both the test being assessed as well as the "gold standard". In a systematic review of the sources of bias and variation in diagnostic test accuracy studies, Whiting and colleagues found that use of a case-control design, observer variability, availability of clinical information, choice of reference standard, disease prevalence, and severity as well as verification biases were the major sources with generally greater impact on the estimate of sensitivity than specificity [18]. Methods for determining sample size for studies of the accuracy of diagnostic tests are tailored to the particular indices which are being studied. Sample size estimates can be calculated for several accuracy indices including sensitivity and specificity, the area under the receiver operating characteristic curve, the sensitivity at a fixed false positive rate, and the likelihood ratio [19].

The reproducibility of the test should also be evaluated particularly when it involves a subjective interpretation of the results. Both the inter-observer and intra-observer variation should be examined and evaluated with an appropriate measure, such as a kappa statistic, which reveals the degree of agreement between test readers. The test procedure should be well described so that it can be replicated by others. As well, there may be a significant learning curve associated with the interpretation of a new diagnostic test and this must be taken into account as the test is evaluated.

Given the plethora of studies that may exist evaluating the accuracy of a given diagnostic test, there has been interest in completion of diagnostic test accuracy systematic reviews and meta-analyses. The challenges involved have been addressed by a Cochrane Methods group [20]. Tools were developed to assess the quality of the constituent studies [21, 22]. Challenges are often posed by heterogeneity in the design, setting, and results of the various primary studies. Care needs to be taken when formulating the questions for the systematic review.

4   Factors Relevant to the Choice of Diagnostic Tests

The choice of diagnostic tests is certainly influenced by test performance, but this is not the only important factor to be considered. Although a Ferrari may outperform the competition, its cost and seating capacity may make it unsuitable for the job at hand. In choosing a diagnostic test one must consider, in addition to test performance, the cost, availability, acceptability, and utility of the diagnostic test. A practical hierarchy can be defined based on (1) diagnostic power or performance, (2) availability and acceptability where considered relevant, and (3) cost [23].

Cost and availability are obvious concerns when one considers the choice of diagnostic tests. A very expensive test with limited availability would have to outperform standard tests by a wide margin before it could be considered for routine use. The acceptability of the diagnostic test is also a major concern, particularly for the patient. An invasive test with potentially serious complications will not be accepted readily by patients, particularly if there is a safer, noninvasive alternative. One must also consider that information produced in research about diagnostic tests is utilized by several different types of decision makers who are interested in different types of information [24]. Policy-making organizations will be more concerned with the "evidence-based" assessment and cost of testing, while patients may place more emphasis on anecdotal experience and the reassurance value of testing. Physicians will typically find themselves acting as representatives of the medical profession and its body of knowledge, and as advocates for each patient [24].

The final arbiter in the choice of diagnostic tests is the clinical utility of the test under scrutiny. Studies of diagnostic test accuracy may, on their own, provide sufficient information to infer clinical value if a new diagnostic test is safer or more specific than the old test, provided both are of similar sensitivity and that treatment based on results of the old test has been shown to improve patient outcomes in clinical trials [25]. Establishing whether a new test improves patient outcomes beyond the outcomes achieved using an older test or maybe no test prior to treatment may require the completion of randomized trials. A randomized trial can assess the outcomes of patients undergoing testing, document adverse effects, and assess impact on management decision making and measure patient satisfaction and the cost-effectiveness of testing [26]. A variety of randomized designs have been proposed with the choice among them depending upon the objective of testing and whether alternative test/treat strategies are to be compared [27]. A framework for evaluating the links and mechanisms whereby outcomes are impacted in diagnostic test/treat trials has been proposed [28]. Concerns have been raised about the efficiency of some designs proposed for test/treat trials. It has been suggested that in the case where two tests are being compared in terms of clinical utility, a paired design in which each participant undergoes both tests with subsequent treatment only randomly assigned when the test results are discordant may be more efficient [29]. Sample size formulae for binary and continuous outcomes have also been proposed by the same authors [29]. Ethical issues that arise in relation to these trials include the need for equipoise, not so much with regard to the relative accuracy of tests, but rather with regard to the comparative health impact of alternative test/ treat strategies. In addition if a clustered design is followed, there is a need for those who decline participation to be aware that the whole diagnostic process in a particular clinic or hospital, for example, may be influenced by the assignment of that site to a novel test/treat strategy for the trial [30].

As commonly done in economic analyses, decision models can also be used to compare various test/treat strategies, but the results depend critically on the accuracy of the assumptions and estimates used to build and inform the models [3].

5 Conclusion

Diagnostic test performance can be measured using a number of different instruments which assess the accuracy and predictive value of the tests. The choice of diagnostic tests, however, is more complex than a simple assessment of performance, and consideration of broader issues such as patient outcomes, acceptability, and cost-effectiveness of testing is necessary. By using the appropriate criteria to assess diagnostic test performance, followed by randomized trials to measure clinical utility, the choice of the best diagnostic test to solve a diagnostic problem can be made.

References

1. Moons KGM, deGroot JAH, Linnet K, Reitsma JB, Bossuyt PMM (2012) Quantifying the added value of a diagnostic test or marker. Clin Chem 58(10):1408–1417

2. Linnet K, Bossuyt PMM, Moons KGM, Reitsma JB (2012) Quantifying the accuracy of a diagnostic test or marker. Clin Chem 58(9):1292–1301

3. Bossuyt PMM, Reitsma JB, Linnet K, Moons KGM (2012) Beyond diagnostic accuracy: the clinical utility of diagnostic tests. Clin Chem 58(12):1636–1643

4. Guyatt G, Drummond R, Meade MO, Cook DJ (eds) (2008) Users' guides to the medical literature: a manual for evidence-based clinical practice, 2nd edn. McGraw Hill, New York, NY

5. Haynes RB, Sackett DL, Guyatt GH, Tugwell P (2005) Clinical epidemiology: how to do clinical practice research, 3rd edn. Lippincott, Williams and Wilkins, Philadelphia, PA

6. Grimes D, Schulz K (2005) Refining clinical diagnosis with likelihood ratios. Lancet 365: 1500–1505

7. Obuchowski NA (2003) Receiver operating characteristic curves and their use in radiology. Radiology 229:3–8

8. Hanley JA, McNeil BJ (1983) A method of comparing the areas under receiver operating characteristic curves derived from the same cases. Radiology 148:839–843

9. DeLong ER, DeLong DM, Clarke-Pearson DL (1988) Comparing the areas under two or more correlated receiver operating curves: a nonparametric approach. Biometrics 44:837–845

10. Glas SG, Lijmer JG, Prins MH et al (2003) The diagnostic odds ratio: a single indicator of test performance. J Clin Epidemiol 56: 1129–1135

11. Shiu S-Y, Gatsonis C (2012) On ROC analysis with nonbinary reference standard. Biom J 54(4):457480

12. Reibnegger G (2013) Beyond the 2×2 contingency table: a primer on entropies and mutual information in various scenarios involving m diagnostic categories and n categories of diagnostic tests. Clin Chim Acta 425:97–103

13. Joseph L, Gyorkos TW, Coupal L (1995) Bayesian estimation of disease prevalence and the parameters of diagnostic tests in the absence of a gold standard. Am J Epidemiol 141(3): 263–272

14. Limmathurotsakul D, Turner EL, Wuthiekanun V, Thaipadungpanit J, Suputtamongkol Y, Chierakul W et al (2012) Fool's gold: why imperfect reference tests are undermining the evaluation of novel diagnostics: A reevaluation of 5 diagnostic tests for leptospirosis. CID 55:322–331

15. Pan-ngum W, Blacksell SD, Lubell Y, Pukrittayakamee S, Bailey MS, deSilva HJ et al (2013) Estimating the true accuracy of diagnostic tests for Dengue infection using Bayesian latent class models. PLoS One 8(1):1–7

16. Lim C, Wannapinij P, White L, Day NPJ, Cooper BS, Peacock SJ et al (2013) Using a web-based application to define the accuracy of diagnostic tests when the gold standard is imperfect. PLoS One 8(11):1–8

17. Mullherin SA, Miller MC (2002) Spectrum bias or spectrum effect? Subgroup variation in diagnostic test evaluation. Ann Intern Med 137:598–602

18. Whiting PF, Rutjes AWS, Westwood ME, Mallett S, QUADAS-2 Steering Group (2013) A systematic review classifies sources of bias and variation in diagnostic test accuracy studies. J Clin Epi 66:1093–1104

19. Obuchowski NA (1998) Sample size calculations in studies of test accuracy. Stat Methods Med Res 7:371–392

20. Leeflang MMG, Deeks JJ, Takwoingi Y, Macaskill P (2013) Cochrane diagnostic accuracy reviews. Syst Rev 2(82):1–6

21. Schünemann HJ, Oxman AD, Brozek J, Glasziou P, Jaeschke R, Vist GE, Williams JW Jr, Kunz R, Craig J, Montori VM, Bossuyt P, Guyatt GH, GRADE Working Group (2008) Grading quality of evidence and strength of recommendations for diagnostic tests and strategies. BMJ 336(7653):1106–10

22. Whiting PF, Rutjes AWS, Westwood ME, Mallett S, Deeks JJ, Reitsma JB et al (2011) QUADAS-2: A revised tool for the quality assessment of diagnostic accuracy studies. Ann Intern Med 155:529–536

23. Knottnerus JA, Muris JW (2003) Assessment of the accuracy of diagnostic tests: the cross-sectional study. J Clin Epidemiol 56:1118–1128

24. Ransohoff DF (2002) Challenges and opportunities in evaluating diagnostic tests. J Clin Epidemiol 55:1178–1182

25. Lord SJ, Irwig LE, Simes RJ (2006) When is measuring sensitivity and specificity sufficient to evaluate a diagnostic test, and when do we need randomized trials? Ann Intern Med 144: 850–855

26. Rodger M, Ramsay T, Fergusson D (2012) Diagnostic randomized controlled trials: the final frontier. Trials 13(137):1–7

27. Lijmer J, Bossuyt PMM (2009) Various randomized designs can be used to evaluate medical tests. J Clin Epidemiol 62:364–373

28. di Ruffano LV, Hyde CJ, McCaffrey KJ, Bossuyt PMM, Deeks JJ (2012) Assessing the value of diagnostic tests: a framework for designing and evaluating trials. BMJ 344(e686):1–9

29. Lu B, Gatsonis C (2012) Efficiency of study designs in diagnostic randomized clinical trials. Stat Med 32(9):1451–1466

30. Dowdy DW, Gounder CR, Corbett EL, Ngwira LG, Chaisson RE, Merritt MW (2012) The ethics of testing a test: randomized trials of the health impact of diagnostic tests for infectious diseases. CID 55:1522–1526

Chapter 18

Qualitative Research in Clinical Epidemiology

Deborah M. Gregory and Christine Y. Way

Abstract

This chapter has been written to specifically address the usefulness of qualitative research for the practice of clinical epidemiology. The methods of grounded theory to facilitate understanding of human behavior and construction of monitoring scales for use in quantitative studies are discussed. In end-stage renal disease patients receiving long-term hemodialysis, a qualitative study used grounded theory to generate a multilayered classification system, which culminated in a substantive theory on *living with end-stage renal disease and hemodialysis*. The qualitative data base was re-visited for the purpose of scale development and led to the Patient Perception of Hemodialysis Scale (PPHS). The quantitative study confirmed that the PPHS was psychometrically valid and reliable and supported the major premises of the substantive theory.

Key words Clinical epidemiology, Grounded theory, Instrument development, Qualitative research

---

1 Using Qualitative Research Methods in Clinical Epidemiology

Over the past decade, the discipline of clinical epidemiology focused on evidence-based medicine and evidence-based health policy themes. Greater interest in qualitative research methods accompanied this trend [1] and can be partially attributed to the increased recognition given the role of psychosocial factors in shaping health outcomes. Focusing on physiological manifestations of disease to the exclusion of the total illness experience—behavioral, social, psychological, and emotional—is a rather limited view of what it means to live with a chronic illness. The primary objective of qualitative inquiry is to reconstruct the richness and diversity of individuals' experiences in a manner that maintains its integrity (i.e., the truth value). As such, qualitative findings may be used to identify clinical areas requiring consideration and, in turn, facilitate the development of appropriate and timely interventions for modifying or resolving problem areas.

Certain basic assumptions differentiate qualitative from quantitative modes of inquiry. Although both types of inquiries use a variety of methodological approaches to generate data about

Patrick S. Parfrey and Brendan J. Barrett (eds.), *Clinical Epidemiology: Practice and Methods*, Methods in Molecular Biology, vol. 1281, DOI 10.1007/978-1-4939-2428-8_18, © Springer Science+Business Media New York 2015

individuals' experiences with events and situations, quantitative studies are concerned with explaining a phenomenon, whereas qualitative studies are interested in understanding and interpreting it. As well, objectivity and generalizability are the goals of quantitative science versus the subjectivity and contextualization goals of qualitative science.

For researchers committed to the scientific paradigm of knowledge development, concerns with interpretive methods relate to the perceived shortcomings of objectivity, reliability, and validity versus the espoused rigor of the experimental method. A guarded acceptance of evidence from qualitative studies has been recommended until better guidelines are devised for data collection and analysis [2]. However, this is an inaccurate representation because there are explicit rules for enhancing the rigor and adequacy of qualitative inquires [3, 4].

Divergent philosophical traditions guiding qualitative researchers is one reason why one group may argue for precise quality criteria to assess rigor [5] and another group view such restrictions as limiting access to the full richness and diversity of individuals' experiences [6, 7]. Most qualitative researchers operate somewhere in between this divide. In a review of validity criteria for qualitative research, Whittemore, Chase, and Mandle [4] argued that rigor can be combined with subjectivity and creativity if flexible criteria exist to support the basic tenets of interpretive research. Relevant criteria highlighted by the authors included credibility and authenticity (accurate reflection of experiences and differing or comparable subtleties within groups), criticality and integrity (critical appraisal that involves checking and rechecking to ensure data interpretations are true and valid), auditability or explicitness (specification of a decision trial in method and interpretation for other researchers to follow), vividness (capturing the richness of the data while striving for parsimony, so informed readers can appreciate the logic), creativity (imaginative but grounded in the data), thoroughness (sampling and data adequacy to ensure full development of themes and connectedness among them), congruence (logical link between question, method, and findings), and sensitivity (ethical considerations). The authors also highlighted techniques that could facilitate application of these criteria and lessen validity threats during study design (method and sampling decisions), data collection, and analysis (clarity and thoroughness, member checks, and literature reviews, among others), and presentation of findings (audit trail, rich, and insightful descriptions).

2 Grounded Theory Methodology

Grounded theory methodology was developed by Glaser and Strauss [8] and later refined by Glaser [9, 10] and Strauss and Corbin [11]. The primary objective of this method is to facilitate greater understanding of human behavior and interactions within variant and similar contexts. The inductive-deductive approach to studying phenomena is focused on generating as opposed to testing theory. As conceptualized by Glaser and Strauss, substantive theory is seen as emerging from a substantive area of inquiry. For example, a substantive theory could be generated from exploring common perceptions shared by individuals comprising distinct clinical groups: patients with end-stage renal disease (ESRD) on long-term hemodialysis or members of families with the germ-line mutation for hereditary nonpolyposis colorectal cancer (HNPCC).

The strength of grounded theory is that the interest is not on merely describing how individuals experience a particular phenomenon like some qualitative approaches. What makes it unique is the emphasis placed on identifying and describing the social–psychological processes grounded in the emergent data. That is, the focus is not solely with how illnesses, diagnostic procedures, or treatment protocols are experienced but rather how information about them is received and assimilated into existing belief structures in a way that becomes a stimulant for desired behavior, and makes it possible to achieve optimal health functioning.

The key differentiating features of the method warrant consideration. First, grounded theory involves the simultaneous collection of data through interviews and its analysis. This concurrent approach allows the researcher to use the constant comparative method of analysis to compare and interpret each piece of data with other pieces within and among interview transcripts until codes are refined and collapsed, outlier cases considered and rejected, and the groundwork laid for formulating substantive theory. Second, theoretical sampling is an important tool for data collection and analysis. This form of sampling involves the deliberate selection of participants based on their experience with the area of interest and the needs of the emerging theory [12]. Third, a limited review of the relevant literature is completed prior to the research. To avoid prejudgments, an in-depth review is delayed until critical junctures in the analysis to help refine emerging constructs and position them, if possible, within existing theory (i.e., thematic categories guide the search for relevant studies).

Glaser and Strauss [8] used category labels to describe groups of events or situations with common attributes. Categories are composed of properties, with incidents defining descriptors used to define properties. Transcripts are analyzed line by line and open codes, based on participants own words, inserted in relevant margins to help reduce researcher bias. These substantive codes are aligned with similar and dissimilar ideas, thoughts, or beliefs.

In the second stage of analysis, open codes are collapsed, without altering identified themes, into key properties aligned with emerging categories. Descriptors (i.e., grouping and collapsing of substantive codes from incidents in the data), properties, and categories are constantly reassessed for validity. As the categories approach saturation (no new insights are produced), theoretical sampling ceases. With further analysis, it is possible to delineate interrelationships among the categories, which eventually culminate into a theory's propositions. A final step involves reflecting on the data and emergent categories for a core construct (dominant social–psychological process) that links things into a meaningful whole while accounting for most of the variation observed in the data.

Researchers often revisit the thematic categories, defining a substantive theory for the purpose of scale construction. Within these categories are rich data clusters that enable the generation of items for scales that represent specific content or domains. Following scale validation through psychometric analysis, useful operational measures are available to test the theory's propositions. For example, items for quality-of-care [13] and quality-of-life [14, 15] scales were generated from qualitative data bases.

---

3   Example of Using Grounded Theory to Generate Substantive Theory

3.1   Background

Clinicians and researchers have been interested in documenting how experiences with end-stage renal dialysis (ESRD) and hemodialysis influence overall adjustment and the achievement of quality outcomes. The research evidence suggests that individuals on long-term maintenance hemodialysis are required to adapt to highly volatile illness and treatment experiences, a changing support base, and significant losses and lifestyle restrictions. Emotionally, psychologically, physically, socially, and spiritually, there is a constant search for a sense of balance or normalcy. There is also evidence of a constant struggle to obtain a quality-of-life standard which can provide a benchmark for evaluating unpredictable events.

3.2   Design

A grounded theory study was designed to grasp an understanding of the meaning and significance of events and situations as defined by the "dialysis culture" for patients with ESRD. The primary purpose was to provide evidence for an interactive paradigm that views patients as free human beings who interact with all aspects of dialysis care. A secondary purpose was to identify periods of "critical interactive moments" during hemodialysis and determine their impact on perceived care quality.

3.3   Sample and Procedure

From a population of 71 patients receiving hemodialysis at the study site during data collection (April–September 1996), 44 met the inclusion criteria (minimum of 12 weeks on dialysis, able to understand the interview process and study purpose and give informed consent, fluent in the English language, 19 years of age and over, and not experiencing an acute illness episode or significant decline in health). Semi-structured interviews of 60–90 min duration were conducted with all participants. Initial question content focused on the total illness trajectory (personal reactions to illness, treatment, and critical events; informal and formal supports). Many additional questions were generated by the thematic content emerging during the concurrent data analysis (supportive role of organizations, institutions, and predialysis clinics; suggestions to help prepare new patients for dialysis; decision-making about or availability of transplant and home dialysis options; conduciveness of physical environment; exposure to varying acuity levels of fellow patients). A second interview was scheduled 6–8 weeks following the first to confirm interpretive summaries constructed from each participant's transcript, clarify identified gaps in the data, and confirm conceptual categories and properties.

3.4 Data Analysis

Data analysis proceeded in several phases. Taped interviews were first transcribed verbatim within 48 h and checked for accuracy. Immersion in the data was facilitated by listening to participants' interviews while reading the transcripts. At the second step, the focus was on interpreting the meaning of words and sentences through reading and rereading each transcript. Integral to this process was assigning substantive codes to recurrent themes. This served two purposes: becoming immersed with each narrative to help construct interpretive summaries and identifying further probes and questions.

Theoretical sampling indicated that common themes were emerging after completion of 15 interviews and first-level coding (i.e., substantive codes). At this point, interviewing was temporarily stopped and the constant-comparative method of analysis applied to the data sets by two independent raters. The objective was to create a meaning context by forging determinate relationships between and among codes (i.e., substantive codes highlighting the major processes present in the data). The result was a multilayered classification system of major categories and associated properties, descriptors, and indicators. As potential relationships between the categories were tested within the data, a substantive theory began to emerge.

Additionally, each transcript was perused for critical events or "turning points" of sufficient magnitude to send a powerful message to participants at different points in the hemodialysis cycle. The data suggested that critical turning points could potentially alter attitudes toward treatment. Because turning points surfaced across all the thematic categories, each transcript was subsequently perused to identify critical incidents that seemed integral to the category. Validity was assured by having two researchers construct independent interpretive summaries of each transcript and achieve consensus on the final version. An important focus was to capture the weight and importance of critical events for study participants. Participants were given an opportunity to read, or receive a verbal presentation on, their interpretive summaries. All participants confirmed their interpretive summaries, adding a further element of credibility to the findings.

Following initial application of the constant-comparative method and construction of interpretive summaries, debriefing sessions were held regularly to clarify the themes and emerging conceptual categories. This additional time with the data was intensive, resulting in multiple revisions of the initial categories and their properties and thematic descriptors (eight drafts). Category saturation (i.e., no new data emerging) and the beginnings of a substantive theory (i.e., theoretical constructs and tentative linkages) was achieved following coding of 30 data sets. Because the team wanted to ensure that all consenting patients were given an opportunity to share their views, data collection proceeded until interviews were completed with all 36 patients.

At the final step the focus shifted to enhance the credibility and accuracy of the classification system by subjecting it to examination by independent consultants. The initial verification session led to the collapsing of properties and categories into a more parsimonious set (i.e., from 10 to 7 categories and 48 to 36 properties) and descriptor labels added to differentiate meaningful divisions within properties. The revised classification system was then applied to 20 data sets; however, difficulties with overlapping categories continued to impede the coding process. Further discussions between the consultants and research team culminated in a further collapsing of categories and properties (i.e., from 7 to 3 categories and 36 to 18 properties). All data sets were subsequently recoded with the revised classification system and an interrater agreement of 95 % achieved.

3.5 Findings

The findings suggested that the experiences of patients with ESRD and on long-term hemodialysis could be captured with three categories (meaning of illness and treatment, quality supports, and adjustment to a new normal). Adjustment to a new normal emerged as the core construct defining the social–psychological process. The substantive theory, living with end-stage renal disease and hemodialysis (LESRD-H), proposes that illness and treatment experiences and social supports exert a direct impact on adjustment to a new normal (*see* Fig. 1). It is also conjectures that critical turning points (i.e., meanings attributed to positive and negative critical events that surface periodically to exert a singular and cumulative effect) link the constructs. Finally, all the constructs exert a direct impact on quality outcome with adjustment to a new normal also mediating the impact of illness and treatment experiences and social supports on outcome.

All components of the substantive theory constantly change in response to alterations in health status, perceived usefulness of supports, and an evolving new normal. Adjustment to a new normal encompasses how people view themselves and their roles in relation to life on dialysis. Patients had to contend with ongoing

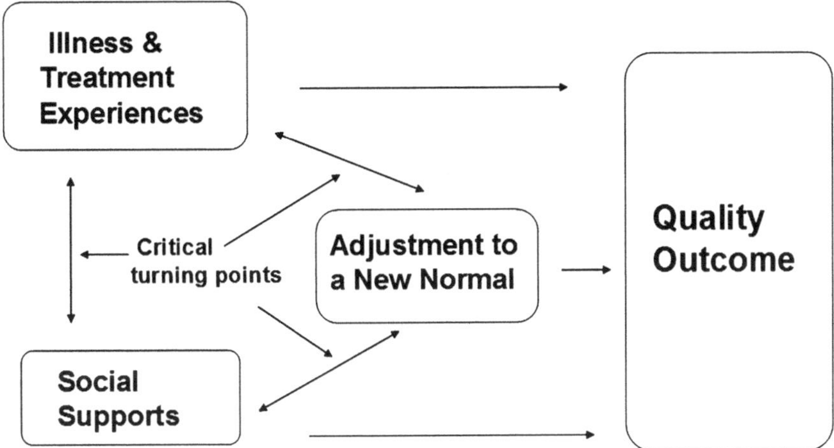

Fig. 1 Living with end-stage renal disease and hemodialysis

emotional, psychological, social, and spiritual struggles as they attempted to maintain a semblance of normalcy. The meaning of illness and treatment category captures the stress of dealing with the concurrent effects of ESRD, comorbid conditions, and hemodialysis treatment, as well as the ambiguity resulting from the tension between knowing what is needed to maximize health versus what is actually done about it. The supports category reflects the perceived availability and usefulness of support from informal and formal network members. It refers to the caring approaches (i.e., technical, emotional, and psychological) used by significant others (family, friends, health care providers, and fellow patients) during dialysis and on nondialysis days. Quality outcome is an evolving end point with subjective (i.e., satisfaction with life) and objective (i.e., morbidity and mortality) components that are constantly changing in response to illness and treatment events, social supports, and adjustment.

The thread linking the theory's constructs was labeled *critical turning points* because of their import for shaping attitudes and behavior. Critical turning points ebbed and flowed in importance and impact in response to changing contextual factors (i.e., the physical environment: space, atmosphere; health status: perceived, actual; technical care: machine functioning, monitoring, response) and state of preparedness of the person for the event (i.e., aware of possibility for their unanticipated occurrence, knowing what to do, actual doing). As well, critical turning points in one area could shape subsequent perceptions of another area, and occurrences during a specific dialysis session, whether early or later in the treatment cycle, might or might not affect acceptance of this treatment type. Although isolated critical incidents early in the hemodialysis cycle (i.e., acute illness episode precipitating renal failure, loss of transplant or alternate treatment modality, loss of access site, and loss of meaningful employment) were highly impressionable, the cumulative effects of a series of critical incidents over time seemed to have far greater implications for how patients rated the quality of supports and potential health outcomes.

It might be helpful to work through an example to clarify what these separate but connected forces mean for a person living with dialysis. A *sudden drop in blood pressure* while on hemodialysis was identified by a number of respondents as a critical event. Although a physiological event that may be anticipated or unanticipated, depending on the track record of the person on dialysis, it is also a psychological event appraised cognitively first and emotionally second. Psychologically, one is driven to search for a causal factor. The search may attribute responsibility to the mistakes of others (i.e., removal of too much fluid or its removal too quickly, malfunctioning equipment: *quality of care or social support,* the way that the person chooses to be in the world (i.e., not adhering to fluid and diet restrictions) or changing physical health status (i.e., comorbid illnesses such as coronary artery disease, diabetes: *meaning of illness and treatment.* Emotionally, one identifies the feeling states of fear, anxiety, and uncertainty (i.e., a terrifying experience comparable to dying, fearing for one's life, inability to control the event's inception but possibly its severity). The emotional reaction may empower some individuals to assume actions that ideally reduce the severity of the event (i.e., be attentive to feeling states that constitute warning signs, alerting the nurse when detecting a change in physical status, ensuring that blood pressure readings are taken regularly). In contrast, other individuals may be so terrified and anxious about the uncertainty of event occurrences that they are in a constant state of tension while on dialysis (i.e., over-attentive to feeling states, constantly seeking attention from the nurses, too demanding): *adjustment to a new normal.*

What do these critical turning points mean for dialysis patients? First, it is a dawning of sorts, because the person must confront his or her own vulnerability. Second, it speaks to the "fragility" or limitations of technical care. Third, it impresses upon the person the need to be more vigilant about changing feeling states, healthy behavior, and the actions of health care providers. What is clear is that the person experiencing critical turning points is taken to a new level of awareness regarding the responsibilities of the self and others.

3.6 Implications of Qualitative Findings

The substantive theory's constructs on meaning of illness and quality supports have been discussed extensively in the chronic illness literature and so augment theoretical work in this area. The challenge facing health care providers is to identify care modalities capable of facilitating high-quality outcomes. As supported by study findings, appropriate care strategies are contingent on the social psychological processes defining patients' experiences with illness and variant treatments.

4   An Example of Using a Qualitative Database for Scale Construction

4.1   Justification for Developing a Clinical Monitoring Tool

Irreversible kidney failure is a condition affecting increasing numbers of individuals, especially the elderly. Without treatment, the condition is fatal. Life can be prolonged with dialysis, but in accepting it, the person confronts many challenges. Prior research into patient experiences with ESRD and hemodialysis assessed physical and psychological stressors, methods of coping, quality of life, quality of supports, and satisfaction with care in a piecemeal fashion.

This phase of the project was designed to develop reliable and valid scales for generating a descriptive database that would support the major premises of the model and, ultimately, provide health care workers with useful information at various points in the hemodialysis cycle. As noted in the preceding qualitative discussion, the findings supported the presence of a multidimensional construct. Therefore, items had to be generated that would capture how individuals interpret illness and treatment experiences, evaluate the quality of support systems (formal and informal), and adjust to an evolving normal state. The importance of critical turning points suggested that the scales had to be capable of differentiating among individuals experiencing and not experiencing problems within the identified thematic areas, as well as capturing responsiveness to change over time through natural evolution or planned intervention. This work culminated in the development of a testable version of the Patient Perception of Hemodialysis Scale (PPHS).

4.2   Item Generation

A set of disease- and treatment-specific items were generated from the qualitative database. This phase involved the following steps:

1. Identification of an initial set of items from the three major thematic categories constituting the substantive theory.

2. Reduction of initial items and determination of the best rating scale format for this population.

3. Validation (content and face) of generated items by experts and ESRD patients.

4.2.1   Step 1. Identification of an Initial Set of Items from a Qualitative Database

Initially, coded transcripts were entered into a Paradox database file and transferred into the Statistical Program for the Social Sciences for descriptive analysis. This step led to the creation of a descriptive profile of frequency and priority ratings of categories, properties, descriptors, and indicators by subject and group. Based on the priority ratings within and across data sets, the research team, composed of members from different professional backgrounds, once again reviewed the coded transcripts to identify phrases to guide formulation of item stems. This step resulted in the generation of 164 stems. As item construction proceeded, the emphasis was placed on conciseness and avoidance of negative wording, ambiguous terminology, jargon, value-laden words and double-barreled questions.

4.2.2 Step 2. Reduction of the Initial Set of Items and Rating Scale Selection

The first draft of the items was reviewed and modified by the researchers to increase clarity and diminish redundancy. This resulted in the elimination of 46 items. The revised version was content validated by two hemodialysis patients who had participated in the qualitative study and expressed an interest in this phase of the research. These individuals were also asked to comment on item clarity and relevancy. A direct outcome of this step was a further reduction of items from 118 to 98.

The research team then proceeded to develop a rating scale to subject the items to a more rigorous pretest. The initial rating scales focused on frequency of occurrence (never, rarely, sometimes, often, or almost always), as well as importance of select events and situations (not at all, a little bit, moderately, quite a bit, considerably). Although it was recognized that a five-point scale might not be sufficient for maximum reliability, the consensus was that it would be difficult to devise unambiguous additional ordinal adjectives.

4.2.3 Step 3. Content and Face Validation

The four content experts in the field who were asked to review the scale confirmed the appropriateness of items for the identified domains. An adult literacy expert was also consulted to ensure that the scale was at the appropriate reading level for the target population. Finally, three hemodialysis patients were asked to participate in the rating of each item. One of the investigators was present to identify difficulties in administration, ambiguities in wording, and the time required to complete the task. It was determined that patients experienced difficulty discerning between the frequency and importance scales, adding considerably to the administration time. Following patient input, scale items were reduced to 64, ambiguous items reworded, and the rating scale modified to facilitate ease of application.

The final version of the PPHS comprises 64 items, with 42 of the items positively worded and 22 negatively worded. The rating scale format that seemed to facilitate patients' response was a five-point Likert-type scale ranging from 0 (never, not at all) to 4 (almost always, extremely) with the lead-ins of how often, how satisfied, how concerned, or how confident.

4.3 Pilot Study and Preliminary Psychometric Analysis

This phase of the research was primarily focused on generating data to conduct a preliminary psychometric analysis of the PPHS. The PPHS was pilot tested in a sample of patients receiving in-center hemodialysis at all provincial dialysis sites. One of the investigators trained an individual to administer the PPHS and the dialysis version of the Ferrans and Powers' Quality of Life Instrument (QLI) [16]. Initially, interviews were conducted face to face with 112 patients during the first 2 h of hemodialysis treatment and ranged from 60 to 90 min.

The psychometric analysis of the data generated from the administration of the PPHS and the QLI in the pilot study proceeded as follows: validity analysis of the PPHS, and reliability analysis of the PPHS.

<table>
<tr><td>

4.3.1 Step 1. Validity Analysis of the PPHS

</td><td>

Construct validity of the PPHS was assessed in a number of ways. First, exploratory factor analysis was used to generate a factor structure. With this analysis, it was possible to determine if scale items that formed factor structures aligned in a logical fashion with the thematic categories comprising the substantive theory. Second, correlational analysis (i.e., Pearson's r and Spearman's ρ) was used to examine the associations among the major subscales (i.e., constructs in the theoretical model). Third, correlation matrixes were generated to determine the intercorrelations among the components of each subscale, as well as the association of each component to its relevant subscale. The final step involved assessing the criterion-related validity (i.e., concurrent validity) of the PPHS with the QLI.

</td></tr>
</table>

Exploratory factor analysis tentatively supported the construct validity of the PPHS (i.e., generated three major item clusters—illness and treatment experiences, social supports, and adjustment to a new normal—that supported the theoretical constructs comprising the substantive theory induced from the qualitative database). The analysis confirmed the following: (a) Illness and treatment experiences comprise four interrelated domains—physiological stressors, knowledge, performance of activities of daily living, and self-health management. (b) Social supports comprise two separate but interrelated domains—formal (nurses, physicians, and allied healthcare workers) and informal (i.e., family) networks. (c) Adjustment to a new normal consisted of two separate but interrelated domains—psychological distress and emotional well-being.

Construct validity is also supported by the statistically significant, strong, positive correlations observed between the major subscales and the total scale: adjustment to a new normal ($r=0.91$), illness and treatment experiences ($r=0.77$) and social supports ($r=0.71$). As hypothesized, the highest correlation is for the adjustment to a new normal subscale. These findings indicate that each major subscale measures separate but interconnected aspects of the whole patient experience. The subscales also depict low to moderate, statistically significant correlations with each other (r values range from 0.34 to 0.54).

Construct validity is further supported by statistically significant, moderate to strong, positive correlations of minor subscales with the relevant major subscale. The score ranges within each major subscale are as follows: illness and treatment experience subscale (r values range from 0.41 to 0.78), social supports subscale (r values range from 0.43 to 0.82) and adjustment to a new normal subscale (r values range from 0.80 to 0.90).

Concurrent validity of the PPHS with the QLI is only partially supported with the pilot study data. Statistically significant, positive relationships are observed among most major components of the PPHS and the QLI, but many of these are in the low to moderate range (r values from 0.23 to 0.62). Despite the logical alignment between the major subscales of the PPHS and the QLI, closer scrutiny reveals differences in a number of content areas. This suggested that the QLI may not have been the most appropriate scale for assessing the concurrent validity of the PPHS.

4.3.2 Step 2. Reliability Analysis of the PPHS

Once a preliminary list of factors was generated by exploratory factor analysis and validated for theoretical consistency, the next step was to assess the reliability of the scale structures. A Cronbach's (α) test was used to assess subscale and total PPHS internal consistency.

The total instrument has an alpha coefficient of $r = 0.91$. Alpha coefficients for the three major subscales are as follows: adjustment to a new normal ($r = 0.88$), social supports ($r = 0.84$) and illness and treatment experiences ($r = 0.71$). The pilot study analysis reveals that internal consistency is high for the total scale and slightly lower, but within acceptable ranges, for each of the subscales. Finally, alpha coefficients for the components of each major subscale range from $r = 0.43$ to 0.89. The findings indicate that the individual components of the illness and treatment experience, supports, and adjustment subscales have a fair to very good internal consistency. The low reliability scores for some components (i.e., self-management, allied health, and family) could be attributed to the small number of items.

5 Summary

Qualitative research methods facilitate greater understanding of human behavior and interactions within variant and similar contexts. Grounded theory is a useful qualitative approach for generating theory to capture basic psychosocial processes that can be formulated into a substantive theory. In turn, the major theoretical constructs of the theory can be used for scale development. Scales developed in this manner are more sensitive because they are firmly grounded in the patients' own experiences. Useful monitoring tools can be developed for identifying significant changes in individuals' experiences with illness and treatment, social supports, and long-term adjustment, which have important implications for the quality of survival for patients with chronic disease in the short- and long term.

References

1. Jones R (2007) Strength of evidence in qualitative research. J Clin Epidemiol 60:321–323
2. Poses RM, Isen AM (1998) Qualitative research in medicine and health care questions and controversy. J Gen Intern Med 13(1):32–38
3. Popay J, Rogers A, Williams G (1998) Rationale and standards for the systematic review of qualitative literature in health services research. Qual Health Res 8(3):341–351
4. Whittemore R, Chase SK, Mandle CL (2001) Validity in qualitative research. Qual Health Res 11(4):522–537
5. Morse JM, Barrett M, Mayan M, Olson K, Spiers J (2002) Verification strategies for establishing reliability and validity in qualitative research. Int J Qual Meth 1(2):1–19
6. Horsburgh D (2003) Evaluation of qualitative research. J Clin Nurs 12:307–312
7. Rolfe G (2006) Validity, trustworthiness and rigour: quality and the idea of qualitative research. J Adv Nurs 53(3):304–310
8. Glaser B, Strauss A (1967) The discovery of grounded theory. Aldine, Chicago
9. Glaser B, Strauss A (1978) Theoretical sensitivity. Sociology, Mill Valley, CA
10. Glaser BG (1992) Basics of grounded theory analysis. Sociology, Mill Valley, CA
11. Strauss A, Corbin J (1990) Basics of qualitative research: grounded theory procedures and techniques. Sage, Newbury Park, CA
12. Morse JM, Field PA (1996) Nursing research: the application of qualitative approaches. Chapman & Hall, London
13. Wilde B, Starrin B, Larsson G, Larsson M (1993) Quality of care from the patient perspective: a grounded theory study. Scand J Caring Sci 7(2):113–120
14. Tarlov AR, Ware JE Jr, Greenfield S, Nelson EC, Perrin E, Zubkoff M (1989) The medical outcomes study: an application of methods for monitoring the results of medical care. JAMA 262(7):925–930
15. Paget L, Tarlov AR (1996) The medical outcomes trust: improving medical outcomes from the patient's point of view. J Outcome Manage 3(3):18–23
16. Ferrans C, Powers MJ (1993) Quality of life of hemodialysis patients. Psychometric assessment of the quality of life index. Am Neph Nur Assoc J 20(5):575–582

Chapter 19

Health Economics in Clinical Research

Braden J. Manns

Abstract

The pressure for health care systems to provide more resource intensive health care and newer, more costly, therapies is significant, despite limited health care budgets. As such, demonstration that a new therapy is effective is no longer sufficient to ensure that it is funded within publicly funded health care systems. The impact of a therapy on health care costs is also an important consideration for decision-makers who must allocate scarce resources. The clinical benefits and costs of a new therapy can be estimated simultaneously using economic evaluation, the strengths and limitations of which are discussed herein. In addition, this chapter includes discussion of the important economic outcomes that can be collected within a clinical trial (alongside the clinical outcome data) enabling consideration of the impact of the therapy on overall resource use, thus enabling performance of an economic evaluation, if the therapy is shown to be effective.

Key words Economic evaluation, Cost-effectiveness, Costs, Health economics

1 Overview

The pressure for health care systems to provide more resource intensive health care and newer, more costly, therapies is substantial, but health care budgets are limited. For example, nephrology programs caring for patients with ESRD are faced with numerous harsh realities: sicker patients requiring more medical interventions, newer and more expensive technology, and fixed budgets [1]. In 2011 in the USA, almost $50 billion was spent by all payers to care for patients with ESRD [2], and in economically developed countries, it has been estimated that nearly 3 % of overall health budgets are spent on ESRD care [1, 3–5] This is despite the fact that less than a quarter of a percent of the Canadian and US populations have ESRD [3, 5]. Given these cost pressures, demonstrating that a new therapy is effective is no longer sufficient to ensure its uptake in practice within publicly funded health care. The impact of the therapy on health care costs must also be considered by decision-makers who then

Patrick S. Parfrey and Brendan J. Barrett (eds.), *Clinical Epidemiology: Practice and Methods*, Methods in Molecular Biology, vol. 1281, DOI 10.1007/978-1-4939-2428-8_19, © Springer Science+Business Media New York 2015

decide how scarce resources should be allocated. If considered during the trial planning stages, important economic outcomes can be collected alongside clinical outcome data in a clinical trial. This enables the performance of an economic evaluation which measures the impact of a therapy on clinical outcomes and overall resource use.

In this chapter, we discuss the basics of health economics, outlining important concepts that clinicians and other health professionals should understand. Also highlighted is the role and use of economic evaluations, including the various types, and a general overview of how economic evaluations can be performed and interpreted. The strengths and weaknesses of economic evaluation are discussed along with how to avoid common pitfalls. Finally, information that could be collected alongside a clinical trial or that is often required from clinical research studies that would enable performance of a full economic evaluation is highlighted. Throughout the chapter, examples are highlighted to facilitate comprehension of the basic principles of economic evaluation.

2   Health Economics: The Basics

Whenever the term "economics" is mentioned in the context of caring for patients requiring dialysis, most clinicians likely assume that the intent is to limit expenditure. In reality, economics is about the relationship between resource inputs (the labor and capital used in treatment) and their benefits (improvements in survival and quality of life) [6]. The magnitude of such costs and benefits and the relationships between them are analyzed by use of "economic evaluation." A full economic evaluation compares the costs and effectiveness of all the alternative treatment strategies for a given health problem.

Most clinicians are comfortable interpreting and applying clinical studies that compare therapies and report the relative occurrence of a medical outcome of interest. In truth, if there was no scarcity of resources in health care, then such evidence of effectiveness would be all that would be required in medical decision-making. As we move into the twenty-first century, there is no denying that rationing of health care occurs, and that scarcity of resources is a reality in all publicly funded health care systems, including the USA.

2.1   Basic Concepts: Opportunity Cost and Efficiency

2.1.1   Opportunity Cost

The concept of opportunity cost, which is central to health economics, rests on two principles, scarcity of resources and choice [6]. As noted, even in societies with great wealth, there are not enough resources to meet all of societies' desires, particularly in the face of expensive technological advancement. This brings up the concept of choice, where society, due to the presence of scarcity, must make choices about what health programs to fund and which ones to forgo. It is the benefits associated with a forgone health care program or opportunity that constitutes opportunity costs. In the planning of health services, the aim of economic evaluations has been to ensure that the benefits from health care programs implemented are greater than the "opportunity costs" of such programs. For example, in the absence of a budgetary increase, use of resources to establish a nocturnal hemodialysis program would result in less resources being available for a second program, such as a multidisciplinary chronic kidney disease (CKD) clinic for predialysis patients. Allocation of resources to the nocturnal hemodialysis program would only be reasonable if the health gains per dollar spent exceeded those of the forgone opportunity, in this case a multidisciplinary CKD clinic. Thus, one way to help determine which is the better use of resources is to estimate the resources used (or costs) and health outcomes (or benefits) of each competing program.

2.1.2 What Is Meant by Efficiency?

Efficiency is about the relationship between inputs (i.e., resources) and outcomes (i.e., improvements in health). In health economics there are two types of efficiency, allocative and technical [6]. Allocative efficiency deals with the question of whether to allocate resources to different groups of patients with different health problems (i.e., should a health region direct resources towards a rehabilitation clinic for patients with chronic obstructive pulmonary disease, or to a nocturnal hemodialysis program for end-stage renal disease (ESRD) patients). This is in contrast to technical efficiency where the resources are being distributed among the same patient population, in an attempt to maximize health gains for that patient group within the budget available (i.e., for patients with acute renal failure, should an intensive care unit (ICU) provide intermittent hemodialysis or continuous renal replacement therapy) [7]. Choosing the proper type of economic evaluation depends on understanding what type of efficiency question is to be addressed.

3   The Different Types of Economic Evaluations

There are three main types of economic evaluation that follow from the concepts of opportunity cost and efficiency. Which one is used will depend on the question being addressed. If the question is one of "technical efficiency" (i.e.: *with a fixed amount of resource available, what is the most efficient way of treating people with acute renal failure in the ICU, intermittent hemodialysis or continuous renal replacement therapy?* [7]), then a cost-effectiveness or cost–utility study is most appropriate. If the question is one of "allocative efficiency" (i.e.: *an ESRD program hoping to develop a nocturnal hemodialysis program competes for funding with a respiratory program wishing to establish a rehabilitation program for patients with chronic obstructive pulmonary disease*), then a cost–utility or possibly cost–benefit study is more appropriate. When addressing technical efficiency, the same group of patients will be treated, but the question becomes one of "how". Allocative efficiency questions inevitably involve comparisons of different groups of patients (i.e., how many resources to *allocate* to each). All economic evaluations compare a specific technology (or policy) to another, whether it is the status quo or a comparable technology.

3.1 Cost-Effectiveness Analysis

Cost-effectiveness analyses assess health benefits in naturally occurring units such as life years gained, cases prevented, or units of blood pressure reduction achieved using an intervention and can be used to evaluate technical efficiency. Early studies examining the cost-effectiveness of statins (cholesterol-lowering drugs) assessed the cost to prevent a heart attack [8], among other outcomes. Studies found that the cost to prevent a heart attack averaged $5,000, while the cost per life year saved was $27,000. This highlights a challenge associated with the use of cost-effectiveness analysis; that is, there is no consensus as to what constitutes good value for money in the prevention of hearts attacks. Moreover, comparing the results of this study with other cost-effectiveness studies that report health benefits using a different metric, or for treatments for patients with other health conditions, is not possible.

A subset of cost-effectiveness analysis is cost-minimization analysis, which can be used when clinical outcomes between treatment strategies in the same patient population are known to be equivalent. In cost-minimization analysis, the cost of the treatments being compared, as well as the associated costs (or savings) in other areas of health care (such as outpatient visits) are estimated, but clinical outcomes are excluded as they do not differ. For example, if different dialysis modalities were known to be equivalent in survival and quality of life, then a cost-minimization analysis could be used to compare the alternate modalities. Canadian micro-costing studies have noted that total health care costs of treating dialysis patients with in-center hemodialysis (hospital and satellite), home hemodialysis, and peritoneal dialysis is approximately $95,000 to $107,000, $71,000 to $90,000, and $56,000 per year, respectively ($2013 CAD) [9–11]. Assuming that the clinical outcomes associated with the different therapies are equal [12–15], then using cost-minimization analysis, one could conclude that treating eligible patients with home-based dialysis could save significant resources without impacting outcomes.

3.2 Cost–Utility Analysis

Comparisons often need to be made between therapies for which clinical success may be measured in very different units. When such an "allocative decision" needs to be made, it is important to express health benefits in an equivalent fashion. This can be done using either a cost–benefit analysis or cost–utility analysis. In a cost–benefit analysis, medical outcomes are valued in dollars, often using a method called "willingness-to-pay" [6]. Cost–benefit studies are most often used as a research tool and interested readers are referred elsewhere for more detail [6].

Cost–utility analysis, on the other hand, is commonly used by decision-makers to address issues of technical or allocative efficiency. This type of analysis is perhaps the most familiar to clinicians since it is the basis of "QALY league tables" [16, 17]. Clinical outcomes are usually considered in terms of healthy years. Healthy years can be measured using a "utility-based" index, which incorporates effects on both quantity and quality of life; the most widely used scale is the "quality-adjusted life year" (QALY). The QALY is determined as the product of the number of years of life gained (or remaining) multiplied by the "utility" or "quality" of those years (rated from zero—a state equivalent to death—to one—equivalent to a state of full health) [18]. In practice, the utility score can be determined using either direct or indirect measures. Direct measures include the standard gamble or the time trade-off, which can be assessed in the relevant patient group. Although these measures are felt to be the most theoretically valid measures of utility, they are difficult to include in a study, often requiring the help of an administrator [18]. Alternatively, utility scores can be derived from indirect measures, like the Euroqol EQ-5D or the Health Utilities Index, which are both questionnaire-based measures that are easy and quick for patients to complete. As such, these measures can easily be incorporated into a clinical trial, along with other relevant measures of health-related quality of life (HRQOL), enabling estimation of the expected QALYs associated with a treatment strategy. Details on the different methods that can be used to elicit such utilities are available elsewhere [18].

An example of a cost–utility analysis is that by Cameron et al., where the authors sought to clarify the costs and benefits of blood glucose self-monitoring in patients with type 2 diabetes who do not use insulin [19]. A meta-analysis of randomized controlled trials comparing self-monitoring with no self-monitoring showed that HbA1C was 0.25 % (95 % CI 0.15–0.36 %) lower in patients who were randomized to blood glucose self-monitoring [20]. Though the difference was statistically significant, it was uncertain whether this would translate into clinically significant health benefits. Moreover, the cost associated with blood glucose test strips was estimated to be over $370 million in Canada in 2006, more than 50 % of which was for patients not taking insulin [19]. An economic evaluation was performed to better inform decisions regarding prescribing and reimbursement of blood glucose test strips [19]. The authors began with an estimate of the effect of self-monitoring on HbA1C and, based on this effect, they used modeling techniques to derive the difference in both diabetes-related end points and life expectancy that would be expected given the achieved difference in HbA1C. The life-years of hypothetical patients were then weighted by the utility associated with the various health states modeled (all based on the occurrence of diabetes-related complications). The primary clinical outcome of the analysis was QALYs and the cost per QALY gained. They found that, compared with no self-monitoring, self-monitoring was associated with a cost per QALY gained of CDN $113,643. In the patient subgroup receiving only lifestyle interventions the cost–utility ratio was less favorable at $292,144 per QALY. This introduces the next topic. What does $113,643 per QALY mean? Does that represent good value for money?

4   How to Interpret the Results of Economic Evaluations

Of course, before evaluating the results of any study, whether it is an economic evaluation, a clinical trial or observational research, it is important to determine whether the study is valid. While this is a key step, the details of how to determine if an economic evaluation is valid or not are beyond the scope of this chapter. As with other areas of clinical research, good practice in economic evaluation is guided by several published guidelines [21–24] and adherence to these guidelines increases the likelihood of a published evaluation being valid.

When interpreting the results of an economic evaluation comparing a new intervention with standard care, it is often helpful to first compare the treatments on the basis of clinical outcomes and costs separately (Fig. 1) [25]. As noted in Fig. 1, there are some situations where an intervention should clearly be introduced (i.e., less expensive and superior clinical outcomes (cell A1)) and others where the therapy should clearly not be used (i.e., more expensive and less effective (cell C3)). The use of economic evaluation is considered most important in cell C1, where a new therapy is judged more effective, but is also more expensive than a comparator. In these situations, judgment is required as to whether the extra resources represent "good value for money." Returning to the notion of opportunity cost, in these situations, one must consider whether the required expenditure could be used to support other unfunded treatments that would improve health to a greater extent, either for the same group of patients (technical efficiency) or another group of patients (allocative efficiency).

In practice, it is often difficult to perform such comparisons between "competing interventions" since decision-makers often consider funding for new interventions at discrete (and different) points in time. In these situations, decision-makers may compare the cost per QALY for the intervention being considered with the

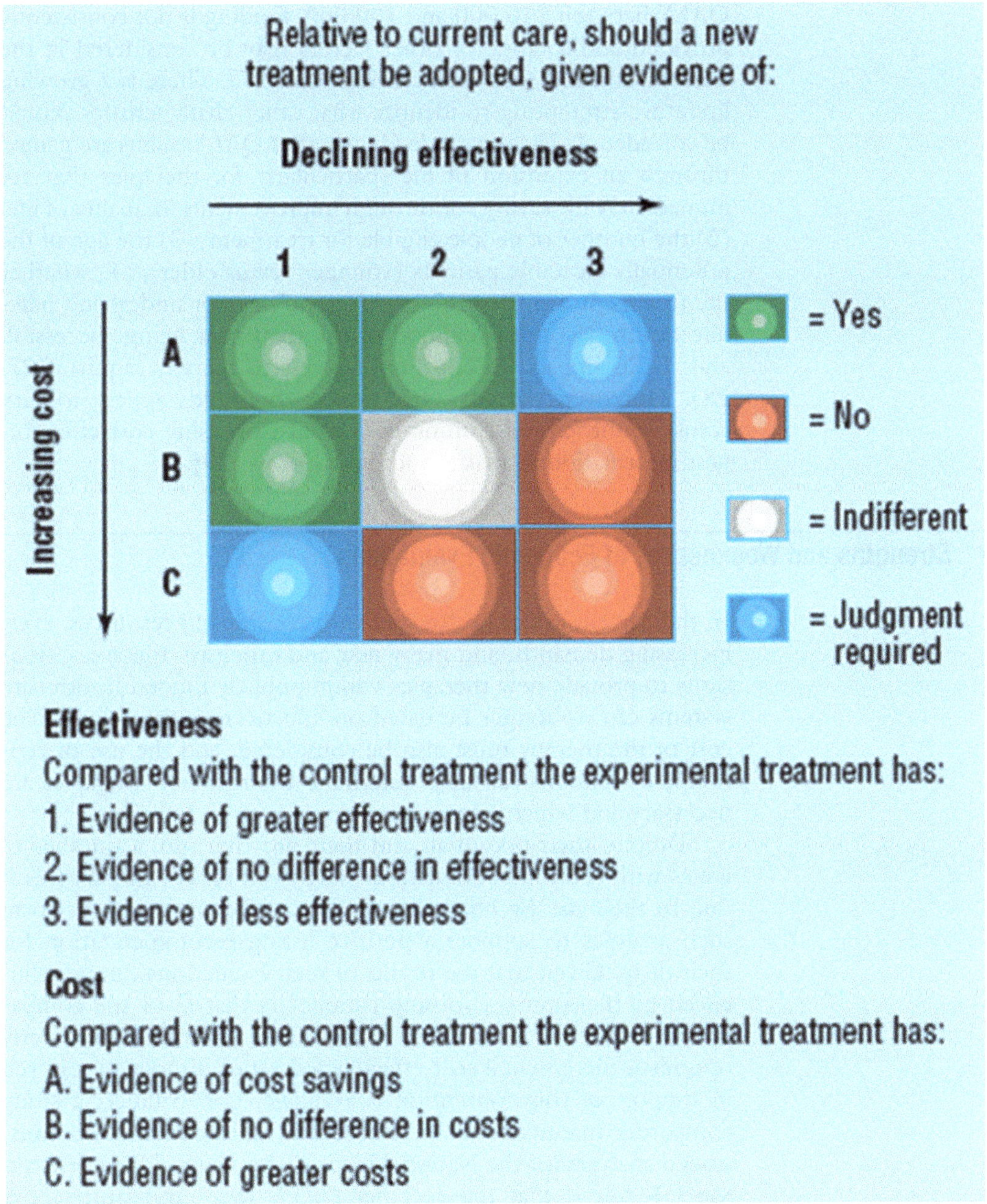

Effectiveness

Compared with the control treatment the experimental treatment has:

1. Evidence of greater effectiveness
2. Evidence of no difference in effectiveness
3. Evidence of less effectiveness

Cost

Compared with the control treatment the experimental treatment has:

A. Evidence of cost savings
B. Evidence of no difference in costs
C. Evidence of greater costs

Fig. 1 Assessing the cost of effectiveness of a new therapy relative to current care (with permission from C. Donaldson [25])

cost per QALY of therapies that have been previously rejected or accepted for funding. Using such a strategy, it has been observed that most therapies with a cost per QALY below \$20,000 are funded within Canadian Medicare [26], and that most therapies with a cost per QALY above \$100,000 are not funded within Canadian publicly funded health care. For therapies with a cost per

QALY between \$20,000 and 100,000, funding is not consistently provided and a range of other factors may be considered in the decision to fund such interventions [26, 27]. There is a growing literature attempting to identify what other characteristics should be considered. These include (1) whether QALYs gains are gained through an extension of life (particularly for therapies that are immediately life saving) or through improvements in quality of life, (2) the number of people eligible for treatment, (3) the age of the potentially treatable patients (younger versus older), (4) whether the treatment was for people with good or poor underlying baseline health, (5) the likelihood of the treatment being successful, and (6) its impact on equality of access to therapy (equity) [27, 28]. Moreover, the cost-effectiveness thresholds appear to vary across countries and committees tasked with using cost-effectiveness information to make funding decisions [29].

5   Strengths and Weaknesses of Economic Evaluations

In the current era of health care with constrained resources, ever-increasing demands, and many new and expensive therapies, decisions to provide new therapies within publicly funded health care systems can no longer be based on effectiveness data alone. The cost of the therapy must also be considered, and the use of economic evaluations can help determine whether new therapies are necessary and which ones to provide.

Despite their potential, and their growing use, a number of issues with economic evaluations have been raised. In part this is due to their use by pharmaceutical manufacturers who perform such analyses to support a positive listing recommendation for their drug. Given that the results of such evaluations can be influenced by the inputs, choosing parameters that favor the company's product is commonly undertaken, resulting in overly optimistic incremental cost-effectiveness ratios. Empirical research in support of this contention is available. For instance, a study comparing manufacturer-sponsored and independently commissioned analyses for the National Institute for Clinical Excellence in the UK found that the cost per QALY was significantly more attractive in nearly 50 % of manufacturer-sponsored submissions [30]. Requiring manufacturers to adhere to published guidelines on the conduct of economic evaluations may minimize such bias [21, 23, 24].

The quality of the data also limits the validity of an economic evaluation, including accurate assessments of the impact of the therapy on clinical outcomes, quality of life, and the costs associated with the therapy. This commonly happens when clinical trials of a new intervention are performed without regard to the eventual requirement for conducting an economic evaluation.

First, the impact of a new therapy on clinical end points may be unknown. This may occur in situations when randomized trials have not been conducted or are ethically impossible to perform. In the absence of RCTs, and hence not knowing whether a new therapy is effective, the performance of an economic evaluation is unlikely to inform decision-making since it will be unable to determine whether a therapy represents good value for money. The impact of a new therapy on clinical end points is also unknown when randomized trials have been done but the outcomes studied have included only putative surrogate outcomes. For instance, in the assessment of blood glucose self-monitoring in patients with type 2 diabetes who do not use insulin, only the impact of this testing on HbA1C (a putative surrogate end point for clinical outcomes) was studied. The authors began with an estimate of the effect of self-monitoring on HbA1C and, based on this effect, they used modeling techniques to derive the difference in both diabetes-related end points (i.e., heart attacks, strokes, and kidney failure) and life expectancy that would be expected given the achieved difference in HbA1C. Some antidiabetic agents that lower HbA1C have been shown in clinical trials to be associated with improved clinical outcomes, while other agents that lower HbA1C have been shown to increase the risk of cardiovascular outcomes. Given this, the cost-effectiveness of blood glucose self-monitoring is sensitive to an assumption of clinical benefit (on heart attacks and strokes) associated with lowering HbA1C.

Second, an accurate assessment of the impact of the therapy on quality of life may not be available, as quality of life measures may not have been included in the randomized trials. Lastly, the impact of the therapy on other health care costs may not have been measured or was not measured adequately. In these situations, the impact of the therapy on costing outcomes must be estimated, and the uncertainty in these variables leads to uncertainty in the overall cost-effectiveness of the new therapy. When planning an RCT, these three limitations can all potentially be addressed by measuring clinical end points, the impact of the therapy on overall quality of life and health care costs. Although some of these methodological challenges may be present in many analyses, it is important to minimize their impact through careful planning and conduct of the analysis, as described below.

6 How to Conduct an Economic Evaluation

Economic evaluations can either be done alongside a clinical trial or by using decision analysis [31]. Perhaps the best example of an economic evaluation done alongside a clinical trial was that of lung volume reduction surgery for patients with severe emphysema [32]. In this study, investigators randomized patients with emphysema to lung volume reduction surgery or medical care and followed them for 3 years, examining survival, quality of life, and health care costs. Investigators found that in certain predefined subgroups, surgery improved survival and quality of life, but increased costs significantly. By combining the impact of the therapy on survival and quality of life into QALYs, the authors were able to estimate a cost per QALY of US $190,000 over a 3-year time horizon (Table 1) [32].

Given the minimization of bias that occurs during the randomization process, data collected alongside an RCT is likely to be of high quality, and valid. Moreover, given the timely nature of RCTs that are required for medication licensing, conducting an economic evaluation alongside a clinical trial also ensures that the results are available in a timely fashion. Moreover, if the authors of the RCT have collected resource use data, then an additional advantage is that information on cost and outcomes is available from the same patients, increasing the transparency and accuracy of the analysis.

There are several limitations, however, including that RCTs are often performed under very strict conditions and the results may not be representative of those that would be seen under usual clinical conditions [31]. Moreover, RCTs may not use the appropriate comparator, or may use surrogate (i.e., non-clinical) rather than clinical end points, which, as noted above, makes performance of a valid economic evaluation challenging. Moreover, one of the main problems associated with doing an economic evaluation alongside a clinical trial exclusively is that clinical trials typically have a short time horizon, rather than a longer time horizon as recommended by practice guidelines [31]. With specific reference to the example discussed above, by using only a 3-year time horizon, it assumes that the additional survivors who survived because they had lung surgery, rather than receiving medical care, died at 3 years, when in reality, these survivors would be likely to survive for several more years.

In reality, most economic evaluations are performed using decision analysis. Decision analysis is a systematic approach to decision-making under conditions of uncertainty, where information is combined from a variety of sources, including clinical trials, observational studies and costing studies. Using data on health outcomes and costs from an observational cohort of patients, a mathematical model is usually constructed to simulate what happens to patients with the condition of interest who are treated using the new treatment or standard of care. The ability of a new treatment to avert adverse clinical outcomes can then be overlaid on this model using the results from the relevant RCTs, and the long-term impact of this therapy on outcomes and costs, compared with standard care, can be determined. In the economic evaluation of lung-volume reduction surgery, investigators subsequently used decision analysis to model the impact of lung

Table 1

Total health care costs, and QALYs gained for patients with emphysema randomized to lung-volume reduction surgery, or supportive medical care alone

Variable	No. of patients	Surgery group Mean (95 % CI)	No. of patients	Medical-therapy group Mean (95 % CI)	P Value	Cost-effectiveness ratio for surgery ($)
All patients Total costs ($) Quality-adjusted life-years gained	531	98,952 (91,694–106,210) 1.46 (1.46–1.47)	535	62,560 (56,572–63,547) 1.27 (1.27–1.28)	<0.001 <0.001	190,000
Patients with predominantly upper-lobe emphysema and low exercise capacity Total costs ($) Quality-adjusted life-years gained	137	110,815 (93,404–128,226) 1.54 (1.53–1.55)	148	61,804 (50,248–73,359) 1.04 (1.03–1.05)	<0.001 <0.001	98,000
Patients with predominantly upper-lobe emphysema and high exercise capacity Total costs ($) Quality-adjusted life-years gained	204	84,331 (73,699–94,962) 1.54 (1.54–1.55)	212	55,858 (47,161–64,555) 1.42 (1.42–1.43)	<0.001 <0.001	240,000
Patients with non-upper-lobe emphysema and low exercise capacity Total costs ($) Quality-adjusted life-years gained	82	111,986 (93,944–130,027) 1.25 (1.23–1.26)	65	65,655 (52,075–79,236) 1.10 (1.09–1.12)	<0.001 <0.001	330,000

With permission from Ramsey et al. [32]

surgery on longer term clinical outcomes and costs at 10 years and determined that the cost per QALY was $53,000 (i.e., significantly more attractive than noted using a 3-year time horizon).

7   What to Consider When Planning Your Clinical Trial?

Since proving evidence of effectiveness in a well-conducted clinical trial no longer ensures the uptake of a new therapy, it is important to build an economic argument for the new therapy in question as well, enabling decision-makers to make a more informed decision regarding funding. The information required can be collected alongside randomized trials in many situations, but this must be planned in advance. Conducting an economic sub-study within a clinical trial is acknowledged as important by many agencies who fund large clinical trials—in fact, acquiring funding for such studies is more likely if an economic sub-study is proposed.

So what is important to consider in the planning of a clinical trial? Firstly, determining the impact of the therapy on clinical end points is crucial since if only putative surrogate end points are measured, the impact of the therapy on clinical end points will remain unknown. Where appropriate, the impact of the therapy on quality of life should be measured using disease specific and generic quality of life measures [6, 18]. As noted above, one of the generic quality of life measures should include a utility measure, which can be directly incorporated into an economic evaluation.

Assessing the impact of the therapy on costs is also important. Sometimes, when the study is limited in duration, or sample size, an accurate assessment of the impact of the therapy on costs is not possible. Where possible though, it is important to not only accurately measure the cost of the new intervention (particularly when the intervention is costly, complicated or requires hospital admission), but to also measure the impact of the therapy on the occurrence of costly adverse health outcomes that may differ between the treatment strategies. For instance, if the therapy is designed to prevent an adverse health outcome, such as arteriovenous fistula failure, or dialysis line sepsis, both of which may require hospital admission and/or surgery, measuring the cost of this complication is important [33]. The types of costs that should be included in an economic evaluation (and should therefore be measured in an RCT) have been reviewed and are discussed in recently released guidelines for conduct of economic evaluations [21]. While there are different methods of measuring costs, this discussion is outside the scope of this article—interested readers are referred elsewhere [18].

Finally, there may be certain variables that can be measured accurately within a clinical trial that will impact the economic attractiveness of a new therapy and that need to be considered within the context of the disease and the treatment. For instance, the frequency or severity of adverse events may have a significant impact on the attractiveness of the therapy, and in certain situations, adherence with the new therapy may be important. Measuring these alongside the trial will enhance the validity of the accompanying economic evaluation.

8 How Can Health Care Professionals Use the Results of Economic Evaluations When Caring for Their Patients?

Confronted with fiscal and demographic challenges, publicly funded health care systems face increasing pressure to constrain resource use without impacting health care services. Health care managers continually decide how to allocate scarce health care resources, including determining what tests and treatments will be made available. However, prioritizing health care resources is not the sole responsibility of managers and decision-makers, and to be successful in maximizing population health, active physician engagement is required. With less than one half of one percent of the nation's population determining how over 10 % of the GDP is spent, clinical decisions are "purchasing decisions" and should be made within the context of competing uses of finite resources to ensure that the most effective interventions are available for the patients who are most likely to benefit. While most clinicians have been trained to consider only the needs of the patient in front of them when making recommendations and providing care, given fiscal realities, this position may not be sustainable in the long term.

Physicians make value-based decisions about other finite resources such as their time and use of beds in a hospital or intensive care unit [34]—and need to apply this same skill set to other health care resources. Although health care decision-makers may limit access to tests or therapies that do not provide reasonable value for money, in many situations, the physician is the gate keeper to tests or treatments, which is appropriate given that they use complementary information to make informed decisions about their patients. This section is meant to help physicians incorporate the notion of value for money into routine clinical care.

Faced with a patient with a health issue, a physician considers the work up and/or treatment needed. It is important, however, for the physician to first consider whether the intervention (or test) is truly effective. Is there evidence that it improves clinical outcomes (or only that it improves nonclinical outcomes), and was the comparison against standard of care, or placebo. If it was placebo, do you expect that the new intervention will have a significant benefit in comparison to what is already standard of care. This is particularly true if the effectiveness of the intervention is marginal at best, or has only been shown to impact nonclinical end points [35] (in other words, when significant clinical uncertainty exists). In these circumstances, physicians should not feel compelled to routinely offer such therapies or tests, particularly when they are notably more expensive than current therapy.

Assuming the test or therapy has been shown to improve clinical outcomes with respect to the standard of care, it is important to next consider the resource implications of the new treatment. Are there other less expensive treatments that could be tried first? In many situations, there are less expensive, or generic medications that many patients will respond to. If other therapies have been tried, consideration as to whether the medication or treatment provides value for money is important, and physicians need to begin to integrate and routinely consider cost and "value for money" in clinical practice. While it may be difficult to operationalize the use of economic evaluations during every patient encounter, if costs were integrated within clinical practice guidelines, incorporating the consideration of cost into usual physician practice would become easier. In situations where physicians deal with this issue on a daily basis, and where cost has not been considered in clinical practice guidelines, then groups of physicians could consider developing local standards of care with which their practice is consistent.

The uncomfortable truth is that resources are limited and choices must be made. While physicians have an obligation to their patient, they must also consider their obligation to society and to their other patients. If the goal of a health care system is to maximize the health of all of its population under the constraint of a fixed budget, then considering cost-effectiveness is a reasonable tool to help make these choices. While physicians may be reluctant to incorporate the consideration of cost in their daily care, their role in allocating scarce resources cannot be avoided. Indeed, since one of the roles of publicly funded health care is to maximize health gains within a restricted budget, considering "value for money" and limiting expensive therapies to those who can benefit most seems a reasonable and equitable approach. Modifying and adhering to physician-developed clinical practice guidelines that take cost into account could help ease the tension between a physician's clinical decision-making and health system objectives.

9   Conclusion

Given financial constraints and cost pressures that exist within publicly funded health care systems, it is not surprising that the demonstration of effectiveness of a new therapy is no longer enough to ensure that it can be used in practice within publicly funded health care systems. The impact of the new therapy on costs is important and is considered by decision-makers who decide how and whether scarce resources should be invested. When planning a clinical trial, important economic outcomes can be collected alongside the clinical data, permitting the evaluation of the impact of the therapy on overall resource use, and thus enabling the performance of an economic evaluation, if appropriate.

References

1. Manns B, Taub K, Donaldson C (2000) Economic evaluation and end-stage renal disease: from basics to bedside. Am J Kidney Dis 36:12–28
2. U.S. Renal Data System, USRDS (2013) Annual Data Report: Atlas of Chronic Kidney Disease and End-Stage Renal Disease in the United States, National Institutes of Health, National Institute of Diabetes and Digestive and Kidney Diseases, Bethesda, MD
3. Hirth RA (2007) The organization and financing of kidney dialysis and transplant care in the United States of America. Int J Health Care Finance Econ 7(4):301–318
4. Tomson CR (2000) Recent advances: nephrology. BMJ 320(7227):98–101
5. Manns BJ, Mendelssohn DC, Taub KJ (2007) The economics of end-stage renal disease care in Canada: incentives and impact on delivery of care. Int J Health Care Finance Econ 7(2–3):149–169
6. Donaldson C, Shackley P, Detels R, Holland WW, McEwan J, Omenn GS (1997) Economic evaluation. Oxford textbook of public health. (3 edn). Oxford: Oxford University Press, pp 849–870
7. Manns B, Doig CJ, Lee H, Dean S, Tonelli M, Johnson D, Donaldson C (2003) Cost of acute renal failure requiring dialysis in the intensive care unit: clinical and resource implications of renal recovery. Crit Care Med 31(2):449–455
8. Johannesson M, Jonsson B, Kjekshus J, Olsson AG, Pedersen TR, Wedel H (1997) Cost effectiveness of simvastatin treatment to lower cholesterol levels in patients with coronary heart disease. Scandinavian Simvastatin Survival Study Group. N Engl J Med 336(5):332–336
9. Lee H, Manns B, Taub K, Ghali WA, Dean S, Johnson D, Donaldson C (2002) Cost analysis of ongoing care of patients with end-stage renal disease: the impact of dialysis modality and dialysis access. Am J Kidney Dis 40(3):611–622
10. Klarenbach S, Tonelli M, Pauly R, Walsh M, Culleton B, So H, Hemmelgarn B, Manns B (2014) Economic evaluation of frequent home nocturnal hemodialysis based on a randomized controlled trial. J Am Soc Nephrol 25(3):587–594
11. Chui BK, Manns B, Pannu N, Dong J, Wiebe N, Jindal K, Klarenbach SW (2013) Health care costs of peritoneal dialysis technique failure and dialysis modality switching. Am J Kidney Dis 61(1):104–111
12. Fenton SS, Schaubel DE, Desmeules M, Morrison HI, Mao Y, Copleston P, Jeffery JR, Kjellstrand CM (1997) Hemodialysis versus peritoneal dialysis: a comparison of adjusted mortality rates. Am J Kidney Dis 30(3):334–342
13. Foley RN, Parfrey PS, Harnett JD, Kent GM, O'Dea R, Murray DC, Barre PE (1998) Mode of dialysis therapy and mortality in end-stage renal disease. J Am Soc Nephrol 9(2):267–276
14. Bloembergen WE, Port FK, Mauger EA, Wolfe RA (1995) A comparison of mortality between patients treated with hemodialysis and peritoneal dialysis. J Am Soc Nephrol 6(2):177–183
15. Collins AJ, Hao W, Xia H, Ebben JP, Everson SE, Constantini EG, Ma JZ (1999) Mortality risks of peritoneal dialysis and hemodialysis. Am J Kidney Dis 34(6):1065–1174
16. Gerard K, Mooney G (1993) QALY league tables: handle with care. Health Econ 2(1):59–64
17. Mauskopf J, Rutten F, Schonfeld W (2003) Cost-effectiveness league tables: valuable guidance for decision makers? Pharmacoeconomics 21(14):991–1000
18. Drummond M, O'Brien B, Stoddart G, Torrance G (1997) Methods for the economic evaluation of health care programmes, 2nd edn. Oxford University Press, Oxford
19. Cameron C, Coyle D, Ur E, Klarenbach S (2010) Cost-effectiveness of self-monitoring of blood glucose in patients with type 2 diabetes mellitus managed without insulin. Can Med Assoc J 182(1):28–34
20. McIntosh B, Yu C, Lal A, Chelak K, Cameron C, Singh SR, Dahl M (2010) Efficacy of self-monitoring of blood glucose in patients with

type 2 diabetes mellitus managed without insulin: a systematic review and meta-analysis. Open Med 4(2):e102–e113

21. Guideliness for the economic evaluation of health technologies: Canada [3rd edition]. Ottawa: Canadian Agency for Drugs and Technologies in Health; 2006

22. McGhan WF, Al M, Doshi JA, Kamae I, Marx SE, Rindress D (2009) The ISPOR good practices for quality improvement of cost-effectiveness research task force report. Value Health 12(8):1086–1099

23. Drummond MF, Jefferson TO (1996) Guidelines for authors and peer reviewers of economic submissions to the BMJ. The BMJ Economic Evaluation Working Party. BMJ 313(7052):275–283

24. Gold R, Siegel J, Russell L, Weinstein M (1996) Cost-effectiveness in health and medicine. Oxford University Press, New York

25. Donaldson C, Currie G, Mitton C (2002) Cost effectiveness analysis in health care: contraindications. BMJ 325(7369):891–894

26. Laupacis A, Feeny D, Detsky AS, Tugwell PX (1992) How attractive does a new technology have to be to warrant adoption and utilization? Tentative guidelines for using clinical and economic evaluations. CMAJ 146(4):473–481

27. Schwappach DL (2003) Does it matter who you are or what you gain? An experimental study of preferences for resource allocation. Health Econ 12(4):255–267

28. Shrive FM, Ghali WA, Lewis S, Donaldson C, Knudtson ML, Manns BJ (2005) Moving beyond the cost per quality-adjusted life year: modeling the budgetary impact and clinical outcomes associated with the use of sirolimus-eluting stents. Can J Cardiol 21(9):783–787

29. Clement FM, Harris A, Li JJ, Yong K, Lee KM, Manns BJ (2009) Using effectiveness and cost-effectiveness to make drug coverage decisions: a comparison of Britain, Australia, and Canada. JAMA 302(13):1437–1443

30. Miners AH, Garau M, Fidan D, Fischer AJ (2005) Comparing estimates of cost effectiveness submitted to the National Institute for Clinical Excellence (NICE) by different organisations: retrospective study. BMJ 330(7482):65

31. O'Brien B (1996) Economic evaluation of pharmaceuticals. Frankenstein's monster or vampire of trials? Med Care 34(12 Suppl):DS99–DS108

32. Ramsey SD, Berry K, Etzioni R, Kaplan RM, Sullivan SD, Wood DE (2003) Cost effectiveness of lung-volume-reduction surgery for patients with severe emphysema. N Engl J Med 348(21):2092–2102

33. Tonelli M, Klaarenbach S, Jindal K, Manns B (2006) Economic implications of screening strategies in arteriovenous fistulae. Kidney Int 69(12):2219–2226

34. Stelfox HT, Hemmelgarn BR, Bagshaw SM, Gao S, Doig CJ, Nijssen-Jordan C, Manns B (2012) Intensive care unit bed availability and outcomes for hospitalized patients with sudden clinical deterioration. Arch Intern Med 172(6):467–474

35. Manns B, Owen WF Jr, Winkelmayer WC, Devereaux PJ, Tonelli M (2006) Surrogate markers in clinical studies: problems solved or created? Am J Kidney Dis 48(1):159–166

Part V

Clinical Genetic Research

Chapter 20

Clinical Genetic Research 1: Bias

Susan Stuckless and Patrick S. Parfrey

Abstract

Clinical epidemiological research in genetic diseases entails assessment of phenotypes, the burden and etiology of disease, and the efficacy of preventive measures or treatments in populations. In all areas, the main focus is to describe the relationship between exposure and outcome and to determine one of the following: prevalence, incidence, cause, prognosis, or effect of treatment. The accuracy of these conclusions is determined by the validity of the study. Validity is determined by addressing potential biases and possible confounders that may be responsible for the observed association. Therefore, it is important to understand the types of bias that exist and also to be able to assess their impact on the magnitude and direction of the observed effect. The following chapter reviews the epidemiological concepts of selection bias, information bias, and confounding and discusses ways in which these sources of bias can be minimized.

Key words Genetic diseases, Epidemiology, Selection bias, Information bias, Confounding, Validity

1 Introduction

The scope of clinical epidemiology is broad, ranging from the study of the patterns and predictors of health outcomes in defined populations to the assessment of diagnostic and management options in the care of individual patients. Moreover, the discipline encompasses such diverse topics as the evaluation of treatment effectiveness, causality, assessment of screening and diagnostic tests, and clinical decision analysis [1]. No matter what topic you are addressing, there are two basic components to any epidemiological study: exposure and outcome. The exposure can be a risk factor, a prognostic factor, a diagnostic test, or a treatment, and the outcome is usually death or disease [2]. In inherited diseases, mutated genes are the risk factors which predispose to autosomal dominant, autosomal recessive, x-linked and complex disorders. Clinical Epidemiology methods are used to describe associations between exposures and outcomes.

The best research design for the investigation of causal relationships is the randomized clinical trial. However, it is not always

Patrick S. Parfrey and Brendan J. Barrett (eds.), *Clinical Epidemiology: Practice and Methods*, Methods in Molecular Biology, vol. 1281, DOI 10.1007/978-1-4939-2428-8_20, © Springer Science+Business Media New York 2015

feasible or ethical to perform such a study and under these circumstances, observational studies may be the best alternatives. Observational studies are hypothesis-testing analytic studies that do not require manipulation of an exposure [3]. Participants are simply observed over time and their exposures and outcomes are measured and recorded. Three main study designs are used in observational studies: cohort, case-control, and cross-sectional. While these studies cannot prove causality, they can provide strong evidence for and show the strength of an association between a disease and putative causative factors [4]. Consequently, these research designs are frequently used to determine the phenotype associated with particular genotypes [5–7] and to assess the impact of interventions on the outcomes of inherited diseases [8]. The limitations imposed by these research designs are often compounded by lack of power due to the reality of small sample sizes for some disorders.

Epidemiologic studies have inherent limitations that preclude establishing causal relationships [4]. While an appropriate research question, or hypothesis, is the foundation of a scientific study, proper methodology and study design are essential to interpret and, ultimately, to have clinical relevance [9]. Assessing the quality of epidemiological studies equates to assessing their validity [10]. To assess whether an observed association is likely to be a true cause-effect relationship, you need to consider three threats to validity: bias, confounding, and chance [10, 11]. Bias occurs when there is a deviation of the results of a study from the truth and can be defined as "any systematic error in the design, conduct or analysis of a study that results in a mistaken estimate of an exposure's effect on the risk of disease" [4]. Confounding is considered a "mixing of effects." It occurs when the effect of exposure on the outcome under study is mixed with the effect of a third variable, called a confounder [12]. Chance can lead to imprecise results and are an inevitable consequence of sampling, but the effects can be minimized by having a study that is sufficiently large. The role of chance is assessed by performing statistical tests and calculating confidence intervals [11]. It is only after careful consideration of these threats to validity that inferences about causal relationships can be made. In inherited diseases, multiple biases frequently influence the results of cohort studies, confounding may be present, and chance is more likely to occur because of small sample sizes.

Evaluating the role of bias as an alternative explanation for an observed association, or lack of one, is vital when interpreting any study result. Therefore, a better understanding of the specific types of bias that exist and their implication for particular study design is essential. The remainder of this chapter will be devoted to (a) describing various types of bias and how they relate to the study of inherited diseases, (b) discussing bias in relation to specific study designs, and (c) reporting general methods used to minimize bias.

2   Types of Bias Common in Epidemiologic Studies

It is impossible to eliminate all potential sources of error from a study, so it is important to assess their magnitude. There are two types of error associated with most forms of research: random and systematic. Random error is caused by variations in study samples arising by chance and systematic error refers to bias. Random error affects the precision of a study and may be minimized by using larger sample sizes. This may be impossible in rare genetic conditions. Systematic errors (bias) can affect the accuracy of a study's findings and must be addressed by good study design [13]. This may also be difficult in inherited diseases particularly because of ascertainment bias, survivor bias, volunteer bias, lead-time bias, and so forth. Bias is not diminished by increasing sample size.

Each of the major parts of an investigation is at risk of bias, including selection of subjects, performance of the maneuver, measurement of the outcome, data collection, data analysis, data interpretation, and even reporting the findings [13]. Bias has been classified into three general categories: selection bias, information bias, and confounding [1, 14, 15]. Others include a fourth category of bias referred to as intervention bias [16–18]. Types of bias are listed in Table 1.

Table 1
Bias in clinical studies

Selection bias
Ascertainment bias
Competing risks bias
Volunteer bias
Nonresponse bias
Loss to follow-up bias
Prevalence-incidence bias
Survivor treatment selection bias
Overmatching bias
Information bias
Recall bias
Lead-time bias
Length-time bias
Diagnostic bias
Will Rogers phenomenon
Family information bias
Intervention bias
Compliance bias
Proficiency bias
Contamination bias

2.1   Selection Bias: Are the Groups Similar in All Important Respects?

Selection bias is a distortion in the estimate of association between risk factor and disease that results from how the subjects are selected for the study [19, 20]. It occurs when there is a systematic difference between the characteristics of the people that are selected for the study and those that are not [21]. Selection biases will ultimately affect the applicability and usefulness of findings and make it impossible to generalize the results to all patients with the disorder of interest. Many types of biases occur in the study of inherited disorders, and the following are just a few of the more common biases that fall under the category of selection bias.

2.1.1   Ascertainment Bias

Ascertainment bias can occur in any study design. It is introduced by the criteria used to select individuals and occurs when the kind of patients selected for study are not representative of all cases in the population [16]. This is especially relevant to studies which examine risk associated with the inheritance of a mutated gene. Ascertainment bias is further complicated by the tendency of families with more severe disease to be identified through hospital clinics (often called referral bias), rather than through population-based research strategies [6].

Example
In Lynch syndrome families with a mismatch repair gene mutation, the lifetime risk of colorectal cancer has been determined using families that have been selected for genetic testing based on the Amsterdam criteria. These criteria require that CRC be present in three relatives, one of whom is a first degree relative of the other two, that at least two generations be affected, and that CRC occur in one of the family members before the age of 50 years. The use of these very restrictive criteria were helpful in the search for causative genes but were bound to cause an ascertainment bias towards multiple case families and towards a more severe phenotype. Smaller families with only one or two CRC cases and families with other Lynch syndrome-related cancers would not be selected leading to an overrepresentation of families with multiple CRC cases in the study sample. Furthermore, families in which cancer occurred at a later age were excluded. The estimates of penetrance obtained in this manner would not be representative of all mutation carriers in the general population [5, 22].

2.1.2   Competing Risks Bias

Competing risks occur commonly in medical research. Often times, a patient may experience an event, other than the one of interest, which alters the risk of experiencing the actual event of interest. Such events are known as competing risk events [23] and may produce biased risk estimates.

Example

Carriers of MSH2 (a mismatch repair gene) mutations are at risk of developing a number of different cancers, such as CRC, endometrial cancer, uterine cancer, stomach cancer, transitional cell cancers of the kidney, ureter, bladder, and others. Therefore, estimates of risk obtained may be biased because multiple events are related to the genetic mutation. An individual who develops stomach cancer, for example, and who dies from it, will no longer be at risk for another type of cancer, such as CRC. Thus, when examining the incidence of CRC, stomach cancer would be a competing risk because those who die of it are no longer at risk of CRC.

2.1.3   Volunteer Bias

Volunteer bias is also referred to as "self-selection" bias. For ethical reasons, most studies allow patients to refuse participation. If those who volunteer for the study differ from those who refuse participation, the results will be affected [9, 13]. Volunteers tend to be better educated, healthier, lead better lifestyles, and have fewer complications given similar interventions than the population as a whole [14]. Research into genetic-environmental interactions has shown the control group (those without the disease of interest) to have higher educational levels and higher annual income than the diseased group [24].

Example

Those who volunteer to enter genetic screening programs may be healthier than those who refuse. This would lead to an incorrect assumption that the screening protocol favorably affects outcome. It may be that disease severity is responsible for the observed difference, not the actual screening test.

2.1.4   Nonresponse Bias

Nonresponse bias occurs when those who do not respond to take part in a study differ in important ways from those who respond [13, 25, 26]. This bias can work in either direction, leading to overestimation or underestimation of the risk factor/intervention.

Example

Prevalence of disease is often estimated by a cross-sectional survey or questionnaire. If for example, you are trying to determine the prevalence of disease associated with a genetic mutation, family members may be contacted and sent a questionnaire to obtain the necessary information. If those who return the questionnaire differ from those who do not return it, then estimates of disease prevalence will be biased. It may be that those who failed to return the questionnaire were sicker, therefore underestimating the true prevalence of disease.

2.1.5   Loss
to Follow-Up Bias

Loss to follow-up bias can be seen in cohort studies and occurs when those who remain in the study differ from those "lost," in terms of personal characteristics and outcome status [9, 14, 18, 21].

When the losses/withdrawals are uneven in both the exposure and outcome categories, the validity of the statistical results may be affected [16].

Example
In order to determine the effectiveness of an intervention in reducing disease risk, it may also be necessary to look at the potential side effects of the intervention to get an accurate picture. For example, if patients drop out of a study because of side effects of the intervention, then the results will be biased. Excluding these patients from the analysis will result in an overestimate of the effectiveness of the intervention.

2.1.6 Prevalence-Incidence (Neyman) Bias

Selective survival may be important in some diseases. For these diseases the use of prevalent instead of incident cases usually distorts the measure of effect [27] due to the fact that a gap in time occurs between exposure and selection of cases. A late look at those exposed early will miss fatal, mild, or resolved cases [13, 15, 25, 26].

Example
If cases for a particular disease are taken from hospital wards, they may not be representative of the general population. For example, if one wanted to look at the relationship between myocardial infarction (MI) and snow shoveling, hospitalized patients would not include patients with a mild, undetected MI, or fatal cases that died on scene or on route to hospital. Therefore, the relationship between MI and snow shoveling would be underestimated.

2.1.7 Survivor Treatment Selection Bias

Survivor treatment selection bias occurs in observational studies when patients who live longer have more probability to receive a certain treatment [16].

Example
Arrhythmogenic right ventricular cardiomyopathy (ARVC) is a cause of sudden cardiac death, usually due to tachyarrhythmias. Patients with tachyarrhythmias are treated with antiarrhythmic drugs and implantable cardioverter-defibrillator (ICD) therapy [8]. However, in order for patients with ARVC to receive an ICD, they have to live long enough to have the surgery. Therefore, patients who receive an ICD may differ in disease severity from those who died before treatment, leading to an overestimation of the effect of the intervention.

2.1.8 Overmatching Bias

Overmatching bias occurs when cases and controls are matched on a nonconfounding variable (associated with the exposure but not the disease) and can underestimate an association [16].

2.2 Information Bias

Information bias is also referred to as "measurement bias." Information bias is a distortion in the estimate of association between risk factor and disease that is due to systematic measurement error or misclassification of subjects on one or more variables, either risk factor or disease status [19]. It occurs if data used in the study are inaccurate or incomplete, thus influencing the validity of the study conclusions [20, 21]. The effect of information bias depends on its type and may result in misclassification of study subjects. Misclassification can be "differential" if it is related to exposure or outcome and differs in the groups to be compared, or "nondifferential" if it is unrelated to exposure and outcome and is the same across both groups to be compared [9, 16]. The following biases are all considered to be a particular type of information bias.

2.2.1 Recall Bias

Recall or memory bias may be a problem if outcomes being measured require that subjects (cases and controls) recall past events. Questions about specific exposures may be asked more frequently of cases than controls, and cases may be more likely to intensely search their memories for potential causative exposures [13, 25–27]. The recall of cases and controls may differ both in amount and accuracy and the direction of differential recall cannot always be predicted [20, 26]. However, in most situations, cases tend to better recall past exposures leading to an overestimation of the association between outcome and prior exposure to the risk factor [19]. This is particularly important in family studies of genetic disease, where there is usually a cross-sectional start point and phenotypic information is obtained using retrospective and prospective designs. Retrospective chart reviews are unlikely to contain the detailed clinical information that can be obtained by prospective evaluation, thus requiring patients to recall past events to ensure complete information.

Example
Mothers of children with birth defects/abnormalities may recall exposure to drugs or other toxins more readily than mothers of healthy born children. This may lead to an overestimation of the association between a particular drug/toxin and birth defects.

2.2.2 Lead-Time Bias

Lead-time bias is produced when diagnosis of a condition is made during its latency period, leading to a longer duration of illness [16] (*see* Fig. 1). If study patients are not all enrolled at similar, well-defined points in the course of their disease, differences in outcome over time may merely reflect this longer duration [28]. It falsely appears to prolong survival.

Example
This is particularly relevant in studies evaluating the efficacy of screening programs as cancer cases detected in the screened group

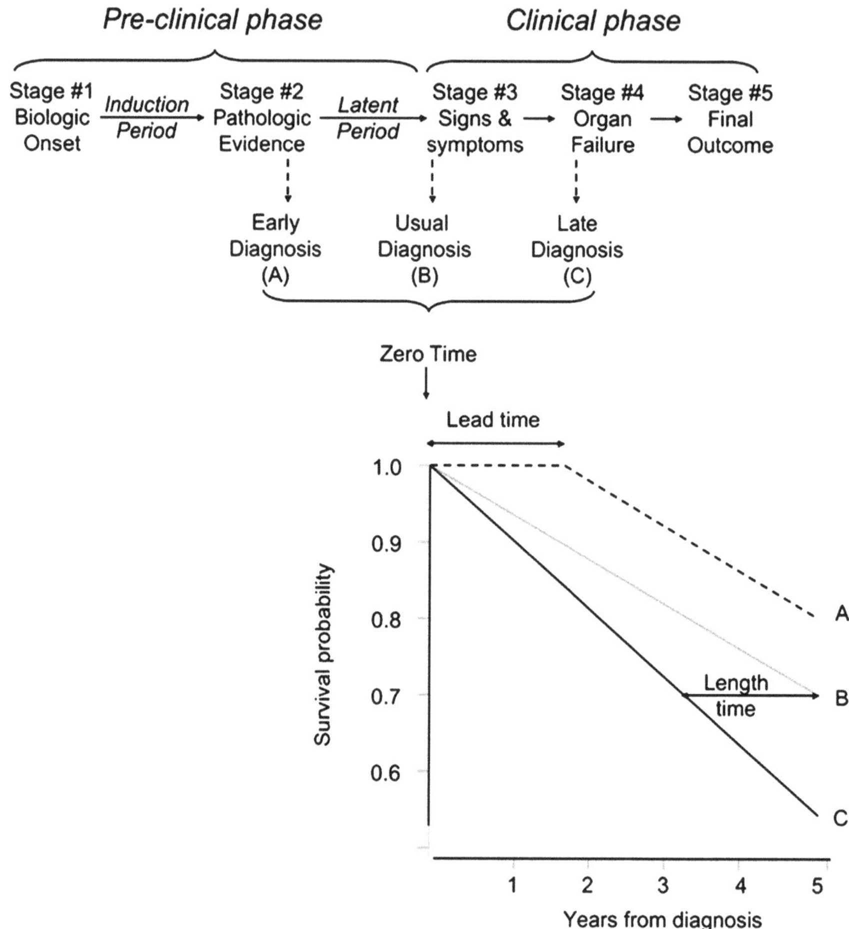

Fig. 1 Natural course of a disease and possible biases related to the timing of diagnosis. The course of a disease is represented as a sequence of stages, from biologic onset to a final outcome such as death. Disease diagnosis can be made as soon as pathologic lesions are detectable (stage #2); when initial signs and symptoms occur (stage #3); or later on (stage #4). Lead-time bias occurs when subjects are diagnosed earlier (**a**) than usual (**b**) independent of the speed of progression of the disease. If group A, for example, contains more subjects diagnosed in stage #2, the apparent observed benefit is due to a zero-time shift backward from the time of usual diagnosis leading to a longer observed duration of illness. Length-time bias occurs when more severe forms of the disease (**c**), characterized by shorter induction and/or latent periods and lower likelihood of early or usual diagnosis, are unbalanced by group. The apparent difference in prognosis is due not only to differences in disease progression (*slope*) but also to differences in timing of diagnosis. With permission from ref. 32

will have a longer duration of illness than those diagnosed through routine care. For example, it may appear that cancer cases detected through screening have a 10-year survival as compared to a 7-year survival for those detected symptomatically. However, the apparent increase in survival may be due to the fact that the screening procedure was able to detect the cancer 3 years prior to the development of symptoms. Therefore, the overall survival time, from disease onset to death, is the same for both groups.

2.2.3 Length-Time Bias

Length-time bias occurs when a group of patients contains more severe forms of the disease characterized by shorter induction periods or includes patients who have progressed further along the natural course of the disease and are in a later phase of disease (*see* Fig. 1).

Example

The apparent worse prognosis in one group of ADPKD patients compared to another may not be due to faster progression of the disease but that more cases with chronic kidney disease (who are further on in the natural course of the disease) have been enrolled in one group compared to the other.

2.2.4 Diagnostic Bias

Diagnostic bias is also referred to as surveillance bias and tends to inflate the measure of risk. This bias occurs when the disease being investigated is more likely to be detected in people who are under frequent medical surveillance as compared to those receiving routine medical attention [25]. Screening studies are prone to this type of bias [9].

Example

Carriers of mutations which predispose to cancer may undergo more intensive follow-up than those with undetected mutations allowing for earlier cancer detection among the former group.

2.2.5 Will Rogers Phenomenon

In medicine, the Will Rogers phenomenon refers to improvement over time in the classification of disease stages: if diagnostic sensitivity increases, metastases are recognized earlier so that the distinction between early and late stages of cancer will improve [29]. This produces a stage migration from early to more advanced stages and an apparent higher survival [16].

Example

This bias is relevant when comparing cancer survival rates across time or even among centers with different diagnostic capabilities. For example, Hospital A may have a more sensitive diagnostic test to detect cancer than Hospital B. Patients deemed to have early stage cancer at Hospital B would actually be deemed later stage cancer patients at Hospital A because of the sensitivity of the test at Hospital A to detect even earlier stage cancers. Therefore, Hospital A will appear to have better survival for its early stage cancer patients when compared to early stage cancer patients at Hospital B. However, the increased survival at Hospital A is due to a more sensitive measure which allows for better definition of an early stage cancer.

2.2.6 Family Information Bias

Within a family, the flow of information about exposure and disease is stimulated by a family member who develops the disease [9, 13, 25, 26]. An affected individual is more likely than an unaffected family member to know about the family history for a particular disease.

Example
An individual with a particular disease is more likely to recall a positive family history of disease than a control subject who does not have the disease. Therefore, risk estimates for the effect of family history on disease may be overestimated when obtained from a case as opposed to a control.

2.3 Intervention (Exposure) Bias

This group of biases involves differences in how the treatment or intervention was carried out, or how subjects were exposed to the factor of interest [17, 18]. Three common intervention biases are compliance bias, proficiency bias, and contamination bias.

2.3.1 Compliance Bias

Compliance bias occurs when differences in subject adherence to the planned treatment regimen or intervention affect the study outcomes [13, 16, 26].

Example
Patients who enter clinical screening programs following genetic testing may not always be compliant with guidelines established for appropriate screening intervals. Therefore, patients who do not follow the protocol guidelines will tend to have worse outcomes than compliant patients and this will lead to an apparent decrease in the effectiveness of screening.

2.3.2 Proficiency Bias

Proficiency bias occurs when treatments or interventions are not administered equally to subjects [13]. This may be due to skill or training differences among personnel and/or differences in resources or procedures used at different sites [17].

Example
Colorectal cancer screening protocols may differ between facilities. For example, one hospital may use barium enema as the screening procedure whereas another may use colonoscopy. Colonoscopy is more efficient at detecting polyps than barium enema, leading to better outcomes. Therefore, comparing the impact of screening between these two hospitals, without taking into account the different screening procedures, would lead to a biased result.

2.3.3 Contamination Bias

Contamination bias occurs when control group subjects inadvertently receive the intervention or are exposed to extraneous treatments, thus potentially minimizing the difference in outcomes between the cases and controls [13, 16, 26].

Example
To determine the effectiveness of ICD therapy in patients with ARVC as opposed to ARVC patients without an ICD, drug therapy should also be taken into consideration. If those in the control group are receiving antiarrhythmic drugs and those in the intervention group are not, then contamination bias may exist. This may lower survival benefit estimates for the ICD group.

2.4 Confounding: Is an extraneous factor blurring the effect?

This is part of the section heading and should not be written here.

All associations are potentially influenced by the effects of confounding, which can be thought of as alternative explanations for an association. To be a confounder, a variable must meet the following three characteristics:

1. It must be a risk factor for the disease in question.

2. It must be associated with the exposure under study, in the population for which the cases were derived.

3. It must not be an intermediate step in the causal pathway between exposure and disease [30].

To accurately assess the impact of confounding, you must consider the size and direction of the effect modification. It is not merely the presence or absence of a confounder that is the problem; it's the influence of the confounder on the association that is important [21]. Confounding can lead to either observation of apparent differences between study groups when they don't really exist (overestimation), or, conversely, observation of no differences when they do exist (underestimation) [21].

Age and sex are the most common confounding variables in health-related research. They are associated with a number of exposures, such as diet and smoking habits, and are also independent risk factors for most diseases [11]. Confounding cannot occur if potential confounders do not vary across groups [10]. For example, in a case-control study, for age and sex to be confounders, their representation should sufficiently differ between cases and controls [27].

3 Biases Linked to Specific Study Designs

While some study designs are more prone to bias, its presence is universal. There is no ideal study design: different designs are appropriate in different situations and all have particular methodological issues and constraints [1, 9].

Selection biases relate to the design phase of an observational study and are the most difficult to avoid [20]. They can be minimized in prospective cohort studies but are problematic in retrospective and case-control studies, because both disease outcome and exposure have already been ascertained at the time of participant selection [9]. Bias in the choice of controls is also a major issue in case-control studies. Ensuring that controls are a representative sample of the population from where the cases came is difficult and can be time consuming [14].

Loss to follow-up bias is a major problem in prospective cohort studies especially if people drop out of a study for reasons that are related to the exposure or outcome [31]. If the duration of follow-up is shorter than the time required for a particular exposure to have its effect on an outcome, then risks will be underestimated [14, 21].

Recall bias is major issue for case-control and retrospective cohort studies where exposure status may be self-reported [9]. Subjects who know their disease status are more likely to accurately recall prior exposures. This bias is particularly problematic when the exposure of interest is rare [26]. Prevalence-incidence bias is also problematic for case-control studies, especially if cases are identified in the clinical setting because mild cases who do not present to clinic or those who have died at a young age are likely to be missed [25].

Cross-sectional studies are particularly vulnerable to volunteer bias and nonresponse bias. This type of study requires participants to fill out a questionnaire/survey and is likely to be biased as those who volunteer are unlikely to be representative of the general population and those who respond likely differ from those who do not respond.

4   Methods to Minimize the Impact of Bias and Confounding in Epidemiologic Studies

Issues of bias and confounding are challenges that researchers face, especially in observational studies. Techniques exist to prevent and adjust for these biases analytically, and an understanding of their characteristics is vital to interpreting and applying study results [12].

4.1   Strategies for Dealing with Bias

The causes of bias can be related to the manner in which study subjects are chosen, the method in which study variables are collected or measured, the attitudes or preferences of an investigator, and the lack of control of confounding variables [9]. The key to decreasing bias is to identify the possible areas that could be affected and to change the design accordingly [18, 21].

Minimizing selection biases requires careful selection of a study population for whom complete and accurate information is available [21]. To ensure this, clear and precise definitions should be developed for populations, disease, exposure, cases and controls, inclusion and exclusion criteria, methods of recruiting the subjects into the study, units of measurement, and so forth. Comparison of baseline characteristics is important to ensure the similarity of the groups to be compared. Paying careful attention to the willingness of subjects to continue with the study and employing multiple methods of follow-up can be useful in reducing loss [30]. Some loss is almost inevitable, depending on the length of the study, and as such it can be useful to perform sensitivity analyses. Here the missing group are all assumed to have a good or bad outcome and the impact of these assumptions on the outcome is evaluated [18].

Minimizing information biases requires appropriate and objective methods of data collection and good quality control. Information bias can be reduced by the use of repeated measures, training of the researchers, using standardized measures, and using more than one source of information [18]. Blinding of subjects, researchers, and statisticians can also reduce those biases where knowledge of a subject's treatment, exposure, or case-control status may influence the results obtained [14, 20].

4.2 Strategies for Dealing with Confounding

Confounding is the only type of bias that can be prevented or adjusted for, provided that confounding was anticipated and the requisite information was collected [15]. In observational studies, there are two principle ways to reduce confounding:

1. Prevention in the design phase by restriction or matching

2. Adjustment in the analysis phase by either stratification or multivariate modeling [2, 10–12, 15, 21, 27]

At the time of designing the study, one should first list all those factors which are likely to be confounders, and then decide how to deal with each in the design and/or analysis phase [30].

4.2.1 Prevention in the Design Phase

The simplest approach is *restriction*. Restriction occurs when admission to the study is restricted to a certain category of a confounder [2, 21, 27]. For example, if smoking status is a potential confounder, the study population may be restricted to nonsmokers. Although this tactic avoids confounding it leads to poorer external validity, as results are limited to the narrow group included in the study, and also, potential shrinking of the sample size [12, 15].

A second strategy is *matching*, so that for each case one or more controls with the same value for the confounding variable are selected. This allows all levels of a potential confounder to be included in the analysis and ensures that within each case-control stratum, the level of the confounder is identical [2, 21, 27]. A common example is to match cases and controls for age and gender. Matching is most commonly used in case-control studies, but it can be used in cohort studies as well and is very useful when the number of subjects in a study is small. However, when the number of possible confounders increases, matching cases and controls can be difficult, time consuming, and therefore expensive. A number of potential controls may have to be excluded before one is found with all the appropriate characteristics. Also, by definition, one cannot examine the effect of a matched variable [15, 21, 27].

4.2.2 Adjustment in the Analysis Phase

Adjusting for confounding will improve the validity but reduce the precision of the estimate [20]. It is only possible to control for confounding in the analysis phase if data on potential confounders were collected during the study. Therefore, the extent to which confounding can be controlled for will depend on the completeness and accuracy of this data [11].

Stratification is one option commonly used to adjust for confounding after the study has been completed. It is a technique that involves the evaluation of association between the exposure and disease within homogeneous categories (strata) of the confounding variable [10, 15, 21]. For example, if gender is a confounding variable, the association between exposure and disease can be determined for men and women separately. Methods are then available for summarizing the overall association, by producing a weighted average of the estimates obtained for each stratum. One such method is the Mantel-Haenszel procedure [21]. If the Mantel-Haenszel adjusted effect differs substantially from the crude effect, then confounding is deemed present [15]. Stratification is often limited by the size of the study and its ability to only control for a small number of factors simultaneously. As the number of confounders increases, the number of strata greatly increases and the sample size within each strata decreases. This in turn, may lead to inadequate statistical power [2, 21].

The second option is *multivariate modeling*. This approach uses advanced statistical methods of analysis that simultaneously adjust (control) for several variables while examining the potential effect of each one [2, 10, 15, 21]. In epidemiological research, the most common method of multivariate analysis is regression modeling which includes linear regression, logistic regression, and Cox's regression, to name a few. Linear regression is used if the outcome variable is continuous, logistic regression is used if the outcome variable is binary, and Cox's regression is used when the outcome is time dependent. Multivariate modeling can control for more factors than stratification but care should still be taken not to include too many variables. Also, the appropriateness and the fit of the model should be examined to ensure accurate conclusions [21].

Each method of control has its strengths and limitations and in most situations, a combination of strategies will provide the best solution [21].

5   Conclusions

In epidemiologic research, it is essential to avoid bias and to control for confounding. However, bias of some degree will always be present in an epidemiologic study. The main concern, therefore, is how it relates to the validity of the study. Selection biases make it impossible to generalize the results to all patients with the disorder

Table 2
Questions to aid in the identification of biases [14]

- Is the study population defined?
- Does the study population represent the target population?
- Are the definitions of disease and exposure clear?
- Is the case definition precise?
- What are the inclusion or exclusion criteria?

- Do the controls represent the population from which the cases came?
- Could exposure status have influenced identification or selection of cases or controls?
- Are the cohorts similar except for exposure status?
- Are the measurements as objective as possible?
- Is the study blinded as far as possible?

- Is the follow-up adequate?
- Is the follow-up equal for all cohorts?
- Is the analysis appropriate?
- Are the variable groups used in the analysis defined a priori?
- Is the interpretation supported by the results?

of interest, while the measurement biases influence the validity of the study conclusions [20]. Key questions to ask to identify biases when planning, executing, or reading a study are identified in Table 2 [14]. If answers to these questions are unsatisfactory, then careful consideration should be given to the quality and clinical relevance of the study's results.

The previous discussion is just an overview of some of the main types of biases inherent in observational research. For a more detailed and comprehensive list, refer to articles by Sackett [26], Delgado-Rodríquez and Llorca [16], and Hartman et al. [13].

References

1. Young JM, Solomon MJ (2003) Improving the evidence base in surgery: sources of bias in surgical studies. ANZ J Surg 73:504–506

2. Jepsen P, Johnsen SP, Gillman MW, Sorensen HT (2004) Interpretation of observational studies. Heart 90:956–960

3. Blackmore CC, Cummings P (2004) Observational studies in radiology. AJR 183: 1203–1208

4. Barnett ML, Hyman JJ (2006) Challenges in interpreting study results: the conflict between appearance and reality. JADA 137:32S–36S

5. Stuckless S, Parfrey PS, Woods MO, Cox J, Fitzgerald GW, Green JS, Green RC (2007) The phenotypic expression of three MSH2 mutations in large Newfoundland families with Lynch Syndrome. Fam Cancer 6:1–12

6. Dicks E, Ravani P, Langman D, Davidson WS, Pei Y, Parfrey PS (2006) Incident renal events and risk factors in autosomal dominant polycystic kidney disease: a population and family based cohort followed for 22 years. Clin J Am Soc Nephrol 1:710–717

7. Moore SJ, Green JS, Fan Y, Bhogal AK, Dicks E, Fernandez BF, Stefanelli M, Murphy C, Cramer BC, Dean JCS, Beales PL, Katsanis N, Bassett A, Davidson WS, Parfrey PS (2005) Clinical and genetic epidemiology of Bardet-Biedl syndrome in Newfoundland: a 22-year prospective, population-based cohort study. Am J Med Genet 132A:352–360

8. Hodgkinson KA, Parfrey PS, Bassett AS, Kupprion C, Drenckhahn J, Norman MW, Thierfelder L, Stuckless SN, Dicks EL, McKenna WJ, Connors SP (2005) The impact of implantable cardioverter-defibrillator therapy on survival in autosomal-dominant arrhythmogenic right ventricular cardiomyopathy (ARVD5). J Am Coll Cardiol 45:400–408

9. Sica GT (2006) Bias in research studies. Radiology 238:780–789

10. Zaccai JH (2004) How to assess epidemiological studies. Postgrad Med J 80:140–147

11. Moles DR, dos Santos Silva I (2000) Causes, associations and evaluating evidence; can we trust what we read? Evid Base Dent 2:75–78

12. Dore DD, Larrat EP, Vogenberg FR (2006) Principles of epidemiology for clinical and formulary management professionals. P&T 31:218–226

13. Hartman JM, Forsen JW, Wallace MS, Neely JG (2002) Tutorials in clinical research: part IV: recognizing and controlling bias. Laryngoscope 112:23–31

14. Sitthi-amorn C, Poshyachinda V (1993) Bias. Lancet 342:286–288

15. Grimes DA, Schulz KF (2002) Bias and causal associations in observational research. Lancet 359:248–52

16. Delgado-Rodríguez M, Llorca J (2004) Bias. J Epidemiol Community Health 58:635–641

17. Major types of research study bias. http://www.umdnj.edu/idsweb/shared/biases.htm

18. Clancy MJ (2002) Overview of research designs. Emerg Med J 19:546–549

19. Bayona M, Olsen C (2004) Observational studies and bias in epidemiology. YES—The Young Epidemiology Scholars Program; Copyright 2004. http://www.collegeboard.com/prod_downloads/yes/4297_MODULE_19.pdf

20. World Health Organization (2nd ed.) (2001) Health research methodology: A guide for training in research methods. http://www.wpro.who.int/NR/rdonlyres/F334320C-2B19_4F38-A358-27E84FF3BC0F/0/contents.pdf

21. Hammal DM, Bell CL (2002) Confounding and bias in epidemiological investigations. Pediatr Hematol Oncol 19:375–381

22. Carayol J, Khlat M, Maccario J, Bonaiti-Pellie C (2002) Hereditary non-polyposis colorectal cancer: current risks of colorectal cancer largely overestimated. J Med Genet 39:335–339

23. Satagopan JM, Ben-Porat L, Berwick M, Robson M, Kutler D, Auerbach AD (2004) A note on competing risks in survival data analysis. Br J Cancer 91:1229–1235

24. Wang PP, Dicks E, Gong X, Buehler S, Zhao J, Squires J, Younghusband B, McLaughlin JR, Parfrey PS (2009) Validity of random-digit-dialing in recruiting controls in a case—control study. Am J Health Behav 33:513–20

25. Manolio TA, Bailey-Wilson JE, Collins FS (2006) Genes, environment and the value of prospective cohort studies. Nat Rev Genet 7:812–820

26. Sackett DL (1979) Bias in analytic research. J Chron Dis 32:51–63

27. Dorak MT (2012) Bias and confounding. http://www.dorak.info/epi/bc.html

28. EBM Definitions (2014) Clinical epidemiology definitions. http://www.fammed.ouhsc.edu/robhamm/UsersGuide/define.htm

29. Vineis P, McMichael AJ (1998) Bias and confounding in molecular epidemiological studies: special considerations. Carcinogenesis 19:2063–2067

30. Mother and Child Health: Research Methods (2014) Chapter 13: Common pitfalls. http://www.oxfordjournals.org/our_journals/tropej/online/ce_ch13.pdf

31. Okasha M (2001) Interpreting epidemiological findings. Student BMJ 9:324–325

32. Ravani P, Parfrey PS, Dicks E, Barrett BJ (2007) Clinical research of kidney diseases II: problems of study design. Nephrol Dial Transpl 22:2785–2794

Chapter 21

Clinical Genetic Research 2: Genetic Epidemiology of Complex Phenotypes

Darren D. O'Rielly and Proton Rahman

Abstract

Genetic factors play a substantive role in the susceptibility to common diseases. Due to recent and rapid advancements in characterization of genetic variants and large-scale genotyping platforms, multiple genes and genetic variants have now been identified for common, complex diseases. The most efficient method for gene identification at present appears to be large-scale association-based studies, which integrate genetic and epidemiological principles. As the strategy for gene identification studies has shifted towards genetic association-based methods rather than traditional linkage analysis, epidemiological methods are increasingly being integrated into genetic investigations. Consequently, the disciplines of genetics and epidemiology, which historically have functioned separately, have been integrated into a discipline referred to as genetic epidemiology. In this chapter, we review methods for establishing the genetic burden of complex genetic disease, followed by methods for gene and/or genetic variant identification and when appropriate we highlight the epidemiological issues that guide these methods.

Key words Genetic epidemiology, Linkage studies, Association studies, Whole genome-wide association scans, Genotyping, Linkage disequilibrium

1 Introduction

Despite many advances in medicine, the basis for most common, complex disorders still remains elusive [1]. Complex disorders, assumed to be of multifactorial etiology, exhibit non-Mendelian inheritance and arise from an interplay of genetic, epigenetic, and environmental factors. Cumulative evidence implicates a substantive role for genetic factors in the etiology of common diseases [1]. Recent evidence suggests that common genetic variants will explain at least some of the inherited variation in susceptibility to common disease [2]. These variants may impact disease susceptibility, expression, or drug response. For most traits, there is evidence that rare Mendelian mutations, low-frequency segregating variants, and copy number variants (CNVs) may also contribute toward complex phenotypes. The elucidation of the genetic determinants

Patrick S. Parfrey and Brendan J. Barrett (eds.), *Clinical Epidemiology: Practice and Methods*, Methods in Molecular Biology, vol. 1281, DOI 10.1007/978-1-4939-2428-8_21, © Springer Science+Business Media New York 2015

is of great importance as it can suggest mechanisms that can lead to a better understanding of disease pathogenesis, and improved prediction of disease risk, diagnosis, prognosis, and therapy.

The contribution of genetics to complex disease is usually ascertained by conducting population-based genetic-epidemiological studies followed by carefully planned genetic analyses [3]. Specifically, these include family- and population-based epidemiological studies that estimate the genetic burden of disease followed by molecular studies that investigate candidate gene, genome-wide linkage, or genome-wide association studies, which set out to identify the specific genetic determinants.

As the strategy for gene identification studies has shifted towards genetic association methods rather than traditional linkage analysis, epidemiological methods are increasingly being integrated into genetic concepts [4]. As a result, the disciplines of genetics and epidemiology, which historically have functioned separately, have been integrated into a discipline referred to as genetic epidemiology. In this chapter, we review methods for establishing the genetic burden of complex genetic disease, followed by methods for gene and/or genetic variant identification. We end with a discussion on genome-wide association analysis, the so-called "missing heritability" of complex disease, and finally we discuss strategies to elucidate this "missing heritability" in future genomic investigations.

2 Establishing a Genetic Component of a Complex Trait

For complex traits, it is necessary to prove claims of genetic determination. The obvious way to approach this is to show that the trait segregates in families. Segregation analysis is the main statistical tool for analyzing the inheritance of any trait, and it can provide evidence for or against a major susceptibility locus.

Complex genetic diseases are considered to be heritable as they clearly cluster in families. However, these traits do not demonstrate a clear Mendelian pattern of inheritance (i.e., dominant or recessive). The strength of the genetic effect in any particular disease varies significantly and is not necessarily intuitive, as familial clustering, from a clinical perspective, occurs more frequently in highly prevalent diseases. If the contribution of the genetic variation is small, then a gene identification project becomes very difficult if not impossible, as large sample sizes will be required in order to identify genetic factors. As a result, it is important to carefully examine all epidemiological data to determine the genetic burden of a complex trait or disease.

One of the most compelling methods to implicate genetics in complex disease is through the use of twin studies [5]. Twin studies typically estimate the heritability of a disorder, which refers to the proportion of variability of a trait attributed to genetic factors.

An increased disease concordance between monozygotic twins as compared to dizygotic twins, strongly implicates genetic factors. This is indeed the case in psoriasis, where there is a threefold increased risk of psoriasis in identical twins as compared with fraternal twins [6, 7]. However, as the concordance for psoriasis among monozygotic twins is 35 %, this suggests that environmental factors also play an important role in disease susceptibility. Importantly, genetic epidemiologists must be mindful that parents give their children their environment as well as their genes and consequently, many traits segregate in families because of shared family environment.

Evidence for genetic variation of a complex trait can also be obtained from population-based studies by estimating the risk ratio. The magnitude of genetic contribution is estimated by assessing the relative proportion of disease in siblings (or other relatives) as compared with the prevalence of disease in the general population. This parameter, originally formulated by Risch, is denoted as λ_R, where "R" represents the degree of relatedness, with higher λ values indicating a greater genetic effect [8]. By convention, any λ value greater than two is generally considered to indicate a significant genetic component. It is important to acknowledge however that λ_R can be influenced by shared environmental factors and thus cannot be solely attributed to genetic factors [8]. Moreover, the prevalence of a particular trait in relatives and the general population can affect its size. Therefore, a strong genetic effect in a very common disease will yield a smaller λ value, compared with an equally strong genetic effect in a rare disease. Consequently, the λ value is not an ideal measure for highly prevalent complex diseases as it can underestimate the genetic component [8].

3   Determining the Mode of Inheritance

Most biological traits of interest to humans have a multifactorial pattern of inheritance in that they are determined by many mutations at multiple loci, as well as by many nongenetic factors [8]. Some traits demonstrate classical Mendelian patterns of inheritance and segregate within families [9–12]. For example, there are reports that propose an autosomal dominant inheritance pattern and others that suggest an autosomal recessive pattern of inheritance for psoriasis [10].

Formal segregation analysis has historically been used as the method for identifying the presence of a major genetic effect. However, due to the expense and time required, segregation analysis is now routinely overlooked. Risch has developed criteria for using risk ratios among relatives of differing relatedness to obtain information about genetic models [8]. When the risk ratio $(\lambda_R - 1)$ decreases by a factor of greater than 2 between the first and second degrees of relatedness, the data are consistent with a multi-locus model [8].

Increasingly, alternative non-Mendelian inheritance patterns are now being proposed for complex disorders. These include triplet expansion mutations (anticipation), genomic imprinting, and mitochondrial-related inheritance [11]. Anticipation is characterized by a dynamic trinucleotide repeat sequence mutation and is associated with an increase in severity and decrease in age of onset in successive generations [11]. Myotonic dystrophy is a classic example of a trait that demonstrates anticipation [12].

Genomic imprinting refers to an epigenetic effect that causes differential expression of a gene depending on the sex of the transmitting parent [13]. The imprinting process dictates that the gene can be transmitted from a parent of either sex and is expressed only when inherited from one particular sex. Imprinting is a normal development process that regulates gene expression and is thought to affect a limited number of genes [13]. The first human disorder recognized to be a consequence of genomic imprinting is the Prader–Willi syndrome [14]. This phenomenon has also been reported in autism and multiple autoimmune diseases including psoriatic arthritis, where the proportion of probands with an affected father (0.65) is significantly greater than the expected proportion of 0.5 [15–17].

Mitochondria contain their own genome and mitochondrial DNA controls a number of protein components of the respiratory chain and oxidative phosphorylation system. Since mitochondria are transmitted maternally, a pattern of matrilineal transmission of a disorder is suggestive of mitochondrial inheritance. The strongest evidence for a mitochondrial DNA mutation in a genetic disease is in Leber's optic atrophy, which is characterized by late-onset bilateral loss of central vision and cardiac dysrhythmias [18]. Mitochondrial DNA (mtDNA) mutations have been linked to several complex diseases including Alzheimer's disease and Parkinson's disease [19–22].

4 Strategies for Gene Identification

Once the genetic burden of a trait has been confirmed, attention is then directed to identifying the specific genetic factors underpinning disease pathogenesis. Two commonly used strategies for genetic identification are linkage and association analyses. Linkage methods are based on a positional cloning strategy, where the disease gene is isolated by its chromosomal location without any knowledge of the function of the gene. Association analysis, on the other hand, assesses the relationship between a particular allele, genotype or haplotype in a gene and a given trait or disease. The underlying assumption in association studies is that the causative allele is relatively more common among individuals with a given trait as compared to a healthy control population. While both methods are meritorious in gene identification, careful consideration of the benefits and limitations of each method must be considered when selecting a method for gene identification.

4.1 Linkage Studies

Linkage methods were initially used for identification of susceptibility determinants across the entire genome. Positional cloning has been very successful for identifying disease-related genes for multiple single gene disorders and select complex disorders. There are three basic steps involved in positional cloning. The first is localization of the relevant genes to candidate regions where susceptibility loci are suspected to reside. The next step involves isolation of the candidate genes. The third step involves demonstration of gene mutations within the suspected disease genes, thus proving that the candidate gene is indeed the true susceptibility gene. Genetic epidemiologists are intimately involved with the first two steps, whereas the third step, functional characterization of a gene, is usually carried out by a molecular biologist.

The immediate appeal of linkage studies is the ability to identify novel genes which may not have been initially considered as potential targets. The initial step of positional cloning requires collection of families with multiple affected individuals so that linkage analysis can be performed.

4.1.1 Design of Linkage Studies

There are two established approaches for linkage analysis. A recombinant-based method (also referred to as the traditional or parametric method) and an allele sharing method (also referred to as the model independent or noparametric method) [1, 3].

Parametric Linkage Analysis

The recombinant-based method has been very successful in elucidating the genetic basis of Mendelian disorders where the mode of transmission is known. However, application of this method to determine susceptibility loci for complex traits has proven much more difficult. This method is based on the biological phenomenon of crossing over, termed "recombination." Crossovers take place randomly along a chromosome and the closer two loci are to one another, the less likely a crossover event will occur. The recombination fraction is denoted as (θ) for a given pedigree, and is defined by the probability that a gamete is recombinant. The recombination fraction is a function of distance, when certain assumptions (e.g., mapping functions) are considered. Unfortunately, given that the number of recombination events cannot be directly counted, the recombination fraction must be estimated. This is performed by the maximum likelihood method based on a likelihood ratio statistic, which requires extensive computations and is performed using specialized statistical packages.

Estimates of the recombination fraction, along with the linkage statistic are central parameters in the traditional linkage method.

The ideal setting for the traditional linkage approach involves ascertaining multigenerational families with multiple affected members. All family members are genotyped to determine the number of recombinants. Subsequently, various assumptions are made regarding the mode of inheritance of the disease, frequency of disease alleles, disease penetrance as well as other prespecified parameters. Based on these assumptions and the pedigree structure of the family, a likelihood function for the observed data is constructed. This likelihood is a function of the recombination fraction. Using this likelihood function, a test of the hypothesis of no linkage between a marker and disease can be performed. This is based on the likelihood ratio statistic:

$$\text{Ho: } \theta = 0.5 \text{ (no linkage) Ha: } \theta < 0.5$$

Then "Z" is equivalent to $Z = \log[L(\theta)/L(\theta = 0.5)]$ where $L(\theta)$ is the likelihood function. The null hypothesis of no linkage is rejected if the value of Z maximized over θ (0, 0.5) is greater than 3.0.

Numerous problems occur when using this method for complex diseases as the following specifications need to be estimated for the traditional method: disease gene frequency, mode of transmission, penetrance of disease genes, phenocopy rate, and marker allele frequency [9]. Estimation of the recombination fraction is also sensitive to pedigree structure and certainty of the diagnosis. Model misspecification can result in a biased estimate of the recombination fraction leading to detrimental effects regarding the power to detect linkage.

Nonparametric Linkage Analysis

An alternative approach to linkage studies for complex traits is the allele sharing or nonparametric method [23]. This refers to a set of methods which are based on the following premise: in the presence of linkage between a marker and disease, sets of relatives who share the same disease status will be more similar at the marker locus than one would expect if the two loci were segregating independently. The similarity at the marker locus is measured by counting the number of alleles shared, or identical by descent (IBD), in two relatives. Alleles are considered IBD if they are descendants of the same ancestral lines. For example, the expected frequency of IBD sharing of two alleles for mating of heterozygous parents is 25, 50, and 25 % for 0, 1, and 2 alleles, respectively. The closer the marker locus is to the disease locus, the more likely these proportions will be skewed.

Linkage is stated to occur if there is a significant distortion of these proportions. The recombinant-based method is always more powerful than the allele sharing method to identify susceptibility regions when the correct model is specified. However, these models are often mis-specified. In the allele sharing method, penetrance is not a confounder as it only includes siblings that share the same status. However, this method may lack power as compared with the traditional method. In order to overcome this limitation, a larger number of affected families are required in the allele sharing method as compared with the traditional method. In other cases, there is little to distinguish between the recombinant-based and allele sharing method, even though the allele sharing method is currently favored among statistical geneticists for linkage-based studies.

A successful genome-wide scan will result in the identification of candidate region(s) where the susceptibility gene(s) is suspected to reside. Genome-wide linkage studies initially used microsatellite markers with an average spacing of about 10 cM. It has largely been superseded by the use of single nucleotide markers (SNPs). The advantage of microsatellite markers is that they are more polymorphic than diallelic SNPs and consequently are more informative. However, given that there are many more SNPs than microsatellites, even with just 10,000 SNPs covering the genome (an approximate marker density of 0.3 cM), the information content for SNP genotyping is greater than microsatellite mapping. Currently, microarrays consisting of over a million SNPs, essentially blanketing the genome, are commercially available for linkage studies within families.

4.1.2 Analysis and Interpretation of Linkage Studies	In recombinant-based linkage analysis, standard practice is to summarize the results of a linkage analysis in the form of a LOD score function (log to the base 10 of the likelihood function). The results from the allele-sharing method may be summarized using various methods (e.g., p value, chi-square, Z value), but can be transformed into a LOD score as well. The threshold for the traditional recombinant based method was set by Morton in 1955 [24] at a LOD score of 3 for simple Mendelian traits. In 1995, Lander and Kruglyak [25], considering genetic model constraints, suggested that the LOD score threshold be raised to achieve the genome-wide significance level of 5 %. They proposed that significant linkage be reported if the LOD score reaches at least 3.3–3.8 (p value 0.000045–0.000013, respectively), depending on the pedigree structure. Suggestive linkage can be reported if the LOD score is at least 1.9–2.4 (p value 0.0017–0.00042, respectively), depending on the pedigree structure.

Overall, replication studies for complex disease have been very disappointing in confirming the initial linkage. Commonly cited reasons for this include the possibility that the results of the initial findings were false positive or that the disease exhibits genetic (locus) heterogeneity [26]. It should be acknowledged that failure to replicate does not necessarily disprove a hypothesis unless the study is adequately powered. Therefore, replication studies should clearly state the power of the study to detect the proposed effect. Since replication studies involve testing an established prior hypothesis, the issues regarding multiple testing in a genome scan may be overlooked. As a result, a point-wise comparison p value of 0.01 is sufficient to declare confirmation of linkage at the 5 % level [25].

The number of false-positive results increases with the number of tests performed, which poses a problem for genome-wide linkage studies. Bonferroni's correction, which is used extensively in epidemiological studies, is too conservative for genetic studies. As a result, two stipulations account for multiple testing prior to establishing definite linkage: a high level of significance, and a replication study using an independent sample cohort.

The power of a hypothesis test is the probability of correctly rejecting the null hypothesis given that the alternate hypothesis is true. The following factors may influence the power to detect linkage in a complex disease: (1) the strength of genetic contribution; (2) the presence of epistasis or locus heterogeneity between genes; (3) the recombination fraction between the disease gene and marker locus; (4) the heterozygosity markers used; (5) the relationships of the relatives studied; and (6) the number of families or affected relative pairs available [3, 9, 26]. The calculation of sample size is not straightforward in linkage studies. Although simulation studies have estimated the number of sibling pairs to detect linkage for various degrees of genetic contribution to a disease, these are based on the assumption that the markers are fully informative and tightly linked (i.e., no recombination) to the disease locus [27].

4.1.3 Challenges and Limitations of Linkage Studies

Difficulties encountered in linkage analysis of complex traits include: incomplete penetrance (i.e., phenotype is variably expressed despite having the genotype); phenocopies (i.e., disease phenotype results from causes other than the gene being mapped); genetic (locus) heterogeneity (i.e., when two or more loci can independently cause disease); epistasis (i.e., interacting genotypes at two or more unlinked loci); gene–environment interactions (i.e., where environmental factors can also contribute to disease susceptibility); and insufficient recruitment of family members [3].

The ability to successfully identify a susceptibility region using the positional cloning approach, in part, depends on how well one is able to overcome these limitations. Phenocopies can be reduced by strict adherence to diagnostic criteria and with minimal inclusion of patients with atypical features. Incomplete penetrance can be overcome by using the allele sharing method as all relatives analyzed in this method express the phenotype. Sufficient number of families can be ascertained through extensive international collaborations [3]. Gene–gene interactions (i.e., epistasis) and gene–environment interactions are present challenges that have been difficult to address in the identification of the susceptibility genes.

Genetic heterogeneity is a serious obstacle to overcome in linkage studies. Due to a wide spectrum of clinical features within a disease, at times, evidence for linkage to a locus in one family may be offset by evidence against linkage in another family. Even a modest degree of heterogeneity may significantly weaken the evidence for genetic linkage [9]. A potential solution to limit genetic heterogeneity involves transforming the complex disease into a more homogenous subset. This can be done by splitting the disorder based on the phenotype, studying a single large pedigree, focusing on one ethnic group, or by limiting the study to a single geographic region. Further characterization of the phenotypes usually increases the recurrence risk for relatives and reduces the number of contributing loci [26]. These measures may also enhance the identification of a subset of families that show a Mendelian pattern of disease transmission, allowing more powerful model-based methods to be used in the linkage analysis. Unfortunately, there is no uniformly accepted method for correctly splitting a disease into the various genetic forms.

The successful cloning of the *APC* gene for colon cancer on chromosome 5 was found when the phenotype was restricted to extreme polyposis [28]. In this case an apparent complex trait was narrowed to a simple autosomal one. Early age of onset has also been used as a method to limit genetic heterogeneity. For instance, in a subset of non-insulin dependent diabetes (NIDDM) patients with an earlier age of onset (as reviewed in [3]), segregation analysis revealed an autosomal dominant transmission pattern. Subsequent studies revealed that a mutation in the glucokinase gene accounts for 50 % of cases of NIDDM in the young. Susceptibility genes for breast cancer and Alzheimer's have also been identified by stratifying patients according to the age of onset of the clinical disorder. Studying families with multiple affected members or "high genetic load" can limit heterogeneity such was the case with hereditary nonpolyposis colon cancer (HNPCC), which was mapped by selecting probands with two other affected relatives (as reviewed in [3]). Finally, disease severity has been exploited in genetic studies, focusing on extreme ends of a trait, whether it be mild or severe. This approach works especially well for continuous traits [9, 26].

4.2 Association-Based Studies

Association is not a specifically genetic phenomenon; rather it is simply a statistical statement about the co-occurrence of allele or phenotypes. In principle, linkage and association are totally different phenomena. Linkage is a relation between loci, but association is a relation between alleles or phenotypes. Linkage is a specifically genetic relationship, while association is simply a statistical observation that might have various causes. Linkage creates associations within families, but not among unrelated people.

Association-based studies have gained much popularity and have become the method of choice for identification of genetic variants for complex diseases. Association studies are easier to conduct than linkage analysis because no multigenerational families or special family structures are required. Moreover, association-based methods are more efficient for identifying common variants for modest to weak genetic effects, which is the typical effect size for a complex trait. Association studies have also immensely benefited from the characterization of a large number of SNP markers, linkage disequilibrium (LD) data from the HapMap project, and the development of high throughput genotyping technologies. Although association-based genetic studies have rapidly increased in number, it is important to appreciate the assumptions, results, and challenges using this approach.

4.2.1 Design of Association-Based Studies

Association studies can either be direct or indirect. For direct association studies, the marker itself plays a causative role. The topology of the SNP is helpful for selecting variants, as those that alter function through non-synonymous protein-coding changes, or through effects on transcription or translation are more valuable. In an indirect association, the association is due to a marker locus being in close proximity to a causative locus, so that there is very little recombination between them. The specific gene or region of interest is usually selected on a positional basis. Haplotypes are important in the indirect approach, because regions within some markers are non-randomly associated. Accordingly, SNPs are prioritized not only on their potential function but also with respect to their position. Tag-SNPs serve as efficient markers as they are within blocks displaying strong LD. Haplotype length and allele frequencies from different populations are available from public databases such as the International HapMap Project [29].

The candidate gene approach focuses on associations between genetic variation within prespecified genes of interest and phenotypes or disease states. Candidate genes are most often selected for study based on a priori knowledge of the functional impact of the gene on the trait or disease in question. This approach usually uses the case–control study design and once investigators have selected a candidate gene, they must decide which polymorphism would be most useful for testing in an association study. Candidate gene association studies are better suited for detecting genes underlying common complex diseases where the risk associated with any given candidate gene is relatively small [30]. The major difficulty with this approach is that in order to choose a potential candidate gene, researchers must already have an understanding of the mechanisms underlying disease pathophysiology.

When genotypes are determined at SNPs throughout the genome of each individual, the study is called a genome-wide association study (GWAS) [31]. The most common approach of GWAS studies is the case–control setup which compares two large groups of individuals, one healthy control group and one case group affected by a disease. Individuals in each group are genotyped for the majority of common known SNPs with the exact number depending on the genotyping technology [32]. For each SNP, it is then investigated if the allele frequency is significantly altered between the case and the control group [33].

A driving assumption for GWAS is that common diseases are likely caused by common variants [34, 35]. Because the phenotypic effect of any one variant is expected to be small, these alleles may reach sufficiently high frequencies to be considered common (at least 5 %). The HapMap Project has allowed the development of high-throughput approaches to ascertain the genotype for individuals at 1 million SNPs across the genome, giving a good resolution for GWAS. Since their debut in 2005, GWAS have identified thousands of SNPs associated with hundreds of different complex traits and phenotypes [32].

Conducting a GWAS for complex traits has been a formidable challenge because the contribution of any one locus to the phenotype is expected to be small compared with the sizable effects of variants causing monogenic disorders. Furthermore, the mapping experiments need to cover the entire human genome at a sufficiently high resolution for discovery. Of course, the fact that the diseases are common means that large cohorts of individuals can be recruited for case–control studies, with thousands of affected and non-affected persons enrolled in a study, thus providing substantial power.

Regardless of whether the study is a candidate gene or genome-wide association approach, key elements of any association-based study are selection of the disease trait, identification of the cases and controls, selection of markers and genotyping platform, and finally the genetic analysis and interpretation.

Selection of Disease Trait

As in linkage studies, the phenotype is critical for association-based genetic studies. Before initiating a genetic association study, it is important to verify the genetic burden of the disease. Similar to linkage studies, most of the traits for association studies are dichotomous, from a clinical perspective, as this best reflects a disease versus a healthy state. However, there are advantages to studying quantitative traits, especially ones that demonstrate high heritability. In general, quantitative traits are measured more accurately and retain substantially more power than qualitative traits. An important consideration for quantitative traits is the distribution of the trait, as most gene mapping methods assume a normal distribution.

Endophenotypes, which are broadly defined as the separable features of a disease, are very helpful for gene mapping initiatives. An endophenotype-based approach has the potential to enhance the genetic dissection of complex diseases because endophenotypes may be a result of fewer genes than the disease entity, and may be more prevalent and more penetrant [36]. They suggest that the endophenotype should be heritable, be primarily state-independent (i.e., manifest in an individual whether or not illness is active), co-segregate with illness within families, and be found in non-affected family members at a higher rate than in the general population [36]. Unfortunately, the identification of such phenotypes has often been elusive for many complex diseases.

Choice of Population for Association-Based Studies

The most cost-efficient method for association-based studies is the traditional case–control design, where unrelated probands are compared with unaffected, unrelated controls [37]. Most of the cases for association-based studies are ascertained from disease registries or are retrieved from hospital or clinic visits. The unrelated controls are usually healthy individuals from the community or hospital-based controls. As population stratification can hamper the results of a genetic association study, attempts are made to match the ethnicity of cases and controls. Appropriately ascertained controls are essential to case–control studies and this is accomplished by matching the ancestry of cases and controls (up to the level of the grandparents if possible). While some investigators feel that this is sufficient, significant stratification can still occur, especially in populations with historical admixture such as African Americans. As summarized in an editorial from Ehm et al. [38], understanding of the criteria used to select the case and control samples should be clearly articulated. It is important to indicate the geographic location, population- or clinic-based selection, and source of controls. Other designs for association-based methodologies include family-based case–control (e.g., parent offspring trios), multiplex case–control (i.e., multiple cases from one pedigree), or prospective cohort designs.

Of the family association-based methods, the trio design (i.e., two parents and an offspring) is the most popular. Importantly, there is no issue of population stratification using this method and the analysis of trios is conducted via a transmission disequilibrium test, where the non-transmitted parental alleles are used as control alleles [9, 26]. The use of trios is not without limitations; there may be difficulties in recruiting parents, particularly for late-onset diseases, and there is some inefficiency compared with the case–control design due to the genotyping of more individuals.

Selection of Markers and Genotyping Technology

Single nucleotide polymorphisms (SNPs) are the marker of choice for association-based studies due to being sufficiently numerous to define LD blocks (unlike microsatellites) and SNPs are less mutable than microsatellites. SNP markers are selected using various criteria including: the potential function of the SNP, extent of LD of the SNP (i.e., tag-SNPs), and technological considerations (i.e., ability to be multiplexed in a single reaction) [2].

Huizinga et al. recommended that authors specify the quality measures used for genotyping analysis, in order to minimize genotyping errors and allow the results to be more easily replicated with similar genotyping protocols [39]. The quality measures include: internal validation, blinding of laboratory personnel of the affected status, procedures for establishing duplicates, quality control from blind duplicates, and blind or automated data entry. Assurance regarding the satisfaction of the Hardy–Weinberg equilibrium is also important. Hardy–Weinberg or genetic equilibrium is a basic principle of population genetics, where there is a specific relationship between the frequencies of alleles and the genotype of a population. This equilibrium remains constant as long as there is random mating and absence of selection pressures associated with the alleles.

Due to the rapid advances in marker selection and genotyping technologies, SNP genotyping for association-based studies has improved remarkably over the last decade. These advancements have identified the genetic variants responsible for the genetic component of phenotype directly via GWAS, which have revolutionized the identification of genomic regions associated with complex diseases. The identification of ~2,000 robust associations has been made in more than 300 complex diseases and traits [40]. These numbers are orders of magnitude greater than those of replicable linkage and candidate gene association findings to date for complex diseases.

4.2.2 Analysis and Interpretation of Association-Based Studies

Caution must be used when interpreting the results of a genetic association study. This notion is best exemplified by the fact that so few genetic association studies are replicated. In a review of 166 putative associations that had been studied three times or more, only six were reproduced at least 75 % of the time [41]. The major reasons for the lack of replication include false-positive associations, false-negative associations, and a true association that is population-specific (i.e., relatively rare). The most robust results from an association study will have a significance that is maintained after careful scrutiny for population stratification and multiple testing issues. The results should be replicated independently in another separate population. A replicated association may be as a result of a SNP being the causative mutation, or being in LD with the true disease allele. Finally, the results should be supported by functional data, if the variant is predicted to be causative.

The greatest problem with association studies is the high rate of false-positive associations. The use of a p-value below 0.05 as a criterion for declaring success in association-based studies is not appropriate. Multiple testing must be taken into account due to the large number of markers being analyzed, but, the traditional Bonferroni's correction that is often used in epidemiological studies, is far too harsh for genetic epidemiology [34]. This is because the selected markers are often in LD (thus not independent) and some of the characteristics of the disease entity are closely correlated. Permutation tests are increasingly used to correct p-values for multiple testing. This process generates a distribution of the best p-value expected in the entire experiment under the null hypothesis of no association between genotype and phenotype. Bayesian methods have also been proposed that take into account pretest estimates of likelihood but this approach is often difficult to interpret.

Population stratification can result in false positives. Controlling for ancestry as noted above is one method to minimize this effect. Methods have also been proposed to detect and control population stratification by genotyping dozens of random unlinked markers (as reviewed in [34]). Ideally, these markers should be able to distinguish between the subpopulations. Most studies that have attempted to use this genomic control have themselves been underpowered and the ability to detect modest stratification has been limited. The impact on population stratification after matching for ethnicity solely based on a family history is presently being debated, and needs to be better elucidated. A false-positive result can also occur if the cases and controls are genotyped separately, especially if the genotyping of the cases and controls are done at different centers.

False-negative results can arise from an inadequate sample size to detect a true difference. When reporting a negative replication study, attempts must be made to assess the power of the study to exclude a genetic effect of a certain magnitude. Occasionally, true heterogeneity will exist within populations; however, this is relatively rare.

Due to the difficulties in interpreting genetic association studies, Freimer and Sabatti [42] published suggested guidelines for future submissions to *Human Molecular Genetics*. For candidate gene analysis, they suggest that a distinction be made between a candidate with previous statistical evidence and those proposed solely on biological hypotheses. Investigators should also specify the p-value, the phenotypes, and the genomic region, and quantitative estimate of the prior probability. There must be a rational attempt to account for multiple testing and in a conservative, least favorable scenario, it has been proposed that the p-value be less than 10^{-7}, to declare an association. For higher p-values, the authors should justify why the association is noteworthy.

4.2.3 Challenges of Association-Based Studies

A surprising finding which was evident from some of the earliest GWAS investigations for complex diseases was small associated odds ratios. Moreover, the total fraction of the phenotypic variation explained for most phenotypes remains small (often 10 % or less) relative to the published heritability estimates, which are estimated using the trait covariance among relatives (i.e., familial clustering) [43–45].

Of particular interest is the distribution of causal variants along the genome, their number, and their frequency spectrum. GWAS are particularly suited to capture common variants (i.e., Minor Allele Frequency ≥ 5 %) and depends on the common disease common variant model. The "missing heritability" is the proportion of the estimated heritability of a complex disease that is not presently accounted for by known genetic variants [46, 47]. For many complex traits and diseases, it appears that one half to one third of the genetic variance is not tagged by current and past SNP chips [44, 48]. These findings suggest that many lower-frequency variants are also needed to explain the genetic variance that is not tagged by SNP chips. In Fisher's infinitesimal model there are expected to be a large number of rare variants (i.e., <1 % MAF) associated with disease. The rare-allele model proposes that rare variants of large effect account for a significant fraction of phenotypic variation [45, 49]. The combined contribution of multiple rare loci to the population-level genetic variance remains an open question because association studies that focus on rare variants remain underpowered.

Many explanations for the sources of "missing heritability" have been proposed including imperfect SNP-tagging (producing weak GWAS signals), structural variations, gene–environment interactions, epigenetics (e.g., methylation analysis), epistatic interactions, parent-of-origin effects, phenotype misclassification, exclusion of the mitochondrial genome, and errors in narrow-sense heritability estimates [43, 44, 50–52]. This "missing heritability," which is also reflected in the generally small odds ratios and limited predictive value [53, 54] of these variants, has raised questions about the ultimate applicability of these findings to risk prediction in particular to those variants that will be clinically actionable [55, 56].

4.3 Future Direction

In order to elucidate additional genetic variation in complex disease and account for the "missing heritability," researchers will need to improve on genome-wide study designs, phenotyping, and data analysis, as well as combining complementary data collected from multiple investigations.

Deeper sequencing-based characterization of genomic variation, fine mapping, imputation, and denser SNP arrays are extending the reach of GWAS to ever lower ranges of minor allele frequency [57–60]. As genomic technologies improve, detection of associations with variants of lower frequency is increasingly becoming possible. As large-scale parallel-sequencing studies of many thousands of individuals become commonplace, then sufficient power is likely to be gained, allowing both rare and common variants to be dissected to a greater extent.

Improving on current study designs (i.e., sample size, extreme phenotypes, better phenotyping, and inclusion of family-based studies) may help shed light on fundamental genes, pathways, and cell types involved in disease, and help explain some of the so-called "missing heritability" associated with complex disease.

As sample sizes increase, so too do the number of identified genomic regions and the amount of variation explained by association studies. Increasing sample size will have the greatest effect on power. Replacing high-density SNP chips with full sequencing will tag low-frequency loci, but it will not be enough alone to capture the effects of rare variants, because many rare variants will be at such low number that large data sets are required for their detection. Another general strategy for increasing power is to focus on samples with extreme phenotypes and whose relatives have similarly extreme phenotypes [61–63].

Misclassifying a phenotype, especially when multiple distinct phenotypes are influenced by different sets of underlying causal variants, can reduce power in a GWAS investigation. Phenotyping may be inaccurate, thus combining phenotypes or diseases that have partially or even completely distinct underlying causal variants. This will average effect sizes across groups of individuals, who could be better separated on the basis of better phenotyping or a combination of information from different sources.

Overlapping GWAS results with other genomic sources of information is likely to explain additional variation and identify novel pathways. The targeting of expression SNPs and the linking of GWAS, gene expression, and methylation data have uncovered additional variants and provided direct information on the underlying biology of complex phenotypes [64]. Finally, one cannot assess a single gene in isolation. Careful consideration should be given to developing a genetic risk score involving multiple loci as demonstrated by Chen et al. [65]. It will be necessary to integrate relevant clinical information and environmental risk factors. The inclusion of disease-specific, environmental, and genetic information will likely enhance the predictive capacity of any model. Ideally, these predictive algorithms require prospective evaluation in randomized controlled trials to assess the utility of including genetic information [66].

5   Conclusion

The identification of genes of a complex trait remains a difficult task that requires substantial resources, including a large collection of samples (including families), highly informative markers, technical expertise, and high-throughput genotyping, as well as sophisticated statistical approaches. However, due to the wealth of data which emanated from the Human Genome Project and HapMap project, as well as the experience attained from the numerous linkage and association studies, gene variant identification is now possible for complex genetic disease.

The two most common approaches are genetic linkage and association studies with the latter having greater power than linkage studies to detect genotype relative risk of modest effect. With advances of genotyping technology and well-validated SNPs extensively covering the genome, there is great promise for this method for identification of genetic determinants for complex disease. However, because this approach requires many more samples and markers its interpretation should be viewed with caution until it is independently replicated.

GWAS have identified many thousands of significant associations across several hundred human phenotypes, and it is clear that, for any given trait, genetic variance is likely contributed from a large number of loci across the entire allele frequency spectrum. The proposed framework for future studies briefly outlined above will likely result in the identification of rare variants, which will help elucidate the genetic variation of a range of complex traits and hopefully solve the mystery of "missing heritability." Moreover, these steps will improve our ability to predict disease risk and identify new drug targets.

References

1. Lander ES, Schork NJ (1994) Genetic dissection of complex traits. Science 265:2037–2048
2. Newton-Cheh C, Hirschhorn JN (2005) Genetic association studies of complex traits: design and analysis issues. Mutat Res 573: 54–69
3. Ghosh S, Collins FS (1996) The geneticist's approach to complex disease. Ann Rev Med 47:333–353
4. Hirschhorn JN (2005) Genetic approaches to studying common diseases and complex traits. Pediatr Res 57:74R–77R
5. Risch N (1997) Genetic linkage from an epidemiological perspective. Epidemiol Rev 19: 24–32
6. Bandrup F (1982) Psoriasis in monozygotic twins. Variations in expression of individuals with identical genetic constitution. Acta Derm Venereol 62:229–236
7. Farber EM, Nail L et al (1974) Natural history of psoriasis in 61 twin pairs. Arch Dermatol 109:207–211
8. Risch N (1990) Linkage strategies for genetically complex traits. 1. Multi locus model. Am J Hum Genet 46:222–228
9. Sham P (1998) Statistics in human genetics. Wiley, London
10. Heneseler T (1997) The genetics of psoriasis. J Am Acad Dermatol 37:S1–S11
11. Sherman SL (1997) Evolving methods in genetic epidemiology. IV. Approaches to non-Mendelian inheritance. Epidemiol Rev 19:44–51
12. Harper PS, Harley HG, Reardon W et al (1992) Anticipation in myotonic dystrophy: new insights on an old problem. Am J Hum Genet 51:10–16
13. Hall JG (1990) Genomic imprinting: review and relevance to human diseases. Am J Hum Genet 46:857–873
14. Langlois S, Lopez-Rangel E, Hall JG (1995) New mechanisms for genetic disease and non-traditional modes of inheritance. Adv Pediatr 42:91–111
15. Rahman P, Gladman DD, Schentag CT, Petronis A (1999) Excessive paternal transmission in psoriatic arthritis. Arthritis Rheum 42:1228–1231
16. Fradin D, Cheslack-Postava K, Ladd-Acosta C, Newschaffer C, Chakravarti A, Arking DE et al (2010) Parent-of-origin effects in autism identified through genome-wide linkage analysis of 16,000 SNPs. PLoS One 5(9), pii: e12513
17. Fransen K, Mitrovic M, van Diemen CC, Thelma BK, Sood A, Franke A et al (2012) Limited evidence for parent-of-origin effects in inflammatory bowel disease associated loci. PLoS One 7:e45287
18. Wallace DC (1992) Disease of the mitochondrial DNA. Annu Rev Biochem 61:1175–1212
19. Swerdlow RH, Burns JM, Khan SM (2013) The Alzheimer's disease mitochondrial cascade hypothesis: progress and perspectives. Biochim Biophys Acta, S0925-4439(13)00289-5
20. Kuan WL, Poole E, Fletcher M, Karniely S, Tyers P, Wills M et al (2012) A novel neuroprotective therapy for Parkinson's disease using a

viral noncoding RNA that protects mitochondrial complex I activity. J Exp Med 209:1–10

21. Swerdlow RH, Parks JK, Davis JN 2nd, Cassarino DS, Trimmer PA, Currie LJ et al (1998) Matrilineal inheritance of complex I dysfunction in a multigenerational Parkinson's disease family. Ann Neurol 44:873–881

22. Samuels DC, Li C, Li B, Song Z, Torstenson E, Boyd Clay H et al (2013) Recurrent tissue-specific mtDNA mutations are common in humans. PLoS Genet 9:e1003929

23. Kruglyak L, Daly MJ, Reeve-Daly MP et al (1996) Parametric and nonparametric linkage analysis: a unified multipoint approach. Am J Hum Genet 58:1347–1363

24. Morton NE (1955) Sequential tests for detection of linkage. Am J Hum Genet 7:277–318

25. Lander E, Kruglyak L (1995) Genetic dissection of complex traits: guidelines for interpreting and reporting linkage results. Nat Genet 11:241–247

26. Ott J (1999) Analysis of human genetic linkage, 3rd edn. Johns Hopkins University Press, Baltimore

27. Risch N (1990) Linkage strategies for complex traits. II. The power of affected relative pairs. Am J Hum Genet 46:219–221

28. Nagase H (1993) Mutations of the APC gene. Hum Mut 2:425–434

29. The international HapMap Consortium (2003) The International HapMap project. Nature 426:789–796

30. Collins FS, Guyer MS, Charkravarti A (1997) Variations on a theme: cataloging human DNA sequence variation. Science 278:1580–1581

31. Giardine B, Riemer C, Hefferon T, Thomas D, Hsu F, Zielenski J et al (2007) PhenCode: connecting ENCODE data with mutations and phenotype. Hum Mutat 28:554–562

32. Hindorff LA, Sethupathy P, Junkins HA, Ramos EM, Mehta JP, Collins FS et al (2009) Potential etiologic and functional implications of genome-wide association loci for human diseases and traits. Proc Natl Acad Sci U S A 106:9362–9367

33. Clarke GM, Anderson CA, Pettersson FH, Cardon LR, Morris AP, Zondervan KT (2011) Basic statistical analysis in genetic case-control studies. Nat Protoc 6:121–133

34. Hirschhorn JN, Daly MJ (2005) Genome-wide association studies for common diseases and complex traits. Nat Rev Genet 6:95–108

35. Bodmer W, Bonilla C (2008) Common and rare variants in multifactorial susceptibility to common diseases. Nat Genet 40:695–701

36. Gottesman II, Gould TD (2003) The endophenotype concept in psychiatry: etymology and strategic intentions. Am J Psychiatry 160:636–645

37. Cordell HJ, Clayton DG (2005) Genetic epidemiology 3: genetic association studies. Lancet 366:1121–1131

38. Ehm MG, Nelson MR, Spurr NK (2005) Guidelines for conducting and reporting whole genome/large scale association studies. Hum Mol Genet 14:2485–2488

39. Huizinga TWJ, Pisetsky DS, Kimberly RP (2004) Associations, populations, truth. Arthritis Rheum 50:2066–2071

40. Manolio TA (2013) Bringing genome-wide association findings into clinical use. Nat Rev Genet 14:549–558

41. Hischhorn JN, Lohmueller K, Byrne E, Hischhorn K (2002) A comprehensive review of genetic association studies. Genet Med 4:45–61

42. Freimer NB, Sabatti C (2005) Guidelines for association studies. Hum Mol Genet 14:2481–2483

43. Eichler EE, Flint J, Gibson G, Kong A, Leal SM, Moore JH et al (2010) Missing heritability and strategies for finding the underlying causes of complex disease. Nat Rev Genet 11:446–450

44. Manolio TA, Collins FS, Cox NJ, Goldstein DB, Hindorff LA, Hunter DJ et al (2009) Finding the missing heritability of complex diseases. Nature 461:747–753

45. Dickson SP, Wang K, Krantz I, Hakonarson H, Goldstein DB (2010) Rare variants create synthetic genome-wide associations. PLoS Biol 8:e1000294

46. McClellan J, King MC (2010) Genetic heterogeneity in human disease. Cell 141:210–217

47. Bustamante CD, Burchard EG, De la Vega FM (2011) Genomics for the world. Nature 475:163–165

48. Visscher PM, Brown MA, McCarthy MI, Yang J (2012) Five years of GWAS discovery. Am J Hum Genet 90:7–24

49. Gibson G (2012) Rare and common variants: twenty arguments. Nat Rev Genet 13:135–145

50. Tuzun E, Sharp AJ, Bailey JA, Kaul R, Morrison VA, Pertz LM et al (2005) Fine-scale structural variation of the human genome. Nat Genet 37:727–732

51. Spencer C, Hechter E, Vukcevic D, Donnelly P (2011) Quantifying the underestimation of relative risks from genome-wide association studies. PLoS Genet 7:e1001337

52. McCarroll SA (2008) Extending genome-wide association studies to copy-number variation. Hum Mol Genet 17(R2):R135–R142

53. Jakobsdottir J, Gorin MB, Conley YP, Ferrell RE, Weeks DE (2009) Interpretation of genetic association studies: markers with replicated highly significant odds ratios may be poor classifiers. PLoS Genet 5:e1000337

54. Aschard H, Chen J, Cornelis MC, Chibnik LB, Karlson EW, Kraft P (2012) Inclusion of gene-gene and gene-environment interactions unlikely to dramatically improve risk prediction for complex diseases. Am J Hum Genet 90:962–972

55. Manolio TA (2010) Genomewide association studies and assessment of the risk of disease. N Engl J Med 363:166–176

56. Lopes MC, Zeggini E, Panoutsopoulou K (2011) Do genome-wide association scans have potential for translation? Clin Chem Lab Med 50:255–260

57. 1000 Genomes Project Consortium, Abecasis GR, Altshuler D, Auton A, Brooks LD, Durbin RM et al (2010) A map of human genome variation from population-scale sequencing. Nature 467:1061–1073

58. Tennessen JA, Bigham AW, O'Connor TD, Fu W, Kenny EE, Gravel S et al (2012) Evolution and functional impact of rare coding variation from deep sequencing of human exomes. Science 337:64–69

59. Mohlke KL, Scott LJ (2012) What will diabetes genomes tell us? Curr Diab Rep 12: 643–650

60. Servin B, Stephens M (2007) Imputation-based analysis of association studies: candidate regions and quantitative traits. PLoS Genet 3:e114

61. Li D, Lewinger JP, Gauderman WJ, Murcray CE, Conti D (2011) Using extreme phenotype sampling to identify the rare causal variants of quantitative traits in association studies. Genet Epidemiol 35:790–799

62. Guey LT, Kravic J, Melander O, Burtt NP, Laramie JM, Lyssenko V et al (2011) Power in the phenotypic extremes: a simulation study of power in discovery and replication of rare variants. Genet Epidemiol. doi:10.1002/gepi.20572

63. Li M, Boehnke M, Abecasis GR (2006) Efficient study designs for test of genetic association using sibship data and unrelated cases and controls. Am J Hum Genet 78:778–792

64. Edwards SL, Beesley J, French JD, Dunning AM (2013) Beyond GWASs: illuminating the dark road from association to function. Am J Hum Genet 93:779–797

65. Chen H, Poon A, Yeung C, Helms C, Pons J, Bowcock AM et al (2011) A genetic risk score combining ten psoriasis risk loci improves disease prediction. PLoS One 6:e19454

66. Pirmohamed M, Burnside G, Eriksson N, Jorgensen AL, Toh CH, Nicholson T et al (2013) A randomized trial of genotype-guided dosing of warfarin. N Engl J Med 369:2294–2303

Clinical Genetic Research 3: Genetics ELSI (Ethical, Legal, and Social Issues) Research

Daryl Pullman and Holly Etchegary

Abstract

ELSI (Ethical, Legal, and Social Issues) is a widely used acronym in the bioethics literature that encompasses a broad range of research areas involved in examining the various impacts of science and technology on society. In Canada, GE^{3}LS (Genetics, Ethical, Economic, Environmental, Legal, Social issues) is the term used to describe ELSI studies. It is intentionally more expansive in that GE^{3}LS explicitly brings economic and environmental issues under its purview. ELSI/GE^{3}LS research has become increasingly important in recent years as there has been a greater emphasis on "translational research" that moves genomics from the bench to the clinic. The purpose of this chapter is to outline a range of ELSI-related work that might be conducted as part of a large scale genetics or genomics research project, and to provide some practical insights on how a scientific research team might incorporate a strong and effective ELSI program within its broader research mandate. We begin by describing the historical context of ELSI research and the development of GE^{3}LS research in the Canadian context. We then illustrate how some ELSI research might unfold by outlining a variety of research questions and the various methodologies that might be employed in addressing them in an area of ELSI research that is encompassed under the term "public engagement." We conclude with some practical pointers about how to build an effective ELSI/GE^{3}LS team and focus within a broader scientific research program.

Key words Ethical, Legal, Social issues (ELSI), GE^{3}LS, Clinical genetics, Mixed methods

1 Introduction: What Is ELSI Research?

ELSI (Ethical, Legal, and Social Issues) is a widely used acronym in the bioethics literature that encompasses a broad range of research areas involved in examining the various impacts of science and technology on society more generally. GE^{3}LS (Genetics, Ethical, Economic, Environmental, Legal, Social issues) is a made in Canada variation on ELSI studies; it is intentionally more expansive in that GE^{3}LS explicitly brings economic and environmental issues under its purview. In this chapter we use the ELSI acronym generally as it is more commonly found in the wider scientific literature. However, we occasionally refer to GE^{3}LS

Patrick S. Parfrey and Brendan J. Barrett (eds.), *Clinical Epidemiology: Practice and Methods*, Methods in Molecular Biology, vol. 1281, DOI 10.1007/978-1-4939-2428-8_22, © Springer Science+Business Media New York 2015

when discussing how some of these activities have developed in Canada in particular.

In the past decade, there has been an increasing interest in "translational research" that moves the outputs of bench science to the bedside or the marketplace in an effective, economical and ethical manner [1, 2]. This translational emphasis sometimes means that scientific teams must focus more of their attention and resources on the product delivery end of the research pipeline, and comparatively less on the discovery end. While ELSI arise at each phase of the research pipeline process, they are especially acute in the translational context when broader issues of science policy, technology assessment, user preparedness to adopt new technologies, and consumer willingness to utilize them, all become more immediate. ELSI research is often instrumental in the translational aspect of scientific research and many research teams are actively engaging ELSI experts to assist with this translational mandate [3]. Working closely with an appropriate team of ELSI researchers can assist translational genomics teams to identify and address potential barriers to the uptake of the products of their work. The purpose of this chapter is to outline a range of ELSI-related work that might be conducted as part of a large scale genetics or genomics research project, and to provide some practical insights on how a scientific research team might incorporate a strong and effective ELSI program within its broader research mandate.

At its heart, ELSI research in genomics is interdisciplinary; it brings together researchers from a wide range of academic disciplines spanning the life, clinical, and social sciences. It may also include a range of other stakeholder or user groups (e.g., policymakers, commercial partners, special interest groups, or research populations). ELSI research includes philosophers, bioethicists, legal scholars, policy experts, economists, geographers, communications experts, humanities scholars, and social scientists from virtually every social science discipline (anthropology, archaeology, psychology, sociology, to name only a few). In short, ELSI research is as diverse as the range of disciplines represented and it draws upon the research methodologies that each of these disciplines brings to the issues under investigation.

In this chapter, we begin with a brief historical overview of the advent of ELSI research in general and GE³LS research in particular as the latter has evolved over the past decade in the Canadian context. We then discuss the important distinction between descriptive and normative research that is important to understand when determining the kinds of ELSI questions that need investigation in relation to a particular scientific or clinical research project, or in assessing the outputs of ELSI research. We then illustrate how some of this work might unfold by outlining a variety of research questions and the various methodologies that might be employed in an area of ELSI research encompassed under the term "public engagement." We conclude with some practical pointers about how to build an effective ELSI/GE³LS team and focus within a broader scientific research program.

2 Advent of ELSI/GE³LS Research

The modern era of genetics and genomics research can be traced to the inception of the Human Genome Project which was proposed in the 1980s and formally initiated in 1990. From the outset there was an emerging concern about what the implications of the genomics era might mean for humankind more generally. Very early on, the Human Genome Organization—an international oversight body that was instituted at the first meeting on genome mapping and sequencing at Cold Spring Harbor in April 1988 [4]—established an ELSI committee to identify and attend to broader ethical, legal and social issues that were anticipated to arise. That committee issued a "Statement on the Principled Conduct of Genetics Research" in 1995 [5] and the committee continues to provide ELSI oversight as new issues arise. While HUGO's mandate was international in scope, a number of national bodies also evolved in the succeeding years. In the USA the National Human Genome Research Institute (NHGRI) was established in 1989 to support and facilitate genomics research. The NHGRI has embraced an ELSI mandate and continues to support research in this area [2, 3].

In Canada, the major impetus for genomics research came with the creation of Genome Canada, a not-for-profit government agency established in 2000 to leverage research in genomics and proteomics for the benefit of all Canadians. Genome Canada's mandate includes not only human genetics research, but also genetic and genomics research in forestry, agricultural, aquaculture and related biosciences. Hence the ELSI mandate expanded accordingly to include economic and environmental concerns. The GE³LS acronym captures this broader mandate more explicitly.

While Genome Canada was not unique in recognizing the relevance of ELSI/GE³LS research to the genomics enterprise, it was unique in that it made the inclusion of a GE³LS research component a mandatory requirement for all of the large scale science projects it funded. At least three different models of GE³LS research evolved over the early years of Genome Canada's mandate which came to be known respectively as "stand-alone," "embedded," and "integrated" GE³LS research. "Stand-alone projects," as the name suggests, were GE³LS projects that were funded directly by Genome Canada through one of its regional genomics research centers and which operated independently of any science related project. Such stand-alone projects are similar to what other genomic research organizations might fund under their ELSI programs. "Embedded projects" is GE³LS research that is funded within a larger genomics science project but in which there is no necessary connection between the science and the GE³LS research being conducted. For all intents and purposes stand-alone and embedded projects are essentially the same; it is only the manner in which they are funded that differs (i.e., stand-alone projects are funded directly by Genome Canada while embedded projects are funded indirectly through a science platform). The most interesting, challenging, but also often the most rewarding GE³LS research projects are those that are integrated into the science project from which it draws its funding. In actuality a properly integrated GE³LS project is not separate from a science project but is part and parcel of the project from its inception. What this means is that from the beginning of the project when researchers are deciding upon the research questions they want to explore and the manner in which they will construct their research proposal for funding purposes, appropriate GE³LS researchers are involved in drafting the research proposal to identify specific GE³LS issues that arise out of the proposed scientific or clinical research, and to develop appropriate methods for addressing them. Thus, it is not uncommon that one of the co-principal investigators on a large scale genomics project would be a GE³LS expert responsible for working closely with the lead scientists and clinicians and for over-seeing the potentially broad ranging GE³LS mandate.

While integrated GE³LS research can be the most rewarding, it is also often the most challenging as considerable energies must often be invested to overcome disciplinary barriers. Thus, Collins et al. [3] observe: "New mechanisms for promoting dialogue and collaboration between the ELSI researchers and genomic and clinical researchers need to be developed; such examples might include structural rewards for interdisciplinary research, intensive summer courses or mini-fellowships for cross-training, and the creation of centers of excellence in ELSI studies to allow sustained interdisciplinary collaboration." A first step in promoting dialogue and collaboration between ELSI and genomic and clinical researchers is for those from disparate research orientations to understand something of the other's perspective. In point of fact, as already noted, there is no particular ELSI perspective as ELSI encompasses a wide and diverse range of research methodologies. Nevertheless, there are some basic distinctions that help to navigate the ELSI domain and which can inform decisions about the kinds of ELSI questions that might be explored. The first of these is the distinction between descriptive and normative research.

2.1 "Descriptive" Versus "Normative" Research

Descriptive and normative research both figure prominently in ELSI work. While the outputs of each type of investigation are often complementary, the general methodologies can differ considerably. "Descriptive" research, as the name implies, sets out to examine the world as we encounter it and to understand the way things actually are. This type of research is most familiar to basic scientists and clinical researchers as they set out to understand various physical phenomena such as gene functions and clinical manifestations of a disease, for example. ELSI researchers who focus primarily on descriptive work do much the same thing, although the phenomena they describe are generally social. If we are interested in knowing whether the public is concerned about the privacy of their genetic information, for example, or if there is general anxiety about whether life insurers might require them to have a genetic test before being considered for insurance purposes, social scientists might develop a survey or conduct focus groups with the goal of understanding what people actually feel or believe about genetic privacy or genetic discrimination issues (see our discussion of "public engagement" outlined later in this chapter). This kind of work is descriptive; it aims simply to ascertain what people are thinking or feeling without making any judgment about whether such views or beliefs are good or bad, right or wrong. Researchers have found, for example, that people who suffer from Huntington's disease experience discrimination when seeking life insurance [6]. While this may be descriptively true, we still don't know what follows from it normatively. That is, should life insurance companies be prohibited from asking questions about family history? Should they be required to insure people with terminal illnesses? These latter questions are "normative," and no amount of empirical work will provide definitive answers on such issues.

Normative or prescriptive work aims to provide arguments in support of some preferred view of how things ought to be. Put otherwise, the normative challenge is to derive an "ought" from an "is." Such normative work is generally more conceptual than empirical in nature, and at times a normative conclusion about how things ought to be might go contrary to a descriptive observation about what is actually the case. That being said, normative conclusions are generally responsive to empirical realities. In 2008, for example, the USA introduced federal legislation (the "Genetic Information Nondiscrimination Act," better known as "GINA") to prohibit discrimination with regard to employment and health [7]. Insofar as the vast majority of American's receive health insurance through their employers (descriptively true), the US Congress decided it was necessary to have a law that prohibited employers from using genetic information when screening potential employees (a normative process). Canada does not have any legislation similar to GINA, although there have been some that have lobbied for it. The reality is, however, that because Canada has a program of universal health care Canadians do not rely upon their employers for health insurance. This empirical difference results in a different normative conclusion for Canada [8].

Generally ELSI research spans both the descriptive and normative domains. It includes both social scientists with expertise in exploring the social world which will be impacted by the outputs of genetic research, as well as normative researchers like ethicists, health policy experts, and legal scholars who are charged with addressing the most appropriate ways for translating that research to the greater social good. The methodologies involved vary considerably but all are essential to the translational task. ELSI researchers have generally developed good working relationships across the various disciplines involved in addressing these descriptive and normative tasks. The effectiveness of their work increases exponentially when they can engage genomics and clinical researchers directly in the ELSI process as well.

3 Public Engagement with Genomics: An Instructive Case Study of ELSI Research Topics and Methods

A significant portion of ELSI genetics research over the last two decades has focused on public attitudes towards, and engagement with, new genomic developments. This research is instructive in both the number of ELSI topics and content areas highlighted, as well as the variety of research methods employed. In this section we describe a number of empirical research studies that highlight significant ELSI concerns in clinical genetics research, as well as the breadth of mixed methods employed in ELSI research designs.

3.1 Why Is Public Engagement a Significant ELSI Focus in Genetics Research?

While promoting public participation in policy decisions is not new, there is a growing emphasis in both academic and policy circles on the importance and *necessity* of public involvement [9, 10], particularly in health contexts [11], and most recently, in the area of genetics and personalized medicine [12–14]. Community engagement is endorsed by many federal agencies as a way to "build trust, enlist new resources and allies, create better communication and improve health outcomes" [9]. At the same time, research efforts to improve population and individual health increasingly rely on large-scale collections of individuals' genetic information, linked with other health, lifestyle, and administrative data. Such collections or "biobanks," are often used in prospective, longitudinal cohort studies and have become standard research tools to investigate the interactive effects of genes, environment, and lifestyle on health and disease [12, 13, 15]. New genomic sequencing technologies such as whole-genome sequencing (which measures variation across an individual's entire genome) and whole-exome sequencing (which measures variation only in the portion of DNA that encodes for proteins) are increasingly guiding clinical practice for a number of disorders [16–18]. While such developments offer the potential for genomic information to improve health outcomes, they are also associated with a number of significant ELSI (e.g., clinical validity and utility of the information generated, data management and sharing, and informed consent models for such research). These new developments in genomics continue to increase the number of disorders for which genetic testing is available, whether through the primary health-care system, direct to consumer (DTC) testing via the internet [19, 20], or as part of expanded newborn screening panels [21]. Not surprisingly, there is a growing interest on the part of policy-makers and scholars alike (i.e., those responsible for the normative outputs of ELSI studies) in public attitudes towards these continued developments and the ELSI issues they raise.

3.2 An Overview of Pubic Engagement Approaches in Genetics ELSI Research

A variety of methods have been employed to engage communities in genomics consultation initiatives including surveys, focus groups, town hall meetings, citizens' juries, and Web or community forums, to name just a few. Engagement can have a number of different levels and has been described as existing on a continuum or ladder, ranging from simply providing information, to more substantial community consultation, through to communities having an equal share in the decision-making power [11, 22]. Early ELSI research was largely at the public information level and aimed to explore public interest and uptake in biobank research and their attitudes towards the associated ELSI (such as informed consent processes and the return of individual research results). These studies largely employed national, random surveys of the general public.

ELSI studies at times employ large random surveys of the general public, even at the national level. For example, there was widespread support in the USA (84 %) for the creation of a large genetic cohort study with 60 % of Americans indicating they would become donors [23]. Interest in the study and willingness to participate did not significantly vary among demographic groups. Notably, however, features of the research such as study burden and whether individual results would be returned to participants did affect willingness to participate. Similarly, majority (83 %) of patients in a large Veterans Affairs' patient database indicated their support for the creation of a large genomic research study, and 71 % indicated they would likely participate [24]. Similar support for genomics and biobanking research has been observed in national surveys across Canada [13, 25], other US locales [15], Sweden [26], Scotland [27], as well as in large international efforts (e.g., the International HapMap Project) [28].

Other ELSI research efforts have moved beyond merely soliciting information from communities and assessing their research participation interest to provide more substantive consultation opportunities. These ELSI research studies have used a variety of methods, including town hall meetings, the creation of community advisory boards, and engagement forums, to name a few. In an instructive report, Lemke and colleagues [29] described community engagement activities undertaken by six biobanks in the USA, highlighting a range of public engagement mechanisms. Biobank governance was informed by community surveys and focus groups with patient and specialist groups, but also by consensus development panels, community advisory panels, and deliberative democracy events. Case studies such as these are especially informative; they reveal the pragmatic and policy outcomes of ELSI engagement efforts (e.g., influencing the choice of biobank consent processes or the policy on the return of individual research results) showing again how the descriptive informs the normative. These research efforts also reveal the challenges of community engagement (e.g., engaging the public on a topic about which many claim they are uninformed, or recruiting a diverse range of stakeholders for advisory groups and panels).

ELSI research in public engagement with genetics has highlighted a key area of concern about genetic health literacy. At least some knowledge (and perhaps prior thought) about many of the ELSI in genomics and personalized medicine (e.g., clinical utility of tests, policies on data sharing, biobank governance) are necessary if the public is to participate in policy discussions in a meaningful way. In order to raise awareness about personalized medicine, the NHGRI hosts a series of ELSI community engagement programs including the Family History Demonstration projects and the Community Genetics Forum that have been well received [30]. These efforts represent novel ELSI research approaches and are designed to facilitate community dialogue about the connections between genetics and health. Pragmatically, they also provide educational curricula and materials for community groups and others wishing to engage with issues around genetics and personalized medicine. Ongoing ELSI research efforts in the authors' local jurisdiction are also intended to raise public awareness about genetics and health. In Newfoundland, for example, we have conducted public surveys, as well as delivered community education and consultation sessions about newborn screening, genomics research and specific issues related to biobanking (e.g., consent models) [31–33]. These projects employed a number of ELSI methods including both qualitative (focus groups, open survey items) and quantitative (e.g., conjoint analysis) approaches. In accordance with prior research [34, 35], all these public engagement efforts revealed a largely positive attitude towards the potential for genomic medicine to improve health, but also areas ELSI of public concern such as the privacy of genetic information, storage of and access to the information, as well as questions about the clinical utility of genomic information for health. Notably, these are the very ELSI with which policy makers and health-care systems will continue to grapple as genomic medicine is integrated into current health-care systems.

On the end of the continuum of public engagement methods are those that are far more ambitious than projects described thus far. The deliberative democracy approach employed by the British

Columbia biobank in Canada has been well described [13, 36]. In this stand-alone ELSI project, a diverse group of citizens committed to a two-weekend deliberation on the values that should guide biobanking in their province. Participants were charged with reaching consensus (if possible) on a range of important ELSI such as consent procedures, biobank governance, and access to biobank data. Consensus was reached in several areas (e.g., public support for the biobank, an independent governing body, and standardization in biobank tools and procedures). However, several areas of disagreement remained (e.g., one-time blanket consent, donor compensation, and the ownership of biobank biological samples). The results of the deliberations were provided to the BC Biobank and ongoing dialogue will assist with incorporating the results into the review of policies of the biobank and future community engagement efforts [13].

A similarly ambitious and novel community engagement approach was employed with a group of young offenders in South Wales [37]. In that ELSI project, a mock jury trial engaged youth with ELSI raised by the creation of a National DNA database. Still other ELSI research developed a "Genome Diner" community engagement approach which brought together scientific experts, as well as school children and their parents to deliberate ELSI associated with genomic research [38]. Interactive discussions were held in school cafeterias, arranged as a "menu": Appetizers (warm up questions), Main Course (specific discussion topics) and Dessert (summary of discussions from each table). Participants evaluated the program highly, and geneticists in particular demonstrated a greater knowledge about and more favorable attitudes toward the public's ability to contribute to genomics policy and discussion.

In Canada, a deliberative workshop approach was used to explore issues raised by the inclusion of genomic profiling in two routine health-care contexts—risk assessment for colorectal cancer or type 1 diabetes as part of newborn bloodspot screening [39]. Workshops lasted for 2–3 h and included three components: an information component, a deliberation component, and a data collection component. The information component provided descriptions of the genomic technology of interest, as well as its possible implications (both positive and negative), in standard PowerPoint format. The deliberation component provided an opportunity for questions, discussion and debate about the information presented. The data collection component used multiple approaches to capture participants' reactions and attitudes (e.g., free form booklet responses, Likert-type attitude items, and group discussion field notes). In total, eight workshops ($n = 170$) in two provinces (NL and ON) were completed. Results were consistent with existing ELSI literature in that attitudes were generally positive, but with notable areas of concern. For example, community members were concerned about the clinical utility and validity of genomic information, access to biobank data, and the potential for negative psychosocial effects such as undue worry about uncertain disease-risk estimates.

These ELSI research efforts reveal that the public is open to discussion about genomics and personalized medicine and tend to rate public engagement efforts on these topics highly. Public information studies in particular (e.g., surveys, focus groups, opinion polls) reveal that the public has a largely positive attitude about the potential for genomics to improve health, and most indicate they would participate in biobanks and other large genetic cohort studies. These ELSI studies also reveal, however, that critical elements such as informed consent processes, data protection and sharing regulations, biobank and data registry governance, as well as the validity and utility of genomic information for medical decision making must be addressed to assure the public of the potential worth of personalized medicine. They are also instructive in highlighting the range of ELSI that have been the focus of much genomics research in the last two decades, as well as the range of methodologies employed by ELSI researchers.

4 Practical Considerations When Undertaking an ELSI Initiative

ELSI research is an inherently complex undertaking, particularly for first-time interdisciplinary researchers. Tait and Lyall note that "Interdisciplinary research often requires more resources of time, effort, imagination, and money than single discipline research (and may also involve higher risks of failure) but the rewards can be substantial, in terms of advancing the knowledge base and helping to solve complex societal problems" [40]. In this final section we outline some practical considerations for those wishing to engage in interdisciplinary ELSI research in genomics.

1. Accept that ELSI research will likely require more time upfront and a preliminary research phase that is somewhat open-ended. Extra time will be needed to promote the formation of a cohesive research team with the correct disciplines represented given the nature of the research question. The ELSI questions themselves may take some time to negotiate. Initial discussions with team members will involve specifying the parameters on research questions and methodological approaches that are relevant. Stokols and colleagues [41] note that teams need to develop "shared conceptual frameworks that integrate and transcend the multiple disciplinary perspectives represented among team members" (p. S97).

    In an integrated ELSI project, it is essential that ELSI team members are engaged very early on. This includes the integration of ELSI researchers during the funding proposal stage as they will be instrumental in drafting portions of the proposal to identify specific ELSI that arise from the scientific or clinical research. Avoid contacting an ELSI researcher a few days before the funding deadline and asking him or her to provide a page or two on some of the issues that might arise out of the project. Given the broad range of ELSI research that might be undertaken with any large scale genomics project, the ELSI lead researcher will need time to identify both the key ELSI objectives and the kinds of expertise necessary to address them.

2. Choose team members with interdisciplinary characteristics such as flexibility, adaptability, creativity, and a real willingness to keep an open mind and be curious about ideas from other disciplines and backgrounds [40, 41]. It follows that good communication and listening skills are essential.

3. Allow an adequate budget for ELSI research in genomics. This might include the standard costs of ELSI research descriptive methodologies (e.g., survey administration, transcription of interviews), but might also include other ELSI activities that are part of the broader normative research plan (e.g., expert consensus meetings, educational tool development). An ELSI budget like any research budget will depend on the questions one hopes to answer, and the outputs to be achieved. As ELSI methodologies vary widely, budgets will vary as well. As a rule of thumb, however, it is our experiences that an integrated ELSI budget should comprise approximately 5–8 % of the overall scientific or clinical project.

4. Schedule regular team meetings that include not only ELSI team members, but also members of the broader scientific or clinical project. In our experience, monthly (or at least quarterly) team meetings provide a relatively informal opportunity for team members to interact, which can promote team cohesion and function [41]. Practically, these are useful venues to keep all team members informed of the various stages of the research project and provide excellent training opportunities for students and other trainees. Non-ELSI students become exposed early to the idea of integrated ELSI research and learn in an active way about the facilitators and barriers to interdisciplinary research. In addition, ELSI students will gain some familiarity with the process and content of scientific and clinical research. Finally, regular meetings also promote networking opportunities that may be important when putting together a team for a future research project.

5. Discuss publication process and authorship requirements up-front. Determine a systematic way to ensure that all and only legitimate contributors are listed on each publication and that contributions are acknowledged appropriately. Different

disciplines have different standards and these need to be acknowledged and negotiated from the outset. For example, multiauthored papers are common in the basic and social sciences, but less so in the humanities. In the basic sciences first and last author are generally considered the most significant, while in the social sciences the order of authorship is often more important; contributors are often arranged in a descending order. If two or three contributors did the bulk of the work while the remaining coauthors contributed equally, the first two or three authors are ordered according to their relative contributions while the rest would be added in alphabetical order. In the humanities, by contrast, multiauthored works (i.e., more than two or three co-authors) are rare, although it is common to have a lengthy acknowledgement section at the end of a paper. Given the importance of a publication record to the careers of most academics, sorting out how these procedural details will be managed at the outset will be important. Even when authorship criteria are determined it is often advisable to have a publication subcommittee that evaluates each publication produced in the project before it goes out for review. Who should be included as authors and in what order their names should appear may depend to some degree on the journal in which the team hopes to place the publication.

5   Conclusion

Given the continuing emphasis on genomic research in general and the increasing pressure to do translational research in particular, the question is not whether one should engage in ELSI research, but rather when and how to do so most effectively. Our hope is that this chapter has provided a useful overview of the nature and scope of ELSI research, and some practical pointers on how to engage in it successfully.

References

1. Rubio D, Schoenbaum E, Lee L et al (2010) Defining translational research: implications for training. Acad Med 85:470–475

2. Green ED, Guyer MS, National Human Genome Research Institute (2011) Charting a course for genomic medicine from base pairs to bedside. Nature. doi:10.1038/nature09764

3. Collins FS, Green ED, Gutmacher AE et al (2003) A vision for the future of genomics research. Nature 422:1–13

4. McKusick VA (1989) HUGO: history, purposes and membership. http://hugo-international.org/abt_history.php. Accessed 15 Apr 2014

5. HUGO ELSI Committee (1995) Statement on the principled conduct of genetics research. http://www.hugo-international.org/img/statment%20on%20the%20principled%20conduct%20of%20genetics%20research.pdf. Accessed 17 March 2014

6. Bombard Y, Veenstra G, Friedman JM et al (2009) Perceptions of genetic discrimination among people at risk for Huntington's disease: a cross sectional survey. BMJ 338:b2175

7. United States Congress (2008) Genetic Information Nondiscrimination Act of 2008. https://www.govtrack.us/congress/bills/110/hr493/text. Accessed 17 Apr 2014

8. Pullman D, Lemmens T (2010) Keeping the GINA in the bottle: assessing the current need for genetic non-discrimination legislation in Canada. Open Med 4(2):95–97

9. McCloskey D, McDonald M, Cook J et al (2011) Community engagement: definitions and organizing concepts from the literature. http://www.atsdr.cdc.gov/communityengagement/pdf/PCE_Report_Chapter_1_SHEF.pdf. Accessed 10 March 2014

10. Daudelin G, Lehoux P, Abelson J et al (2010) The integration of citizens into a science/policy network in genetics: governance arrangements and asymmetry in expertise. Health Expect 14:261–271

11. Attree P, French B, Povall S, Whitehead M, Popay J (2011) The experience of community engagement for individuals: a rapid review of evidence. Health Soc Care Community 19(3):250–260

12. Haldeman K, Cadigan R, Davis A et al (2014) Community engagement in US biobanking: multiplicity of meaning and method. Public Health Genomics. doi:10.1159/000357958

13. Burgess M, O'Doherty K, Secko D (2008) Biobanking in British Columbia: discussions of the future of personalized medicine through deliberative public engagement. Per Med 5(3):285–296

14. Henderson G, Juengst E, King NM, Kuczynski K, Michie M (2012) What research ethics should learn from genomics and society research: lessons from the ELSI Congress of 2011. J Law Med Ethics 40(4):1008–1024

15. Lemke A, Wolf W, Herbert-Beirne J, Smith M (2010) Public and biobank participant attitudes toward genetic research participation and data sharing. Public Health Genomics 13:368–377

16. Burke W, Trinidad S, Clayton E (2013) Seeking genomic knowledge: the case for clinical restraint. Hastings Law J 64(6):1650–1664

17. Ginsburg G, Willard H (2009) Genomic and personalized medicine: foundations and applications. Trans Res 154(6):277–287

18. Manolio T, Chisholm R, Ozenberger B, Roden DM, Williams MS, Wilson R, Bick D, Bottinger EP, Brilliant MH, Eng C, Frazer KA, Korf B, Ledbetter DH, Lupski JR, Marsh C, Mrazek D, Murray MF, O'Donnell PH, Rader DJ, Relling MV, Shuldiner AR, Valle D, Weinshilboum R, Green ED, Ginsburg GS (2012) Implementing genomic medicine in the clinic: the future is here. Genet Med 15(4):268–269

19. Borry P, Cornel M (2010) Where are you going, where have you been: a recent history of the direct-to-consumer genetic testing market. J Community Genet 1:101–106

20. McBride C, Wade C, Kaphingst K (2010) Consumers' views of direct-to-consumer genetic information. Annu Rev Genomics Hum Genet 11:427–446

21. Tarini B, Goldenberg J (2012) Ethical issues with newborn screening in the genomics era. Annu Rev Genomics Hum Genet 13:381–393

22. Rowe G, Frewer L (2005) A typology of public engagement mechanisms. Sci Tech Hum Values 30(2):251–290

23. Kaufman D, Murphy J, Scott J et al (2008) Subjects matter: a survey of public opinions about a large genetic cohort study. Genet Med 10:831–839

24. Kaufman D, Murphy J, Erby L, Hudson K, Scott J (2009) Veterans' attitudes regarding a database for genomic research. Genet Med 11:329–337

25. Godard B, Marshall J, Laberge C (2007) Community engagement in genetics research: results of the first public consultation for the Quebec CARGaGENE project. Community Genet 10:147–158

26. Hoeyer K, Olofsson B, Mjorndal T, Lynöe N (2004) Informed consent and biobanks: a population-based study of attitudes towards tissue donation for genetic research. Scand J Public Health 32:224–229

27. Haddow G, Cunningham Burley S, Bruce A, Parry S (2008) Generation Scotland: consulting publics and specialists at an early stage in a genetic database's development. Crit Publ Health 18(2):139–149

28. Rotimi C, Leppert M, Matsuda I, Zeng C, Zhang H, Adebamowo C, Ajayi I, Aniagwu T, Dixon M, Fukushima Y, Macer D, Marshall P, Nkwodimmah C, Peiffer A, Royal C, Suda E, Zhao H, Wang VO, McEwen J, International HapMap Consortium (2007) Community engagement and informed consent in the International HapMap project. Community Genet 10:186–198

29. Lemke A, Wu J, Waudby C, Pulley J, Somkin C, Trinidad S (2010) Community engagement in biobanking: experiences from the eMERGE network. Genomics Soc Policy 6(3):35–52

30. National Human Genome Research Institute. Community Genetics Forum (2007) http://www.genome.gov/19518473. Accessed 16 Apr 2014, Accessed 2 Apr 2014

31. Etchegary H, Dicks E, Hodgkinson K, Pullman D, Green J, Parfrey P (2010) Public attitudes about genetic testing in the newborn period. J Obstet Gyne Neonatal Nurs 41(2):191–200

32. Etchegary H, Green J, Dicks E, Pullman D, Street C, Parfrey P (2013) Consulting the community: public expectations and attitudes

about genetics research. Eur J Hum Genet 21:
1338–1343

33. Pullman D, Etchegary H, Gallagher K, Hodgkinson K, Keough M, Morgan D, Street C (2012) Personal privacy, public benefits, and biobanks: a conjoint analysis of policy priorities and public perceptions. Genet Med 14(2): 229–235

34. Hahn S, Letvak S, Powell K, Christianson C, Wallace D, Speer M, Lietz P, Blanton S, Vance J, Pericak-Vance M, Henrich VC, Genomedical Connection (2010) A community's awareness and perceptions of genomic medicine. Public Health Genomics 13:63–71

35. Haga S, Barry W, Mills R, Ginsburg GS, Svetkey L, Sullivan J, Willard HF (2013) Public knowledge and attitudes towards genetics and genetic testing. Genet Test Mol Biomarkers 17(4):327–335

36. O'Doherty K, Hawkins A (2010) Structuring public engagement for effective input in policy development on human tissue biobanking. Public Health Genomics 13:197–206

37. Anderson C, Stackhouse R, Shaw A, Iredale R (2011) The National DNA database on trial: engaging young people in South Wales with genetics. Public Underst Sci 20(2):146–162

38. O'Daniel J, Rosanbalm K, Boles L, Tindall GM, Livingston TM, Haga SB (2012) Enhancing geneticists' perspectives of the public through community engagement. Genet Med 14(2): 243–249

39. Nicols S, Wilson B, Cragie S, Etchegary H, Castle D, Carroll JC, Potter BK, Lemyre L, Little J (2013) Personalizing public health: public attitudes towards genomic risk profiling as a component of routine population screening. Genome 56:626–633

40. Tait J, Lyall C (2007) Short guide to developing interdisciplinary research proposals. Institute for the Study of Science Teaching and Innovation Briefing Note. http://www.issti. ed.ac.uk/__data/assets/file/0005/77603/ ISSTI_Briefing_Note_1.pdf. Accessed 16 Apr 2014

41. Stokols D, Misra S, Moser R, Hall KL, Taylor BK (2008) The ecology of team science: understanding contextual influences on transdisciplinary collaboration. Am J Prev Med 35(2S):96–115

Part VI

Methods in Evidence-Based Decision Making

Evidence-Based Decision-Making 1: Critical Appraisal

Laurie K. Twells

Abstract

This chapter provides an introduction to the concept of Evidence-based Medicine (EBM) including its history, rooted in Canada and its important role in modern medicine. The chapter both defines EBM and explains the process of conducting EBM. It includes a discussion of the hierarchy of evidence that exists with reference to common methods used to assess the levels of quality inherent in study designs. The focus of the chapter is on how to *critically appraise* the medical literature, as one step in the EBM process. Critical appraisal requires an understanding of the strengths and weaknesses of study design and how these in turn impact the validity and applicability of research findings. Strong critical appraisal skills are critical to evidence-based decision-making.

Key words Evidence-based medicine, Critical appraisal, Study design

1 Introduction

Evidence-based medicine (EBM) is "the conscientious, explicit and judicious use of current best evidence in making decisions about the care of individual patients" [1]. It means integrating individual clinical expertise with the best available external clinical evidence from systematic research [1, 2]. More recently, it has been further defined as the integration of best research evidence with clinical expertise and *patient values* [3]. The process of EBM involves formulating a clinical question, searching and obtaining the best evidence to answer the question, critically appraising the evidence to ensure its validity and applicability, and implementing the findings in practice [1]. Dr. David Sackett is often regarded as the "father of evidence-based medicine" although the term is said to have been first used by Dr. Gordon Guyatt in the 1990s [4, 5]. EBM is a process that grew out of the need for medical education to move away from patient care based solely on "expert opinion" to that based on best evidence [3]. Although now just one step in the process, it is interesting that EBM grew out of critical appraisal—the assessment of the validity of scientific literature

Patrick S. Parfrey and Brendan J. Barrett (eds.), *Clinical Epidemiology: Practice and Methods*, Methods in Molecular Biology, vol. 1281, DOI 10.1007/978-1-4939-2428-8_23, © Springer Science+Business Media New York 2015

and its practical relevance to patient care [1]. Critical appraisal of the scientific literature was advanced by David Sackett and Brian Haynes at McMaster University in the early 1980s when they published a series of articles in the *Canadian Medical Association Journal* (CMAJ) entitled "How to read clinical journals" with various subtopics that included: the etiology or causation of disease, quality of care, the usefulness or harm associated with therapy, and the utility of diagnostic tests [6]. Following these articles, Sackett wrote the seminal text for students "Clinical Epidemiology: A Basic Science for Clinical Medicine" now in its 3rd edition and often referred to as "the bible" of EBM [3, 7, 8]. Over the next two decades, the *CMAJ* articles were further refined and led to the establishment of an EBM Working Group that subsequently developed a series of 25 papers known as the *JAMA User's Guide to the Medical Literature*. These guides were initially developed for clinicians to help them interpret the medical literature and support clinical decision-making [9]. The success of this series of papers provided the impetus for both the *JAMA User's Guide to the Medical Literature*, a textbook (in its 6th printing), as well as the development of a user-friendly, publically available website that houses numerous resources for supporting the practice of EBM (http://www.jamaevidence.com). The articles, text and website include a number of EBM resources, structured guides on how to appraise papers on topics such as therapy, diagnosis, prognosis, quality of care, economic analysis and overviews, and are considered by many as the definitive checklists for critical appraisal [10].

2   The Process of Evidence-Based Medicine

In the opening editorial of the very first issue of the journal *Evidence-Based Medicine*, the essential steps in this emerging science of EBM were summarized. These included: to convert information needs into answerable questions (i.e., to formulate the problem); to track down, with maximum efficiency the best evidence to answer these questions; *to appraise the evidence critically in order to assess its validity (or truthfulness) and its applicability (or usefulness)*; to implement the results of the appraisal into clinical practice and to evaluate performance [11, 12].

This process is often illustrated using Steps or an A's approach shown in Table 1. This chapter is an introduction to **Step 4**, to "*Appraise*" the medical literature in order to assess its validity and applicability. The process of critical appraisal is a very important part, albeit one step, in the EBM process due to two key principles. First, not all evidence is considered equal, and second, a hierarchy of evidence exists linked to its design and inherent methodology.

Table 1
The process of evidence-based medicine

Step 1	Assess important patient or policy problems
Step 2	Ask well-defined clinical questions from case scenarios, the answer to which will inform decision-making.
Step 3	Acquire information by selecting and searching the most appropriate resources
Step 4	Appraise the medical literature for its validity (closeness to the truth) and its applicability (usefulness in clinical practice)
Step 5	Apply the results of the appraisal of medical literature to make sound, reasoned clinical decisions taking into account patient preferences and values
Step 6	Assess or evaluate performance in applying the evidence

Appraising evidence requires an understanding of the strengths and weaknesses of epidemiological study design and how these in turn affect the validity and applicability of study findings [10].

3   Levels of Scientific Evidence

A number of classification systems have been developed to assess and describe the varying levels of evidence associated with different study designs. Although there is some debate over the strengths of individual study methods, there is a general consensus that a hierarchy of evidence exists. Various study designs will provide differing levels of evidence to support a treatment effect or causal relationship by limiting systematic bias [3, 8, 10]. This hierarchy of evidence is most often illustrated by a pyramid or similar graphic that places the types of evidence in the following order of decreasing strength:

1. Systematic reviews and Meta-analysis.
2. Randomized Controlled Trials.
3. Cohort studies.
4. Case–control studies.
5. Cross-sectional studies.
6. Case series/Case reports.
7. Expert opinion.

A very brief summary of these main study designs is provided here. For more detailed information please refer to other chapters in this textbook. Epidemiological research studies are divided into experimental/intervention or observational studies and with the exception of randomized controlled trials, the only experimental study, most are observational in nature. At the top of the pyramid are studies that summarize other studies. Systematic reviews (SR) are produced by systematically searching, critically appraising, and synthesizing available literature on a specific topic (e.g., the difference between parental perception and actual weight status of children: a systematic review). A SR and meta-analysis includes a quantitative summary of all study results, the benefit being an increased power to assess the effectiveness (or lack of) of an intervention (e.g., the effectiveness and risks of bariatric surgery: an updated systematic review *and meta-analysis*). Clearly, the quality of the meta-analysis is dependent on the quality of the RCT's included. In some instances a high quality RCT will dominate the evidence base. In other instances, a meta-analysis will reveal a weak evidence base with few trials homogenous for the intervention, design, patient groups and outcomes. An RCT, considered the gold standard in study design, is the only study design whereby participants are randomly allocated to an intervention/experimental arm (e.g., new cancer treatment) or a control arm (e.g., standard of care + placebo). Follow-up takes place over time to measure one or more outcomes of interest. Within a cohort study, a group of individuals exposed to a risk factor (e.g., diabetes mellitus) is compared to a similar unexposed group and an outcome(s) (e.g., premature mortality) is assessed over a specific time period. Cohort studies can be either prospective or retrospective in nature depending on the nature of data collection. In a case–control study, a group of individuals with a disease/outcome of interest (e.g., birth limb defects) are identified and compared to a control group with respect to their past exposure status (e.g., medication use such as Thalidomide). Cross-sectional studies or prevalence studies classify subjects according to disease and exposure status. Data is often collected through health surveys and questionnaires (e.g., a health survey reports the prevalence of obesity and diabetes in a target population). A case report consists of a detailed report of a single patient while a case series provides information on more than one patient with the same features (e.g., four young men described with rare form of pneumonia, led to the discovery of AIDS) [7, 10, 11].

3.1 Methods Used to Evaluate Scientific Evidence

There are many examples of methods used by organizations to delineate the quality of evidence. Some of these include those developed by the: US Preventive Services Task Force (USPSTF); the Oxford Centre for Evidence-Based Medicine (CEBM) and the Grading of Recommendations Assessment, Development and Evaluation or GRADE working group.

<table>
<tr><td>

3.1.1 The US Preventive Services Task Force

</td><td>

Varying levels of evidence are used to rank the effectiveness of treatments or screening tools relevant to the primary care environment and are classified using the following levels:

</td></tr>
</table>

- Level I: Evidence obtained from at least one properly designed randomized controlled trial, well-conducted systematic review or meta-analysis of homogeneous RCTs.

- Level II-1: Evidence obtained from well-designed controlled trials without randomization.

- Level II-2: Evidence obtained from well-designed cohort or case–control analytic studies.

- Level II-3: Evidence obtained from multiple time series designs with or without the intervention; dramatic results from uncontrolled experiments.

- Level III: Opinions of respected authorities, based on clinical experience, descriptive studies, or reports of expert committees.

Prior to the grading of levels, individual studies are critically appraised for internal validity based on specific criteria unique to each study design. Ultimately each study will be described as good (if a study meets all criteria), fair (if a study does not meet one criterion but does not have a fatal flaw) or poor (the study has a fatal flaw) in terms of methodological quality. For example, when critically appraising an RCT the following descriptors could apply. A study could be described as (1) *Good:* if comparable groups were initially recruited and maintained throughout the study (follow-up at least 80 %); if reliable and valid measurement instruments were used and applied equally to the groups; if interventions were described clearly; if all important outcomes were reported, if confounders were taken into consideration and intention-to-treat (ITT) analysis was conducted. (2) *Fair:* although comparable groups were recruited at the start of the study period, questions in differences in follow-up exist; measurement instruments are acceptable and have been applied equally but may not be the best choice; some but not all important outcomes are considered; and some but not all potential confounders are accounted for. ITT is conducted. (3) *Poor:* groups recruited at the start of the study are not close to being comparable or maintained throughout the study; unreliable/invalid measurement instruments are used or not applied consistently among groups (including not blinding outcome assessment); key confounders are not accounted for; and ITT analysis is absent. ((http://www.uspreventiveservicestaskforce.org/uspstf08/methods/procmanual4.htm))

<table>
<tr><td>

3.1.2 The Oxford Centre for Evidence-Based Medicine

</td><td>

The Oxford Centre for Evidence-Based Medicine (CEBM) provides a grading system (http://www.cebm.net/) to evaluate evidence for different types of questions that include those on therapy,

</td></tr>
</table>

etiology, prevention, harm, prognosis, diagnosis, and economic analysis. The highest level of evidence is classified as 1a and refers to a SR with homogeneity (similar study methods) with the lowest level of evidence a 5 being expert opinion. An evaluation of evidence using these levels results in a recommendation by a grading system (A to D), with a Grade A recommendation suggesting consistent level 1 studies are available through to a Grade D recommendation that suggests only level 5 evidence is available or that alternate evidence is inconclusive.

3.1.3 The Grading of Recommendations Assessment, Development, and Evaluation

The GRADE working group (http://www.gradeworkinggroup.com) has further refined and developed the process of assessing the strength of a study by addressing more than just the quality of the research but also the impact other factors have on the confidence in study results. Similar to other systems, the quality of evidence is assessed on four levels (i.e., high, moderate, low, very low) while *the confidence factor* is based on judgments assigned in five different domains in a structured manner. For example, an RCT may be considered a high quality study with a low risk of bias, but depending on its assessment in other domains, it may be downgraded due to: risk of bias (e.g., no allocation concealment); imprecision (i.e., random error); indirectness (e.g., population, interventions or outcomes differ from those of interest). A body of evidence may be downgraded due to inconsistency (e.g., different point estimates with nonoverlapping confidence intervals) or publication bias (e.g., small sample sizes with large treatment effects, commercially funded research). Alternatively, an observational study of moderate quality could be upgraded due to a large effect size or evidence of a dose–response relationship and would further support inferences of a treatment effect.

4 Critical Appraisal: Basics

Critical appraisal is the process of systematically assessing the validity, usefulness, and relevance of the evidence [12]. The process can be divided into an examination of extrinsic and intrinsic factors. *Extrinsic factors* include taking note of the authors and their affiliations, the journal, the funder, and the stated conflicts of interest [13]. Examining the intrinsic factors requires a rigorous assessment of study design and methodology- the focus of critical appraisal. A number of excellent resources have been developed to support the critical appraisal process (see EBM Resources at end of chapter), and all use a very similar template that involves asking three main questions followed by a subset of specific questions associated with a particular type of question (e.g., therapy) or study design (e.g., cohort study). These questions include:

1. Are the results of the study valid?
2. What are the results?
3. Will the results help in caring for my patients? Are the results applicable or generalizable to my patient population?

For each main question, a number of publicly available EBM resources (e.g., JAMA User's Guides, Clinical Evidence-Based Medicine (CEBM, Cochrane Collaboration) provide checklists, templates, and worksheets to help health professionals and students learn how to effectively appraise the scientific literature in relation to its validity and applicability. In the section below, examples of the types of questions that should be addressed during the appraisal process are provided. This is not an inclusive list but an overview of the types of questions you would expect to answer when appraising an article. References throughout the chapter and in the reference section provide readers with some of the key resources that should be used in the process of critical appraisal.

I. Are the results of the study valid?
   The following questions are relevant for the appraisal of all research studies.
   i. Why is the research being conducted?
       a. Is a brief background or context provided as to why the study was conducted?
       b. What is the study about?
   ii. What is the research question being addressed?
       a. Is there a hypothesis being tested?
       b. Is the question described in a PICO format? (Population, Intervention, Control, Outcome)
       c. If, after I conduct a methodological assessment, the results are valid, are they applicable to my question, my patient or patient population? If yes, keep reading if no move to another paper.
   iii. What type of study has been conducted?
       a. Primary studies present original research, while secondary research summarizes or integrates primary research. A brief descriptor of the main types of studies and their objective is provided in Table 2.
   iv. Was the research study design appropriate to the type of question?

a. The clinical area and/or type of question will normally inform the appropriate choice of study design. Table 3 provides some examples to illustrate these choices.

For each type of study question and/or study design, a set of questions has been developed to assess the validity of the study methods. These questions help to assess whether selection biases (e.g., the groups being compared are different), or information biases (e.g., ascertainment of exposure status) exist as well as to determine the level of confounding that exists and how the authors have chosen to adjust for it.

v. Do the methods used increase the validity of the results? Broad questions for each study design include:

a. Systematic reviews and/meta-analysis—search details, comprehensivness and rigor of review, quality assessment, appropriate synthesis of results, heterogeneity

b. Randomized controlled trials—success of the randomization process (e.g., evidence of allocation concealment, equal groups), follow-up of patients, blinding, statistical analysis (e.g., ITT, per protocol), groups treated equally other than intervention

c. Cohort studies—recruitment of the cohort (e.g., is it representative of a defined population), the measurement of the exposure and outcome (e.g., subjective or objective measures), blinding (e.g., of the assessor), confounding (e.g., restriction, multivariate modelling, sensitivity analysis), loss to follow-up

d. Case–control studies—recruitment of cases (e.g., case definition, representative, prevalent vs. incident, sufficient sample size) and controls (e.g., representative, sufficient sample, matched), exposure ascertainment

e. Diagnostic studies—reference standard, disease status (e.g., level of severity), blinding.

II. What are the results?

i. What are the main results of the study? How are they presented? (e.g., Relative Risk, Odds Ratio, Hazard Ratio, % change, mean difference, sensitivity, specificity, likelihood ratios, Number Needed to Treat).

ii. Is the analysis appropriate to the study design?

    iii. Are the results statistically significant? (e.g., p-values, Confidence Interval (CI))

    iv. What is the treatment effect? Strength of effect?

        a. How precise is it? (e.g., width of CI)

    v. Have the results been adjusted for confounding? (e.g., crude and adjusted analysis)

    vi. Have drop-outs or lost to follow-up been accounted for? (e.g., ITT, per protocol analysis, sensitivity analysis)

    vii. Do you believe the results? Could they be due to chance, bias or confounding?

    viii. Do the results suggest a causal relationship?

        a. Guidelines have been developed to help assess the likelihood of a cause–effect relationship (see Assessing Causation below)

    viii. Are you concerned about publication bias?

III. Are the results from the study applicable/relevant to my research question, patient or population of interest?

    i. Can the results (or test) be applied to my patient/ local population? (e.g., similar socio-demographic, health status, gender, age, country, health system)

        a. Are the results statistically significant and/or clinically significant?

    ii. Were all relevant outcomes included in the study?

    iii. Do the benefits outweigh the harms (if any)?

Table 2
Study design and its major objective

Study design	Major objective
Meta-analysis	To provide an overall summary statistic of multiple primary studies using an a priori protocol and integration of quantitative data from studies identified by a systematic review
Randomized Controlled Trial	To study the efficacy of a treatment or intervention
Cohort Study	To study prognosis, natural history of a disease or causation
Case–control Study	To identify potential causal factors for a disease or to study adverse effects
Cross-sectional Studies	To determine the prevalence of disease or risk factors

Table 3
The relationship between clinical area/type of question and research study

Clinical area	Type of question	Research study
Diagnosis	What disease is responsible for the abnormal findings?	Prospective, blind comparison to a gold standard Cross-sectional study
Therapy	What therapy is appropriate for a disease?	RCT Prospective cohort
Prognosis	What are the expected outcomes of a disease?	Longitudinal studies Retrospective/prospective cohort studies
Prevention	How can a disease be prevented or delayed?	RCT Cohort Case–control Case series
Harm	What intervention or other factor may be contributing to a disease?	RCT Cohort Case–control/Case series

4.1 Assessing Causation

Knowing what causes a disease or adverse outcome may be critical for understanding how to prevent, diagnose, treat or provide a prognosis. According to the Oxford Dictionary, a cause is defined as "something that gives rise to an action, phenomenon or condition" [14]. In the mid 1900s, Austin Bradford Hill and Richard Doll, who were responsible for the seminal studies on smoking and lung cancer, developed a guide to assess the causal relationship between an exposure and an outcome [8]. This is not a list of criteria or rules that have to be met, but a guide to help examine the strength of the available evidence in the context of a causal relationship between an exposure and an outcome (Table 4).

5   Concluding Remarks

The above types of questions and suggested resources will help to support critical appraisal of the scientific literature. These are the tools needed to systematically assess the validity, usefulness and relevance of available evidence. Evidence-based medicine has become synonymous with evidence-based health care or evidence-based practice. Critical appraisal is an important, albeit, one step in this process. Understanding the strengths, weaknesses and quality of study designs, and their inherent ability to provide high grade evidence for health interventions, will inform evidence-based decision-making and evidence-based practice.

Table 4
Austin Bradford Hill's guide for assessing causation [8]

Temporality	Exposure precedes disease
Experimental evidence	Evidence from true experiments
Strength	Exposure strongly associated with disease frequency
Biological gradient or dose–response	More exposure associated with higher disease frequency or severity
Consistency	The association is observed by different persons in different places during different circumstances
Coherence	The association is consistent with the natural history and epidemiology of the disease
Biologic plausibility	Causation is consistent with biological knowledge of the time
Specificity	One cause leads to one effect
Analogy	Cause and effect relationship has been established for a similar risk factor or disease

References

1. Sackett DL, Rosenberg WMC, Gray JAM, Haynes RB, Richardson WS (1996) Evidence based medicine: what it is and what it isn't. BMJ 312:71–72

2. Sackett DL, Rennie D (1992) The science of the art of the clinical examination. JAMA 267(19):2650–2652

3. Sackett DL, Straus SE, Richardson WS, Rosenberg W, Haynes RB (2000) Evidence-based medicine: how to practice and teach EBM, 2nd edn. Churchill Livingstone, Edinburgh

4. Smith R, Drummond R (2014) Evidence-based medicine-an oral history. JAMA 311(4):365–367

5. Guyatt G. (1991). Evidence-based medicine. *ACP J Club 114*:A-16.

6. Sackett DL (1981) How to read clinical journals, I: why to read them and how to start reading them critically. CMAJ 124(5):555–558

7. Sackett DL, Haynes RB, Guyatt GH, Tugwell P (1991) Clinical epidemiology—a basic science for clinical medicine, 2nd edn. Little, Brown and Company, Boston

8. Haynes RB, Sackett DL, Guyatt GH, Tugwell P (2006) Clinical epidemiology- how to do clinical practice research, 3rd edn. Lippincott Williams & Wilkins, Philadelphia

9. Guyatt GH, Rennie D (1993) Users' guides to the medical literature. JAMA 270(17): 2096–2097

10. Greenhalgh T (2001) How to read a paper. The basics of evidence-based medicine. BMJ Books, London

11. Fletcher RW, Fletcher SW (2005) Clinical epidemiology: the essentials, 4th edn. Lippincott Williams & Wilkins, Baltimore

12. Sackett DL, Haynes B (1995) On the need for evidence based medicine. Evidence-Based Medicine 1: 4–5

13. Booth A, Brice A (2004) Evidence-based practice for information professionals: a handbook. Facet Publishing, London

14. Oxford Dictionary. (2014). Oxford University Press. http://www.oxforddictionararies.com

Additional EBM Resources: Online Resources

JAMA User Guides. http://www.jamaevidence.com

Centre for Evidence-Based Medicine (CEBM) Oxford, UK. http://www.cebm.net/

Critical Appraisal Skills Programs (CASP) Oxford, UK. http://www.Students4bestevidence.net/

Greenhalgh T. (1997). How to Read a Paper. *BMJ* 315 (Series of ten articles)

The Cochrane Collaboration. http://www.cochranelibrary.com

CIHR KT learning modules. http://www.cihr-irsc.gc.ca/e/39128.html

KT clearing house (supported by CIHR and St. Michaels' Hospital and University of Toronto). http://ktclearinghouse.ca/cebm/

Evidence updates from the BMJ Evidence Centre: a collaboration between McMaster University and the BMJ Group. https://plus.mcmaster.ca/evidenceupdates/Default.aspx

Additional EBM Resources: Textbook Resources

Sackett DL, Straus S, Richardson S, Rosenberg W, Haynes RB (2000) Evidence-based medicine: how to practice and teach EBM, 2dth edn. Churchill Livingstone, London

Strauss S, Glasziou P, Scott Richardson W, Brian Hayes R (2011) Evidence-based medicine: How to practice and teach it, 4th edn. Churchill Livingstone, London

Guyatt G, Rennie D. eds. (2002). Users' Guides to the Medical Literature: A Manual for Evidence-Based Clinical Practice. Chicago, IL: American Medical Association (3rd edition due out in September 2014])

Guyatt G, Rennie D (eds) (2002) Users guides: essentials of evidence-based clinical practice. American Medical Association, Chicago, IL

McKibbon A, Wilczynski N (2009) PDQ evidence-based principles and practice, 2nd edn. McGraw-Hill, Europe

Chapter 24

Evidence-Based Decision-Making 2: Systematic Reviews and Meta-analysis

Aminu Bello, Natasha Wiebe, Amit Garg, and Marcello Tonelli

Abstract

The number of studies published in the biomedical literature has dramatically increased over the last few decades. This massive proliferation of literature makes clinical medicine increasingly complex, and information from multiple studies is often needed to inform a particular clinical decision. However, available studies often vary in their design, methodological quality, populations studied and may define the research question of interest quite differently, which can make it challenging to synthesize their conclusions. In addition, since even highly cited trials may be challenged over time, clinical decision-making requires ongoing reconciliation of studies which provide different answers to the same question. Because it is often impractical for readers to track down and review all the primary studies, systematic reviews and meta-analyses are an important source of evidence on the diagnosis, prognosis, and treatment of any given disease. This chapter summarizes methods for conducting and reading systematic reviews and meta-analyses, as well as describing potential advantages and disadvantages of these publications.

Key words Meta-analysis, Systematic review, Literature synthesis, Random effects, Forest plot

1 Introduction

The number of studies published in the biomedical literature has dramatically increased over the last few decades—there are now over 21 million citations in MEDLINE from 1964 to 2014 with nearly 4,000 new citations added daily [1]. These citations are from over 5,600 journals worldwide in about 40 languages (~93 % published in English) [1]. This massive proliferation of literature makes clinical medicine increasingly complex, and information from multiple studies is often needed to inform a particular clinical decision [2]. However, available studies often vary in their design, methodological quality, populations studied and may define the research question of interest quite differently, which can make it challenging to synthesize their conclusions. In addition, since even highly cited trials may be challenged over time [3], clinical decision-making requires ongoing reconciliation of studies which

Patrick S. Parfrey and Brendan J. Barrett (eds.), *Clinical Epidemiology: Practice and Methods*, Methods in Molecular Biology, vol. 1281, DOI 10.1007/978-1-4939-2428-8_24, © Springer Science+Business Media New York 2015

provide different answers to the same question. Because it is often impractical for readers to track down and review all the primary studies [4], review articles are an important source of summarized evidence on the diagnosis, prognosis, and treatment of any given disease.

Review articles have traditionally been written as "narrative reviews" where a content expert provides a personal interpretation of available evidence [5–9]. Although potentially useful, a narrative review typically uses an implicit process to compile evidence to support the statements being made. The reader often cannot tell which recommendations were based on the author's unsubstantiated clinical experience versus published clinical studies, and the reasons why some studies were given more emphasis than others. It is possible some narrative reviews preferentially cite evidence that reinforces the preconceived opinions of the authors on the topic in question. In addition, narrative reviews generally do not provide a quantitative summary of the literature.

2 How Do Systematic Reviews Differ from Narrative Reviews?

In contrast, a systematic review uses an explicitly defined process to comprehensively identify all studies pertaining to a specific focused question, appraise the methods of the studies, summarize their results, identify reasons for different findings across studies, and cite limitations of current knowledge [10–14]. Unlike a narrative review, the structured and transparent process used to conduct a properly done systematic review allows the reader to gauge the quality of the review process and the potential for bias. Meta-analyses usually combine the aggregate level data reported in each primary study (point and variance estimate of the summary measure). On occasion a review team will obtain individual patient data from each of the primary studies [15–20]. Although some authors consider a meta-analysis the best possible use of all available data—others regard the results with skepticism and question whether they add anything meaningful to scientific knowledge.

3 Why Are Systematic Reviews and Meta-analyses Clinically Relevant?

There are key advantages of systematic reviews and meta-analyses in clinical decision-making as compared to the traditional narrative reviews [21–23]:

1. *Providing robust data for clinical decisions:* Reading a well-conducted systematic review is an efficient method by which to learn about all previous studies on a given topic, and why some studies may differ from others in their results (a finding referred

to as heterogeneity among the primary studies). Such evidence summaries often form the knowledge base used to support clinical decisions, evidence-based practice guidelines, economic evaluations, and future research agendas. The assessment of the expected effect of an intervention or exposure provided by a systematic review can be integrated with information about other relevant treatment options, patient preferences and health care system factors. Reviewing the evidence summary allows the reader to establish whether the scientific findings are consistent and valid across populations, settings, and treatment variations, and whether findings vary significantly by particular subgroups.

2. *Minimizing bias*: Meta-analysis and systematic reviews overcome some of the biases and natural variation inherent with small studies where results may not be robust against chance variation—especially for small treatment effects. Further, the predefined and explicit methodology of a systematic review includes steps to minimize bias in all parts of the process: identifying relevant studies, selecting them for inclusion, and summarizing their data, and (for meta-analysis) statistically combining data across studies.

3. *Enhancing generalizability of findings into practice*: Systematic reviews overcome the lack of generalizability inherent in studies conducted in one particular type of population by including many trials conducted in varying populations. Reasons for a difference in study findings can also be explored, which can yield new insights.

4. *Increasing statistical power*: Single studies viewed separately, may reach inconclusive results due to relatively small sample size and wide confidence intervals. Statistical power and estimate precision can be improved with meta-analysis.

4   How Are Systematic Reviews Conducted?

A series of guidelines has been published describing how to report systematic reviews on therapy [24], screening or diagnosis [25], cost-effectiveness [26], or prognosis [27]. In 1996; the Quality of Reporting of Meta-Analyses (QUORUM) statement was published to improve specifically the quality of reporting meta-analyses of RCTs [28]. In the year 2000 there was the publication of Meta-analysis of Observational Studies in Epidemiology (MOOSE) guidelines for reporting systematic reviews of observational studies [29]. These statements include a checklist, which describes the preferred way to report a systematic review/meta-analysis. Recently, these guidelines have been updated by the publication of

PRISMA (Preferred Reporting Items for Systematic reviews and Meta-Analyses), which have been updated to address several conceptual and practical advances in the science of systematic reviews [30].

Conducting a systematic review/meta-analysis involves a number of steps that start with protocol development and research question formulation, design and study selection criteria, followed by retrieval of potentially relevant studies, selection of those studies to be included and evaluation of study risk of bias [21, 31, 32] (Table 1). Thereafter, the actual meta-analysis is performed and the primary studies evaluated for heterogeneity (qualitative and quantitative). Finally the results are evaluated for reproducibility (sensitivity testing) to ensure that bias did not influence the result, and implications for practice and/or policy [12, 33, 34] (Table 1).

Table 1
Steps to undertake a systematic review

Step	Description
Defining a research question	The problems to be addressed by the review should be identified, with the objectives of the review clearly stated. A prospective protocol defines the populations, inclusion/exclusion criteria, interventions, study designs, and outcomes
Literature search	The published and unpublished literature should be carefully searched for relevant studies required to answer the research question of interest. A professional librarian should help to design the search, where possible
Study selection	Once all possible studies have been identified, they should be independently assessed by two reviewers for eligibility (against inclusion criteria) with retrieval of full text papers for those that met the inclusion criteria (or for which eligibility cannot be initially assessed). Eligible articles should be processed for methodological quality (using a critical appraisal framework)
Data abstraction	Of the remaining studies, relevant characteristics and results should be abstracted onto a data abstraction form. Some studies will be excluded even at this late stage. A list of included studies should then be created
Synthesis, exploration for heterogeneity, and reporting of the results	The findings from the individual studies should be aggregated, synthesized, and reported—all according to the initially proposed protocol. Deviations to or addition from the protocol should be clearly noted and mentioned in the report
Placing the findings in context	The findings from the evidence synthesis should then be put into the context of the existing literature. This will address issues such as the quality and heterogeneity of the included studies, the likely impact of bias, as well as the applicability of the findings to practitioners

Reproduced with permission from ref. [32]

5 How Should the Quality of a Systematic Review or Meta-analysis Be Appraised?

Users of systematic reviews need to assure themselves that the underlying methods are sound. Before considering the results, or how the information can be appropriately applied in patient care, there are few questions that readers can ask themselves when assessing the methodological quality of a systematic review [10] (Table 2).

5.1 Was the Review Conducted According to a Prespecified Protocol?

It is reassuring if a review was guided by a written protocol (prepared in advance) which describes the research question(s), hypotheses, review methodology, and plan for how the data will be extracted and compiled. Such an approach minimizes the likelihood that the results or the expectations of the reviewing team influenced study inclusion or synthesis. Although most systematic reviews are conducted retrospectively, reviews and meta-analyses can in theory be defined at the time several similar trials are being planned or under way. This allows a set of specific hypotheses, data collection procedures, and analytic strategies to be specified in advance before any of the results from the primary studies are known. Such a prospective effort may provide more reliable answers to medically relevant questions than the traditional retrospective approach [35].

5.2 Was the Question Focused and Well Formulated?

Clinical questions often deal with issues of treatment, etiology, prognosis, and diagnosis. A well-formulated question usually specifies the patient's problem or diagnosis, the intervention or exposure of interest, as well as any comparison group (if relevant), and the primary and secondary outcomes of interest [36].

Table 2
Assessing the methodological quality of a systematic review

1. Was the review conducted according to a prespecified protocol?
2. Was the question focused and well formulated?
3. Were the right types of studies eligible for the review?

4. Was the method of identifying all relevant information comprehensive?
  (a) Is it likely that relevant studies were missed?
  (b) Was publication bias considered?

5. Was the data abstraction from each study appropriate?   (a) Was the methods used in each primary study appraised?
6. Was the information synthesized and summarized appropriately?   (a) If the results were mathematically combined in meta-analysis, were the methods described in sufficient detail and was it reasonable to do so?

Reproduced with permission from ref. [32]

Adapted from Oxman AD, Cook DJ, Guyatt Users' Guides to Evidence-based Medicine, How to Use an Overview [10]

5.3 Were the "Right" Types of Studies Eligible for the Review?

Different study designs can be used to answer different research questions. Randomized controlled trials, observational studies, and cross sectional diagnostic studies may each be appropriate depending on the primary question posed in the review. When examining the eligible criteria for study inclusion, the reader should feel confident that a potential bias in the selection of studies was avoided. Specifically, the reader should ask whether the eligibility criteria for study inclusion were appropriate for the question asked. Whether the best types of studies were selected for the review also depends on the depth and breadth of the underlying literature search. For example, some review teams will only consider studies published in English. There is evidence that journals from certain countries publish a higher proportion of positive trials than others [37]. Excluding non-English studies appeared to change the results of some reviews, but not others [38–40]. Some review teams use broad criteria for their inclusion of primary studies (i.e., effects of agents which block the renin–angiotensin system on adverse cardiovascular outcomes), while other teams use more narrow inclusion criteria (i.e., restricting the analysis to only those patients with diabetes with kidney failure) [41]. There is often no single correct approach. However, the conclusions of any meta-analysis which is highly sensitive to altering the entry criteria of included studies should be interpreted with some caution [42]. For example, two different review teams considered whether synthetic dialysis membranes resulted in better clinical outcomes compared to cellulose based membranes in patients with acute kidney injury. In one meta-analysis [43], but not the other [44], synthetic membranes reduced the chance of death. The discordant results were due to the inclusion of a study which did not meet eligibility for the second review [45].

5.4 Was the Method of Identifying All Relevant Information Comprehensive?

Identifying relevant studies for a given clinical question amongst the many potential sources of information is usually a laborious process [46]. Biomedical journals are the most common source of information, and bibliographic databases are used to search for relevant articles. MEDLINE currently indexes about 5,600 medical journals and contains 21 million citations [1]. As a supplementary method of identifying information, searching databases such as the Science Citation Index (which identifies all papers which cite a relevant article), as well as newer Internet search engines like Google Scholar and Elsevier's Scirus can be useful for identifying articles not indexed well in traditional bibliographic databases [47]. Searching bibliographies of retrieved articles can also identify relevant articles which were missed. Whatever bibliographic database was used, the review team should have employed a search strategy which maximized the identification of relevant articles [48, 49]. Because there is some subjectivity in screening databases, citations should be reviewed independently and in duplicate by two members of the reviewing team, with the full text article retrieved for any citation deemed relevant by any of the reviewers. There is also some subjectivity in assessing the eligibility of each full text article, and the risk that relevant reports were discarded is reduced if two reviewers independently perform each assessment [50].

Important sources of information other than journal articles should also be considered. Conference proceedings, abstracts, books, as well as inquiries to relevant industrial organizations can all yield potentially valuable information. Inquiries to experts, including protocols listed in trial registries, may have also proved useful [51]. A comprehensive search of available literature reduces the possibility of publication bias, which occurs when studies with statistically significant results are more like to be published and cited [52, 53]. It is interesting that some reviews of *n-acetylcysteine* for the prevention of contrast nephropathy analyzed as few as five studies, despite being submitted for publication almost 1 year after publication of a review of 12 studies [54]. While there are many potential reasons for this, one cannot exclude the possibility that some search strategies missed eligible trials. In addition to a comprehensive search method which makes it unlikely that relevant studies were missed, it is often reassuring if the review team used graphical (funnel plot) and statistical methods (Begg test; Egger test) to confirm there is little chance that publication bias influenced the results [39].

5.5 Was the Data Abstraction from Each Study Appropriate?

In compiling relevant information the review team should have used a rigorous and reproducible method of abstracting all relevant data from the primary studies. Often two reviewers abstract key information from each primary study including study and patient characteristics, setting, and details about the intervention, exposure or diagnostic test as is appropriate. Language translators may be needed. Teams who conduct their review with due rigor will indicate they contacted the primary authors from each of the primary studies, to confirm the accuracy of abstracted data as well as to provide additional relevant information not provided in the primary report. Some authors will go through the additional effort of blinding or masking the results from other study characteristics, so that data abstraction is as objective as possible [55, 56].

Data on the methodological risk of bias of each primary study should always be extracted (recognizing this is not always as straightforward as it may first seem) [57–62]. The question to be posed by the reader is whether the reviewing team considered if each of the primary studies was designed, conducted, and analyzed in a way to minimize or avoid biases in the results. For randomized controlled trials, lack of concealment of allocation, inadequate generation of the allocation sequence, and lack of double blinding can exaggerate estimates of the treatment effect [61, 63]. The value of abstracting such data is that it may help explain important differences in the results amongst the primary studies [61]. For example, long-term risk estimates can become unreliable when participants are lost to study follow-up—those who participate in follow-up often systematically differ from non-participants. For this reason, prognosis studies are vulnerable to bias, unless the loss to follow-up is less than 20 % [64].

5.6 How Was the Information Synthesized and Summarized?

Several types of figures are commonly used to summarize information in a systematic review: a flow diagram of study selection (Fig. 1) [65], a forest plot depicting individual and most often an overall pooled estimate of effect (Fig. 2) [33, 66], and a funnel

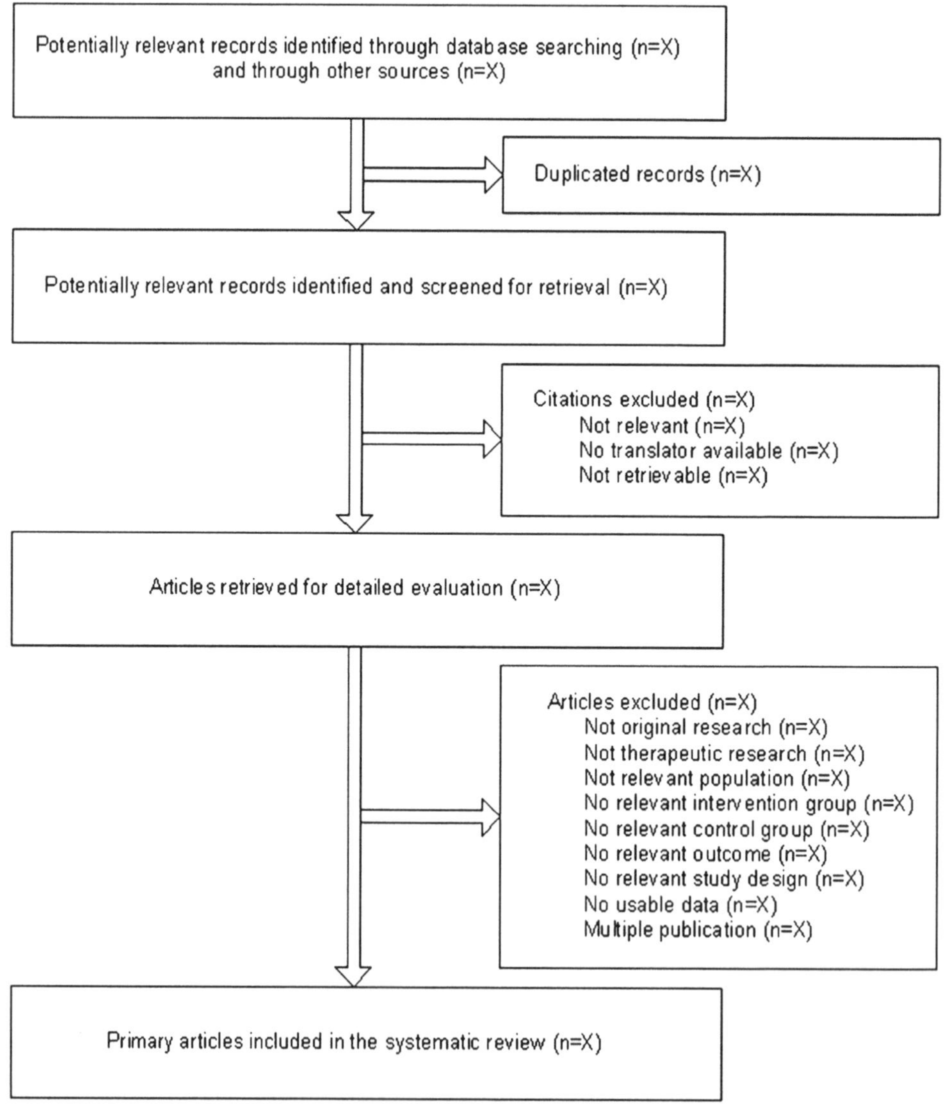

Fig. 1 Example of a PRISMA flowchart for study selection. X represents the number of studies in each category. Reproduced with permission from ref. [32]

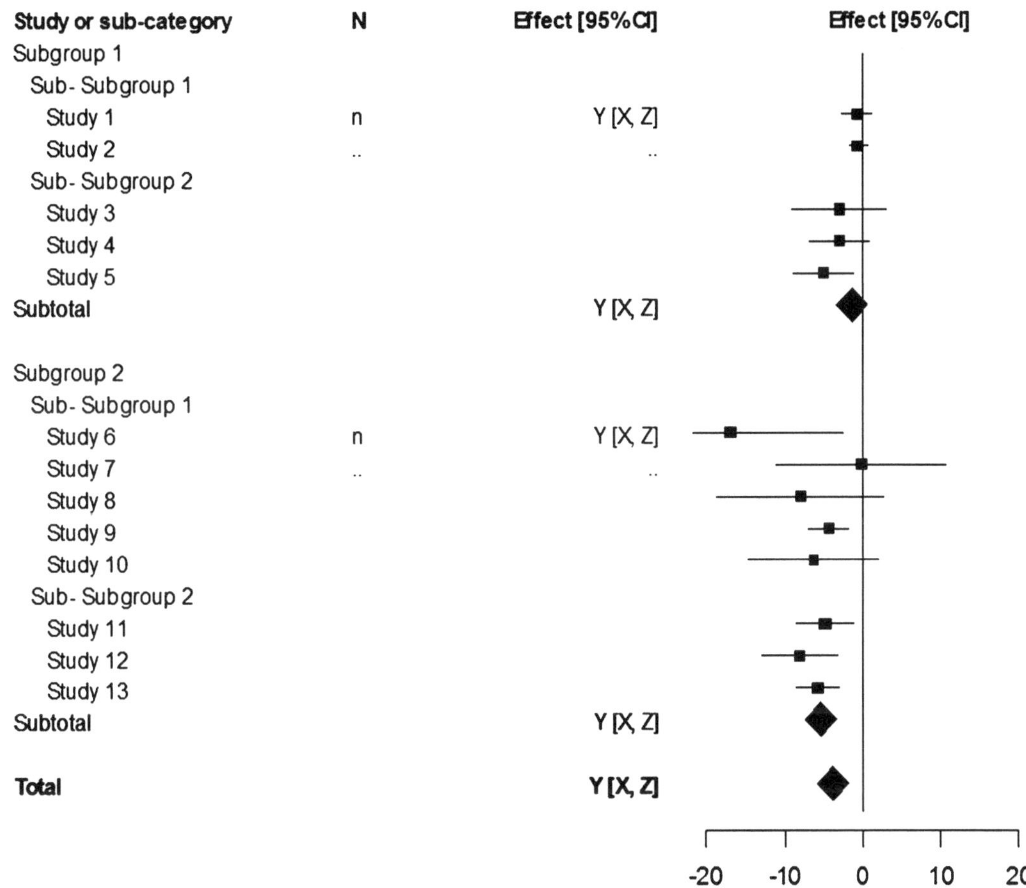

Fig. 2 Example of a forest plot. Each row of a forest plot (also called meta-graph) represents information pulled from one study or the total or a subgroup of pooled studies. The marker represents the point estimate of effect. The width of the bar represents the 95 % confidence limits. A *diamond marker* usually indicates the total or a subgroup total of pooled results. In this example Y is the point estimate of effect for each trial, and X, Z are the 95 % confidence limits. To the left of the plot is tabular information for each study, often the sample size of each group or study and the numerical point and interval estimates. Reproduced with permission from ref. [32]

plot showing an assessment of publication bias (Fig. 3). Other figures such as a meta-regression plot (Fig. 4) and a network meta-analysis plot (Fig. 5) are more complex and not commonly used. A forest plot contains the individual study point estimates and their associated 95 % confidence intervals. Confidence limits may also include differences too small to be clinically important [67] and should be deemed as neither evidence of an "important effect" nor evidence of "no difference" in effect. The forest plot also allows one to appreciate the heterogeneity of results, allowing for a visual comparison of the point estimates and 95 % confidence intervals for the effect of each study, and the overall pooled result. A funnel plot is a simple scatter plot of each study's precision (inversion of

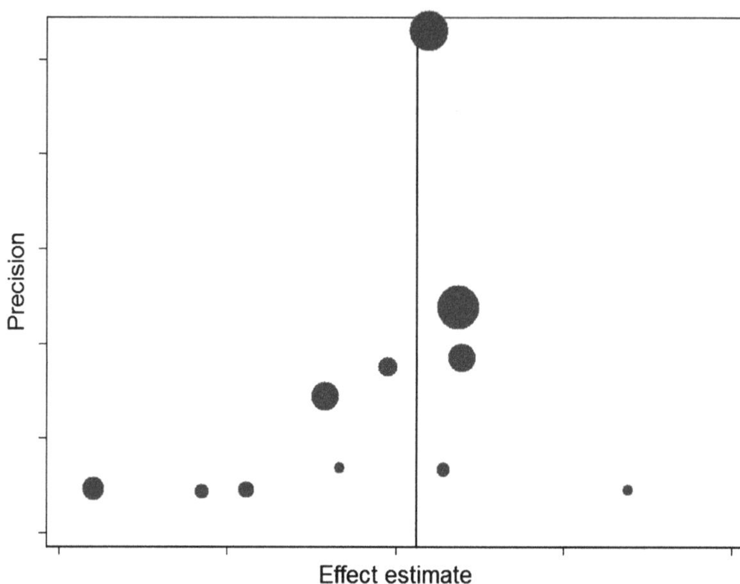

Fig. 3 Example of a funnel plot. Each study's precision (the inverse of the standard error of each study's effect estimate) is plotted against each study's effect estimate. These markers are sized according to the study's sample size; larger studies are marked with *larger circles*. A *vertical line* is drawn through our overall pooled estimate of effect to aid the eye in detecting symmetry (an inverted funnel) or asymmetry. This funnel plot appears mildly asymmetric. The emptier right side of the inverted funnel may indicate small missing studies. Reproduced with permission from ref. [32]

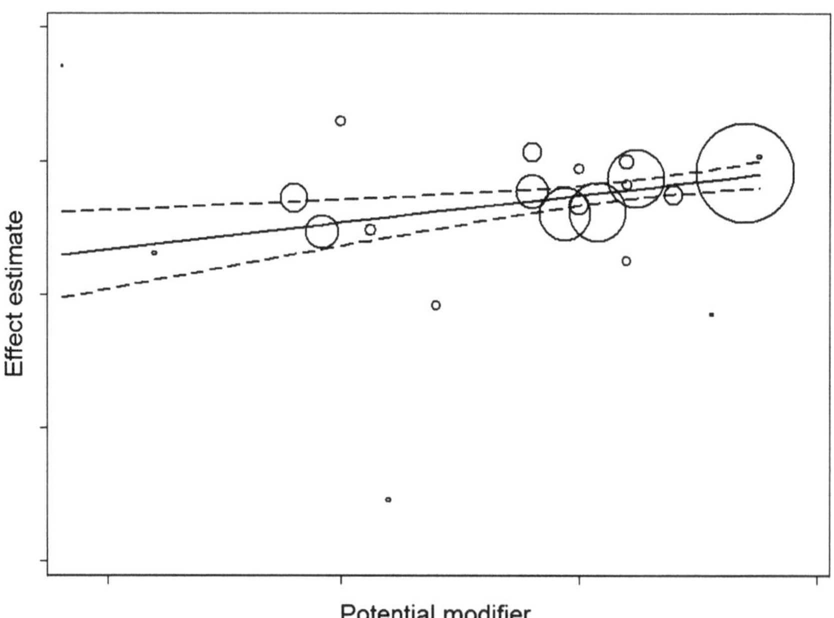

Fig. 4 Example of a meta-regression plot. Each primary study's estimate of effect is plotted against a variable that may potentially modify the relationship between outcome and intervention (or exposure). The markers (*circles*) are sized according to precision—the inverse of the standard error of each study's effect estimate. The three lines are the fitted (*solid*) and the upper and lower bounds (*dashed*) of the 95 % confidence intervals. Reproduced with permission from ref. [32]

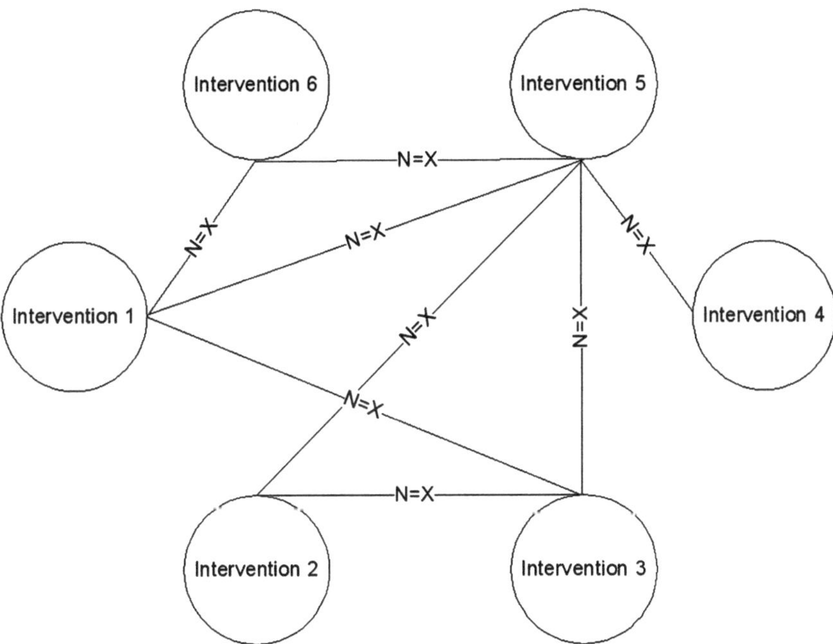

Fig. 5 Example of a network meta-analysis figure. Reproduced with permission from ref. [32]

standard error) on the *y*-axis against each study's effect on the *x*-axis. Because small studies have less precision and large studies have more, scatter should form an inverted funnel when there are no systematic missing studies. A line is often drawn through the overall pooled effect to aid the eye in detecting symmetry (an inverted funnel) or asymmetry. Asymmetry suggests missing evidence—often small unpublished studies.

The meta-regression plot is not widely used (Fig. 4). Because the unit of analysis in this form of regression is the study rather than the participant or patient, the analysis is typically underpowered and statistical significance is rare. The meta-regression plot is both a scatter and line plot. Each study's estimate of effect is plotted against the value of the potential modifier and a regression line is drawn through the scatter of observations. A slope indicates the direction and whether there is an association between the potential modifier and the effect estimate. In publications of network meta-analyses, due to multiple intervention groups and the complexity therein, a figure depicting the number of comparisons between each set of interventions is usually provided (Fig. 5). Often a matrix of direct and mixed evidence for each comparison is reported, rather than a forest plot showing the pooled and each individual study's estimate. The matrix, a square table with the intervention labels running along the center diagonal, allows one to appreciate what direct evidence is absent and where the mixed evidence does not agree with the direct evidence (Fig. 6). The row-column cell of

Intervention 6	Y (X,Z)	Y (X,Z)	Y (X,Z)	Y (X,Z)	Y (X,Z)
Y (X,Z)	Intervention 5	Y (X,Z)	Y (X,Z)	Y (X,Z)	Y (X,Z)
-	Y (X,Z)	Intervention 4	Y (X,Z)	Y (X,Z)	Y (X,Z)
-	Y (X,Z)	-	Intervention 3	Y (X,Z)	Y (X,Z)
-	Y (X,Z)	-	Y (X,Z)	Intervention 2	Y (X,Z)
Y (X,Z)	Y (X,Z)	-	Y (X,Z)	-	Intervention 1

Fig. 6 Example of a direct and mixed evidence matrix. The mixed evidence appears in the *shaded upper triangle* and the corresponding direct evidence appears in the *unshaded lower triangle*. A *dash* indicates no available direct evidence (meaning that trials specifically comparing this pair of treatments were not identified in the review). In this example Y is the point estimate of effect for each trial, and X, Z are the 95 % confidence limits. Reproduced with permission from ref. [32]

the available direct evidence corresponds to the column-row cell of the mixed evidence. A good understanding of the common statistical terms used in meta-analyses is also important (Table 3).

However, these measures are not always required in cases where the primary studies are very heterogeneous (differ in the design, populations studied, interventions and comparisons used, or outcomes measured). In those situations, it may be more appropriate to simply report the results descriptively using text and tables. When the primary studies are similar in characteristics, and the studies provide a similar estimate of a true effect, then meta-analysis may have been used to derive a more precise estimate of this effect [68]. In meta-analysis, data from the individual studies are not simply combined as if they were from a single study. Rather greater weights are given to the results from studies that provide more information, because they are likely to better reflect the true effect of interest. Quantitatively, the calculation of a summary effect estimate can be accomplished under the assumption of "fixed" effects or "random" effects model. Although a thorough description of the merits of each approach is described elsewhere [69], it is fair to say that a random effects model is more conservative than the fixed effects approach, and that a finding which is

Table 3
Common statistical terms used in meta-analyses

Measure	Description	For all examples assume that the value of each measure = 2
For pooling …		
Relative risk or Risk ratio (RR)	Risk of the experimental group divided by the risk of the control group. Risk is another term for probability	Participants with the experimental therapy had two times the risk of experiencing the outcome than participants with the control therapy
Odds ratio (OR)	Odds of the experimental group divided by the odds of the control group. The OR will appear to exaggerate the estimate of RR	Participants with the experimental therapy had two times the odds of experiencing the outcome than participants with the control therapy
Risk difference (RD)	Risk of the experimental group minus the risk of the control group	Participants with the experimental therapy had 2 % more risk of experiencing the outcome than participants with the control therapy
Number needed to treat (NNT)	The NNT is not used to pool results from individual studies because its variance is difficult to estimate. It may be calculated from RD, RR, or OR along with an estimate of control risk to clarify the degree of effect	In order to prevent one poor outcome two participants need to be treated with the experimental therapy rather than with the control therapy
Mean difference (MD)	Mean of the experimental group minus the mean of the control group. It is a difference of means rather than a mean of differences	Participants with the experimental therapy had 2 units more, on average, of the outcome than participants with the control therapy
For exploring heterogeneity …		
I^2	The percent of variance due to between study variance as opposed to between participant (or within study) variance	2 % of the total variance is due to between study differences. Since this value is much smaller than 25 %, there is very little between-study heterogeneity in this effect estimate
Relative risk ratio (RRR)	The relative risk of studies with the potential modifier divided by the relative risk of the studies without the potential modifier	Studies with the potential modifier had a relative risk of experiencing the outcome two times as large as studies without the potential modifier
Difference of mean difference (MDD)	The mean difference of studies with the potential modifier minus the mean difference of the studies without the potential modifier	Studies with the potential modifier had a mean difference that was 2 units greater than studies without the potential modifier

Reproduced with permission from ref. [32]

statistically significant with the latter but not the former should be viewed with skepticism. Whenever individual studies were pooled in meta-analysis, it is important for the reader to determine whether it was reasonable to do so. One way of determining whether the results are similar enough to pool across studies is to inspect the graphical display of the results.

Some review teams may also report a statistical test for heterogeneity [70], to help prove that primary study results were no different than what would have been expected through statistical sampling. The most commonly used technique for quantification of heterogeneity is the Q statistic, which is a variant of the chi-square test. Although a nonsignificant result (by convention a $p \geq 0.1$) is often taken to indicate that substantial heterogeneity is not present, this test is statistically underpowered, especially when the number of studies being pooled is small. The magnitude of the heterogeneity can be quantified with a new statistic referred to as the I^2, which describes the percentage of variability beyond that expected by statistical sampling. Values of 0–30 %, 31–50 %, and greater than 50 % represent mild, moderate, and notable heterogeneity respectively [71]. As mentioned above, a careful exploration of the sources of heterogeneity can lead to new insights about mechanism or subgroups for future study.

6   What Are the Strengths of Systematic Reviews and Meta-analyses?

Physicians make better clinical decisions when they understand the circumstances and preferences of their patients, and combine their personal experience with clinical evidence underlying the available options [72]. The public and professional organizations (such as medical licensing boards) also expect that physicians will integrate research findings into their practice in a timely way. Thus, sound clinical or health policy decisions are facilitated by reviewing the available evidence (and its limitations), understanding reasons why some studies differ in their results (a finding sometimes referred to as heterogeneity amongst the primary studies), coming up with an assessment of the expected effect of an intervention or exposure (for questions of therapy or etiology), and then integrating the new information with other relevant treatment, patient and health care system factors. Therefore, reading a properly conducted systematic review is an efficient way of becoming familiar with the best available research evidence for a particular clinical question.

In cases where the review team has obtained unpublished information from the primary authors, a systematic review can also extend the available literature. The presented summary allows the reader to take account a whole range of relevant findings from research on a particular topic. The process can also establish whether the scientific findings are consistent and generalizable across populations, settings, and treatment variations, and whether findings vary significantly by particular subgroups. Again, the real strength of a systematic review lies in the transparency of each phase of the synthesis process, allowing the reader to focus on the merits of each decision made in compiling the information, rather than a simple contrast of one study with another as in other types of reviews.

A well-conducted systematic review attempts to reduce the possibility of bias in the method of identifying and selecting studies for review, by using a comprehensive search strategy, and specifying inclusion criteria which ideally have not been influenced by knowledge of the primary studies. If this is not done, bias can result. For example, studies demonstrating a significant effect of treatment are more likely to be published than studies with negative findings, are more likely to be published in English, and are more likely to be cited by others [42, 73–76]. Therefore, systematic reviews with cursory search strategies (or those restricted to the English language) may be more likely to report large effect sizes associated with treatment.

Mathematically combining data from a series of well-conducted primary studies may provide a more precise estimate of the underlying "true effect" than any individual study [51]. In other words, by combining the samples of the individual studies, the overall sample size is increased, enhancing the statistical power of the analysis and reducing the size of the confidence interval for the point estimate of the effect. Sometimes, if the treatment effect in small trials shows a nonsignificant trend towards efficacy, pooling the results may establish the benefits of therapy. For example, ten trials examined whether angiotensin converting enzyme (ACE) inhibitors were more effective than other antihypertensive agents for the prevention of nondiabetic kidney failure [77]. Although some of the individual trials had nonsignificant results, the overall pooled estimate was more precise, and established that ACE inhibitors are beneficial for preventing progression of kidney disease in the target population. For this reason, a meta-analysis of well-conducted randomized controlled trials is often considered the strongest level of evidence [78]. Alternatively, when the existing studies have important scientific and methodological limitations including smaller sized samples, the systematic review may identify where gaps exist in the available literature. In this case an exploratory meta-analysis can provide a plausible estimate of effect that can be tested in subsequent studies [79, 80]. Ultimately, the effect estimates obtained from systematic reviews are more likely to prove robust in larger multicenter randomized controlled trials than other forms of medical literature, including animal experiments, observational studies, and single randomized trials [81, 82].

7 What Are the Limitations of Systematic Reviews and Meta-analyses?

Although well-done systematic reviews and meta-analyses have important strengths, they also have potential limitations. First, the summary provided in a systematic review and meta-analysis of the literature is only as reliable as the methods used to estimate the effect in each of the primary studies. In other words, conducting a meta-analysis does not overcome problems inherent in the design and execution of the primary studies. Meta-analysis also does not correct biases due to selective publication, where studies reporting dramatic effects are more likely to be identified, summarized, and subsequently pooled in meta-analysis than studies reporting smaller effect sizes. Since more than three quarters of meta-analyses did not report any empirical assessment of publication bias, the true frequency of this form of bias is unknown [83].

Controversies also arise about the interpretation of summarized results, particularly when the results of discordant studies are pooled in meta-analysis [84]. The review process inevitably identifies studies that are diverse in their design, methodological quality, specific interventions used, and types of patients studied. There is often some subjectivity when deciding how similar studies must be before pooling is appropriate. Combining studies of poor quality with those which were more rigorously conducted, may not be useful, and can lead to worse estimates of the underlying truth, or a false sense of precision around the truth [84]. A false sense of precision may also arise when various subgroups of patients defined by characteristics such as their age or sex differ in their observed response. In such cases reporting an aggregate pooled effect might be misleading, if there are important reasons to explain this heterogeneity [84–87].

Finally, simply describing a manuscript as a "systematic review" or "meta-analysis" does not guarantee that the review was conducted or reported with due rigor [32, 35]. Important methodological flaws of systematic reviews published in peer reviewed journals have been well described. The most common flaws are failure to assess the methodological risk of bias of included primary studies, and failure to avoid bias in study inclusion. In some cases, industry supported reviews of drugs have expressed fewer reservations about methodological limitations of the included trials than rigorously conducted Cochrane reviews on the same topic. However, the hypothesis that less rigorous reviews more often report positive conclusions than good quality reviews of the same topic has not been borne out in empirical assessment. Nonetheless, like all good consumers, users of systematic reviews should carefully consider the quality of the product, and adhere to the dictum "caveat emptor": let the buyer beware. These limitations may explain differences in the results of meta-analyses as compared to subsequent large randomized controlled trials, which have occurred in about a third of cases [82].

8   Summary

Like all research, systematic reviews and meta-analyses have both strengths and weaknesses. When performed with methodological rigor, they enhance our understanding of the information available from all relevant studies on a given topic. Many of the perceived limitations of meta-analysis are not inherent to the methodology, but represent deficits in the conduct or reporting of individual primary studies. With the massive proliferation of clinical studies and limited time available for users to fathom the literature, systematic reviews will help to guide clinical decision-making and policy. To maximize their potential advantages, it is essential that future reviews be conducted and reported properly, and be interpreted judiciously by the discriminating reader.

References

1. Anonymous (2014) https://www.nlm.nih.gov/pubs/factsheets/nlm.html. Accessed 20 April 2014

2. Umscheid CA (2013) A primer on performing systematic reviews and meta-analyses. Clin Infect Dis 57(5):725–734

3. Ioannidis JP (2005) Contradicted and initially stronger effects in highly cited clinical research. JAMA 294(2):218–228

4. Garg AX, Iansavichus AV, Kastner M, Walters LA, Wilczynski N, McKibbon KA, Yang RC, Rehman F, Haynes RB (2006) Lost in publication: half of all renal practice evidence is published in non-renal journals. Kidney Int 70(11):1995–2005

5. Barrett BJ, Parfrey PS (2006) Clinical practice. Preventing nephropathy induced by contrast medium. N Engl J Med 354(4):379–386

6. Halloran PF (2004) Immunosuppressive drugs for kidney transplantation. N Engl J Med 351(26):2715–2729

7. Schrier RW, Wang W (2004) Acute renal failure and sepsis. N Engl J Med 351(2):159–169

8. Tonelli M, Lloyd A, Clement F, Conly J, Husereau D, Hemmelgarn B, Klarenbach S, McAlister FA, Wiebe N, Manns B (2011) Efficacy of statins for primary prevention in people at low cardiovascular risk: a meta-analysis. CMAJ 183(16):E1189–E1202

9. Pannu N, Klarenbach S, Wiebe N, Manns B, Tonelli M (2008) Renal replacement therapy in patients with acute renal failure: a systematic review. JAMA 299(7):793–805

10. Oxman AD, Cook DJ, Guyatt GH (1994) Users' guides to the medical literature. VI. How to use an overview. Evidence-based medicine working group. JAMA 272(17):1367–1371

11. Cook DJ, Greengold NL, Ellrodt AG, Weingarten SR (1997) The relation between systematic reviews and practice guidelines. Ann Intern Med 127(3):210–216

12. Bafeta A, Trinquart L, Seror R, Ravaud P (2014) Reporting of results from network meta-analyses: methodological systematic review. BMJ 348:g1741

13. Fowkes FG, Rudan D, Rudan I, Aboyans V, Denenberg JO, McDermott MM, Norman PE, Sampson UK, Williams LJ, Mensah GA, Criqui MH (2013) Comparison of global estimates of prevalence and risk factors for peripheral artery disease in 2000 and 2010: a systematic review and analysis. Lancet 382(9901):1329–1340

14. Tusting LS, Willey B, Lucas H, Thompson J, Kafy HT, Smith R, Lindsay SW (2013) Socioeconomic development as an intervention against malaria: a systematic review and meta-analysis. Lancet 382(9896):963–972

15. Lyman GH, Kuderer NM (2005) The strengths and limitations of meta-analyses based on aggregate data. BMC Med Res Methodol 5:14

16. Simmonds MC, Higgins JP, Stewart LA, Tierney JF, Clarke MJ, Thompson SG (2005) Meta-analysis of individual patient data from randomized trials: a review of methods used in practice. Clin Trials 2(3):209–217

17. Schwingshackl L, Hoffmann G (2014) Dietary fatty acids in the secondary prevention of coronary heart disease: a systematic review, meta-analysis and meta-regression. BMJ Open 4(4):e004487

18. Sorita A, Ahmed A, Starr SR, Thompson KM, Reed DA, Prokop L, Shah ND, Murad MH, Ting HH (2014) Off-hour presentation and outcomes in patients with acute myocardial infarction: systematic review and meta-analysis. BMJ 348:f7393

19. Threapleton DE, Greenwood DC, Evans CE, Cleghorn CL, Nykjaer C, Woodhead C, Cade JE, Gale CP, Burley VJ (2013) Dietary fibre intake and risk of cardiovascular disease: systematic review and meta-analysis. BMJ 347:f6879

20. Kalil AC, Klompas M, Haynatzki G, Rupp ME (2013) Treatment of hospital-acquired pneumonia with linezolid or vancomycin: a systematic review and meta-analysis. BMJ Open 3(10):e003912

21. Gagliardino JJ, Arrechea V, Assad D, Gagliardino GG, Gonzalez L, Lucero S, Rizzuti L, Zufriategui Z, Clark C Jr (2013) Type 2 diabetes patients educated by other patients perform at least as well as patients trained by professionals. Diabetes Metab Res Rev 29(2):152–160

22. Murthy L, Shepperd S, Clarke MJ, Garner SE, Lavis JN, Perrier L, Roberts NW, Straus SE (2012) Interventions to improve the use of systematic reviews in decision-making by health system managers, policy makers and clinicians. Cochrane Database Syst Rev 9:CD009401

23. Durand MA, Carpenter L, Dolan H, Bravo P, Mann M, Bunn F, Elwyn G (2014) Do interventions designed to support shared decision-making reduce health inequalities? A systematic review and meta-analysis. PLoS One 9(4):e94670

24. Moher D, Schulz KF, Altman DG (2001) The CONSORT statement: revised recommendations for improving the quality of reports of parallel group randomized trials. BMC Med Res Methodol 1:2

25. Bossuyt PM, Reitsma JB, Bruns DE, Gatsonis CA, Glasziou PP, Irwig LM, Moher D, Rennie D, de Vet HC, Lijmer JG (2003) The STARD statement for reporting studies of diagnostic accuracy: explanation and elaboration. Ann Intern Med 138(1):W1–W12

26. Drummond MF, Jefferson TO (1996) Guidelines for authors and peer reviewers of economic submissions to the BMJ. The BMJ economic evaluation working party. BMJ 313(7052):275–283

27. von Elm E, Altman DG, Egger M, Pocock SJ, Gotzsche PC, Vandenbroucke JP (2007) The strengthening the reporting of observational studies in epidemiology (STROBE) statement: guidelines for reporting observational studies. Lancet 370(9596):1453–1457

28. Moher D, Cook DJ, Eastwood S, Olkin I, Rennie D, Stroup DF (1999) Improving the quality of reports of meta-analyses of randomised controlled trials: the QUOROM statement. Quality of reporting of meta-analyses. Lancet 354(9193):1896–1900

29. Stroup DF, Berlin JA, Morton SC, Olkin I, Williamson GD, Rennie D, Moher D, Becker BJ, Sipe TA, Thacker SB (2000) Meta-analysis of observational studies in epidemiology: a proposal for reporting meta-analysis. Of observational studies in epidemiology (MOOSE) group. JAMA 283(15):2008–2012

30. Moher D, Liberati A, Tetzlaff J, Altman DG (2009) Preferred reporting items for systematic reviews and meta-analyses: the PRISMA statement. Ann Intern Med 151(4):264–269, W64

31. Sambunjak D, Franic M (2012) Steps in the undertaking of a systematic review in orthopaedic surgery. Int Orthop 36(3):477–484

32. Bello AK, Wiebe N, Garg AX, Tonelli M (2011) Basics of systematic reviews and meta-analyses for the nephrologist. Nephron Clin Pract 119(1):c50–c60, discussion c1

33. Riley RD, Lambert PC, Abo-Zaid G (2010) Meta-analysis of individual participant data: rationale, conduct, and reporting. BMJ 340:c221

34. Wardlaw JM, Warlow CP, Counsell C (1997) Systematic review of evidence on thrombolytic therapy for acute ischaemic stroke. Lancet 350(9078):607–614

35. Yusuf S (1997) Meta-analysis of randomized trials: looking back and looking ahead. Control Clin Trials 18(6):594–601, discussion 61-6

36. Counsell C (1997) Formulating questions and locating primary studies for inclusion in systematic reviews. Ann Intern Med 127(5):380–387

37. Vickers A, Goyal N, Harland R, Rees R (1998) Do certain countries produce only positive results? A systematic review of controlled trials. Control Clin Trials 19(2):159–166

38. Moher D, Pham B, Klassen TP, Schulz KF, Berlin JA, Jadad AR, Liberati A (2000) What contributions do languages other than English make on the results of meta-analyses? J Clin Epidemiol 53(9):964–972

39. Egger M, Davey Smith G, Schneider M, Minder C (1997) Bias in meta-analysis detected by a simple, graphical test. BMJ 315(7109):629–634

40. Gregoire G, Derderian F, Le Lorier J (1995) Selecting the language of the publications included in a meta-analysis: is there a Tower of Babel bias? J Clin Epidemiol 48(1):159–163

41. Strippoli GF, Craig MC, Schena FP, Craig JC (2006) Role of blood pressure targets and specific antihypertensive agents used to prevent diabetic nephropathy and delay its progression. J Am Soc Nephrol 17(4 Suppl 2): S153–S155

42. Egger M, Smith GD (1998) Bias in location and selection of studies. BMJ 316(7124): 61–66

43. Subramanian S, Venkataraman R, Kellum JA (2002) Influence of dialysis membranes on outcomes in acute renal failure: a meta-analysis. Kidney Int 62(5):1819–1823

44. Jaber BL, Lau J, Schmid CH, Karsou SA, Levey AS, Pereira BJ (2002) Effect of biocompatibility of hemodialysis membranes on mortality in acute renal failure: a meta-analysis. Clin Nephrol 57(4):274–282

45. Teehan GS, Liangos O, Lau J, Levey AS, Pereira BJ, Jaber BL (2003) Dialysis membrane and modality in acute renal failure: understanding discordant meta-analyses. Semin Dial 16(5):356–360

46. Dickersin K, Scherer R, Lefebvre C (1994) Identifying relevant studies for systematic reviews. BMJ 309(6964):1286–1291

47. Steinbrook R (2006) Searching for the right search–reaching the medical literature. N Engl J Med 354(1):4–7

48. Wilczynski NL, Haynes RB (2002) Robustness of empirical search strategies for clinical content in MEDLINE. Proc AMIA Symp 904–908

49. Wilczynski NL, Walker CJ, McKibbon KA, Haynes RB (1995) Reasons for the loss of sensitivity and specificity of methodologic MeSH terms and textwords in MEDLINE. Proc Annu Symp Comput Appl Med Care 436–440.

50. Edwards P, Clarke M, DiGuiseppi C, Pratap S, Roberts I, Wentz R (2002) Identification of randomized controlled trials in systematic reviews: accuracy and reliability of screening records. Stat Med 21(11):1635–1640

51. Pogue J, Yusuf S (1998) Overcoming the limitations of current meta-analysis of randomised controlled trials. Lancet 351(9095):47–52

52. Davidson RA (1986) Source of funding and outcome of clinical trials. J Gen Intern Med 1(3):155–158

53. Rochon PA, Gurwitz JH, Simms RW, Fortin PR, Felson DT, Minaker KL, Chalmers TC (1994) A study of manufacturer-supported trials of nonsteroidal anti-inflammatory drugs in the treatment of arthritis. Arch Intern Med 154(2):157–163

54. Biondi-Zoccai GG, Lotrionte M, Abbate A, Testa L, Remigi E, Burzotta F, Valgimigli M, Romagnoli E, Crea F, Agostoni P (2006) Compliance with QUOROM and quality of reporting of overlapping meta-analyses on the role of acetylcysteine in the prevention of contrast associated nephropathy: case study. BMJ 332(7535):202–209

55. Berlin JA (1997) Does blinding of readers affect the results of meta-analyses? University of Pennsylvania Meta-analysis Blinding Study Group. Lancet 350(9072):185–186

56. Jadad AR, McQuay HJ (1996) Meta-analyses to evaluate analgesic interventions: a systematic qualitative review of their methodology. J Clin Epidemiol 49(2):235–243

57. Balk EM, Bonis PA, Moskowitz H, Schmid CH, Ioannidis JP, Wang C, Lau J (2002) Correlation of quality measures with estimates of treatment effect in meta-analyses of randomized controlled trials. JAMA 287(22):2973–2982

58. Balk EM, Lau J, Bonis PA (2005) Reading and critically appraising systematic reviews and meta-analyses: a short primer with a focus on hepatology. J Hepatol 43(4):729–736

59. Moher D, Cook DJ, Jadad AR, Tugwell P, Moher M, Jones A, Pham B, Klassen TP (1999) Assessing the quality of reports of randomised trials: implications for the conduct of meta-analyses. Health Technol Assess 3(12): i–iv, 1–98

60. Verhagen AP, de Vet HC, de Bie RA, Boers M, van den Brandt PA (2001) The art of quality assessment of RCTs included in systematic reviews. J Clin Epidemiol 54(7):651–654

61. Juni P, Altman DG, Egger M (2001) Systematic reviews in health care: assessing the quality of controlled clinical trials. BMJ 323(7303):42–46

62. Devereaux PJ, Choi PT, El-Dika S, Bhandari M, Montori VM, Schunemann HJ, Garg AX, Busse JW, Heels-Ansdell D, Ghali WA, Manns BJ, Guyatt GH (2004) An observational study found that authors of randomized controlled trials frequently use concealment of random-

ization and blinding, despite the failure to report these methods. J Clin Epidemiol 57(12):1232–1236

63. Schulz KF, Chalmers I, Hayes RJ, Altman DG (1995) Empirical evidence of bias dimensions of methodological quality associated with estimates of treatment effects in controlled trials. JAMA 273(5):408–412

64. Laupacis A, Wells G, Richardson WS, Tugwell P (1994) Users' guides to the medical literature. V. How to use an article about prognosis. Evidence-based medicine working group. JAMA 272(3):234–237

65. Jadad AR, Cook DJ, Jones A, Klassen TP, Tugwell P, Moher M, Moher D (1998) Methodology and reports of systematic reviews and meta-analyses: a comparison of Cochrane reviews with articles published in paper-based journals. JAMA 280(3):278–280

66. Buscemi N, Hartling L, Vandermeer B, Tjosvold L, Klassen TP (2006) Single data extraction generated more errors than double data extraction in systematic reviews. J Clin Epidemiol 59(7):697–703

67. Horton J, Vandermeer B, Hartling L, Tjosvold L, Klassen TP, Buscemi N (2010) Systematic review data extraction: cross-sectional study showed that experience did not increase accuracy. J Clin Epidemiol 63(3):289–298

68. Deeks JJ (2002) Issues in the selection of a summary statistic for meta-analysis of clinical trials with binary outcomes. Stat Med 21(11): 1575–1600

69. DerSimonian R, Laird N (1986) Meta-analysis in clinical trials. Control Clin Trials 7(3): 177–188

70. Hardy RJ, Thompson SG (1998) Detecting and describing heterogeneity in meta-analysis. Stat Med 17(8):841–856

71. Higgins JP, Thompson SG (2002) Quantifying heterogeneity in a meta-analysis. Stat Med 21(11):1539–1558

72. Haynes RB, Devereaux PJ, Guyatt GH (2002) Physicians' and patients' choices in evidence based practice. BMJ 324(7350):1350

73. Sterne JA, Egger M, Smith GD (2001) Systematic reviews in health care: investigating and dealing with publication and other biases in meta-analysis. BMJ 323(7304):101–105

74. Simes RJ (1987) Confronting publication bias: a cohort design for meta-analysis. Stat Med 6(1):11–29

75. Easterbrook PJ, Berlin JA, Gopalan R, Matthews DR (1991) Publication bias in clinical research. Lancet 337(8746):867–872

76. Dickersin K, Min YI, Meinert CL (1992) Factors influencing publication of research results. Follow-up of applications submitted to two institutional review boards. JAMA 267(3):374–378

77. Giatras I, Lau J, Levey AS (1997) Effect of angiotensin-converting enzyme inhibitors on the progression of nondiabetic renal disease: a meta-analysis of randomized trials. Angiotensin-converting-enzyme inhibition and progressive renal disease study group. Ann Intern Med 127(5):337–345

78. Guyatt G, Gutterman D, Baumann MH, Addrizzo-Harris D, Hylek EM, Phillips B, Raskob G, Lewis SZ, Schunemann H (2006) Grading strength of recommendations and quality of evidence in clinical guidelines: report from an american college of chest physicians task force. Chest 129(1): 174–181

79. Anello C, Fleiss JL (1995) Exploratory or analytic meta-analysis: should we distinguish between them? J Clin Epidemiol 48(1):109–116, discussion 17-8

80. Boudville N, Prasad GV, Knoll G, Muirhead N, Thiessen-Philbrook H, Yang RC, Rosas-Arellano MP, Housawi A, Garg AX (2006) Meta-analysis: risk for hypertension in living kidney donors. Ann Intern Med 145(3):185–196

81. Hackam DG, Redelmeier DA (2006) Translation of research evidence from animals to humans. JAMA 296(14):1731–1732

82. LeLorier J, Gregoire G, Benhaddad A, Lapierre J, Derderian F (1997) Discrepancies between meta-analyses and subsequent large randomized, controlled trials. N Engl J Med 337(8):536–542

83. Palma S, Delgado-Rodriguez M (2005) Assessment of publication bias in meta-analyses of cardiovascular diseases. J Epidemiol Community Health 59(10):864–869

84. Lau J, Ioannidis JP, Schmid CH (1998) Summing up evidence: one answer is not always enough. Lancet 351(9096):123–127

85. Thompson SG (1994) Why sources of heterogeneity in meta-analysis should be investigated. BMJ 309(6965):1351–1355

86. Berlin JA (1995) Invited commentary: benefits of heterogeneity in meta-analysis of data from epidemiologic studies. Am J Epidemiol 142(4):383–387

87. Davey Smith G, Egger M, Phillips AN (1997) Meta-analysis. Beyond the grand mean? BMJ 315(7122):1610–1614

Chapter 25

Evidence-Based Decision-Making 3: Health Technology Assessment

Daria O'Reilly, Kaitryn Campbell, Meredith Vanstone, James M. Bowen, Lisa Schwartz, Nazila Assasi, and Ron Goeree

Abstract

This chapter begins with a brief introduction to health technology assessment (HTA). HTA is concerned with the systematic evaluation of the consequences of the adoption and use of new health technologies and improving the evidence on existing technologies. The objective of mainstream HTA is to support evidence-based decision- and policy-making that encourage the uptake of efficient and effective health care technologies. This chapter provides a basic framework for conducting an HTA as well as some fundamental concepts and challenges in assessing health technologies. A case study of the assessment of drug eluting stents in Ontario is presented to illustrate the HTA process. Whether HTA is beneficial—supporting timely access to needed technologies—or detrimental depends on three critical issues: when the assessment is performed; how it is performed; and how the findings are used.

Key words Health technology assessment, Health care technology, Economic evaluation, Evidence-based decision-making, Health policy

1 Introduction

Health care technologies can be described as interventions or methods that are used to promote health; prevent, diagnose, or treat disease; or improve rehabilitation [1]. Health care technologies include drugs, biologics, medical devices (e.g., pacemakers), medical and surgical procedures, organizational and managerial systems (e.g., alternative health care delivery methods), and public health programs [1, 2]. Considerable growth in new, innovative health care technologies over the last number of years has brought remarkable improvements in health gains, quality of life, and the organization and delivery of health care. Some health care technologies have the potential to transform health care and alter established ways of delivering health care while improving health outcomes in an efficient and cost-effective manner. For example, the introduction of angioplasty has resulted in improvements in heart

Patrick S. Parfrey and Brendan J. Barrett (eds.), *Clinical Epidemiology: Practice and Methods*, Methods in Molecular Biology, vol. 1281, DOI 10.1007/978-1-4939-2428-8_25, © Springer Science+Business Media New York 2015

attack survival over open-heart surgery. These new health care technologies often come with a high price tag. As a result, there is a challenge of investing in those services that offer the best value for money. Decision-makers must find a balance between providing access to high-quality care and improving health outcomes on the one hand and managing health care budgets on the other.

The difficult decisions surrounding adoption, reimbursement, and means of diffusion have resulted in the increased demand for information to help make more evidence-based decisions [2]. The development and proliferation of many health technology assessment (HTA) producers around the world reflects this demand.

1.1 What Is "Health Technology Assessment"?

HTA means different things to different people in different parts of the world and has been defined and conducted in a variety of ways and thus, it is not possible to provide one clear and comprehensive definition [3]. However, the International HTA Glossary defines HTA as the "The systematic evaluation of the properties and effects of a health technology, addressing the direct and intended effects of this technology, as well as its indirect and unintended consequences, and aimed mainly at informing decision making regarding health technologies" [1]. HTA is conducted by interdisciplinary groups using explicit analytical frameworks and may involve the investigation of one or more of the following attributes of technologies: performance characteristics, safety, clinical efficacy, effectiveness, cost-effectiveness, social, legal, ethical, and economic impacts [2, 4]. The main purpose of HTA is to act as "a bridge" between evidence and policy-making. It seeks to provide health policy-makers with accessible, useable, and evidence-based information to guide their decisions about the appropriate use of new and existing technologies and the efficient allocation of resources [5, 6]. During an assessment, data from research studies and other scientific sources are systematically gathered, analyzed, and interpreted. The findings from this process are then summarized in reports that translate scientific data into information that is relevant to decision-making. HTA has increasingly emerged as a tool for informing more effective regulation of the utilization and diffusion of health technologies at various levels (e.g., patient, health care provider or institution, regional, national, and international level) [2].

HTA information may be particularly useful in supporting decisions when:

- A technology has high unit or aggregate costs.
- Explicit trade-off decisions must be made in allocating resources among technologies.
- A technology is highly complex, precedent-setting, or involves significant uncertainty.

- A proposed provision of a treatment, diagnostic test, or piece of medical equipment is innovative or controversial.
- An established technology is associated with significant variations in utilization and outcomes [4].

HTA is an important analytical tool that is used in an assortment of settings by people with diverse backgrounds, perspectives, and goals. Assessments could be conducted in order to differentiate technology value (e.g., a new drug seeking reimbursement on a formulary) or an academic study of the health consequences of a particular health care practice, such as a randomized trial or a systematic review of any or all aspects of a particular health care practice carried out by an HTA agency. However, there is little uniformity across Canada and elsewhere concerning HTA methodology and application. No doubt this diversity strengthens the results, but it also makes generalization difficult [3].

Technology evaluation is not a single process but varies, depending on what is being evaluated, by whom, and for what purpose. Generally, the evaluation of a new drug proceeds along different lines than that of a medical device or diagnostic test. Furthermore, questions involving technology assessment can be local (e.g., a hospital evaluating the need for a new PET scanner), national (e.g., evaluation of a new drug), or a combination of both. Although there is obviously some variation in how technology assessment is performed, some factors are common to the process [7].

To be effective, HTA should serve as a bridge between scientific evidence, the judgment of health professionals, the views of patients, and the needs of policy-makers. Much is at stake regarding how the results of HTA are interpreted and applied.

In the following section, we provide a basic framework for conducting an HTA. Note that the assessment of health technologies is an iterative process and some of the steps may not occur linearly and some may even overlap.

2 Basic Framework for Conducting an HTA

2.1 Identifying the Topic for Assessment and Setting Priorities

Determining what technologies to assess and setting priorities among them can be difficult given that there are more health technologies in need of evaluation than there are resources required for assessing them. In some instances, the assessment topics may already be determined. For example, the Common Drug Review at the Canadian Agency for Drugs and Technologies in Health (CADTH) conducts objective, rigorous reviews of the clinical, cost-effectiveness, and patient evidence for all new drugs. On the other hand, many new and existing medical devices and surgical procedures have never been assessed and remain unproven. Potential technology assessment topics can be identified through several sources, including informal surveys of advisory committees, health care stakeholders, horizon scanning, or requests from interested parties [8]. Procedures for setting priorities among these candidate technologies are variable. Some HTA agencies have devised processes that use explicit highly systematic and quantitative approaches that incorporate some form of priority-setting criteria (e.g., multicriteria decision analysis (MCDA)) often accompanied by a deliberative process for identifying priorities [2, 8, 9]. Other agencies use ad hoc processes. In many instances, the technologies that get assessed are those with high costs; that have a high potential to improve health outcomes or reduce health risks; that affect a large population base; that may be disruptive to the health care system; and when there is an imminent need to make reimbursement decisions. Having a practical and transparent approach to selecting and prioritizing the most important and policy-relevant topics will help to efficiently allocate resources available for HTA research [8].

2.2 Clear Specification of the Assessment Problem

Once the topic for assessment has been decided, it is imperative to clearly specify the problem(s) or question(s) to be addressed and the target audience for the assessment as these will affect every aspect of the HTA and the usefulness of the results [2]. Assessment problem statements need to consider the patient or population affected; the potential social and ethical issues relevant to the population, context, or society in general; the intervention being considered; what the intervention is being compared to; the relation of the new technology to existing technologies; what the outcome(s) or interest is/are; and the setting [10]. Additionally, those conducting the assessment should have an explicit understanding of the purpose of the assessment and the intended users of the assessment [2].

The intended users or target audiences of the assessment report will influence its content, presentation, and dissemination strategy. Health care professionals, researchers, government policy-makers, and others have different interests and levels of expertise [2]. The scientific or technical level of reports, the presentation of evidence and findings, and the format of reports vary by target audience.

2.3 Evaluation of Social and Ethical Issues

There are different ways of thinking about what a health technology does and what implications it has. In most instances, HTA focuses on whether the technology works for its intended purpose and whether it works better than other technologies. This focus on appropriateness does not usually consider the "side effects" of a technology, or what types of impacts it may have outside of its intended use. Each HTA must consider the social implications of the technology for stakeholder groups such as patients that use the technology, other patients in the system, health care providers, family members, payers, producers/industry, or society [11]. At the same time, a health technology may have some serious ethical issues associated with its use and dissemination which must be identified and evaluated. There have been a number of approaches proposed to assess both the social and ethical dilemmas within an HTA.

A social approach to HTA is concerned with understanding the impacts that a technology has beyond what it is intended to do. Some technologies might have more serious social impacts than others. A social approach to HTA is interested in examining everything a technology might do or affect and integrating those issues into the assessment of the technology's value. This type of approach considers the (positive, negative, unexpected) impacts a technology may have in all spheres of social life, at both the micro and macro level. For instance, the impacts on a person's individual role in their family, community, or job should be considered as well as the impacts to broader groups of society (e.g., particular social groups or society in general) in terms of culture, norms, and values [11]. Technologies with many far-reaching impacts have been called "morally challenging" [12] because they pose moral issues which are broader than the specific technology and people who come into direct contact with that technology (e.g., in vitro fertilization). Other technologies will have fewer ethical or social implications or they may impact smaller groups of people.

2.3.1 Approaches to Identifying Social Impacts

Unlike clinical and economic assessments, which use empirical evidence to correctly explain and predict outcomes of a technology, the first step in assessing social issues is to identify what issues should be considered. There are several ways to approach the identification of issues, including engagement with citizen and patient organizations, primary research, virtual forums, expert consultation, and the synthesis of published qualitative literature [11].

Qualitative research uses interviews, focus groups, observation, and many other approaches to examine the opinions, beliefs, and experiences of different groups of people. Examining published qualitative research about the technology or class of technologies in an HTA can be very helpful in identifying potential issues that should be considered in any recommendations. Looking to see what users, providers, or the public have said about that technology (or class of technologies) can corroborate concerns that the analysts have already identified as well as reveal unexpected issues. It can help to identify and characterize potential problems related to that technology. Qualitative research can also suggest values, goals, and outcomes that matter to patients and could be incorporated into other aspects of the HTA, for instance, with regard to the outcome measures chosen for comparison. Examining existing literature on the technology could be considered due diligence in order to understand the concerns and perspectives of patients, providers, and the public. It can give access to perspectives that may not be easily available to HTA decision-makers, such as the perspectives of marginalized or vulnerable patients who may not be able to easily participate in public engagement exercises.

After identifying potential social impacts of a technology, the next step is to examine who will be affected by those impacts and how they will be affected. This assessment requires an understanding of the values, stakeholders, and domains that may be affected. Values are ideas about what "ought to be" instead of statements about what "is." They may include formal ethical values but may also include broader ideas of what an organization or society thinks is good, what ideals they are committed to upholding, etc. Some agencies have produced lists of core values that they use to guide their consideration of social and ethical issues [13–15]. Values may also be identified from the literature, stakeholders, or experts. These may include explicit values such as autonomy, dignity, equity, patient-centered care, or resource stewardship. HTA is also informed by implicit values such as effectiveness, efficacy, scientific evidence, etc.

2.3.2 Ethical Analysis in HTA

Traditionally ethical analysis is performed through normative reflection on ethical questions around the technology of interest, based on ethical principles and theories. In this approach, the reflection can take place along different philosophical perspectives. For example, utilitarianism promotes maximization of benefits for the greatest number of people; deontological ethics focuses on duties, rules, and obligations; while virtue ethics emphasizes moral character and virtues of individuals [16]. When a principle-based method is used, the ethical reflection is generally directed at the question of whether the consequences resulting from implementation of a specific technology can be justified by the four prima facie bioethical principles of respect for autonomy, beneficence, nonmaleficence, and justice proposed by Beauchamp and Childress [17].

More recently proposed methods promote the use of participatory and interactive approaches in addition to ethical reflection. Participatory models involve diverse stakeholders and citizens in the processes of assessment in order to learn about their personal and societal value positions and obtain their concerns about the technology and its alternatives [18].

Prior to the utilization of an ethical assessment method, it is important to consider its potential limitations. For example, normative approaches require an adequate knowledge of ethics and ethical theories, which may not be available within most HTA organizations. In addition, they can be affected by the ethicists' own prereflective values [19]. Participatory methods, on the other hand, are usually costly, time consuming, and complex to perform. Other challenges that HTA developers might face when attempting to address ethical issues of a health care technology include lack of consensus on a practical method of considering ethical issues in HTA [20, 21], complexity of the collection and processing of qualitative data, the institutional barriers related to the attitudes of researchers, and the availability of required resources. The choice of a method for collection and analysis of ethical data should be based on the context in which technology is being assessed, the purpose of analysis, and availability of required resources [18].

After an examination of relevant issues in light of identified social and ethical values, the next steps vary greatly, depending on the purpose of the HTA, the commissioning agency, and the issues identified. For example, the evaluation of both the ethical and social issues may help to inform the protocol for gathering evidence; to inform other types of assessments; they may suggest particular recommendations about funding or implementation of the technology; or they may be used during deliberation about the evidence presented. As a result, it is recommended that an analysis of the social and ethical issues be performed throughout the HTA process [22].

In summary, social and ethical issues are an important aspect of the HTA process; however, methods for assessing ethical and social implications of health care technologies are still being developed and variable, and the means of translating these implications into policy are often unclear [19].

2.4 Sources of Research Evidence for HTA

One of the great challenges in HTA is to assemble all of the evidence relevant to a particular technology before conducting a qualitative or quantitative synthesis. Although some sources are devoted exclusively to health care topics, others cover the sciences more broadly. Multiple sources should be searched to increase the likelihood of retrieving all relevant reports [23].

A comprehensive search of the literature is a key step in any HTA that relies on the retrieval and synthesis of primary literature as the evidence base. Performing a comprehensive search following accepted practices will help to avoid missing relevant studies; avoid other potential biases such as publication, time lag, and language bias [24–26]; and assist the researcher in the provision of detailed search documentation, aiding transparency and increasing confidence in the assessment. As the literature search is the foundation of most HTAs, it is a reasonable supposition that a poor search would lead to a poor assessment. HTA search methods have, for the most part, been developed based on well-documented search methods employed in systematic review, modified in consideration of the general HTA audience and context [27]. Given the complexity of the methodology, nonprofessional searchers involved in conducting an HTA are advised to seek assistance from a librarian who is experienced in performing HTA or systematic review searching [28].

Table 1
Key and additional databases necessary for HTA

Key databases
PubMed [free, available: http://www.ncbi.nlm.nih.gov/entrez]
Medline [$, available from various vendors]
EMBASE [$, available from various vendors]
The Cochrane Library (includes some/all of the following, depending on vendor: Cochrane Database of Systematic Reviews (CDSR); Database of Abstracts of Reviews of Effects (DARE); Cochrane Central Register of Controlled Trials (CENTRAL); Cochrane Database of Methodology Reviews (CDMR); Cochrane Methodology Register (CMR); Health Technology Assessment Database (HTA); NHS Economic Evaluation Database (NHS EED)) [$ for full text in most of Canada, available from various vendors]
Centre for Reviews and Dissemination, University of York (UK) databases (includes: DARE (Database of Abstracts of Reviews of Effects); NHS EED (Economic Evaluation Database); Health Technology Assessment (HTA) Database; Ongoing Reviews Database) [free, available at: http://www.crd.york.ac.uk/CRDWeb/]
Additional databases that should also be considered based on scope, content, and availability
Cumulative Index to Nursing & Allied Health (CINAHL) [$, available from various vendors]
BIOSIS Previews [$, available from various vendors]
EconLit [$, available from various vendors]
Educational Resources Information Center (ERIC) [free, available at: http://www.eric.ed.gov/; $, available from various vendors]
Health and Psychosocial Instruments (HAPI) [$, available from various vendors]
Health Economic Evaluations Database (HEED) [$, available from John Wiley & Sons, Ltd.]
PsycINFO [$, available from various vendors]

2.4.1 Types of Literature

The two main types of literature and information resources relevant to HTA are published and grey (or fugitive) literature. Bibliographic databases, being the primary source of published literature, are described by the U.S. National Library of Medicine (NLM) as "extensive collections, reputedly complete, of references and citations to books, articles, publications, etc., generally on a single subject or specialized subject area" [29]. The number of databases searched depends on the time, funds, and expertise available and is typically topic-dependant [30]. However, relying on one database exclusively is generally not considered adequate [28]. Table 1 provides key and additional databases necessary for any reasonably comprehensive HTA. When considering which databases to search, consideration should also be given to the availability of special database functions, which might be of use (e.g., automatic updates).

Grey literature consists of "reports that are unpublished, have limited distribution, and are not included in bibliographic retrieval systems" [31] and are usually not easily available. Examples of grey literature include, but are not limited to: book chapters; census, economic, and other data sources; conference proceedings and abstracts; government and technical reports; newsletters; personal correspondence; policy documents; and theses and dissertations. Results from grey literature can make a significant contribution to an assessment, and it has been found that "the exclusion of grey literature from meta-analyses can lead to exaggerated estimates of intervention effectiveness" [32].

Sources of grey literature are abundant, and as with published literature, the number of sources searched depends on resources, topic, and a particular project's or researcher's needs [30]. Certain sources and tools may, however, be considered "core" for any HTA; these include library catalogues; search engines; and websites of HTA organizations, clinical trial registers, professional organizations, and regulatory agencies. A collaboratively produced collection of freely available and up-to-date resources available on the Internet includes many of these core sources and should not be missed [33]. An additional practical grey literature searching resource is produced and regularly updated by the Canadian Agency of Drugs and Technologies in Health (CADTH) [34].

Naturally, there is some crossover between published and grey literature. For example, theses and dissertations are sometimes considered grey literature, as one of their primary routes of access is through library catalogues. However, theses and dissertations from some institutions and countries are also available via bibliographic databases such as Proquest Dissertations and Theses or the Theses Canada Portal [35].

2.4.2 Designing a Search Strategy

Designing a search strategy for the purposes of HTA is both a science and an art; the goal being to develop a strategy which is an optimal balance of *recall* versus *precision* in order to retrieve as many relevant records as possible, without having to sort through an unmanageable number of those which are irrelevant. *Recall* is the ratio of the number of relevant records retrieved to the total number of relevant records in the database, while *precision* is the ratio of the number of relevant records retrieved to the total number of irrelevant and relevant records retrieved; the two are inversely related (Fig. 1) [36].

As stated in Subheading 2.2, the first step in designing an optimum search strategy is to clearly formulate the research question. Identifying key topics and translating them into a clearly focused question using the PICO(S) model (adapted from PICO [37]) is useful, where PICO(S) stands for:

- Patient or population.
- Intervention.
- Comparator.
- Outcome.
- (S)tudy type.

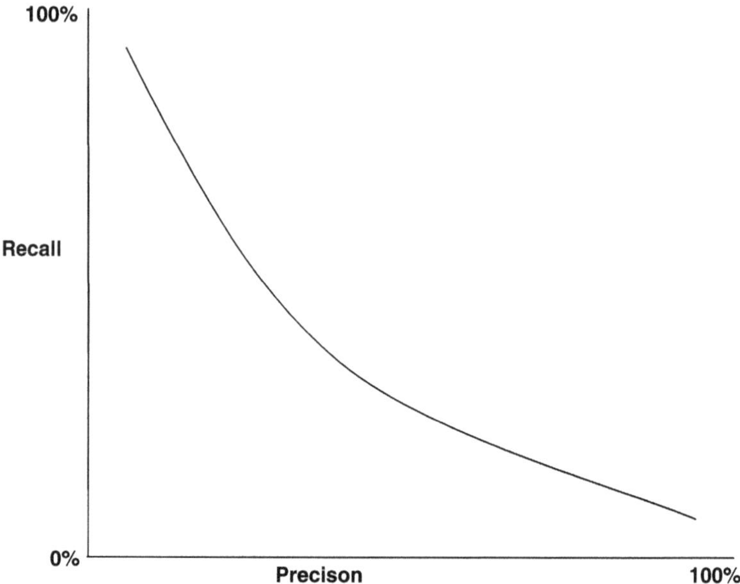

Fig. 1 The relationship between recall and precision

Using this model will not only help in the development of an appropriate search strategy but also help define the study's inclusion and exclusion criteria, and facilitate data extraction from primary studies.

The PICO(S) components can then be "translated" into language appropriate for the resources to be searched. In the case of bibliographic databases, the appropriateness of the language is dependent upon which database and interface is being searched (e.g., PubMed via NLM vs. Embase via OVID). Each database has its own language, or controlled vocabulary, and each interface has its own syntax, or naming system. One should consider how to best combine search terms to make the search most effective (e.g., Boolean operators: OR, AND, NOT).

It is helpful to analyze "seed" documents or articles (previously identified articles which are closely matched representations of the items one wishes to retrieve), if available, to identify search terms of interest. Once developed, the draft search strategy should then be tested and refined as required.

Before running a final search, one should also consider how the results will be managed, as this will impact your record retrieval format. Use of bibliographic management software such as Reference Manager® or RefWorks® is recommended, along with accurate records of databases searched and how many references have been identified through various search methods so that an accurate search result diagram can be completed, according to PRISMA methods [38].

2.5 Assessing the Quality of the Evidence

Evidence interpretation involves classifying the studies, grading the evidence, and determining which studies will be included in the synthesis. Assessors should use a systematic approach to critically appraise the quality of the available studies. Interpreting evidence requires knowledge of investigative methods and statistics [4].

The initial step in interpreting evidence is the establishment of criteria for its inclusion and role in the review; not all data available on a given technology may be suitable or equally useful for the purposes of a specific assessment [39]. The methods and presuppositions of both peer-reviewed publications and other material should be scrutinized on several grounds. Using formal criteria of the methodological rigor and clarity is essential for grading the data and their applicability to the assessment (e.g., User's Guides to the Medical Literature [39, 40]).

A key characteristic of a systematic review is an assessment of the validity of the findings of the included studies in order to minimize bias and provide more reliable findings from which conclusions can be drawn and decisions made [41–43].

2.6 Synthesize and Consolidate Evidence

For many topics in technology assessment, a definitive study that indicates one technology is better than another does not exist. Even where definitive studies do exist, findings from a number of studies often must be combined, synthesized, or considered in broader social and economic contexts in order to respond to the particular assessment question(s) [2].

Data synthesis may be narrative, such as a structured summary and discussion of the studies' characteristics and findings, or quantitative that involves statistical analysis. The statistical combination of results that is most frequently used in HTA is meta-analysis. The combining of studies increases the sample size and therefore more precise estimates of the treatment effects [43]. The Cochrane Collaboration has developed a software program, Review Manager (RevMan), that can perform a variety of meta-analyses, but it must be stressed that meta-analysis is not appropriate in all systematic reviews, for example if the outcomes measured are too diverse [43].

The synthesis of existing data is the most efficient HTA method if high-quality data are available. However, a problem arises when adequate evidence is limited, conflicting, or too uncertain in any or all of the relevant areas (e.g., efficacy, effectiveness, costs, quality of life). This highlights the problem the decision-maker often faces, confronted with the need to make reimbursement decisions and not knowing with certainty whether new health technologies are effective, safe, and cost-effective compared to existing technologies. Uncertainty creates problems for decision-makers because they are charged with choosing between various scenarios when there is insufficient definitive information on which to base decisions [44].

In health care, the stakes for such decisions are high and may carry both high financial and health risks and rewards. For example, the decision-maker could potentially recommend an unfavorable technology or reject a favorable technology, effectively denying access to a potentially beneficial health technology. Furthermore, the overarching imperative and responsibility for decision-makers is to make decisions, even if on poor quality evidence. In these situation, decision-makers then have three options: not implement the technology, fully implement the technology, or conditionally implement the technology [39, 44]. If it is thought that a health technology holds great promise, the decision-maker may also recommend that primary data collection, or a "field evaluation," may be necessary to reduce this informational uncertainty about a technology, thus yielding optimum site-specific recommendations [10, 45, 46].

2.7 Collection of Primary Data (as Appropriate)

If it has been determined that existing evidence will not adequately address the assessment question(s) and that primary data needs to be collected, there are a variety of methods that assessors can use to generate new data on the effects, costs, or patient outcomes of health care technology:

- Experimental or randomized controlled trials (RCTs).
- Nonrandomized trial with contemporaneous controls.
- Nonrandomized trial with historical controls.
- Cohort study.
- Case-control study.
- Cross-sectional study.
- Surveillance (e.g., registries, or surveys).
- Case series.
- Single case report.

These methods are listed in rough order of most to least scientifically rigorous for internal validity (i.e., for accurately representing the causal relationship between an intervention and an outcome). Methods for collecting primary data to answer policy questions are continuing to evolve. While rigorous randomized controlled trials are necessary for advancing research or for achieving market access by regulatory bodies, they do not necessarily address the needs of health policy-makers. There has been an increase in the trend towards "pragmatic" clinical trials that are intended to meet these needs [47]. Pragmatic trials select clinically relevant alternative interventions to compare; recruit participants from heterogeneous practice settings; and collect data on a broad range of health outcomes (e.g., health-related quality of life). Pragmatic trials require that decision-makers become more involved in priority-setting, design, funding, study implementation, etc. [2, 47].

The careful collection of primary data on new technologies raises unique issues since it can be as logistically complex, time consuming, and as expensive as the rest of the assessment combined. The evaluation of technologies early in their life cycle may not be undertaken when the potential return on investment is unknown. Original evaluation consumes resources to such an extent that priority may be given to the assessment of technologies for which substantial data already exist [39]. This creates an ironic cycle in which technologies remain unevaluated until they are widely accepted into practice, at the risk of harmful consequences for patients and financial consequences for institutions and society [39]. As well, there is considerable debate about what kinds of study designs are "good enough" for addressing important HTA questions of effectiveness [48].

Overall, primary data collection for HTA is likely to be most beneficial when idealized efficacy has already been demonstrated in the controlled, but artificial, environment of a randomized clinical trial, and data on effectiveness, feasibility, and cost are needed from a relevant real-world setting [45, 46]. The front-end investment for field evaluations could potentially offset inappropriate larger investments downstream [49].

2.8 Economic Analysis in HTA

Once the benefits and risks are determined from the results of the systematic literature review and, in some cases, the field evaluation, decision makers are often interested in determining whether the benefits of an intervention will be worth the health care resources consumed. In other words, does the technology represent good value for money? In these instances, an economic evaluation will be conducted to measure the incremental costs and benefits of the technology under review compared to one or more other technologies. An economic analysis is a set of formal, quantitative methods used to compare alternative treatments, programs, or strategies in terms of both their costs and consequences [50–52]. Therefore the basic tasks of any economic evaluation are to identify, measure, value, and compare the costs and effects of the alternatives being considered [51]. The overall role of the economic analysis in an HTA is to provide information about the necessary resource consumption from the use of health technologies compared with the health outcome obtained. It is important to remember that economic evaluations seek to inform resource allocation decisions, rather than to make them.

The identification of various types of costs and their subsequent measurement in monetary units is similar across most economic evaluations; however, the nature of the consequences stemming from the alternatives being examined may differ considerably [51].

There are three types of economic analyses that can be relevant to consider as part of an HTA: cost-effectiveness analysis, cost-utility analysis, and cost-benefit analysis.

2.8.1   Cost-Effectiveness
Analysis (CEA)

In the cost-effectiveness analysis, it is necessary to identify, measure, and value both cost and consequences of the compared health technologies. In this type of analysis, the consequences are measured as a single measure or dimension of effect expressed in natural units (e.g., death, life years gained). CEA can be performed on any alternatives that have a common effect (e.g., cost per mmHg drop in diastolic blood pressure obtained). CEA is somewhat limited in decision-making since it cannot be used to compare treatment strategies with different outcomes. From this analysis, it is only possible to conclude which of the alternative technologies is cost-effective in relation to a specified goal [51].

2.8.2   Cost-Benefit
Analysis (CBA)

In cost-benefit analysis, broadest type of economic analysis, consequences are valued in monetary units. The monetary value of an outcome is then compared to the cost of the intervention or its implementation [53]. For example, benefits could include averted medical costs or productivity losses associated with an early diagnosis. Asking about a person's willingness-to-pay for a specific outcome and treating the response as an expression of the preferences for, and the value of, the treatment is another way to value benefits. If the costs of the program are less than the benefits (e.g., costs averted) or societal values (e.g., willingness to pay), the program would be recommended. The clear advantage of this analysis is that the cost and consequences are now both measured in monetary units, from which the net benefit can immediately be calculated and whether the technology is worthwhile can be determined [51, 54]. Due to the methodological challenges associated with CBAs (i.e., placing a monetary value on an outcome), this type of analysis is rarely used [53].

2.8.3   Cost-Utility
Analysis (CUA)

Finally, cost-utility analysis uses health-related quality of life as the measure of treatment effect. The term utility is used here to refer to the preferences individuals or society may have for any particular set of health outcomes (e.g., for a given health state). Utility analysis allows for quality of life adjustments to a given set of treatment outcomes, while simultaneously providing a generic outcome measure for comparison of costs and outcomes of different technologies. The generic outcome, usually expressed as quality-adjusted life years (QALYs), is arrived at in each case by adjusting the length of time spent in a particular health state by the quality of life [55]. Utilities, or preferences, for health states, act as qualitative weights to combine the quantity and quality of life where a utility is measured on a scale from 0 to 1, with 0 representing death and 1 being perfect health. Utility values can be estimated using either direct or indirect methods. Direct measurements of utilities involve using various techniques to elicit a persons' preference for various health states. Some examples of direct elicitation techniques are time trade-off and standard gamble. Because these methods are resource and time intensive, indirect methods are more often employed. Indirect measures of utility values such as the European EuroQoL-5D or the Canadian Health Utility Index self-administered questionnaires are more often used.

CUA is important in instances when the quality of any life years gained is important (e.g., chronic diseases) or when there is a desire for an overall measure of effectiveness enabling comparisons to be made across the heath care sector [51, 54].

Factors like the disease area, the alternative technologies, the measurement and valuation of the consequences, as well as the purpose of the economic analysis are important in deciding which type of economic analysis should be chosen in any given case [54].

To be able to perform an economic analysis of the technology in question, there has to be at least one relevant alternative technology with which it may be compared. The cost-benefit analysis can, however, be conducted for only one technology. An economic analysis aims to answer the questions regarding whether a new health technology is cost-effective compared to current practice, which it is supposed to replace, and whether the technology is cost-effective in general compared to other optimally cost-effective technologies. To be relevant to decision-making, the chosen alternative for the economic analysis should at least represent the current health technology or practice which the new health technology is expected to replace [56].

In some situations it is necessary to model the economic analysis. Extrapolation of short-term clinical data with the purpose of predicting these data in the long run or the extrapolation of intermediate measures of effectiveness to final measures of effectiveness (e.g., high cholesterol as a risk factor for myocardial infarction) might be reasons for the use of modeling in economic analysis. Additionally, economic and clinical data can be missing, especially in the early development phase of a health technology. In such a situation the economic analysis may be entirely modeled and based on the best evidence available. *Decision trees* and *Markov models* are two of the most frequently used types of modeling approaches [54].

The checklist for economic analyses, presented below, can be used as a list for what should be remembered in the conduct of an economic analysis as part of an HTA as well as to provide the reader with an impression of the quality of published economic analyses (Table 2).

Table 2
A checklist for economic analyses (adapted from Drummond et al. [51] and Poulsen [54])

1. Is a there a well-defined question including whose perspective to take during the analysis?
2. Are the relevant competing alternatives included and described in the analysis?
3. Is the effectiveness of the compared technologies documented with sources?
4. Are all relevant costs and consequences, corresponding to the perspective, identified?
5. Are costs and consequences of the technologies measured in appropriate units?
6. Are costs and consequences valued credibly?
7. Are differential timing of costs and consequences handled including discounting?
8. Are sensitivity analyses carried out to test for uncertainty in the economic analysis and to investigate the robustness of this analysis and its conclusion?
9. Are the conclusions in the analysis presented as a ratio of costs and effects?
10. Are the conclusions valid and generalizable, and are all interested parties considered?

2.9 Formulation of Findings and Recommendations

A project's findings and recommendations are the central elements of interest for most readers. Findings are the results or conclusions of an assessment; recommendations are the suggestions or advice that follow from the findings and should be phrased in a format parallel to that of the statement of the original questions. Where conclusions cannot be reached from the evidence considered, some commentary is needed regarding why certain questions cannot be answered [39]. Heath technology assessments should link explicitly the quality of the available evidence to the strength of their findings and recommendations as well as any limitations. Doing so facilitates an understanding of the rationale behind the assessment findings and recommendations. It also provides a more substantive basis on which to challenge the assessment as appropriate. Further, it helps assessment programs and decision-makers determine if a reassessment is needed as relevant evidence becomes available [2].

2.10 Dissemination of Findings and Recommendations

One of the fundamental aspects of an HTA is to translate the scientific data and research results into information that is relevant to health care decision-makers through the dissemination of the findings [10]. The results should be available to others interested in the problem through the published literature and informal collegial communication [39]. Dissemination strategies depend upon the mission or purpose of the organization sponsoring the assessment. Dissemination should be planned at the outset of an assessment along with other assessment activities and should include a clear description of the target audience as well as appropriate mechanisms to reach them [2]. Agencies have been established that provide a forum for HTA agencies and users of HTA reports to exchange information such as the International Network of Agencies for Health Technology Assessment (INAHTA) http://www.inahta.org/Home and Health Technology Assessment international (HTAi) http://www.htai.org/index.php?id=419.

Technology assessments that appear inconclusive should not be withheld from distribution. If they are methodologically sound, such assessments may be both useful to policy-makers and clinicians and also serve as a point of departure for future research [39].

2.11 Monitoring Impact of Assessment Reports	The impact of HTA reports is variable and inconsistently evaluated. Some HTA reports are translated directly into policies with clear and quantifiable impacts (e.g., acquisition or adoption of a new technology; reduction or discontinuation in the use of a technology; or change in third-party payment policy), while the findings of others go unheeded and are not readily adopted into general practice [2]. It is important to keep in mind that HTA results will be only one of the many inputs that determine policy decisions.

Since considerable amounts of scarce resources are invested in HTA, monitoring the impact of an evaluation is essential to maximizing its intended effects and preventing the harmful repercussions of misinterpretation or misapplication [39, 57]. An assessment project should include a plan for the follow-up evaluation of its report [39]. Because technology assessment is an iterative process, new information or changes in the technology may require the re-evaluation of the project's original conclusions [39]. |

3   Case Study: Health Technology Assessment of Drug Eluting Stents Compared to Bare Metal Stents for Percutaneous Coronary Interventions in Ontario

The following HTA was conducted by the Programs for Assessment of Technology in Health (PATH) Research Institute, St. Joseph's Healthcare Hamilton in Hamilton, Ontario. This research group uses an iterative evidence-based framework for reducing uncertainty around a health technology to provide information back to Health Quality Ontario and ultimately to the Ontario Ministry of Health and Long-term Care (MOHLTC) to assist them in making more informed evidence-based health policy recommendations. PATH's Reduction in Uncertainty through Field Evaluations (PRUFE) iterative evidence-based framework is presented in Fig. 2.

3.1 Topic Identification	Prior to 2003, bare metal coronary artery stents (BMS) were commonly being used as part of the percutaneous coronary interventions (PCI) procedure for patients with coronary artery disease

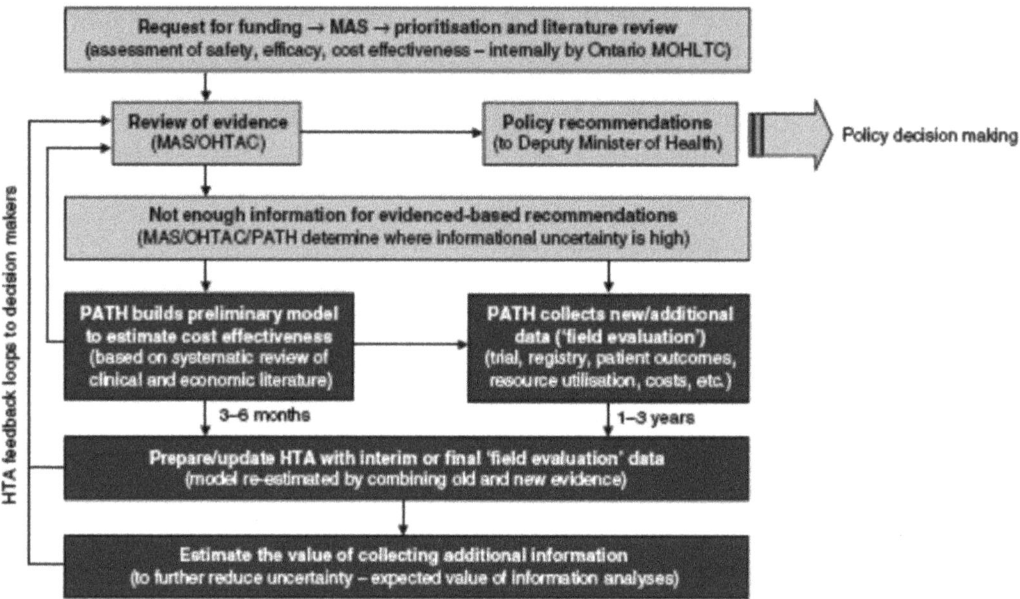

Fig. 2 Programs for Assessment of Technology in Health's (PATH's) reduction of uncertainty through field evaluation (PRUFE) iterative evidence-based decision-making framework

(CAD). However, patients receiving this intervention still had a relatively high restenosis rate (i.e., 15–20 % within a year) [58–60]. The drug eluting stents (DES), licensed in Canada in 2002, held the promise of reducing these rates and thus the potential for increased diffusion throughout the health care system.

3.2 The Assessment Problem

Prior to the introduction of DES in Ontario, the MOHLTC conducted an internal review of the literature pertaining to DES. The review determined that the efficacy of DES compared to Bare Metal Stents (BMS) had been demonstrated in a limited number of published randomized controlled clinical trials, and thus there was uncertainty surrounding the efficacy and cost-effectiveness of DES in a "real-world" setting. These new stents were significantly more costly than the technology they were meant to replace, and the MOHLTC estimated that the budget for coronary artery stents (i.e., BMS and DES) would require an additional $7.5–$28.6 million per year [61]. Due to the informational uncertainty and the high budget impact, the MOHLTC requested that PATH conduct an HTA including a field evaluation and economic analysis to examine the utilization, effectiveness, and costs associated with the introduction of DES into the Ontario health care system in order to make a reimbursement decision.

<table>
<tr><td>

3.3 Sources of Research Evidence for HTA

</td><td>

Due to the lack of Ontario-specific information pertaining to the real-world use of DES, a "field evaluation" and economic analysis was conducted by PATH during the time of introduction. In order to obtain Ontario-specific "real-world" data, the MOHLTC provided 12 Cardiac Care Centres with annual renewable funding for 1 year for DES conditional on data collection for the field evaluation (coverage with evidence development). The resulting prospective population-based registry of all consecutive percutaneous coronary intervention (PCI) procedures in the province of Ontario between 2003 and 2006 provided an unbiased estimate of the effectiveness of this technology in the local environment. This data allowed for the comparison of DES to BMS with respect to repeat revascularization rates (i.e., PCI and coronary artery bypass surgery) and all-cause mortality. Uptake and health care resource utilization data were also collected.

Concurrently, PATH continued the systematic literature review initiated by the MOHLTC to identify any new evidence pertaining to efficacy of DES. The results of the systematic literature review were examined alongside the evidence obtained from the field evaluation.

</td></tr>
<tr><td>

3.4 Interpretation, Synthesis, and Consolidation of Evidence

</td><td>

Only RCTs comparing DES to BMS providing relevant clinical outcomes (i.e., revascularization rates, acute myocardial infarction, and mortality) were included in the systematic literature review. Study results were both qualitatively and quantitatively (i.e., meta-analysis) summarized.

Appropriate statistical methods were employed to measure outcomes for an observational study design to control for potential differences in baseline characteristics (from field evaluation). A naïve economic model was developed and populated with the results from the field evaluation and published literature where data were lacking.

</td></tr>
<tr><td>

3.5 Findings

</td><td>

- The interim results from the field evaluation indicated that DES reduced predicted revascularization rates in some but not all patient cohorts at one year compared to bare metal stents (BMS).

- In non-post-myocardial infarction (MI) patients, DES appeared to be most effective in reducing the need for revascularization in patients with long or narrow lesions ("high-risk" patients). This benefit was magnified in patients with diabetes.

- DES also appeared to be effective in post-MI patients. However, further data collection is required in order to confirm the benefit of DES by lesion type in this patient cohort.

- DES compared to BMS did not appear to provide a reduction in revascularization rates in patients with short and wide lesions, in patients with and without diabetes.

</td></tr>
</table>

3.6 Dissemination

PATH has presented the results of the field evaluation, economic evaluation, and systematic literature review to the Ontario Health Technology Advisory Committee (OHTAC) on a number of occasions. For example, preliminary results for the DES field evaluation were presented on two separate occasions in 2005. Based on these presentations, OHTAC requested more specific analyses of data in patients groups at higher risk of restenosis, in particular patients having diabetes, narrow lesions, or long lesions [62]. These presentations provided the Committee with the opportunity to make recommendations about further analysis. This iterative process ensures that the information provided by the researchers is in line with the needs of decision-makers in order to make reimbursement decisions.

The final HTA report of the field evaluation of the DES was completed and is available through the PATH web site via the following link: http://www.path-hta.ca/Libraries/Reports/DESreportMay2007.sflb.ashx.

The findings of the HTA of DES have also been presented to other provincial governments (e.g., Agence d'évaluation des technologies et des modes d'intervention en santé [AETMIS] in Quebec) and to key stakeholders (e.g., Cardiac Care Network (CCN) of Ontario with representatives from nursing, medical, government, and administrators). Additionally, the results have been presented at national and international peer-reviewed scientific conferences (i.e., Society for Medical Decision Making, Canadian Association for Population Therapeutics, and International Society for Pharmacoeconomics and Outcomes Research).

3.7 Impact of Assessment Results

In March of 2007, OHTAC made the following recommendations to the Deputy Minister of Health of Ontario with regard to DES for PCI interventions in Ontario:

1. DES be offered to those patients considered for stent placement and who have:
   (a) Diabetes.
   (b) Long lesions (greater than 20 mm) and/or narrow lesions (less than or equal to 2.75 mm).
2. That PATH continue to collect data on patients who received DES.
3. That the current support for DES not be increased at this time.
4. These recommendations be provided to hospitals and cardiologists as soon as possible.

4 Discussion

The main purpose of HTA is to consolidate the best available evidence on technologies, so the results can have value in decision-making in which clinical practice and heath policy are concerned. When well-conceived and implemented, HTA can make an important contribution to the proper distribution of resources, to the selection of cost-effective interventions, and to greater efficiency and more effective services [63].

The proper timing of the assessment of a health technology warrants special attention, as it can be very complex. Assessments can be conducted at any stage in a technology's life cycle to meet the needs of a variety of stakeholders (e.g., investors, regulators, payers) and each may need to subsequently reassess technologies [2]. However, a trade-off exists between decision-makers' wish for early assessment prior to widespread diffusion of health technologies and the problem of reliability and certainty of the information available early in the life cycle, thus leading to potential errors in decision-making. At the same time, late assessment runs the risk that the technology has already been used widely and costs have been incurred. Difficulties in convincing providers to discard an intervention once it has been introduced into clinical practice illustrate this dilemma [64, 65]. This quandary in decision-making has been formulated by Martin Buxton as "it's always too early to evaluate until, unfortunately, it's suddenly too late!" [66].

Compounding this problem is the fact that the stages of a technology's life cycle are often not clearly delineated, and technologies do not necessarily mature through them in a linear fashion. A technology may be established for certain applications and may be investigational for others. A technology once considered obsolete may return to established use for a better-defined or entirely different purpose. Technologies often undergo multiple incremental innovations after their acceptance into practice [2]. As a result, HTA must be viewed as an iterative process. It may be necessary to revisit a technology when competing technologies are developed, the technology itself evolves, or new information is introduced. Reassessment may require additional data collection and ongoing assessments may be enhanced with techniques that aggregate results of research [2].

5 Concluding Remarks

This chapter provides a basic framework for conducting an HTA as well as some fundamental concepts and challenges of the dynamic field of health technology assessment with the ultimate goal of encouraging the uptake of efficient and effective health care technologies.

There are no standard methods for conducting HTA and new methods are continuously evolving. In fact, a variety of methods are often used depending on the purpose of the assessment, the resources available, the context and setting, etc. In any event, the general trend in HTA is to call for and emphasize more rigorous methods [2]. There is little argument that RCTs are an accepted high standard for testing efficacy under ideal circumstances, but they may not be the best means to evaluate all interventions and technologies that decision-makers are considering [67]. Observational studies with analyses that consider potential bias offer an opportunity to capture data from community practices costing less than randomized trials. In some cases, the process of performing an effective HTA can also include the process of collecting primary data through pragmatic trials, through local research initiatives [45, 46]. As a result, it is important for decision- and policy-makers to have a basic understanding of the basic research methods, ethical and sociocultural issues that may be taken into consideration in an HTA.

The future of HTA is not easy to predict. One thing is clear, however, HTA is here to stay. The need to contain costs and to target the use of technologies in areas that represent the best value for money will mean that decision-makers need more high-quality information on technologies' impacts [68]. Coverage decisions are already made more and more frequently based on HTA. Still, implementing HTA results into clinical practice remains a formidable challenge [3].

Whether HTA is beneficial—supporting timely access to needed technologies—or detrimental depends on three critical issues: when the assessment is performed; how it is performed; and how the findings are used. Heightened demand for technology assessment arising from private and public organizations' quest for value in health care is pushing the field to evolve keener processes and assessment reports tailored for particular user groups [2].

References

1. Facey K (2006) INAHTA health technology assessment (HTA) glossary. http://htaglossary.net/HomePage. Accessed 15 Apr 2014

2. Goodman CS (2004) Introduction to health technology assessment. The Lewin Group, Falls Church, VA

3. Banta D (2003) The development of health technology assessment. Health Policy 63(2): 121–132

4. Goodman CS, Snider G, Flynn K (1996) Health care technology assessment in VA, 1996. Management Decision and Research Center, Health Services Research and Development Service, Washington, DC, pp 1–5

5. Jonsson E et al (2002) Summary report of the ECHTA/ECAHI project. European collaboration for health technology assessment/assessment of health interventions. Int J Technol Assess Health Care 18(2):218–237

6. Poulsen PB (1999) Economic evaluation and the diffusion of health technology. Health technology assessment and diffusion of health technology. Odense University Press, Odense, pp 183–220

7. Franklin C (1993) Basic concepts and fundamental issues in technology assessment. Intensive Care Med 19(2):117–121

8. Husereau D, Boucher M, Noorani H (2010) Priority setting for health technology assessment at CADTH. Int J Technol Assess Health Care 26(3):341–347

9. Noorani HZ et al (2007) Priority setting for health technology assessments: a systematic review of current practical approaches. Int J Technol Assess Health Care 23(3):310–315

10. Canadian Agency for Drugs and Technologies in Health (2003) CADTH: home page [web site]. The Agency, Ottawa, ON

11. Lampe K et al (2009) The HTA core model: a novel method for producing and reporting health technology assessments. Int J Technol Assess Health Care 25(S2):9–20

12. Hofmann BM (2008) Why ethics should be part of health technology assessment. Int J Technol Assess Health Care 24(04):423–429

13. National Institute for Health and Clinical Excellence (2008) Social value judgments: principles for the development of NICE guidance. National Institute for Health and Care Excellence, London, pp 1–36

14. Giacomini M et al (2012) Social and ethical values for health technology assessment in Ontario. Health Quality Ontario Social Values and Ethics Evaluation Subcommittee, Toronto, ON

15. INAIITA Ethics Working Group (2005) INAHTA's working group on handling ethical issues. Final report, Final report, June 2005

16. Niederstadt C, Droste S (2010) Reporting and presenting information retrieval processes: the need for optimizing common practice in health technology assessment. Int J Technol Assess Health Care 26(4):450–457

17. Beauchamp TL, Childress J (2001) Principles of biomedical ethics, 5th edn. Oxford University Press, New York

18. Assasi N et al (2014) Methodological guidance documents for evaluation of ethical considerations in health technology assessment: a systematic review. Expert Rev Pharmacoecon Outcomes Res 14(2):203–220

19. Van der Wilt GJ, Reuzel R, Banta HD (2000) The ethics of assessing health technologies. Theor Med Bioeth 21(1):103–115

20. Arellano LE, Willett JM, Borry P (2011) International survey on attitudes toward ethics in health technology assessment: an exploratory study. Int J Technol Assess Health Care 27(1):50–54

21. Saarni SI et al (2008) Ethical analysis to improve decision-making on health technologies. Bull World Health Organ 86(8):617–623

22. Hofmann B (2005) On value-judgements and ethics in health technology assessment. Poiesis Prax 3(4):277–295

23. Jadad AR, Moher D, Klassen TP (1998) Guides for reading and interpreting systematic reviews: II. How did the authors find the studies and assess their quality? Arch Pediatr Adolesc Med 152(8):812–817

24. Goodman CS (2004) Retrieving evidence for HTA, in HTA 101: introduction to health technology assessment. Lewin Group, Falls Church, VA

25. Moher D et al (2003) The inclusion of reports of randomised trials published in languages other than English in systematic reviews. Health Technol Assess 7(41):1–90

26. Savoie I et al (2003) Beyond Medline: reducing bias through extended systematic review search. Int J Technol Assess Health Care 19(1):168–178

27. Royle P, Waugh N (2003) Literature searching for clinical and cost-effectiveness studies used in health technology assessment reports carried out for the National Institute for Clinical Excellence appraisal system. Health Technol Assess 7(34):iii, ix-51

28. Higgins JPT, Green S (2011) Searching for studies. In: Higgins JPT, Green S (eds) Cochrane handbook for systematic reviews of interventions version 510. The Cochrane Collaboration, Oxford

29. U.S. National Library of Medicine (1991) Databases, bibliographic, in MeSH database. US National Library of Medicine, Bethesda, MD

30. Centre for Reviews Dissemination University of York (2009) Systematic reviews: CRD's guidance for undertaking reviews in health care. The Centre, York

31. Last JM (2001) A dictionary of epidemiology, 4th edn. Oxford University Press, New York

32. McAuley L et al (2000) Does the inclusion of grey literature influence estimates of intervention effectiveness reported in meta-analyses? Lancet 356(9237):1228–1231

33. Institute of Health Economics, Osteba, and AUnEts (2013) Health technology assessment on the Net international: 2013. Institute of Health Economics (IHE), Edmonton, AB

34. Canadian Agency for Drugs and Technologies in Health (CADTH) Information Services (2014) Grey matters: a practical deep-web search tool for evidence-based medicine. Canadian Agency for Drugs and Technologies in Health, Ottawa, ON

35. Library and Archives Canada (2008) Theses Canada portal. Library and Archives Canada, Ottawa, ON

36. Jizba R (2007) Measuring search effectiveness. In: Creighton University (ed) Creighton University Health Sciences Library and Learning Resources Center. Creighton University, Omaha, NE

37. Straus SE et al (2005) Evidence-based medicine: how to practice and teach EBM, 3rd edn. Elsevier, New York

38. Liberati A et al (2009) The PRISMA statement for reporting systematic reviews and meta-analyses of studies that evaluate healthcare interventions: explanation and elaboration. BMJ 339:b2700

39. Heitman E (1998) Ethical issues in technology assessment. Conceptual categories and procedural considerations. Int J Technol Assess Health Care 14(3):544–566

40. Guyatt G, Rennie D (2002) User's guides to the medical literature, vol 5. American Medical Association Press, Chicago, IL

41. Antman EM et al (1992) A comparison of results of meta-analyses of randomized control trials and recommendations of clinical experts. Treatments for myocardial infarction. JAMA 268(2):240–248

42. Oxman AD, Guyatt GH (1993) The science of reviewing research. Ann N Y Acad Sci 703:125–133, discussion 133-4

43. Higgins JPT, Green S (2011) Cochrane handbook for systematic reviews of interventions. The Cochrane Collaboration, Oxford

44. Coburn D (2007) Managing decision making under uncertainty: perspectives from a central administrator. In: Organization for Economic Co-Operation and Development (ed) OECD Health Project. Health technologies and decision making. Organization for Economic Co-Operation and Development, Paris, pp 119–130

45. Goeree R, Levin L (2006) Building bridges between academic research and policy formulation: the PRUFE framework – an integral part of Ontario's evidence-based HTPA process. Pharmacoeconomics 24(11):1143–1156

46. McIsaac ML, Goeree R, Brophy JM (2007) Primary data collection in health technology assessment. Int J Technol Assess Health Care 23(1):24–29

47. Tunis SR, Stryer DB, Clancy CM (2003) Practical clinical trials: increasing the value of clinical research for decision making in clinical and health policy. JAMA 290(12):1624–1632

48. Lilford RJ et al (2001) Issues in methodological research: perspectives from researchers and commissioners. Health Technol Assess 5(8):1–57

49. Health Technology Assessment Task Group (2004) Health technology strategy 10: final report. Health Canada, Ottawa, ON

50. Detsky AS, Naglie IG (1990) A clinician's guide to cost-effectiveness analysis. Ann Intern Med 113(2):147–154

51. Drummond M et al (2005) Methods for the economic evaluation of health care programmes, 3rd edn. Oxford University Press, Oxford

52. Eisenberg JM (1989) Clinical economics. A guide to the economic analysis of clinical practices. JAMA 262(20):2879–2886

53. Tarride JE et al (2009) Approaches for economic evaluations of health care technologies. J Am Coll Radiol 6(5):307–316

54. Poulsen PB (2001) The economy. In: Kristensen FB, Horder M, Poulsen PB (eds) Health technology assessment handbook. Danish Institute for Health Technology Assessment, Copenhagen, pp 96–121

55. Weinstein M, Stason W (1977) Foundations of cost-effectiveness analysis for health and medical practices. N Engl J Med 296:716–721

56. Canadian Agency for Drugs Technologies in Health (2006) Guidelines for the economic evaluation of health technologies: Canada, vol 3. Canadian Agency for Drugs Technologies in Health, Ottawa, ON

57. Drummond M, Weatherly H (2000) Implementing the findings of health technology assessments. If the CAT got out of the bag, can the TAIL wag the dog? Int J Technol Assess Health Care 16(1):1–12

58. George CJ et al (1998) One-year follow-up of the Stent Restenosis (STRESS I) Study. Am J Cardiol 81(7):860–865

59. Macaya C et al (1996) Continued benefit of coronary stenting versus balloon angioplasty: one-year clinical follow-up of Benestent trial. Benestent Study Group 13. J Am Coll Cardiol 27(2):255–261

60. Stone GW et al (2004) One-year clinical results with the slow-release, polymer-based, paclitaxel-eluting TAXUS stent: the TAXUS-IV trial 14. Circulation 109(16):1942–1947

61. Medical Advisory Service (2003) Review of drug-eluting coronary stents [Internal document]. Ontario Ministry of Health and Long Term Care, Toronto, ON, pp 1–23

62. Ontario Health Technology Advisory Committee (2007) OHTAC recommendation: drug eluting stents (DES). Medical Advisory Secretariat Ministry of Health and Long-term Care, Toronto, ON

63. Pan American Health Organization (1998) Developing health technology assessment in Latin America and the Caribbean. World Health Organization, Geneva
64. Mowatt G et al (1998) When is the 'right' time to initiate an assessment of a health technology? Int J Technol Assess Health Care 14(2):372–386
65. Sculpher M, Drummond M, Buxton M (1997) The iterative use of economic evaluation as part of the process of health technology assessment. J Health Serv Res Policy 2(1):26–30
66. Buxton M (1987) Problems in the economic appraisal of new health technology: the evaluation of heart transplants I the UK. In: Drummond M (ed) Economic appraisal of health technology in the European Community. Oxford Medical Publications, Oxford, pp 103–118
67. Eisenberg JM (1999) Ten lessons for evidence-based technology assessment. JAMA 282(19):1865–1869
68. Stevens A, Milne R, Burls A (2003) Health technology assessment: history and demand. J Public Health Med 25(2):98–101

Chapter 26

Evidence-Based Decision-Making 4: Development and Limitations of Clinical Practice Guidelines

Bruce Culleton

Abstract

Clinical practice guidelines are systematically developed statements to assist practitioners and patients reach appropriate health care decisions. If developed properly, clinical practice guidelines assimilate and translate an abundance of evidence published on a daily basis into practice recommendations and, in doing so, reduce the use of unnecessary or harmful interventions, and facilitate the treatment of patients to achieve maximum benefit and minimum risk at an acceptable cost. Traditionally, clinical practice guidelines were consensus-based statements, often riddled with expert opinion. It is now recognized that clinical practice guidelines should be developed according to a transparent process involving principles of bias minimization and systematic evidence retrieval and review, with a focus on patient-relevant outcomes. The process for the development, implementation, and evaluation of clinical practice guidelines is reviewed in this chapter.

Key words Clinical practice guidelines, Clinical practice recommendations, Critical appraisal, Guideline grading, Implementation, Evaluation

1 Introduction

Clinical practice guidelines (CPG) are systematically developed statements to assist practitioners and patients reach appropriate health care decisions. Their purpose is "to make explicit recommendations with a definite intent to influence what clinicians do" [1]. If developed properly, CPG assimilate and translate the abundance of evidence published on a daily basis into practice recommendations and, in doing so, reduce the use of unnecessary or harmful interventions, and facilitate the treatment of patients to achieve maximum benefit and minimum risk at an acceptable cost. CPG are not meant to replace sound medical decision-making which takes into account critical elements relevant to patient care including patient preferences and clinician experience.

Traditionally, CPG were consensus-based statements, often riddled with expert opinion. Frequently, expert opinion was associated with bias (often nonintentional) and consensus-based

Patrick S. Parfrey and Brendan J. Barrett (eds.), *Clinical Epidemiology: Practice and Methods*, Methods in Molecular Biology, vol. 1281, DOI 10.1007/978-1-4939-2428-8_26, © Springer Science+Business Media New York 2015

recommendations are currently viewed with a certain amount of skepticism. It is now recognized that CPG should be developed according to a transparent process involving principles of bias minimization and systematic evidence retrieval and review, with a focus on clinically relevant outcomes. The process for the development, implementation, and evaluation of CPG is reviewed in this chapter.

2   Principles of Clinical Practice Guideline Development

The National Health and Medical Research Council of Australia has published CPG development principles [2]. Briefly, these principles state:

- Processes for developing and evaluating CPG should focus on outcomes.

- CPG should be based on the best available evidence and graded according to the level, quality, relevance, and strength of evidence.

- CPG development should be multidisciplinary and include consumers.

- CPG should be flexible and adaptable to local conditions. They should include evidence for different target populations and take into account patient preferences.

- CPG should be developed with resource constraints in mind.

- Implementation plans should be developed along with CPG.

- The implementation of CPG should be evaluated.

- CPG should be revised regularly to account for new evidence.

Details to adhere to these principles and other relevant issues in the development of CPG are discussed in the sections that follow.

2.1 Determine the Guideline Topic, Scope, and Target Audience

CPG are often developed by professional medical societies or associations in response to a perceived need, such as variation in the delivery of care by health care providers for the same medical problem. Ideally, a needs assessment is performed with the user of the guidelines in mind. When CPG topics are ultimately selected, there must be a clear purpose and a defined problem to be addressed. The audience is usually obvious but this should be stated in the process of CPG development.

2.2 Convene a Guideline Chair and Committee to Oversee Guideline Development

The committee should consist of members with clinical expertise relevant to the topic and representatives from all pertinent groups including consumers and other allied health professionals, as applicable. If CPG are to be relevant, those who are expected to use them should participate in their development. Although the committee's precise composition will depend upon a number of factors, strong consideration should be given to members with an ability to critically appraise published articles and with experience on other CPG workgroups. Health economists, bioethicists, and representatives of regulatory authorities may be relevant to certain committees.

2.3 Identify the Health Outcomes and the Appropriate Questions

The outcomes and questions will differ depending upon the topic under consideration. Outcome considerations include patient-relevant hard outcomes (e.g., all-cause or cardiovascular mortality), other patient-relevant outcomes (e.g., quality of life, hospitalization rates), surrogate outcomes (e.g., LDL cholesterol lowering, blood pressure reduction), process-related outcomes (e.g., re-admission rates, relapse rates), and patient satisfaction outcomes, to name a few. In general, it is accepted that these outcomes differ and the choice of outcome depends upon the topic, scope, and target audience. Within the realm of CPG, emphasis should be placed on patient-relevant outcomes.

2.4 Retrieve the Scientific Evidence

Recommendations placed in CPG should be based on the best possible evidence. Therefore, if possible, a systematic literature review should be performed very early in the course of guideline generation. The method chosen for the systematic review can range from highly structured quantitative syntheses of the literature (e.g., meta-analyses) to a subjective overview of observational data. The committee must decide between rigor and pragmatism [3] taking into consideration the extra costs and time to perform formalized quantitative reviews. Regardless of choice, the methods used to review the literature must be clearly stated.

2.5 Formulate the Guidelines and/or Recommendations

2.5.1 Phrase the Statement

Although guidelines can be presented as charts or flow diagrams, most often than not, guideline statements are presented as free flowing text. The guideline or recommendation statement should be as clear and concise as possible. Abbreviations should be avoided in the statement itself and statements should be phrased to initiate an action using terms such as "should" or "consider." Negatively phrased statements are frequently avoided.

2.5.2 Grade the Evidence

The grading of evidence is an integral part of any CPG development process. Although there is considerable variation in the grading systems used across and within specialty groups, there are several core factors necessary for the success of grading systems. First, the CPG Workgroup members should have experience in the relevant clinical area and have expertise with critical appraisal. Second, the grading system must be structured, explicit, and above all else, transparent. It should be obvious to the reader how a grade was applied to the evidence. The majority of structured grading schemes take into account study design, methodological quality, and the population studied. Consistency of effects across studies is also an important consideration within grading schemes.

Third, grading schemes should explicitly consider the balance between benefit and harm. Finally, the grading scheme should incorporate and define clinically important patient-relevant outcomes.

Due to the considerable variation among grading systems, several groups have promoted the use and implementation of standardized grading schemes. Using a standardized system, it is argued that comparison of recommendations between groups would be facilitated. A standardized scheme would also lessen the likelihood of several societies producing different evidence grades when using the same evidence base, thereby reducing confusion and promoting effective communication.

At the present time, the GRADE (Grades of Recommendation Assessment, Development and Evaluation) Working Group appears to have momentum for harmonizing grading schemes. The GRADE Working Group is composed of international experts in the field of evidence-based medicine and guideline development. The GRADE approach has the benefits of providing a structured approach to grading the quality of evidence for questions regarding interventions and it explicitly identifies how grades are derived and where judgment is involved. It has also been adopted by other organizations [4–6]. The grading of evidence by this group takes into account four key elements: study design, study quality, consistency, and directness. A summary of the criteria used by the GRADE working group is shown in Table 1 [7].

As one can *see* from Table 1, the level for the quality of the evidence can be "high," "moderate," "low," or "very low." For a question of intervention, the quality grade for an aggregate of

Table 1
Criteria for assigning grade of evidence for questions involving interventions

Type of evidence
  Randomized trial = high
  Observational study = low
  Any other evidence = very low

Decrease grade if
- Serious (–1) or very serious (–2) limitation to study quality
- Important inconsistency (–1)
- Some (–1) or major (–2) uncertainty about directness
- Imprecise or sparse data (–1)
- High probability of reporting bias (–1)

Increase grade if
- Strong evidence of association—significant relative risk of >2 (<0.5) based on consistent evidence from two or more observational studies, with no plausible confounders (+1)
- Very strong evidence of association—significant relative risk of >5 (<0.2) based on direct evidence with no major threats to validity (+2)
- Evidence of a dose–response gradient (+1)
- All plausible confounders would have reduced the effect (+1)

randomized controlled trials would start at the entry level of "high"; a collection of observational studies would start at the entry level of "low" and evidence from studies of other designs at "very low." Subsequently, the level for the quality of evidence for a particular outcome is reduced or downgraded, if there are limitations to the methodological quality of the studies, inconsistencies between studies, limitations of the directness of the evidence (i.e., the evidence does not apply directly to the populations, interventions, or outcomes of interest), imprecise or sparse data, or a high probability of reporting bias. On the other hand, the level of evidence of observational studies would be raised or upgraded if there is evidence of a strong or very strong association between the intervention and the outcome, if a dose–response gradient exists, or if unmeasured confounders are minimal. The final grade for the quality of the evidence cannot move higher than to "high" level, or lower than to "very low" level. More information on the GRADE system can be obtained at http://www.gradeworkinggroup.org.

2.5.3   Report the Rationale for the Guideline Statement and the Applied Grade

The scientific basis on which the guidelines were developed should be clearly stated including the strength and consistency of the evidence. Evidence tables can be helpful particularly when multiple studies are used to generate the guideline statement. In cases in which the evidence is lacking or poor, any uncertainty or disagreement amongst committee members should be documented.

2.6   Address Transparency and Conflict of Interest

In a cross-sectional survey of authors of 44 CPG developed for common adult diseases and published between 1991 and July 1999, 87 % of authors reported some form of interaction with the pharmaceutical industry [8]. On average, CPG authors interacted with 10.5 different companies and 59 % had relationships with companies whose drugs were considered in the guideline they authored. Fifty-five percent of the respondents also indicated that the guideline process with which they were involved had no formal process for declaring these relationships. In another recent report on more than 200 guidelines from various countries, it was found that more than one-third of the authors declared financial links to relevant pharmaceutical companies [9]. These links included research grant support, personal compensation for lectures or advice, or even stock holdings and patents.

It also appears that the majority of consensus and guideline development processes are supported either directly or indirectly (through "unrestricted" grants to medical specialty societies or national disease associations) by pharmaceutical companies with vested interests. For example, Amgen (makers of erythropoietic stimulating agents) and DaVita (a US company that provides dialysis services) have been criticized for their close relations and sponsorship of anemia management guidelines developed by the National Kidney Foundation. It is not surprising, therefore, that guidelines' committees have been criticized for effectively increasing the sales and profits of related companies [10].

Given that any perceived influences lessen the credibility and undermine the impartiality of the CPG process, it is important to minimize inappropriate influence. Several approaches have been suggested including the following:

- Full government or societal sponsorship of guideline development and implementation with no financial connections to companies, partnerships, or individuals who are involved with the manufacture, sale, or supply of health technologies in any way relevant to the guidelines. Such an approach would also restrict committee members to those with no conflicts of interest. Supporters of this approach maintain that practice recommendations will always be viewed with skepticism unless industry ties are completely avoided. Critics of the approach point out that the exclusion of authorities or experts who have received compensation from companies with a vested interest would likely compromise the expertise of the guideline committee [11] and perhaps limit the experienced human judgment necessary to make decisions easier at the practice level. The ability or willingness of governments or national associations to create independent and financially secure committees is also questionable.

- Avoidance of a single corporate sponsor, as suggested by Narins and Bennett [12]. Industry contributions can be placed in a common pool for the development of all guidelines, not just those related to the interests of the contributor.

- A process to minimize conflicts and optimize transparency while ensuring the Chair is free of conflict. The National Institute for Clinical Excellence in the United Kingdom (www.nice.org.uk) requires its members to declare financial and other interests and if identified, "the individuals are required to stand down and not take part in the relevant decision-making process for that project." Although such public disclosure may heighten reader's skepticism, it does not release authors from the potentially comprising ties to industry.

- Policies for individuals with inappropriate influence to stand down from relevant discussions or voting.

- Disclosure statements of sponsorship details for the medical specialty societies or national associations (not just for the CPG process).

- Procedures to ensure the choosing of committee chairs and committee members are transparent.

- Rules to ensure potential conflicts of interest are transparent.

- Regulations for members to recuse themselves from critically evaluating his or her own work that might serve as the basis for a recommendation, especially when that recommendation could have economic implications [13].

2.7 Develop an Implementation Strategy

Dissemination and implementation strategies are critical for the success of any CPG. Unfortunately CPG do not implement themselves [14] and simple dissemination does not impact change. It can be very helpful to develop a committee with expertise in medical education and behavior change. Given that behavior of physicians and other health care providers is difficult to alter, and the knowledge that adult learning is complex and variable, dissemination and implementation should involve multiple strategies including several or all of the following:

- Involve users in the CPG development process.
- Compile short summaries with key messages. These can be web based or in the form of brochures or posters or similar educational materials.
- Use professional journals including peer-reviewed journals and publications by relevant societies or interest groups.
- Use the education processes of relevant annual meetings, CME events, or universities; discuss the CPG at conferences and seminars.
- Ask respected clinical leaders to promote the CPG including the use of academic detailing.
- Develop tools to utilize the CPG within routine procedures such as quality assurance.
- Develop information technology tools to incorporate the CPG within practice-based computer reminder prompts or decision-making algorithms.
- Hire professional communicators.
- Consider economic incentives including differential fees for achieving CPG specified targets.
- Consider end-user (i.e., patient) directed advertising.

No single strategy is effective for all health care providers. To be effective, CPG must become embedded in the day-to-day activities of the user.

2.8 Consultation

Before the guideline document is considered final and widely distributed, the document should be sent for review to a wider group of relevant individuals that did not participate in the development of the document. These individuals might include other members of the society responsible for the guideline development, members of associated societies including allied health groups, consumer groups and patient support groups, and health authorities and regulatory agencies. Comments received from this external review process should be reviewed by the guideline committee members and areas of confusion or significant discord should be appropriately addressed in the guideline document.

2.9 Evaluate the Guidelines

The Appraisal of Guidelines, Research, and Evaluation (AGREE) Collaboration (www.agreetrust.org) has created and validated an instrument for clinicians to assess and rate the quality of the CPG document itself. The assessment of quality involves judging whether the potential biases within the guideline development process have been addressed adequately and that the recommendations are internally and externally valid. Within the AGREE instrument the reader is asked to assess, among other things, the overall aim of the guideline, the target population, the degree of stakeholder involvement, the rigor of the methods used to formulate the recommendations, the clarity of the recommendation statements, the organizational, behavioral and cost implications of the guidelines, and the editorial independence of the guidelines.

In addition to the formal evaluation of the CPG document, it is important to determine whether the guidelines and the implementation process have affected the users' knowledge and behavior and whether the guidelines have impacted the desired health outcomes. Unfortunately, these steps are challenging and, similar to the implementation process, are frequently overlooked. Critical components of this process include the following:

- An assessment of guideline dissemination—this is a relatively simple process of counting the number of copies of guidelines printed or downloaded, the number of presentations at national or local meetings, the number of publications and citations, etc.

- An assessment of the impact of CPG on user awareness, knowledge, and understanding—specifically designed questionnaires directed towards the relevant health care practitioner can be helpful for this component.

- An assessment of whether or not the guidelines have contributed to changes in clinical practice or health outcomes—ideally, analyses of longitudinally collected data should allow for assessment of changes in practice in relation to the guidelines (e.g., antihypertensive medication use for blood pressure CPG) and an assessment of health outcomes (e.g., stroke mortality). Comparisons can be made pre- and post-CPG implementation. However, caution is required when interpreting outcomes with prolonged lag times (e.g., change in blood pressure control and stroke mortality) and with inferring causality in pre/postcomparative studies.

2.10 Assess the Need to Revise the Guidelines

CPG lose value to clinicians with time as new evidence develops. As a result, some guidelines set an arbitrary revision date. In a slowly evolving field, the revision date may be premature leading to wasted time and money on guideline revision. Conversely, in a rapidly evolving field, CPG may become outdated before their scheduled revision date. Shekelle et al. [15] developed criteria for when a guideline needs updating and in a review of 17 CPG published by the US Agency for Healthcare Research and Quality, they found that half the guidelines were obsolete by 5.8 years. As a result, the authors suggested that CPG be assessed for validity every 3 years. Given this relatively brief period, it may be worthwhile to consider CPG development as an ongoing process rather than a discrete event. The Canadian Hypertension Education Program, for example, performs automatic literature searches and reviews new evidence on an annual basis [16]. Areas where the guidelines are deemed invalid are then updated expeditiously. For this process to work, the majority of the guideline work group members remain within the same guideline section on a year-to-year basis. Of course this annual revision is not applicable to a field in which new evidence is slowly evolving. Even in that setting however, the validity of published guidelines should be assessed on a regular basis.

2.11 Recognize the Limitations of the Guidelines and the Guideline Development Process

CPG development is a time-consuming and complex process. The cost of CPG development is also an issue, particularly if the CPG are developed with rigor as suggested above. Subjectivity is inevitable despite the best efforts of committee members to minimize bias and follow published grading schemes. It is also worth emphasizing that medicine is an evolving field. At the time of publication, CPG may be partially outdated particularly in fields that are evolving rapidly. Finally, in many circumstances, high quality valid evidence simply may not exist. Development of CPG in these situations is challenging and sometimes impossible.

3 Legal Considerations

3.1 Liability of Guideline Developers and Societies Supporting Guideline Development

Guideline developers should demonstrate that they have taken the necessary steps to ensure proper preparation of the guidelines. These steps are detailed above. It is critical to be transparent about evidence retrieval and synthesis of this evidence into guideline statements. It is also important to state that CPG are not definitive statements and are not meant to replace sound medical decision-making which takes into account critical elements relevant to patient care including patient preferences and clinician experience. The guideline document should also explicitly state the dates of development and the date of final acceptance by the sponsoring body. In this way, the recommendations made within the document are legally correct only to that date. If these steps are taken, it is very unlikely any legal liability will befall the guideline developers or sponsoring society.

3.2 Liability of Practitioners

It is beyond the scope of this document to review the legal liabilities of practitioners if CPG are not followed. Briefly, guidelines have been produced as evidence of what constitutes appropriate care delivered to a patient. However, other factors, including behavior in comparison to a standard of peers and provision of information around potential risks and benefits, are often considered for actions judged negligent.

4 Conclusion

The development of CPG is a complex time-consuming process involving systemic collection and synthesis of evidence, transparency, bias minimization, and detailed implementation and evaluation strategies. If developed correctly, CPG can facilitate treatment of patients to maximize benefits, reduce harm, and ultimately improve patient-relevant health outcomes.

References

1. Hayward RS, Wilson MC, Tunis SR, Bass EB, Guyatt G (1995) Users' guides to the medical literature. VIII. How to use clinical practice guidelines. A. Are the recommendations valid? The Evidence-Based Medicine Working Group. JAMA 274:570–574

2. The National Health and Medical Research Council of Australia (1999) A guide to the development, implementation, and evaluation of clinical practice guidelines. The National Health and Medical Research Council of Australia, Canberra, ACT

3. Browman GP (2001) Development and aftercare of clinical guidelines: the balance between rigor and pragmatism. JAMA 286:1509–1511

4. World Health Organization (2003) Guidelines for WHO guidelines. Global programme on evidence for health policy. World Health Organization, Geneva

5. Guyatt G, Vist G, Falck-Ytter Y, Kunz R, Magrini N, Schunemann H (2006) An emerging consensus on grading recommendations? Evid Based Med 11:2–4

6. Uhlig K, Macleod A, Craig J, Lau J, Levey AS, Levin A, Moist L, Steinberg E, Walker R, Wanner C, Lameire N, Eknoyan G (2006) Grading evidence and recommendations for clinical practice guidelines in nephrology. A position statement from kidney disease: improving global outcomes (KDIGO). Kidney Int 70:2058–2065

7. Atkins D, Best D, Briss PA, Eccles M, Falck-Ytter Y, Flottorp S, Guyatt GH, Harbour RT, Haugh MC, Henry D, Hill S, Jaeschke R, Leng G, Liberati A, Magrini N, Mason J, Middleton P, Mrukowicz J, O'Connell D, Oxman AD, Phillips B, Schunemann HJ, Edejer TT, Varonen H, Vist GE, Williams JW Jr, Zaza S (2004) Grading quality of evidence and strength of recommendations. BMJ 328:1490

8. Choudhry NK, Stelfox HT, Detsky AS (2002) Relationships between authors of clinical practice guidelines and the pharmaceutical industry. JAMA 287:612–617

9. Taylor R, Giles J (2005) Cash interests taint drug advice. Nature 437:1070–1071

10. Editorial (2005) Clinical practice guidelines and conflict of interest. CMAJ 173:1297–1299

11. Campbell N, McAlister FA (2006) Not all guidelines are created equal. CMAJ 174:814–815

12. Narins RG, Bennett WM (2007) Patient care guidelines: problems and solutions. Clin J Am Soc Nephrol 2:1–2

13. Coyne DW (2007) Influence of industry on renal guideline development. Clin J Am Soc Nephrol 2:3–7

14. Field MJ, Lohr KN (1992) Guidelines for clinical practice: from development to use. Institute of Medicine, National Academy Press, Washington, DC

15. Shekelle PG, Ortiz E, Rhodes S, Morton SC, Eccles MP, Grimshaw JM, Woolf SH (2001) Validity of the agency for healthcare research and quality clinical practice guidelines: how quickly do guidelines become outdated? JAMA 286:1461–1467

16. Zarnke KB, Campbell NR, McAlister FA, Levine M (2000) A novel process for updating recommendations for managing hypertension: rationale and methods. Can J Cardiol 16: 1094–1102

Chapter 27

Evidence-Based Decision-Making 5: Translational Research

Deborah M. Gregory and Laurie K. Twells

Abstract

The delay in turning research into practice for the benefit of patient care has been compared to a "leaky pipeline." In the early 2000s, this delay raised concerns among governmental agencies and other sponsors of health services in many countries. Facilitating the translation of basic and clinical research into clinical practice through evidence-based decision-making and improving population health is now a major goal of health research investment agencies. Translational research or knowledge translation has emerged to bridge the gaps between basic and clinical research, and between clinical research and clinical practice.

Various frameworks and definitions of translational research are presented. We present an example of an Integrated Knowledge Translation Team in Bariatric Care, and explain how an integrated knowledge translation (iKT) approach was created at the program's inception. This led to evidence-based decision-making and subsequent practice change in one area of the health care system. Real-world successes and challenges in moving research to practice are discussed.

Key words Translational research, Translational research frameworks, Integrated knowledge translation

---

1   Introduction

It has been frequently stated that it takes 17 years to turn research into practice for the benefit of patient care [1]. The lack of ability to apply research findings has sometimes been compared to a "leaky pipeline" or funnel between research (scientists) and practice (policy makers and practitioners) [1, 2]. In the early 2000s, the gap between research and practice, characterized as a "chasm" by the Institute of Medicine [3], raised concerns among governmental agencies and other sponsors of health services in many countries including the USA, UK, and Canada [2].

Evidence-based approaches emerged in response to the need to improve the quality of health care and to close the gap between research and practice [3]. *Evidence-based practice*, defined as "the integration of best research evidence with clinical expertise

Patrick S. Parfrey and Brendan J. Barrett (eds.), *Clinical Epidemiology: Practice and Methods*, Methods in Molecular Biology, vol. 1281, DOI 10.1007/978-1-4939-2428-8_27, © Springer Science+Business Media New York 2015

and patient values" [4], and *evidence-based decision-making*, defined as "the formalized process of using the skills for identifying, searching for, and interpreting the results of the best scientific evidence, which is considered in conjunction with the clinician's experience and judgment, the patient's preferences and values, and the clinical/patient circumstances when making patient care decisions" [5] have been utilized by a number of disciplines including medicine, nursing, and psychology.

The importance of translation of research knowledge to effective clinical treatment is well known [6] and considered essential to the public good [7]. Facilitating the translation of basic and clinical research into clinical practice and everyday decision-making to improve population health is a priority of health research investment agencies such as the Canadian Institutes of Health Research (CIHR) [8], the National Institutes of Health [9] and the Agency for Healthcare Research and Quality [10] among others in the USA, and the Medical Research Council [11, 12] of the UK. It has become increasingly important to demonstrate the investment of money spent on health research has moved research into practice and policy. Simply providing research evidence at scientific conferences or meetings and through publications in scholarly journals, while important, is not perceived as being adequate to ensure appropriate knowledge use in decision-making. Brownson et al. [13] stated "...too often, discovery of new knowledge begets more discovery (the next study) with little attention on how to apply research advances in real-world public health, social service, and health care settings."

The process of transferring research evidence from basic science into clinical research and from clinical research into clinical practice has been coined by researchers as translational research, knowledge translation, knowledge transfer and exchange, knowledge to action, research utilization, and dissemination and implementation research. McKibbon et al. [14] identified as many as 100 terms used to describe the process of putting knowledge into action. Although the terminology can be confusing, the underlying rationale for each is comparable and focuses on bridging the gap between research and practice.

2   What Is Transitional Research?

The term "translational research" appeared in the literature as early as 1993, but there was limited reference to the term during the 1990s [15]. It has been referred to as the "new buzzword" in the health care research field [16]. In a commentary published in 2008, Woolf stated "translational research means different things to different people, but it seems important to almost everyone's" [17]. The author suggested that for many it referred to the knowledge generated from "bench to bedside" or from basic science to clinical medicine. For health services and public health researchers it referred to "translating research into practice; i.e., ensuring that new treatments and research knowledge actually reach the patients or populations for whom they are intended and are implemented correctly" [17]. Although translational research has not been clearly defined [15], numerous attempts have been made to do so by various fields [18] including medicine, nursing, and psychology.

2.1 Translational Research Frameworks

Various translational research and knowledge translation frameworks and definitions can be found in the literature. In this section, we present an overview of the frameworks referred to as translational research and in the following section we specifically focus on the framework we use to guide our translational research program. This knowledge translation framework is utilized by Canada's federal health research agency—the Canadian Institutes of Health Research.

Translational research has been referred to as a *process* of taking findings from basic research or clinical research and using them to produce innovation in healthcare settings and is also used to *define* research which involves both basic and applied research [11]. Thus there at least two *levels* of translational research. The first level (T1) was defined as "The transfer of new understanding of disease mechanisms gained in the laboratory into the development of new methods for diagnosis, therapy, and prevention and their first testing in humans" (170). The second level (T2) was described as "Translation of results from clinical studies into everyday clinical practice and health decision making" [17]. Fiscella et al. [19] have referred to T1 research as preclinical and further subdivided it into short-term (lasts up to 5 years) and long-term (lasts from 5 to 10 years). The second level was defined as applied clinical research that is clinician-focused, patient-focused, and community-focused.

Lean et al. [20] suggest three *phases* of translational research. Phase 1 is "from bench to bedside," phase 2 "examines how findings from clinical science function when they are applied routinely in practice," and phase 3 "incorporates research processes to evaluate the complex interacting environmental and policy measures that affect…sustainability of clinical and public health strategies" [20]. Phases 2 and 3 equate to level 2 proposed by Woolf [17].

Westfall et al. [18] proposed further dividing the second phase of translational research, defining T2 as research to develop evidence-based recommendations and policies and T3 as research on implementing and disseminating evidence-based interventions in practice [18]. In a commentary by Dougherty and Conway in 2008, an extension of the translational framework was suggested to include quality improvement research to evaluate how to deliver high-care quality consistently and effectively [21].

In 2007, Khoury et al. [22] presented a framework for the continuum of multidisciplinary translation research which revolved around the development of evidence-based guidelines. The authors presented four phases of translational research: T1: discovery to candidate application; T2: health application to evidence-based guidelines; T3: evidence-based practice guidelines to health practice; T4: practice to population health. The model depicts a logical progression from T1 to T4 research, but the process is not necessarily linear. Augurs-Collins et al. later adapted the translational research framework to obesity genomics research and emphasized the central role that knowledge synthesis plays in translational research [23]. Khoury et al. [24] coined the term "translational epidemiology" to highlight the role of epidemiology in translating scientific discoveries into population health impact. Using human genomics as an example, Khoury suggested that epidemiology has a role to play in each of four phases of translational research. In T1, epidemiology explores the role of a basic discovery (e.g., a disease factor or biomarker) in developing a candidate application for use in practice (e.g., a test to guide interventions). An example from genomics would involve assessing the prevalence, associations, interactions, sensitivity, specificity, and predictive value of testing for genetic risk factors. In T2, epidemiology can help to evaluate the efficacy of the candidate application by using observational or experimental studies. This would involve assessing the clinical utility of genetic risk factors in improving health outcomes. In T3, epidemiology can help to assess facilitators and barriers for uptake and implementation of candidate application in practice, for example, assessing the factors associated with implementation of BRCA testing in practice. In T4, epidemiology can help to assess the impact of using candidate applications on population health outcomes, for example assessing the effectiveness of newborn screening programs. Epidemiology also has a leading role in knowledge synthesis, especially using quantitative methods (e.g., meta-analysis) [24].

Translational research is a process promotes the *multidirectional* and *multidisciplinary* integration of basic research, patient-oriented research, and population-based research, with the long-term aim of improving the health of the public [15].

3   Translation of Research in Canada

Canada's national health research investment agency the Canadian Institutes of Health Research (CIHR) was created in 2000 under the authority of the *CIHR Act* [25]. It consists of four pillars of health research: biomedical, clinical, health systems, and population health. Translation of research is embedded in its mandate. A key focus of the agency is "knowledge translation that facilitates the application of the results of research and their transformation into new policies, practices, procedures, products and services" [8]. To promote the movement of research into practice researchers must incorporate a knowledge translation plan in their funding proposals and dedicate funds for the same. Additionally, knowledge users such as decision-makers must demonstrate the use of evidence in planning and priority setting.

CIHR defines knowledge translation as "a dynamic and iterative process that includes the synthesis, dissemination, exchange, and ethically-sound application of knowledge to improve the health of Canadians, provide more effective health services and products, and strengthen the healthcare system." It involves "interactions between researchers and knowledge users that may vary in intensity, complexity and level of engagement depending on the nature of the research and the findings as well as the needs of the particular knowledge user." (http://www.cihr-irsc.gc.ca/e/39033.html).

Knowledge translation (KT) at CIHR is described by two categories—end-of-grant knowledge translation and integrated knowledge translation (iKT). The first involves initiatives undertaken once the research project has been completed and the second is combined into the research process (http://www.cihr-irsc. gc.ca/e/39033.html). In end of grant KT, the researcher develops and implements a plan for making knowledge users aware of the knowledge that was gained during a research project. Therefore, end of grant KT includes the typical dissemination and communication activities undertaken by most researchers, such as KT to their peers through conference presentations and publications in peer-reviewed journals. End of grant KT can also involve more intensive dissemination activities that tailor the message and medium to a specific audience, such as summary briefings to stakeholders, interactive educational sessions with patients, practitioners and/or policy makers, media engagement, or the use of knowledge brokers (http://www.cihr-irsc.gc.ca/e/39033.html).

According to the CIHR, "The term integrated KT describes a different way of doing research with researchers and research users working together to shape the research process starting with collaboration on setting the research questions, deciding the methodology, being involved in data collection and tool development, interpreting the findings and helping disseminate the research results. This approach also known as collaborative research, action-oriented research, and co-production of knowledge, should produce research findings that are more likely to be relevant to and used by the end-users" (http://www.cihr-irsc.gc.ca/e/39033. html). It is more likely this process will result in knowledge users such as policy and decision-makers, clinicians or the public using the results in everyday decision-making.

CIHR has adopted Graham and colleagues *Knowledge to Action Cycle* for promoting the application of research to ensure that new knowledge generates action to improve health or health care services and a framework for the process of knowledge translation (http://www.cihr-irsc.gc.ca/e/39033.html). The "Knowledge to Action Cycle" requires identifying the problem and selecting the relevant knowledge; adapting the knowledge to the local context; assessing the determinants of knowledge use (barriers and supports); selecting, tailoring, implementing, and monitoring knowledge translation interventions; evaluating outcomes or impact of knowledge use; and determining strategies for ensuring sustained knowledge use.

4   The Newfoundland and Labrador Integrated Knowledge Translation Team in Bariatric Care: A Case Study

4.1   Context

In Newfoundland and Labrador (NL), one in every three adults is obese (BMI ≥ 30); the highest rate of obesity in Canada. Within this group, the prevalence of individuals that are excessively obese, classified as either class II (BMI ≥ 35) or class III obese (BMI ≥ 40) is high and continued increases are projected [26]. These excessive weight categories increase the risk of developing chronic conditions such as hypertension, type 2 diabetes, and cardiovascular disease, impair quality of life, place a substantial burden on the health system, and put individuals at a higher risk of premature mortality [26–30]. In Canada, it is estimated that obesity costs the health care system between \$3.9 and \$4.3 billion dollars in direct and indirect medical costs [31, 32].

4.1.1   Bariatric Surgery in Newfoundland and Labrador

Bariatric or weight loss surgery is recommended as a medically effective treatment for class II (BMI ≥ 35 kg/m² + comorbid condition) and class III obesity (BMI ≥ 40 kg/m²) herein referred to as morbid obesity, for individuals who demonstrate unsuccessful weight loss attempts [27]. It is considered superior as a treatment for morbid obesity when compared to any other intervention (e.g., lifestyle, medical management, behavioral, pharmacologic) resulting in substantial and sustainable weight loss, improved quality of life, and reduced likelihood of premature mortality [33–37].

In May 2011, Eastern Health (EH), the largest of four integrated regional health boards in the province of Newfoundland and Labrador started offering laparoscopic sleeve gastrectomy (LSG), a type of bariatric surgery, to eligible patients from the entire province (population 510,000) estimated at 100–150 surgeries annually. LSG is a non-reversible procedure resulting in the removal of approximately 80 % of the stomach, leaving a much smaller stomach or "sleeve" [27, 38]. LSG is a relatively new type of bariatric surgery, until recently considered "investigational," but now a stand-alone procedure that encompasses almost 20 % of all bariatric surgeries in North America [38, 39].

4.1.2 Establishment of a Multidisciplinary Clinical Team in Bariatric Surgery

According to Canadian Clinical Practice Guidelines, successful treatment for morbid obesity is more likely when multidisciplinary health care providers are involved in patient care pre- and post-surgery [27]. Consequently, a multidisciplinary clinical team was established at EH and is comprised of three general surgeons trained in bariatric surgery, a nurse practitioner (NP), and a dietician with access to other medical specialties via consultation. Potential patients referred by their primary health care provider via a standardized referral form are screened by the NP. If eligible, patients are invited to attend an educational session presented by the NP and dietician on topics that include: overview of obesity and associated comorbidities, program and patient weight loss expectations, review of surgery including risks and dietary teachings. If interested, patients meet with the NP and dietician for further assessment and teaching. If deemed an eligible surgery candidate, patients are booked to meet with the surgeon for official consent. Once surgery has been performed patients are followed up post-surgery: 4–6 weeks, 3, 6, 12, 18, and 24 months and annually thereafter. Patients experiencing challenges are offered follow-up more frequently and have access to the NP and dietician through e-mail and phone contact.

4.2 Opportunity for Research: A Window of Opportunity

In a joint report "Developing a Research Agenda to Support Bariatric Care" published by the CIHR and the Canadian Obesity Network in 2010, the gaps in research related to bariatric surgery were highlighted [40]. Although LSG was not specifically highlighted in the report, compared to other bariatric surgeries, research on LSG as a treatment for morbid obesity is limited due to its relatively recent advent. In 2003, in Canada and the USA there were no LSGs performed compared to 19,486 in 2011 [39]. There is limited research on LSG in Canada and elsewhere on (1) experiences of patients who choose bariatric surgery as a modality for treatment of their morbid/clinical obesity, (2) patient expectations of weight loss as a result of undergoing surgery, (3) mid to long term health outcomes 3–5 years and beyond, and (4) patient-reported health outcomes post-surgery. Although there is an increasing body of research reporting on the short to intermediate time period post-surgery (2–5 years), long-term (>5 years) data is limited [41, 42]. The start-up of a bariatric surgery program offering LSG as a treatment for morbid obesity combined with the limited research on LSG provided an opportunity for research.

4.2.1 Development of an Integrated Knowledge Translation Team in Bariatric Care

Initial contact with academic researchers was initiated by one of the surgeons trained in bariatric surgery (DP). As academic researchers trained in the areas of evidence-based medicine and clinical epidemiology, our approach to working together was based on the belief that research knowledge is more likely to be used by knowledge users (e.g., health professionals, decision- makers, policy makers) if they are engaged early in the process and establish an ongoing relationship with the researchers. With the goal of establishing a sustainable, long-term program of research that would provide relevant information to knowledge users, we decided to use the CIHR iKT approach (http://www.cihr-irsc. gc.ca/e/39033.html) as a guide in establishing our team.

Consequently an Integrated Knowledge Translation Team was established at Memorial University to develop a program of research focused on bariatric care. This team is comprised of academic researchers at Memorial University, health care professionals and decision-makers from the Surgical Program at Eastern Health, and policy makers at the Department of Health and Community Services in the provincial government. In addition, it includes database management experts from Eastern Health and data linkage specialists from the NL Centre for Health Information as well as a number of trainees. A partnership has been developed with researchers from other provinces, as well as, national knowledge translation experts from the Canadian Obesity Network. Extensive consultation with local stakeholders took place. In addition, we applied for and received a CIHR meeting, planning, and dissemination grant [43] to bring experts in the field of bariatric care to Memorial University and Eastern Health in order to advise on future research directions. Subsequently our translational research in bariatric care focused on capturing the patient's total experience of waiting for, undergoing, recovering from, and adjusting to life after bariatric surgery. The program also assesses not only the clinical outcomes post-surgery, but patient-reported outcomes (perceptions of physical, emotional, and psychosocial health and well-being) and how these relate to the overall success of the surgical intervention. This research process is dynamic and iterative and includes:

- Determining research capabilities.
- Identifying gaps in the research literature or those relevant to the health system.
- Deciding on research questions.
- Writing research grants/obtaining funding.
- Conducting research.
- Translating research findings to knowledge users.
- Evaluation of interventions undertaken as a result of the evidence provided.

Our vision is to promote the utilization of integrated KT in the development of a more evidence-informed practice in the area of bariatric care with the goal of improving patient health outcomes and enhancing population health through improved treatment options for morbid obesity in the population.

4.2.2 Research Objectives

Our program of research covers the continuum of bariatric care. Specific research objectives include examining (1) the waiting period for surgery and patients' goals and weight loss expectations post-surgery, (2) health outcomes post-surgery such as weight loss/weight regain, resolution/regression of comorbid conditions, changes in quality of life, and the impact on the health system, (3) patients' perceptions and definitions of success after surgery, (4) developing and implementing interventions, and (5) evaluating interventions and applying new knowledge. Future research will focus on the development of interventions, including an evaluation process that is both formative and summative in order to improve patient outcomes and the effectiveness of health services delivery in bariatric care, and to ensure value for money within the publically funded health care system.

4.2.3 Translational Research in Action

Since its inception in January 2011, our translational team has been engaged in five research projects. Four of the projects are completed to date: a qualitative study on patients' experiences with waiting for bariatric surgery, a qualitative study on patients' perceptions of their health and well-being following surgery and definitions of success, a quantitative study on patients' goals and weight loss expectations post-surgery and a quantitative study on projecting future obesity rates in NL [26, 44–46]. In order to accelerate the use of applicable study findings into practice, early communication was established through regular team meetings, ongoing e-mail correspondence and the development of a SharePoint database. The information flow between researchers and knowledge users is bi-directional. Some information moves from research to clinical while other information moves from the clinical arena to research (*see* examples in Table 1). We have described one example of how clinical practice changed as the result of information sharing between the researchers and knowledge users. During a meeting of the integrated research and clinical team, the clinical team identified an observation that over time patients tended not to attend follow-up appointments. The research evidence on patient compliance with follow-up suggests that patients who do well post-operatively and sustain weight loss are those that continue with long-term follow-up and receive support from a multidisciplinary team compared to those who do not comply with regular follow-up appointments. Although surgery results in short-term weight loss in the majority of patients, attendance at regularly scheduled follow-up appointments may further increase long-term effectiveness. The findings of the qualitative studies undertaken by the team's researchers with patients before and after surgery provided evidence for this clinical finding and also elucidated the problem by explaining that patients were not adhering to the assigned schedule of follow-up visits for several reasons including

Table 1
Integrated knowledge translation activities

Issue/finding	Communication	Outcome/intervention
Over time patients not attending follow-up appointments Ensuring patient follow-up critical to ensuring success of program and research objectives	Early identification by clinical team in team meetings	Introduction of TeleHealth to facilitate follow-up visit for patients Early evaluation—reducing loss to follow-up
Unrealistic post-surgery weight loss expectations (refs. 44, 46)	Finding in qualitative and quantitative studies on waiting for bariatric surgery	Realistic weight loss expectations post-surgery emphasized by NP in formal education sessions
Weight loss appears to be variable Some patients doing really well, others regaining much the weight lost	Identified by clinical team during appointments and by research team during data analysis	Initiated study on changes in ghrelin, a gut hormone that induces hunger pre and post-surgery
Ensure sustainability of program funding Ensure sustainability of research program	Joint concern of the research and clinical teams resulting in an integrated effort to provide evidence to decision-makers and policy makers on the effectiveness of the program	Research funding obtained to develop clinical database to house all program data in order to produce report cards for all knowledge users Linkage with the NL Centre for Health Information to determine long term health outcomes
Research findings take time to be published	Joint concern of research and clinical teams	KT opportunities with decision-makers lead to fast decision-making

abhorrent costs associated with travel, food and lodgings, and the perception that follow-up could be completed within their own health region. The integrated knowledge translation team recognized that ensuring patient follow-up was critical to ensuring the success of the program and the research objectives. As a result potential interventions to promote follow-up visits were explored and identified. One intervention implemented by the provincial bariatric surgery program's NP was the introduction of TeleHealth in a number of locations throughout the province to facilitate follow-up visit for patients, allowing patients to stay in their own health regions and reducing out-of-pocket costs of travel. This intervention will be formally evaluated for its effectiveness in promoting compliance with follow-up; however, early indications are that a reduction in the number of patients lost to follow-up has occurred.

A number of factors or *enablers* help support the success of an integrated knowledge translation team [47]. These enablers include but are not limited to:

- A receptive environment.

- Adequate tools and resources (e.g., IT infrastructure, research staff).

- Formal recognition and rewards.

- Developing processes for timely, relevant information (e.g., regular meetings to disseminate and discuss findings before being presented at local, national and international conferences).

- Building the capacity of decision-makers to better use the research findings (e.g., creation of the clinical database and report cards).

- Access to and regular communication with knowledge users and policy makers.

- A multidisciplinary team of academic/clinical experts.

- Training and mentoring of graduate students and trainees.

Just as there are enablers to a successful team there are *challenges* and these include [48]:

- Becoming a team member.

- Understanding and accepting different agendas and timeframes.

- Building trust.

- Sharing of power and authority.

- Respecting the viewpoints of others.

- Being FLEXIBLE and accommodating unexpected events.

- Working on solutions to issues that emerge requires time and effort to ensure sustainability.

- Changing team composition.

4.2.4 Our Experience to Date

Some of these enablers are out of one's control but others may be under one's influence. For example, our team is fortunate to be part of a receptive environment that sees the value in evidence-based decision-making [48]. As well we, have access to our knowledge users and policy makers, which is more likely in smaller populations or geographical regions like ours. We have made communication with our team a priority. The primary contact for keeping the lines of communication open between researchers, clinicians, decision-makers and policy-makers is the responsibility of the lead investigator. In addition, regular team meetings, ongoing informal interactions with all stakeholders, and early and ongoing sharing of research findings to the entire team supports continued engagement of team members. The biggest challenge we have faced thus far is changing team composition (e.g., key knowledge users moving to different and unrelated positions).

5   Concluding Remarks

For integrated knowledge translation to be successful, researchers must engage and integrate potential knowledge users (researchers from different disciplines, decision-makers, policy makers, clinicians) in the research process from the start, develop a collaborative approach to research that is action-oriented and impact-focused, and be part of a receptive environment that supports evidence-based practice and policy [47].

References

1. Green LW (2008) Making research relevant: if it is an evidenced-based practice, where's the practice-based evidence? Fam Pract 25:i20–i24

2. Green LW, Ottoson JM, García C, Hiatt RA (2009) Diffusion theory and knowledge dissemination, utilization, and integration of public health. Annu Rev Public Health 30: 151–174

3. Committee on Quality of Health Care in America, IOM (2000) Crossing the quality chasm: a new health system for the 21st century. The National Academy of Sciences, Washington, DC

4. Sackett D, Straus S, Richardson W (2000) Evidence-based medicine: how to practice & teach, 2nd edn. Churchill Livingstone, London, England

5. Forrest JL, Miller SA (2009) Translating evidence-based decision making into practice: EBDM concepts and finding the evidence. J Evid Base Dent Pract 9:59–72

6. PLoS Medicine (2008) From theory to practice: translating research into health outcomes. Editorial. PLoS Med 5(1):15

7. Perini C (2011) From bench to bedside and to health policies: ethics in translational research. Clin Ter 162(1):51–59

8. Canadian Institutes of Health Research. http://www.cihr-irsc.gc.ca/e/37792.html. Accessed Apr 2014

9. Zerhouni E (2003) Medicine. The NIH roadmap. Science 302:63–72

10. Agency for Healthcare Research and Quality (2001) Translating research into practice (TRIP-II). Agency for Healthcare Research and Quality, Rockville, MD, AHRQ Publication No. 01-P-017, March 2001. http://www.ahrq.gov/research/findings/factsheets/translating/tripfac/index.html. Accessed Apr 2014

11. Cooksey D (2006) A review of UK health research funding. HMSO, Norwich, https://www.gov.uk/government/uploads/system/…/0118404881.pdf. Accessed Apr 2014

12. Greenhalgh T, Robert G, McFarlene F, Bate P, Kyriakidou O (2004) Diffusion of innovations in service organizations: systematic review and recommendations. Millbank Q 82:581–629

13. Brownson RC, Colditz GA, Proctor EK (eds) (2012) Dissemination and implementation research in health. Translating science into practice. Oxford Press, New York

14. McKibbon KA, Lokker C, Wilczynski N et al (2010) A cross sectional study of the number and frequency of terms to refer to knowledge translation in a body of health literature in 2006: a Tower of Babel? Implement Sc 5:16

15. Rubio DM, Schoenbaum EE, Lee LS, Schteingart DE, Marantz PR, Anderson KE, Platt LD, Baez A, Esposito K (2010) Defining translational research: implications for training. Acad Med 85(3):470–475. doi:10.1097/ACM.0b013e3181ccd618

16. Szilagyi PG (2009) Translational research and pediatrics. Acad Pediatr 9:71–80

17. Woolf SH (2008) The meaning of translational research and why it matters. JAMA 299(2):211–213

18. Westfall JM, Mold J, Fagnan L (2007) Practice-based research-"Blue Highways" on the NIH Roadmap. JAMA 297(4):403–406

19. Fiscella K, Bennett M, Szilagyi PG (2008) Nomenclature in translational research. JAMA 299:2148–2149

20. Lean M, Mann J, Hoek J, Elliot R, Schofield G (2008) Translational research. BMJ 337:a863

21. Dougherty D, Conway PH (2008) The "3T's" roadmap to transform US health care. The "how" of high-quality care. JAMA 299(19): 2319–2321

22. Khoury MJ, Gwinn M, Yoon PW, Dowling N, Moore CA, Bradley L (2007) The continuum of translation research in genomic medicine: how can we accelerate the appropriate integration of human genomic discoveries into health care and disease prevention? Genet Med 9(10):665–674

23. Agurs-Collins T, Khoury MJ, Simon-Morton D, Olster DH, Harris JR, Milner JA (2008) Public health genomics: translating obesity genomics research into population health benefits. Obesity 16(3):s85–s94

24. Khoury MJ, Gwinn M, Ioannidis JPA (2010) The emergence of translational epidemiology: from scientific discovery to population health impact. Am J Epidemiol 172:517–524

25. Canadian Institutes of Health Research (CIHR) Act. http://laws.justice.gc.ca/eng/acts/c-18.1/page-1.html. Accessed Apr 2014

26. Twells L, Gregory DM, Reddigan J, Midodzi W (2014) Current prevalence and future predictions of obesity in Canada: a trend analysis. CMAJ Open 2(1):18–26

27. Lau DC, Douketis JD, Morrison KM et al (2007) 2006 Canadian clinical practice guidelines on the management and prevention of obesity in adults and children [summary]. CMAJ 176:1103–1106

28. Twells LK, Bridger T, Knight JC et al (2012) Obesity predicts primary health care visits: a cohort study. Popul Health Manag 15:29–36

29. Flegal KM, Kit BK, Orpana H et al (2013) Association of all-cause mortality with overweight and obesity using standardized body mass index categories. A systematic review and meta-analysis. JAMA 309:71–82

30. Kolotkin RL, Crosby RD, Williams GR (2002) Health related quality of life varies among obese subgroups. Obesity 10(8):748–756

31. Anis AH, Zhang W, Bansback N, Guh DP, Amasi Z, Birmingham CL (2010) Obesity and overweight in Canada: an updated cost-of-illness study. Obes Rev 11:31–40

32. Public Health Agency of Canada (2011) Obesity in Canada. Public Health Agency of Canada Canadian Institute for Health Information, Ottawa, ON

33. Padwal RS, Rueda-Clausaen CF, Sharma AM, Abhorsangaya CB et al (2014) Weight loss and outcomes in wait listed, medically managed and surgically treated patients enrolled in a population based bariatric program. Med Care 52(3):208–215

34. Sjöström L, Nabro K, Sjöström CD et al (2007) Effects of bariatric surgery on mortality on Swedish obese subjects. N Engl J Med 357: 741–752

35. Chang SH, Stoll CR, Colditz GA (2011) Cost-effectiveness of bariatric surgery: should it be universally available? Maturitas 69(2):230–238

36. Christou NV, Sampalis JS, Liverman M et al (2004) Surgery decreases long-term mortality, morbidity and health care use in morbidly obese patients. Ann Surg 240(3):416–423, discussion 423-424

37. Karlsson J, Taft C, Tyden A, Sjöström L, Sullivan M (2007) Ten year trends in health-related quality of life after surgical and conventional treatment for sever obesity: the SOS intervention study. Int J Obes 31:1248–1261

38. Shi X, Karmali S, Sharma AM, Birch DW (2010) A review of laparoscopic sleeve gastrectomy for morbid obesity. Obes Surg 20:1171–1177

39. Buchwald H, Oien D (2013) Metabolic/bariatric surgery worldwide 2011. Obes Surg 23:427–436

40. CIHR Institute of Nutrition, Metabolism and Diabetes and the Canadian Obesity Network (2010) Developing a research agenda to support bariatric care in Canada. Workshop report. December 8–10 2010, Montreal, QC. CIHR Institute of Nutrition, Metabolism and Diabetes and the Canadian Obesity Network, Ottawa, ON

41. American Society for Metabolic and Bariatric Surgery (2010) Updated position statement on sleeve gastrectomy as a bariatric procedure. Surg Obes Relat Dis 6(1):1–5

42. Klarenbach S, Padwal R, Wiebe N, Hazel M, Birch D, Manns B, Karmali S, Sharma A, Tonnelli M (2010) Bariatric surgery for severe obesity: systematic review and economic evaluation. [Internet]. (CADTH technology report; no.129). Canadian Agency for Drugs and Technologies in Health, Ottawa, ON, http://www.cadth.ca/index.php/en/hta/reports-publications/search/publication/2665. Accessed 28 Feb 2011

43. Canadian Institutes of Health Research (CIHR) funding opportunity: meetings, planning and dissemination grant

44. Temple Newhook JR, Gregory DM, Twells LK (2013) The road to obesity: weight loss surgery candidates talk about their histories of weight gain. J Soc Behav Health Sci 7(1):35–51

45. Gregory DM, Temple Newhook J, Twells LK (2013) Patients' perceptions of waiting for bariatric surgery: a qualitative study. Int J Equity Health 12(1):86. doi:10.1186/10.1186/1475-9276-12-86

46. Price H, Gregory D, Twells LK (2013) Weight loss expectations of laparoscopic sleeve gastrectomy candidates compared to clinically expected weight loss outcomes 1-year post surgery. Obes Surg 23(12):1983–1987. doi:10.1007/s11695-013-1007-y

47. Salsberg P, MacaulayMC (2014) CIHR guide to researcher and knowledge user collaboration in health research. http://www.cihr-irsc.gc.ca/e/44954.html. Accessed Apr 2014

48. Templeton J (2014) Unlocking the evidence: the role of the evidence informed practice council in supporting knowledge translation in Eastern Health. Presentation. http://www.easternhealth.ca/downfile.aspx?fileid=437. Accessed Apr 2014

Resources

Canadian Institutes of Health Research. (2005). About Knowledge Translation and Commercialization. Ottawa: Canada. http://www.cihr-irsc.gc.ca/e/29418.html Accessed April 2014

Canadian Institutes of Health Research. More about Knowledge Translation at CIHR. Ottawa: Canada. http://www.cihr-irsc.gc.ca/e/39033.html Accessed April 2014

Canadian Institutes of Health Research. Guide to Knowledge Translation Planning at CIHR: Integration and End-of-Grant Approaches. (2012). Ottawa: CIHR. http://www.cihr-irsc.gc.ca/e/45321.html Accessed April 2014

Canadian Institutes of Health Research. Knowledge Translation in Health Care. http://www.cihr-irsc.gc.ca/e/40618.html Accessed April 2014

Canadian Institutes of Health Research. (2008). A Knowledge Translation Casebook. http://www.cihr-irsc.gc.ca/e/38764.html Accessed April 2014

Canadian Institutes of Health Research. (2010). An End-of-Grant Knowledge Translation Casebook. http://www.cihr-irsc.gc.ca/e/41594.html Accessed April 2014

Canadian Institutes of Health Research. Knowledge Translation and Commercialization Publications. Learning Modules. http://www.cihr-irsc.gc.ca/e/39128.html Accessed April 2014

Knowledge Translation in Health Care: Moving from Evidence to Practice. 2nd ed. (2013). Straus, S.E., Tetroe, J., Graham, I. (eds). Wiley: BMJ Books

Evidence-Based Decision-Making 6: Utilization of Administrative Databases for Health Services Research

Tanvir Turin Chowdhury and Brenda Hemmelgarn

Abstract

Health-care systems require reliable information on which to base health-care planning and make decisions, as well as to evaluate their policy impact. Administrative data provide important information about health services use, expenditures, clinical outcomes, and may be used to assess quality of care. With increased digitalization and accessibility of administrative databases, these data are more readily available for health service research purposes, aiding evidence-based decision-making. This chapter discusses the utility of administrative data for population-based studies of health and health care.

Key words Administrative databases, Health service research, Population-based studies

1 What Are Administrative Data?

In general terms, a database is any compilation of information on characteristics and events stored in an organized manner, which can be used to analyze and answer a specific question [1–3]. Administrative data are collected for purposes other than research, by governments or specific programs, but can be used for research purposes. Some examples of such data recorded by administrative systems are vital statistics records, census data, worker's compensation records, insurance claim records, etc. Administrative health databases collect information on individuals registered with health-care plans or utilizing health services [4, 5] including—tracking service use, monitoring quality of health-care delivery, as well as tracking payments and health plan enrollment. Depending upon the source, such information may include the characteristics of inpatient and outpatient encounters, physicians' visits, provision of home care, stays in chronic and acute care facilities such as nursing homes and hospitals [6, 7], or prescriptions. While not produced explicitly to examine the health or health care of populations, administrative data nevertheless offer important advantages for research. Administrative health databases represent large groups of

Patrick S. Parfrey and Brendan J. Barrett (eds.), *Clinical Epidemiology: Practice and Methods*, Methods in Molecular Biology, vol. 1281, DOI 10.1007/978-1-4939-2428-8_28, © Springer Science+Business Media New York 2015

the population, sometimes an entire population defined by geographic locality (e.g., all persons hospitalized in a province). These databases allow linkage of information concerning individuals between different databases, and linkage of information over periods of time can allow for longitudinal studies over extended periods and various health-care settings. These types of databases already exist in the governmental infrastructure and are relatively inexpensive to acquire, and can be relatively easily used.

2   Potential Sources of Administrative Health Data

Administrative health data are generally derived from documentation of health status monitoring or health-care delivery. There are generally government registries of various types including population and disease registries. A common registry, which exists in most countries, is the registry of vital events such as births and deaths. These can be used to provide a range of demographic statistics often in combination with census or survey data. Other administrative data may be available from government programs that provide entitlements or benefits (e.g., social security). There are also administrative systems that provide details of transactions regarding health-care expenditures. Data on hospital visits may provide useful information on morbidity for specific diseases. Statistics regarding health-care related costs are generally taken from Government financial statistics, private health-care providers' records, or health insurance records. Table 1 provides an overview of some administrative health databases across regions.

3   Administrative Health Database Creation

As health administrative data are collected for purposes other than research, there are challenges in converting these data for research use while providing accurate and valid estimation of disease and risk. Administrative health data in its raw form may not be suitable for immediate analysis. Researchers and analysts often need to manipulate the data into a more readily analyzable form prior to further use. Depending on the source of the data, raw data may include specific variables such as patient identifiers, demographics, clinical information on diagnosis, comorbidities and prescriptions, service utilization, hospital costs, and physician billing data [2, 6]. These data are used to derive new variables for more sophisticated analyses and evaluations, for instance to define an outcome based on a validated algorithm, the use of patients' postal code to derive travel distance to care facilities [9, 10], frequency of prescription refills to assess therapy adherence [11] and data on race to determine variation and access to care across ethnic groups [7].

Table 1
Examples of administrative databases[a]

Country	Database coverage	Type of database	Type of information available
Canada	Provincial Health Authority Databases	Physicians claims	Date, location of service, diagnostic code, provider specialty, cost
		Inpatient encounters	Admission and discharge dates, diagnostic and procedure costs, costs, case-mix group
		Ambulatory care	Date, nature and location of service, diagnostic and procedure costs, costs, case-mix group
		Medication	Formulary drugs, prescription date, cost, and quantity
		Registry	Date of birth, gender, address
USA	Age 65 and older and younger people with disabilities	Medicare	Diagnoses, procedure codes, costs, length of stay in hospitals, comorbidities, outcomes, ambulatory care, prescription
	American Veterans	Veterans Affairs	Diagnoses, procedure codes, costs, length of stay in hospitals, comorbidities, outcomes, ambulatory care, prescription
	Low income residents	Medicaid	Diagnoses, procedure codes, costs, length of stay in hospitals, comorbidities, outcomes, ambulatory care, prescription
	Regional and privately funded	Kaiser Permanente	Diagnoses, procedure codes, costs, length of stay in hospitals, comorbidities, outcomes, ambulatory care, prescription
UK	Primary care	General Practice Research Database	Demographics, diagnoses, prescriptions, referrals, smoking status, height, weight, immunizations, laboratory results
	Primary care	The Health Improvement Network	Demographics, diagnoses, prescriptions, referrals, smoking status, height, weight, immunizations, laboratory results, physicians' notes
Sweden	National	Swedish National Cause of Death Register	Demographics, underlying cause of death, comorbidities.

(continued)

Table 1
(continued)

Country	Database coverage	Type of database	Type of information available
	National	Swedish Hospital Discharge Register	Diagnoses, procedure codes, costs, length of stay in hospitals
The Netherlands	National	The National Hospital Discharge Register	Patient data, admission and discharge data, diagnoses, surgical procedures, and the medical specialties
Finland	National	Finnish Hospital Discharge Register	Diagnoses, procedure codes, costs, length of stay in hospitals, comorbidities, outcomes
Australia	Regional	Western Australian Health Services Research Linked Database	Birth records, midwives' notifications, cancer registrations, inpatient hospital morbidity, inpatient and public outpatient mental health services data, and death records
	National	National Hospital Morbidity Database	Diagnoses, procedure codes, costs, length of stay in hospitals, comorbidities, outcomes
	National	Medicare Australia	Patient data, claims, provider information, service provided, cost
	National	Pharmaceutical Benefits Scheme	Patient information, prescription, medication description, related cost
Japan	National	Japanese Diagnosis Procedure Combination Inpatient Database	Patients' age and sex, diagnoses, procedures, drugs and devices used, lengths of stay, inhospital mortality

[a]Modified and extended from Bello et al. [8]

The overall quality of information contained in administrative databases varies widely. For some conditions and procedures that are explicitly identifiable, such as stroke and myocardial infarction, coding is reasonably good [12, 13]. On the other hand, it is poor for conditions which are more nonspecific, such as chronic kidney disease [14]. Further, variability of structural components of the data (e.g., number of data fields available for entries) may also influence accuracy. Additionally, complex issues (e.g., filtering of data by those doing the coding) might also influence accuracy. The coding detail may also be influenced by payment procedures. Because health-care providers are paid for specific procedures, procedures are generally coded more accurately and completely than diagnoses. A procedure with a high remunerative value has a greater probability of being coded properly than a less remunerative procedure [15]. Imperfect coding is especially problematical for chronic conditions. It has been reported that hospitals under-code chronic diseases, especially for acutely ill patients [4, 16, 17].

A key step in disease ascertainment using health administrative data is to develop a disease definition that uses the diagnostic and treatment codes from the physician billing and hospital discharge databases to identify individuals with the disease [14, 18, 19]. The combined input of clinical experts and knowledgeable data analysts is used to ensure validity of the definition. This process can often involve several iterations of a given methodology and developing a single case ascertainment definition can be a sizable research project on its own. New case definitions should then be validated using chart review or population health surveys that are considered the gold standard. Thus, the accuracy of health administrative data depends not only on the quality of the data but also on the explicit condition being identified and the validity of the coding algorithm in the patient group [12, 14, 18, 20].

It is important to note that administrative health databases differ across countries, regions and groups due to varying health policies, governance structure, technological facilities, and socio-economic settings [2, 4, 6, 21, 22]. For example, the comprehensiveness of information from administrative databases observed in Canada is mainly due to the existence of universal health-care coverage across all provinces. Available data include measures of disease burden, health-care distribution, prevention activities, outcome measurements and assessment of effectiveness of interventions [5, 23, 24].

4 Using Administrative Data for Research Purposes

Despite their administrative origins, these data have provided important insights into health-care practices. More than four decades ago, Wennberg and Gittlesohn [25, 26] used hospital discharge data to expose wide variations in rates of expensive medical interventions across small geographic areas with ostensibly similar populations. In the late 1980s, these and other previously unexplained variations (e.g., in hospital mortality rates, also identified using administrative data) precipitated an "era of assessment and accountability" in American health care [21, 27]. During the early 1990s Gabriel et al. estimated medical and nonmedical costs incurred among a population-based prevalence cohort of individuals with osteoarthritis where osteoarthritis status for each individual was ascertained from a physician diagnosis variable [28]. Administrative data figured prominently in plans to assess the effectiveness of outcomes of care rendered in communities. The Agency for Health Care Policy and Research stipulated the use of large administrative databases to examine the "outcomes, effectiveness, and appropriateness" of health care services with flagship administrative data projects initiated by the Patient Outcomes Research Teams (PORTs) [29–31]. Also, some European countries, notably Denmark, the Netherlands, Sweden, and Finland, have placed much greater emphasis on developing national register data since the 1980s, to replace national censuses and major surveys. For example, Statistics Denmark bases most of its national statistics on "register data" that can be linked both longitudinally and between registers of different types (e.g., health, education, income). In addition, Danish surveys are frequently supplemented with register data on income, health, welfare benefits, housing, etc. allowing objective information to be compared to the responses from survey responses.

5   Data Linkage with Other Data Sources

Reports in the USA [32], Canada [33], the UK [34], and Australia [35] have recommended increasing the use of existing data, such as administrative source data and clinical registry data, to provide comparative clinical performance on health services, hospitals, clinical units, and clinicians for internal use and to consumers via publicly accessible media. Although a limited number of patient outcomes, such as inhospital mortality, complication, and readmission rates, are currently available from some administrative data sources, obtaining data from several different databases that pertain to a specific individual or participant using data linkage is often necessary to ensure adequate risk-adjustment and examine a more comprehensive range of outcomes for comparison.

Data or record linkage has been defined as "a process of pairing records from two files and trying to select the pairs that belong to the same entity [36]." In the UK, 47 % of multicenter clinical databases surveyed in 2003 by Black et al. reported that they undertook routine data linkage with other databases [37]. A review by Evans et al. reported that 68 % of Australian clinical registries routinely undertook some form of data linkage to obtain outcome information, such as death or disease status, and to assess data quality [38]. The use of data linkage in research studies has increased almost sixfold within the last two decades. This proliferation of data linkage is reflected in the establishment of data linkage research centers and initiatives in Australia [39], Canada [40, 41], and the UK [42, 43].

Merging administrative data with other data sources can efficiently enrich the overall database. There are various ways in which extracts of administrative data can be linked with other data sources to create more comprehensive and effective datasets for analysis. It is not always easy to combine an administrative source with another source of information. This is especially true when a common matching key for both sources is not available and record linkage techniques are used. In this case, the type of linkage methodology (e.g., definitive matching or probabilistic matching) is selected in accordance with the objectives of the research program. Administrative data can be successfully linked with a variety of other data sources, for example:

> Linking individual level administrative data with other individual level administrative data via a unique identifier or probabilistic matching methods (matching personal details like names, date of birth, gender, address, etc.).

> Linking individual level administrative data with cross-sectional or longitudinal survey data usually via matching methods.

> Linking individual level administrative data with contextual information on, for example, the neighborhood (postal code based socioeconomic classification in Canada) or organization relevant to the individual (e.g., hospital or primary care clinic attended).

6 Example of a Population-Based Linkage of Health Records in Alberta, Canada: Development of a Health Services Research Administrative Database

An example of broad application of administrative databases to health-care planning for patients with chronic diseases is the administrative database developed for the Interdisciplinary Chronic Disease Collaboration (ICDC, www.ICDC.ca) [23]. This initiative has been formed by linking multiple data sources which originally were for administrative use; the Alberta Kidney Disease Network (AKDN, www.AKDN.info) [41] and Alberta Health (AH) data sources (Fig. 1) which includes data on >3 million Albertans. Available data allow assessment of risk evaluation, case identification, rate and pattern of disease progression, complication rates, and associated costs—which can all be used to guide policy direction. The ICDC repository was developed by linking laboratory data to administrative and other computerized data sources to allow assessment of socio-demographic characteristics, clinical variables, and health outcomes.

A unique provincial health number, provided to all the residents of Alberta by the provincial government, is used to link Alberta Government data with the pan-province laboratory database and a number of other data sources including the provincial drugs program databases [23, 41]. The Alberta Health (AH) provincial health ministry provides basic health insurance to all residents of the province through a universally available health-care plan and the insured residents are included in the AH database. This database allows the estimation of the prevalence of chronic

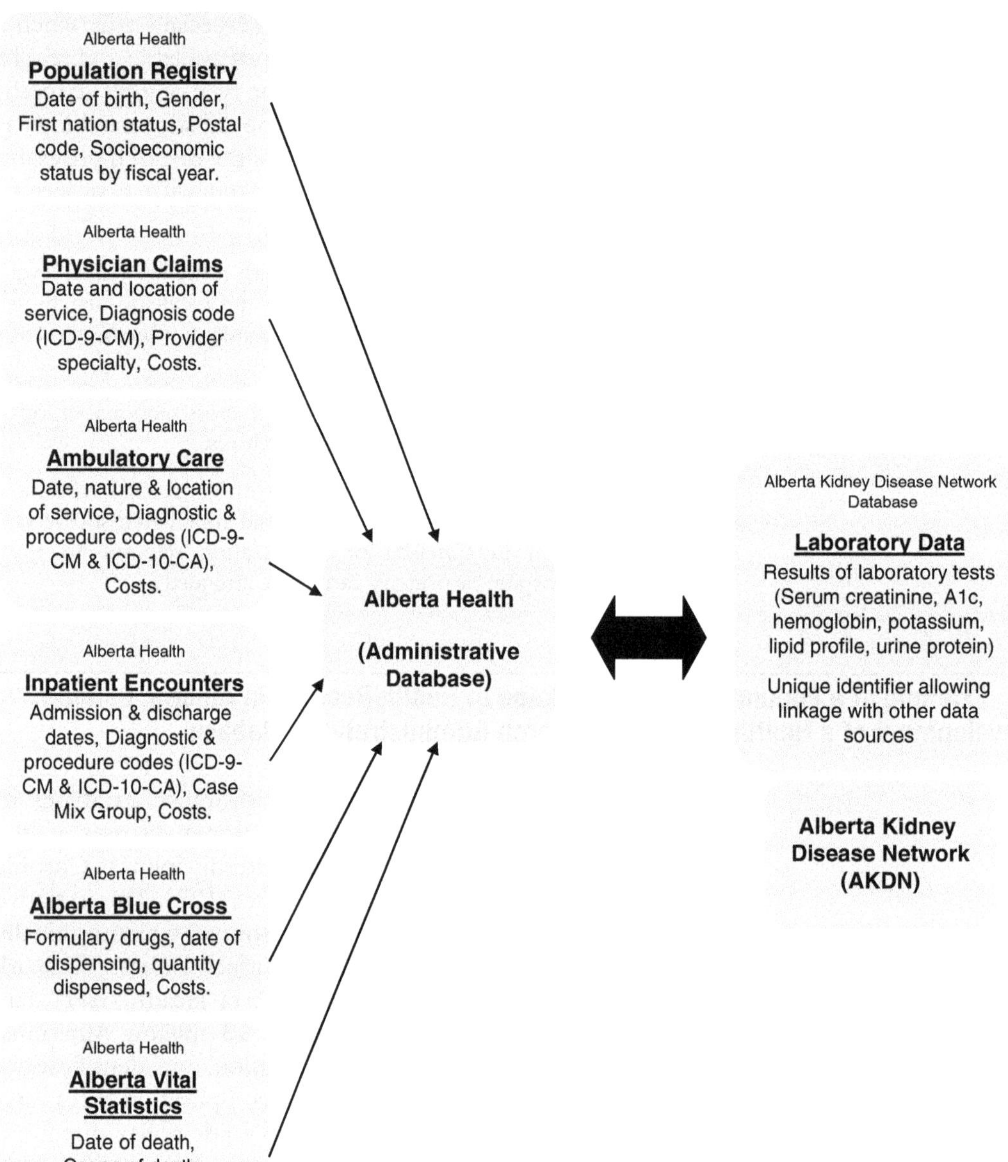

Fig. 1 Example of a Computerized Database. Alberta Health (AH) maintains administrative data for Alberta. The Alberta Kidney Disease Network (AKDN) has developed a process for retrieval, storage, and maintenance of laboratory data and relevant laboratory tests for all patients who have these measurements across the province of Alberta. A data repository is created by linkage between AH administrative data and AKDN lab data and has been used for assessment of outcomes, including health services utilization and mortality for patients with laboratory tests measured. Adapted from Hemmelgarn BR et al. [41]

disease conditions, continuous assessment of health-care utilization, monitoring of the adequacy of the current care through examination of quality indicators, service deliverables, health outcomes, and costs data.

The ICDC databases [13, 26] include basic demographic data for the residents to provide information on the burden of disease and care disparities across various racial and ethnic groups such as First Nations (Aboriginal), Asian (Chinese and South Asian) ethnicity and also by socioeconomic status [44–46]. The database also contains residents' postal code and this enables the unique opportunity for geographic information system analyses on access to care issues (e.g., travel distance or time as factor of health-care access/utilization) [47, 48]. The drug data available from prescription claims enables studies about medication utilization, medication related costs, and clinical outcomes [41, 49]. Table 2 shows

Table 2
Examples of research studies done using ICDC administrative database to address key health issues

Objectives	Authors	Examples of studies conducted using the administrative database
Estimating disease burden	Hemmelgarn et al. [52]	Rates of treated and untreated kidney failure in older vs younger adults
	Turin et al. [51]	Lifetime risk of ESRD
	Turin et al. [50]	Chronic kidney disease and life expectancy
Identification of risk and disease/risk stratification	Hemmelgarn et al. [54]	Relation between kidney function, proteinuria, and adverse outcomes
	Shurraw et al. [55]	Association between glycemic control and adverse outcomes in people with diabetes mellitus and chronic kidney disease: a population-based cohort study
	Turin et al. [56]	Proteinuria and rate of change in kidney function in a community-based population.
	Alexander et al. [57]	Kidney stones and kidney function loss: a cohort study
	Tonelli et al. [58]	Using proteinuria and estimated glomerular filtration rate to classify risk in patients with chronic kidney disease: a cohort study
Case definition and validation	Ronksley et al. [14]	Validating a case definition for chronic kidney disease using administrative data.
	Clement et al. [20]	Validation of a case definition to define chronic dialysis using outpatient administrative data.
Socioeconomic status, First Nations status, ethnicity as risk factor	Chou et al. [59]	Quality of care among Aboriginal hemodialysis patients.

(continued)

Table 2
(continued)

Objectives	Authors	Examples of studies conducted using the administrative database
	Conley et al. [44]	Association between GFR, proteinuria, and adverse outcomes among white, Chinese, and South Asian individuals in Canada
	Samuel et al. [45]	Association between First Nations ethnicity and progression to kidney failure by presence and severity of albuminuria
Geographic location as risk factor	Faruque et al. [48]	Spatial analysis to locate new clinics for diabetic kidney patients in the underserved communities in Alberta
	Ayyalasomayajula et al. [47]	A novel technique to optimize facility locations of new nephrology services for remote areas.
	Tonelli et al. [60]	Association between proximity to the attending nephrologist and mortality among patients receiving hemodialysis.
Quantification of utilization of physician encounters, hospitalization risk and complications.	Ronksley et al. [61]	Patterns of engagement with the health care system and risk of subsequent hospitalization amongst patients with diabetes
	Rucker et al. [9]	Quality of care and mortality are worse in chronic kidney disease patients living in remote areas.
	James et al. [62]	CKD and risk of hospitalization and death with pneumonia.
Health-care costs	McBrien et al. [53]	Health care costs in people with diabetes and their association with glycemic control and kidney function.
	Manns et al. [63]	Population based screening for chronic kidney disease: cost effectiveness study
	Wiebe et al. [10]	Adding Specialized Clinics for Remote-Dwellers with Chronic Kidney Disease: A Cost-Utility Analysis
Resource utilization in health care	Hemmelgarn et al. [64]	Nephrology visits and health care resource use before and after reporting estimated glomerular filtration rate
	Manns et al. [65]	Enrolment in primary care networks: impact on outcomes and processes of care for patients with diabetes.
Knowledge translation	Hemmelgarn et al. [23]	The research to health policy cycle: a tool for better management of chronic non-communicable diseases.

(continued)

Table 2
(continued)

Objectives	Authors	Examples of studies conducted using the administrative database
	Hemmelgarn et al. [66]	Knowledge translation for nephrologists: strategies for improving the identification of patients with proteinuria.
Outcome research	Turin et al. [67]	One-year change in kidney function is associated with an increased mortality risk.
	Turin et al. [68]	Short-term change in kidney function and risk of end-stage renal disease.
	Turin et al. [69]	Change in the estimated glomerular filtration rate over time and risk of all-cause mortality
	Hemmelgarn et al. [54]	Relation between kidney function, proteinuria, and adverse outcomes.

specific examples of studies done using the ICDC administrative data to address key issues in health services research. Data from hospitalizations, health-care expenditures, emergency room records, ambulatory care information, and adverse outcomes are captured for analysis in combination with laboratory data for clinical, population health, as well as policy-relevant research [50–54].

7   Pros and Cons of Using Administrative Data

Table 3 summarizes the advantages and disadvantages of using administrative databases for research. Administrative databases have some advantages over data acquired from primary surveys or primary data collection studies [2, 4, 12, 14, 21]. Generally, administrative data capture a wider population than what is possible in primary studies. Also, administrative databases can be used for a relatively longer follow-up of the study population. Additionally, administrative data are often more cost-effective to obtain than the primarily designed studies or surveys [3, 4]. There are some limitations of administrative database usage that need to be considered for research purposes. First, administrative data are usually not obtained for research purposes [5, 22], thus they may be compromised in terms of data quality as well as generalizability for the observed estimates. Second, administrative data are limited to records obtained for the purposes of reimbursement like physician claims data or drug benefit repayment data, or tracking/monitoring

Table 3
Advantages and disadvantages of administrative data

Advantages of administrative data
• Already collected for operational purposes, thus no additional costs for data collection purposes. Although there are costs for data-management (e.g., extraction, mining, cleaning) activities.
• Data collection process nonintrusive to catchment population.
• These data are generally updated on a regular interval. In some scenarios the update is a continuous process.
• This type of data can provide historical information and allow consistent time-series to be established.
• Collected in a consistent way if part of systematic collection.
• Usually subject to rigorous quality checks for the data collection process.
• Generally a large number of individuals are covered.
• Individuals who may not respond to surveys can be captured.
• Potential for datasets to be linked to various other data sources to develop extensive research resources
Disadvantages of administrative data
• As these are primarily collected for administrative purposes—the data is limited to uses regarding research related to services and administrative questions. For clinical research, this data source has limited usage.
• There is lack of researcher control over contents of the data.
• Proxy indicators sometimes have to be used.
• Any changes to administrative processes could change definitions and this can make comparison over time difficult.
• Quality issues with variables less important to the data vendor (e.g., address details may not be updated).
• Data privacy and protection issues are matter of concern for access of this type of databases.
• Access for researchers is dependent on support of administrative authorities that are the data custodians.

health-care service delivery. Detailed clinical information such as blood pressure and lifestyle related factors such as smoking, drinking, exercise or dietary information, as well as patient-centered potential factors such as patients' satisfaction may not be available. Third, administrative database use for research purposes has been criticized due to the lack of validation for certain characteristics, such as diagnosis of chronic obstructive lung disease and mental health or other clinical outcomes. The researchers focusing on the administrative database usage are working on the development of validated algorithms for case or exposure definitions around the world. Fourth, lack of researchers' control on the population selection may result in variable follow-up and potentially non-generalizable study populations when compared with well-designed population-based cohort studies.

Although administrative databases are primarily intended for health administration and funding, they play an important role in health services research including program management, oversight and policymaking, examining population health and overall disease burden, and quality of care. Recognizing that they may lack some detailed clinical information, administrative data have the potential to provide a relatively cost-effective, less intrusive, and comprehensive resource for research.

References

1. Iezzoni LI (1997) Assessing quality using administrative data. Ann Intern Med 127:666–674

2. Cowper DC, Hynes DM, Kubal JD, Murphy PA (1999) Using administrative databases for outcomes research: select examples from VA health services research and development. J Med Syst 23:249–259

3. Fantini M, Cisbani L, Manzoli L, Vertrees J, Lorenzoni L (2003) On the use of administrative databases to support planning activities the case of the evaluation of neonatal case-mix in the Emilia-Romagna region using DRG and APR-DRG classification systems. Eur J Public Health 13:138–145

4. Malenka DJ, McLerran D, Roos N, Fisher ES, Wennberg JE (1994) Using administrative data to describe casemix: a comparison with the medical record. J Clin Epidemiol 47:1027–1032

5. Ray WA (1997) Policy and program analysis using administrative databases. Ann Intern Med 127:712–718

6. Virnig BA, McBean M (2001) Administrative data for public health surveillance and planning. Annu Rev Public Health 22:213–230

7. Tricco AC, Pham B, Rawson NS (2008) Manitoba and Saskatchewan administrative health care utilization databases are used differently to answer epidemiologic research questions. J Clin Epidemiol 61:192–197.e112

8. Bello A, Hemmelgarn B, Manns B, Tonelli M (2012) Use of administrative databases for health-care planning in CKD. Nephrol Dial Transplant 27:iii12–iii18

9. Rucker D, Hemmelgarn BR, Lin M, Manns BJ, Klarenbach SW, Ayyalasomayajula B, James MT, Bello A, Gordon D, Jindal KK (2011) Quality of care and mortality are worse in chronic kidney disease patients living in remote areas. Kidney Int 79:210–217

10. Wiebe N, Klarenbach SW, Chui B, Ayyalasomayajula B, Hemmelgarn BR, Jindal K, Manns B, Tonelli M (2012) Adding specialized clinics for remote-dwellers with chronic kidney disease: a cost-utility analysis. Clin J Am Soc Nephrol 7:24–34

11. Suissa S, Garbe E (2007) Primer: administrative health databases in observational studies of drug effects—advantages and disadvantages. Nat Clin Pract Rheumatol 3:725–732

12. Kokotailo RA, Hill MD (2005) Coding of stroke and stroke risk factors using international classification of diseases, revisions 9 and 10. Stroke 36:1776–1781

13. Peter CA, Paul AD, Jack VT (2002) A multicenter study of the coding accuracy of hospital discharge administrative data for patients admitted to cardiac care units in Ontario. Am Heart J 144:290–296

14. Ronksley PE, Tonelli M, Quan H, Manns BJ, James MT, Clement FM, Samuel S, Quinn RR, Ravani P, Brar SS (2012) Validating a case definition for chronic kidney disease using administrative data. Nephrol Dial Transplant 27:1826–1831

15. Grimes DA (2010) Epidemiologic research using administrative databases: garbage in, garbage out. Obstet Gynecol 116:1018–1019

16. Iezzoni L, Foley S, Daley J, Hughes J, Fisher E, Heeren T (1991) Comorbidities, complications, and coding bias. Does the number of diagnosis codes matter in predicting in-hospital mortality? JAMA 267:2197–2203

17. Jollis JG, Ancukiewicz M, DeLong ER, Pryor DB, Muhlbaier LH, Mark DB (1993) Discordance of databases designed for claims payment versus clinical information systems: implications for outcomes research. Ann Intern Med 119:844–850

18. Hux JE, Ivis F, Flintoft V, Bica A (2002) Diabetes in Ontario: determination of

prevalence and incidence using a validated administrative data algorithm. Diabetes Care 25:512–516

19. Quan H, Sundararajan V, Halfon P, Fong A, Burnand B, Luthi J-C, Saunders LD, Beck CA, Feasby TE, Ghali WA (2005) Coding algorithms for defining comorbidities in ICD-9-CM and ICD-10 administrative data. Med Care 43:1130–1139

20. Clement FM, James MT, Chin R, Klarenbach SW, Manns BJ, Quinn RR, Ravani P, Tonelli M, Hemmelgarn BR (2011) Validation of a case definition to define chronic dialysis using outpatient administrative data. BMC Med Res Methodol 11:25

21. Jones SS, Adams JL, Schneider EC, Ringel JS, McGlynn EA (2010) Electronic health record adoption and quality improvement in US hospitals. Am J Manag Care 16:SP64–SP71

22. Lillard LA, Farmer MM (1997) Linking Medicare and national survey data. Ann Intern Med 127:691–695

23. Interdisciplinary Chronic Disease Collaboration (2008) The research to health policy cycle: a tool for better management of chronic noncommunicable diseases. J Nephrol 21:621–631

24. Black N (2001) Evidence based policy: proceed with care. BMJ 323:275

25. Wennberg J, Gittelsohn A (1973) Small area variations in health care delivery a population-based health information system can guide planning and regulatory decision-making. Science 182:1102–1108

26. Relman AS (1988) Assessment and accountability: the third revolution in medical care. N Engl J Med 319:1220

27. Roper WL, Winkenwerder W, Hackbarth GM, Krakauer H (1988) Effectiveness in health care. An initiative to evaluate and improve medical practice. N Engl J Med 319:1197

28. Gabriel S, Crowson C, O'Fallon W (1995) Costs of osteoarthritis: estimates from a geographically defined population. J Rheumatol Suppl 43:23–25

29. Clancy CM, Eisenberg JM (1997) Outcomes research at the agency for health care policy and research. Dis Manage Clin Outcomes 1:72–80

30. Lave JR, Pashos CL, AndersonN G, Brailer D, Bubolz T, Conrad D, Freund DA, Fox SH, Keeler E, Lipscomb J (1994) Costing medical care: using Medicare administrative data. Med Care 32:JS77

31. Mitchell JB, Bubolz T, Paul JE, Pashos CL, Escarce JJ, Muhlbaier LH, Wiesman JM, Young WW, EPSTEIN R, Javitt JC (1994) Using Medicare claims for outcomes research. Med Care 32:JS38

32. Institute of Medicine Committee on Quality of Health in America (2001) Crossing the quality chasm: a new health system for the 21st century. National academies press, Washington, DC, pp 1–337

33. Canadian Institute for Health Information (2004) Health care in Canada 2004. Cihi, Ottawa

34. The Bristol Royal Infirmary inquiry: the report of the public inquiry into children's heart surgery at the Bristol Royal Infirmary 1984–1995. London, UK 2001

35. National Health and Hospitals Reform Commission (Australia). Australia. Dept. of health and ageing (2009) A healthier future for all Australians final report June 2009. Dept. of health and ageing, Canberra, a.C.T

36. Winglee M, Valliant R, Scheuren F (2005) A case study in record linkage. Surv Methodol 31:3–11

37. Black N, Barker M, Payne M (2004) Cross sectional survey of multicentre clinical databases in the United Kingdom. BMJ 328:1478

38. Evans S, Bohensky M, Cameron P, McNeil J (2011) A survey of Australian clinical registries: can quality of care be measured? Intern Med J 41:42–48

39. Holman CAJ, Bass AJ, Rouse IL, Hobbs MS (1999) Population-based linkage of health records in Western Australia: development of a health services research linked database. Aust N Z J Public Health 23:453–459

40. Chamberlayne R, Green B, Barer ML, Hertzman C, Lawrence WJ, Sheps SB (1997) Creating a population-based linked health database: a new resource for health services research. Can J Public Health 89:270–273

41. Hemmelgarn BR, Clement F, Manns BJ, Klarenbach S, James MT, Ravani P, Pannu N, Ahmed SB, MacRae J, Jindal K, Quinn R, Culleton BF, Wiebe N, Krause R, Thorlacius L, Tonelli M (2009) Overview of the Alberta kidney disease network. BMC Nephrol 10:30

42. Acheson E, Evans J (1964) The Oxford record linkage study: a review of the method with some preliminary results. Proc R Soc Med 57:269

43. Kendrick S, Clarke J (1993) The Scottish record linkage system. Health Bull (Edinb) 51:72–79

44. Conley J, Tonelli M, Quan H, Manns BJ, Palacios-Derflingher L, Bresee LC, Khan N, Hemmelgarn BR (2012) Association between GFR, proteinuria, and adverse outcomes among White, Chinese, and South Asian individuals in Canada. Am J Kidney Dis 59:390–399

45. Samuel SM, Palacios-Derflingher L, Tonelli M, Manns B, Crowshoe L, Ahmed SB, Jun M, Saad N, Hemmelgarn BR (2013) Association between First Nations ethnicity and progression to kidney failure by presence and severity of albuminuria. CMAJ 186:E86–E94, 130776

46. Deved V, Jette N, Quan H, Tonelli M, Manns B, Soo A, Barnabe C, Hemmelgarn BR (2013) Quality of care for First Nations and non-First Nations People with diabetes. Clin J Am Soc Nephrol 8:1188–1194

47. Ayyalasomayajula B, Wiebe N, Hemmelgarn BR, Bello A, Manns B, Klarenbach S, Tonelli M (2011) A novel technique to optimize facility locations of new nephrology services for remote areas. Clin J Am Soc Nephrol 6: 2157–2164

48. Faruque LI, Ayyalasomayajula B, Pelletier R, Klarenbach S, Hemmelgarn BR, Tonelli M (2012) Spatial analysis to locate new clinics for diabetic kidney patients in the underserved communities in Alberta. Nephrol Dial Transplant 27:4102–4109

49. Schorr M, Hemmelgarn BR, Tonelli M, Soo A, Manns BJ, Bresee LC (2013) Assessment of serum creatinine and kidney function among incident metformin users. Can J Diabetes 37:226–230

50. Turin TC, Tonelli M, Manns BJ, Ravani P, Ahmed SB, Hemmelgarn BR (2012) Chronic kidney disease and life expectancy. Nephrol Dial Transplant 27:3182–3186

51. Turin TC, Tonelli M, Manns BJ, Ahmed SB, Ravani P, James M, Hemmelgarn BR (2012) Lifetime risk of ESRD. J Am Soc Nephrol 23:1569–1578

52. Hemmelgarn BR, James MT, Manns BJ, O'Hare AM, Muntner P, Ravani P, Quinn RR, Turin TC, Tan Z, Tonelli M (2012) Rates of treated and untreated kidney failure in older vs younger adults. JAMA 307:2507–2515

53. McBrien KA, Manns BJ, Chui B, Klarenbach SW, Rabi D, Ravani P, Hemmelgarn B, Wiebe N, Au F, Clement F (2013) Health care costs in people with diabetes and their association with glycemic control and kidney function. Diabetes Care 36:1172–1180

54. Hemmelgarn BR, Manns BJ, Lloyd A, James MT, Klarenbach S, Quinn RR, Wiebe N, Tonelli M (2010) Relation between kidney function, proteinuria, and adverse outcomes. JAMA 303:423–429

55. Shurraw S, Hemmelgarn B, Lin M, Majumdar SR, Klarenbach S, Manns B, Bello A, James M, Turin TC, Tonelli M (2011) Association between glycemic control and adverse outcomes in people with diabetes mellitus and chronic kidney dis-

56. ease: a population-based cohort study. Arch Intern Med 171:1920–1927

56. Turin TC, James M, Ravani P, Tonelli M, Manns BJ, Quinn R, Jun M, Klarenbach S, Hemmelgarn BR (2013) Proteinuria and rate of change in kidney function in a community-based population. J Am Soc Nephrol 24:1661–1667

57. Alexander RT, Hemmelgarn BR, Wiebe N, Bello A, Samuel S, Klarenbach SW, Curhan GC, Tonelli M (2013) Kidney stones and cardiovascular events: a cohort study. Clin J Am Soc Nephrol 04960513

58. Tonelli M, Muntner P, Lloyd A, Manns BJ, James MT, Klarenbach S, Quinn RR, Wiebe N, Hemmelgarn BR (2011) Using proteinuria and estimated glomerular filtration rate to classify risk in patients with chronic kidney disease: a cohort study. Ann Intern Med 154:12–21

59. Chou SH, Tonelli M, Bradley JS, Gourishankar S, Hemmelgarn BR (2006) Quality of care among aboriginal hemodialysis patients. Clin J Am Soc Nephrol 1:58–63

60. Tonelli M, Manns B, Culleton B, Klarenbach S, Hemmelgarn B, Wiebe N, Gill JS (2007) Association between proximity to the attending nephrologist and mortality among patients receiving hemodialysis. Can Med Assoc J 177:1039–1044

61. Ronksley PE, Ravani P, Sanmartin C, Quan H, Manns B, Tonelli M, Hemmelgarn BR (2013) Patterns of engagement with the health care system and risk of subsequent hospitalization amongst patients with diabetes. BMC Health Serv Res 13:399

62. James MT, Quan H, Tonelli M, Manns BJ, Faris P, Laupland KB, Hemmelgarn BR (2009) CKD and risk of hospitalization and death with pneumonia. Am J Kidney Dis 54:24–32

63. Manns B, Hemmelgarn B, Tonelli M, Au F, Chiasson TC, Dong J, Klarenbach S (2010) Population based screening for chronic kidney disease: cost effectiveness study. BMJ 341:c5869

64. Hemmelgarn BR, Zhang J, Manns BJ, James MT, Quinn RR, Ravani P, Klarenbach SW, Culleton BF, Krause R, Thorlacius L (2010) Nephrology visits and health care resource use before and after reporting estimated glomerular filtration rate. JAMA 303:1151–1158

65. Manns BJ, Tonelli M, Zhang J, Campbell DJ, Sargious P, Ayyalasomayajula B, Clement F, Johnson JA, Laupacis A, Lewanczuk R (2012) Enrolment in primary care networks: impact on outcomes and processes of care for patients with diabetes. Can Med Assoc J 184: E144–E152

66. Hemmelgarn BR, Manns BJ, Straus S, Naugler C, Holroyd-Leduc J, Braun TC, Levin A, Klarenbach S, Lee PF, Hafez K, Schwartz D, Jindal K, Ervin K, Bello A, Turin TC, McBrien K, Elliott M, Tonelli M (2012) Knowledge translation for nephrologists: strategies for improving the identification of patients with proteinuria. J Nephrol 25: 933–943

67. Turin TC, Coresh J, Tonelli M, Stevens PE, de Jong PE, Farmer CKT, Matsushita K, Hemmelgarn BR (2012) One-year change in kidney function is associated with an increased mortality risk. Am J Nephrol 36:41–49

68. Turin TC, Coresh J, Tonelli M, Stevens PE, de Jong PE, Farmer CK, Matsushita K, Hemmelgarn BR (2012) Short-term change in kidney function and risk of end-stage renal disease. Nephrol Dial Transplant 27:3835–3843

69. Turin TC, Coresh J, Tonelli M, Stevens PE, de Jong PE, Farmer CK, Matsushita K, Hemmelgarn BR (2013) Change in the estimated glomerular filtration rate over time and risk of all-cause mortality. Kidney Int 83:684–691

Chapter 29

Evidence-Based Decision-Making 7: Knowledge Translation

Braden J. Manns

Abstract

There is a significant gap between what is known and what is implemented by key stakeholders in practice (the evidence to practice gap). The primary purpose of knowledge translation is to address this gap, bridging evidence to clinical practice. The knowledge to action cycle is one framework for knowledge translation that integrates policy-makers throughout the research cycle. The knowledge to action cycle begins with the identification of a problem (usually a gap in care provision). After identification of the problem, knowledge creation is undertaken, depicted at the center of the cycle as a funnel. Knowledge inquiry is at the wide end of the funnel, and moving down the funnel, the primary data is synthesized into knowledge products in the form of educational materials, guidelines, decision aids, or clinical pathways. The remaining components of the knowledge to action cycle refer to the action of applying the knowledge that has been created. This includes adapting knowledge to local context, assessing barriers to knowledge use, selecting, tailoring implementing interventions, monitoring knowledge use, evaluating outcomes, and sustaining knowledge use. Each of these steps is connected by bidirectional arrows and ideally involves healthcare decision-makers and key stakeholders at each transition.

Key words Knowledge translation, Evidence to practice gap

---

1 What Is Knowledge Translation?

Given the volume of medical information published on a daily basis, physicians and other healthcare providers are not able to keep abreast of the generated evidence, including important studies that could potentially impact clinicians' day-to-day practice. This has generated a gap between what is known and what is implemented by key stakeholders in practice (the evidence to practice gap). This gap is relevant to all those who struggle to keep up with evidence: patients, providers, healthcare planners, and funders. The primary purpose of knowledge translation is to address this gap, bridging evidence to practice.

There is much confusion surrounding the various terms used to describe the knowledge translation process, in addition to the theories of practice change, and strategies for implementation [1].

Patrick S. Parfrey and Brendan J. Barrett (eds.), *Clinical Epidemiology: Practice and Methods*, Methods in Molecular Biology, vol. 1281, DOI 10.1007/978-1-4939-2428-8_29, © Springer Science+Business Media New York 2015

Although it is beyond the scope of this review, others have documented the various terms that have been used to describe this process including knowledge transfer, knowledge exchange, implementation science, knowledge dissemination, among others [2]. The term knowledge translation, which has been formally defined by the Canadian Institutes of Health Research as a "dynamic and iterative process that includes synthesis, dissemination, exchange and ethically sound application of knowledge to improve the health of Canadians, provide more effective health services and products, and strengthen the health care system [3]," is now agreed upon by several Canadian and US funders and institutions and thus will be used throughout this chapter.

2   Frameworks for Knowledge Translation

The framework for knowledge translation that has gained popularity recently is the knowledge to action cycle. This framework integrates policy-makers throughout the research cycle, which enhances the likelihood that interventions developed will be feasible and scalable for health system uptake, if they are demonstrated to offer value for money. A Cochrane systematic review demonstrated that interventions tailored to prospectively identified barriers are more likely to improve professional practice than no intervention or dissemination of guidelines [4]. This, in addition to its intuitive appeal and extensive use by Canadian funding agencies, has led to extensive use of the knowledge to action cycle over the past 10 years by researchers and healthcare organizations.

Other theories and frameworks relating to behavior change have been discussed for achieving knowledge translation. Some of these frameworks are more applicable to behavior change in large organizations. For instance, the Institute for Health Care Improvement Collaborative model, which emphasizes change through shared learning and knowledge by experts and senior healthcare leaders, is often used when considering large-scale change within a healthcare organization [5]. Further details on this are available elsewhere [5].

3   Overview of the Knowledge to Action Cycle

An overview of the knowledge to action process is presented in Fig. 1. Graham and colleagues illustrate how the process of knowledge creation and action intersect, with the goal of bridging the evidence to care gap [2].

The cycle usually begins at the bottom of the diagram, with the identification of a problem: either a gap in care provision or because new evidence becomes available suggesting that current

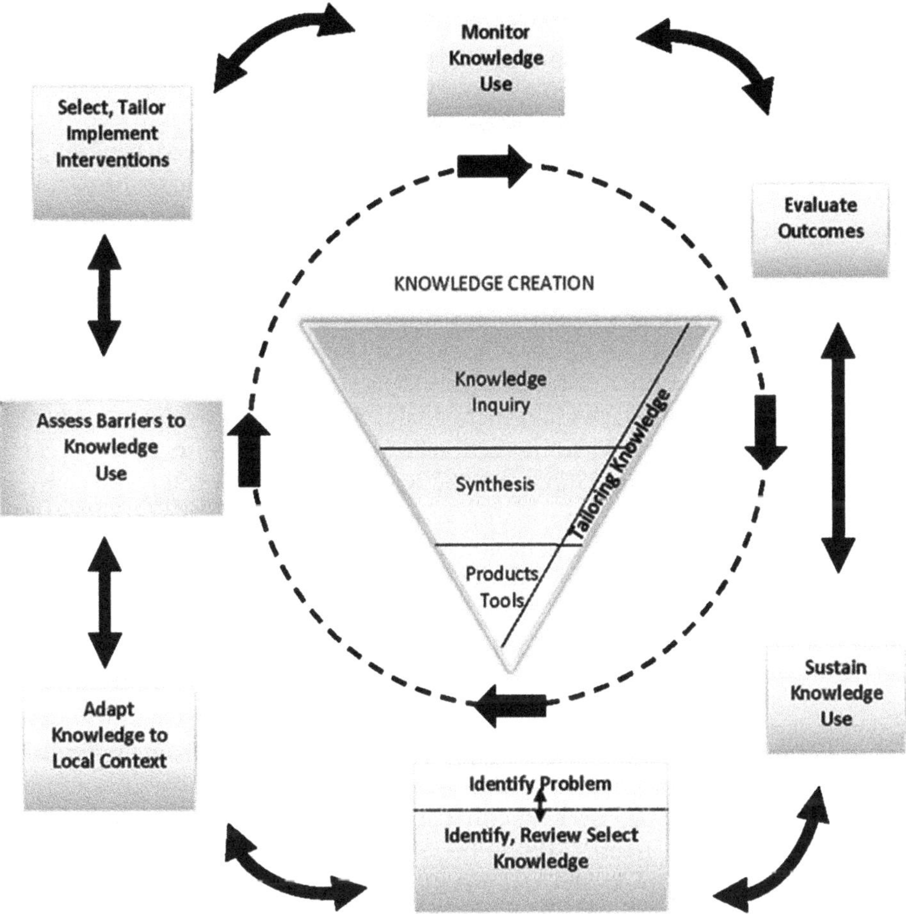

Fig. 1 The knowledge to action cycle [2]

practice is inadequate. Moving in a clockwise fashion, the remaining components of the KTA cycle refer to the action of applying the knowledge. This includes adapting knowledge to local context, assessing barriers to knowledge use, selecting, tailoring implementing interventions, monitoring knowledge use, evaluating outcomes, and sustaining knowledge use. Each of these steps is connected by bidirectional arrows and would ideally involve healthcare decision-makers and key stakeholders at each transition. Stakeholder engagement increases the likelihood that new information will be incorporated into local practice [1].

Knowledge creation is depicted at the center of the KTA cycle, as a funnel. Knowledge inquiry is at the wide end of the funnel and addresses the multitude of primary studies that inform the problem in question. At this stage the data has yet to be organized into a useful format to inform action. Moving down the funnel, the primary data is synthesized, typically through a systematic review or meta-analysis, where the results of relevant studies are combined or considered together. Ideally, knowledge synthesis results in the creation of knowledge products in the form of educational materials, guidelines, decision aids, or clinical pathways. These product tools are clearer and more concise than a full systematic review and can be used to inform stakeholders as they move through the knowledge to action cycle.

Throughout the rest of this chapter, we will use the example of timing of dialysis initiation to illustrate the knowledge to action cycle. Given that the process of evidence generation, including the conduct of randomized trials and the optimal method for systematic reviews and meta-analyses, has been covered elsewhere in this textbook, some sections of the knowledge to action cycle will be presented more succinctly. More attention will be given to the different types of interventions that have been used to influence stakeholder behavior.

4   Timing of Dialysis Initiation: An Example

Many factors are considered when deciding when to start dialysis in outpatients with progressive kidney failure, including lab markers of kidney function and subjectively reported symptoms that develop over time that are related to kidney failure, such as fatigue and nausea. While these symptoms are common in patients with severe kidney failure, they are often difficult to interpret because they can be due to other chronic health conditions common in patients with kidney disease. As such, there is no hard and fast rule and deciding when a patient should start dialysis has been an ongoing controversy for decades. Past clinical guidelines have generally recommended initiation of dialysis when kidney function falls below approximately "10 %" [6].

These guidelines, and the difficulty of attributing patient symptoms to kidney failure, may account for the recent increase in "earlier" (i.e., at a higher level of kidney function) initiation of dialysis in Canada and the United States over the past 10 years. For instance, the proportion of individuals starting dialysis at eGFR > 10 mL/min/1.73 m^2 has increased from 19 % in 1996 to 45 % in 2005 [7]. When patients are started on dialysis early and unnecessarily, this negatively affects patient's quality of life but is also a strain on the healthcare system. Given this, improving timing of dialysis initiation in outpatients with progressive kidney failure was recently selected as a priority for knowledge translation by a Canadian national kidney knowledge translation network [8].

5   Steps in KTA Cycle

5.1   Knowledge Creation: Knowledge Inquiry, Synthesis, and Knowledge Products

As previously discussed and illustrated in Fig. 2, the center of the KTA cycle represents the process of knowledge creation. The wide end of the funnel, knowledge inquiry, encompasses the primary studies (including randomized trials) that inform the problem in question. In order to generate a useable knowledge product, the data needs to be distilled into an organized format that can inform subsequent action.

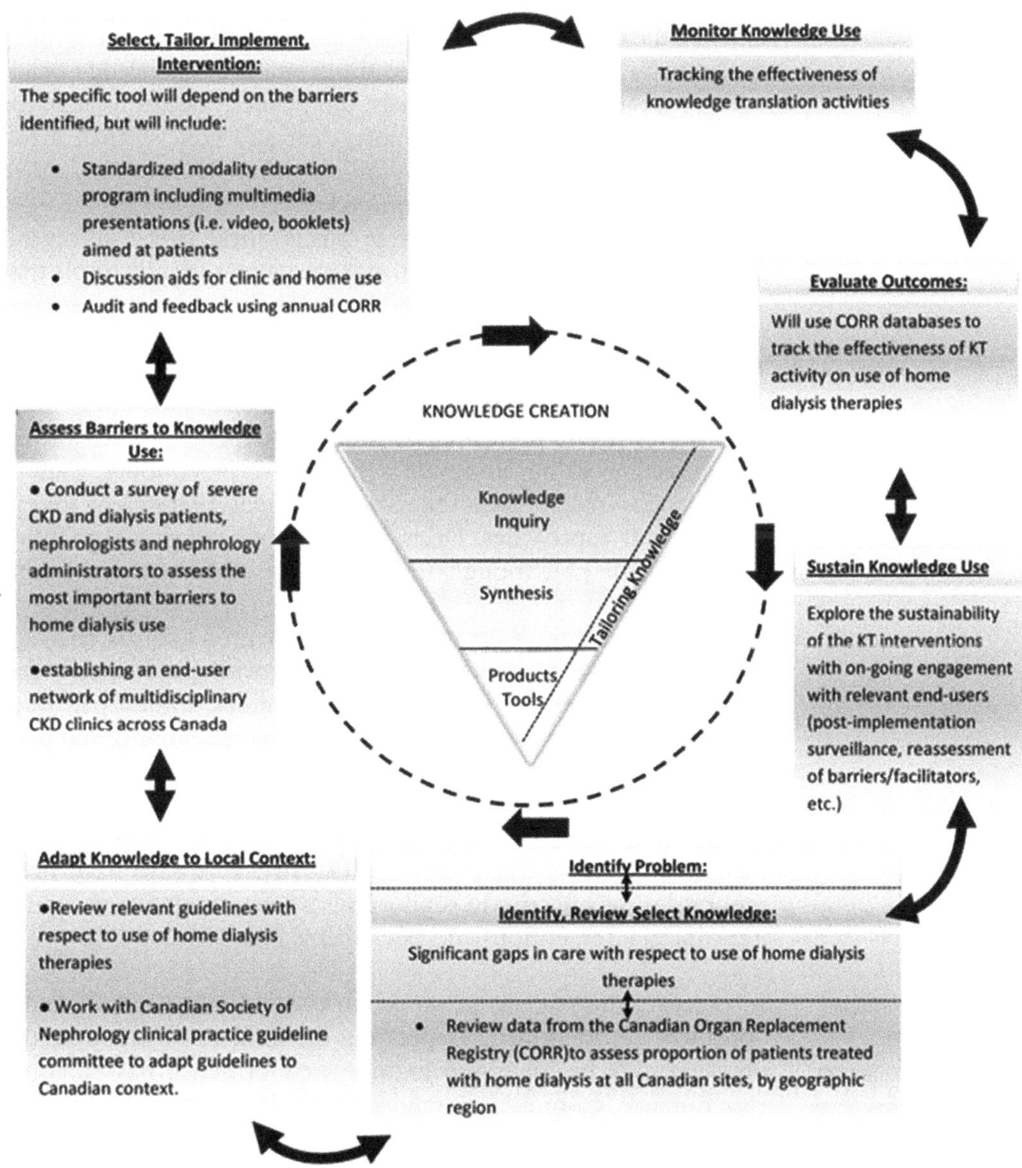

Fig. 2 The knowledge to action cycle for improving timing of dialysis initiation

The process of organizing studies into a usable knowledge product usually involves a systematic review or meta-analysis (*see* Chapter 24), where the results of pertinent studies are combined or considered together to inform action. Some questions, particularly those relating to changes in health policy or complex interventions, are not suited to conventional systematic reviews. In such cases, other approaches are needed—readers are referred to other sources [1].

Although systematic reviews may combine the results of several studies, making it much easier to consider the full breadth of evidence, the results typically are not in a format that are particularly usable by some groups of stakeholders, including patients and healthcare decision-makers. The process of knowledge synthesis, however, ultimately results in the creation of knowledge products (e.g., educational materials, guidelines, decision aids, or clinical pathways), which are more clear and concise than a full systematic review itself, and can inform stakeholders as they move through the knowledge to action cycle.

With respect to knowledge products, these may take several different forms. Patient decision aids are patient friendly tools that are meant to educate patients about their treatment options, including paper-based booklets, internet-based tools and videos. Ideally, they are hinged on high-quality evidence which is summarized in an understandable format for patients. Some patient decision aids are meant to be used by patients independently and others to be used working alongside a healthcare practitioner. Patient decision aids often present the risks and benefits of different testing or treatment approaches. Decision aids have been shown to influence behavior [1], though the impact on other types of health outcomes is less certain.

Clinical pathways are tools for health professionals that are derived from practice guidelines to aid in providing evidence-based health care [9, 10]. While similar to guidelines, clinical pathways differ by being more explicit about the sequence, timing, and provision of interventions and are directly incorporated into routine patient care. Pathways can help to improve the quality, consistency, and continuity of care and ensure that evidence-based and patient-focused care are being provided [11, 12]. Pathways have been reported to be effective in supporting care management and guiding clinical interventions and assessments [13–15].

5.2 The knowledge to action cycle: Selecting Priorities for Knowledge Translation

In practice, the knowledge to action cycle usually begins when a "problem" is identified. Depending on local circumstances, the problem may be identified because new evidence has emerged (for instance, from a large randomized trial) suggesting that the current standard practice is inadequate.

In other situations, evidence to practice gaps will be identified based on routinely measured and reported quality indicators, which may lead stakeholders to have concerns about current health system or provider performance. It should be noted that the strengths and limitations of each quality indicator must be considered. For instance, as quality indicators are often based on healthcare processes (i.e., the proportion of patients with a condition receiving a particular medication or test), they are usually measured with routinely available administrative data, which may have measurement issues, since these databases were not developed for research purposes [1]. Quality indicators should be valid, reliable, and feasible to measure, but importantly, they should be linked to important clinical outcomes and should be based on best evidence.

Researchers may also identify gaps in care from administrative health or other clinical registry data [16]. As above, it is important to consider the validity and reliability of the data, to ensure that the measure relates closely to the outcomes of care and that changes in these measures will improve outcomes. The data should also be representative of the population of interest.

While identifying an evidence to practice gap is critical to justifying a knowledge translation exercise, other factors should be considered before taking on such an exercise. For instance, variation in care is common in health care, particularly when the evidence in an area is weak. As such, in addition to noting variations in care, or suboptimal performance with respect to quality indicators, focusing KT activities in areas where good quality evidence exists to guide care is generally recommended. When choosing among several candidate problems to focus on, in addition to identifying variation in care, and focusing on an area with a strong evidence base, prioritizing areas where change may be most feasible is also important.

5.3 Adapting Knowledge to Local Context

Clinical practice guidelines or other knowledge tools may or may not be available to guide care in an identified problem area, and even if available, tailoring knowledge to local circumstances is often required.

Up until recently, no validated process for adapting clinical practice guidelines to local use existed. However, the ADAPTE collaboration has established a process, including outlining the necessary steps to ensure that guidelines can inform local practice [17]. Importantly, the ADAPTE process engages end users in the guideline adaptation process to make certain that the end products will best serve the stakeholders who will use them. The ADAPTE process consists of three main phases: planning and set up, adaptation of the guideline, and development of the final products. A web-based resource toolkit is available (www.ADAPTE.org).

5.4 Assessing Barriers to Implementation of Evidence

Barriers to implementation of evidence can exist at several levels: the patient, the healthcare professional, team, or organization, or the wider environment.

At the patient level, barriers often prevent patients from obtaining optimal outcomes. Patient barriers may involve both direct and indirect costs: for instance the test or treatment recommended may be too expensive or they may have difficulty getting time off work to attend an appointment. Patients may not understand the importance of a given treatment, or the treatment may not be a priority for them, in comparison to other demands in their life. Society and societal norms can sometimes serve as a barrier for patients. As individuals live within a larger society and lifestyles are generally collective, lifestyle changes (e.g., exercise or changes to a healthy diet) may be hard to implement at an individual level. Finally, barriers to optimal care may relate to patient's expectations of a healthcare encounter. For example, patients may seek medical attention for an upper respiratory tract infection (almost always viral), expecting to receive an antibiotic. However, guidelines do not recommend antibiotics in these situations since they would not be expected to be effective and may cause issues with antibiotic resistance. Leaving the physician's office empty handed may make patients feel like their provider isn't taking their concern seriously; and for physicians, it generally takes longer to explain to patients why an antibiotic is not appropriate compared with writing a prescription. If reducing antibiotic use is the goal of a health system, overcoming patient expectations would be important.

Barriers at the level of the healthcare professional may lie in issues with lack of provider knowledge or uncertainty around how best to manage conditions. With respect to knowledge, it may simply be a lack of awareness of evidence or guidelines, issues with information overload, or difficulties interpreting the quality of all of the evidence that clinicians are required to consider. Finally, there may be a lack of clarity around how to implement a new intervention or self-confidence in skills required in adjusting the doses of treatments—for instance new types of insulin regimens. With respect to uncertainty, in many areas of medicine, only low quality evidence exists. These areas may not be the highest priority for knowledge translation activities since convincing healthcare professionals to change practice in the absence of strong evidence may not only be difficult, for obvious reasons, but can also be met with resistance since key opinion leaders may not be in agreement with best practice. In these areas, in particular, it may be difficult for physicians to go against the usual standard of care they have been practicing.

Barriers may also exist at the level of the healthcare team or healthcare organization. A service, test, or treatment may simply not be available or may be difficult for patients to access. Reimbursement may not be available for some healthcare services.

There may not be enough time to spend with patients to provide information or help them change their behaviors—this may be particularly true for chronic disease management, which typically requires the active involvement of other allied healthcare professionals.

Finally, there may be barriers at the level of the practice environment. For instance, it has been noted that one of the most important barriers to routine handwashing, considered a high priority within hospitals to reduce the spread of hospital-acquired infections, is the availability of sinks. Specifically, the location and number of sinks to permit handwashing between each patient visit may be a significant barrier to proper hand hygiene.

While there are different approaches to determining what barriers are most important within the identified problem area, conducting a survey of the various stakeholder groups is usually required. To inform the survey, an initial focus group may be helpful to generate examples of the barriers that may be playing an important role, followed by a formal survey to determine the most important and modifiable barriers. Patients, healthcare providers, and healthcare administrators should be included as stakeholders when assessing the most important barriers. Of particular interest are barriers that are modifiable, since these may be targets of the KT intervention.

5.5 Selecting, Tailoring, and Implementing Interventions

When considering what interventions might be effective at overcoming the evidence to practice gap, consideration of the most important modifiable barriers is critical. If the most important barrier is at the level of the healthcare organization, then patient and provider education would not be expected to be effective. Moreover, when more than one barrier exists, combinations of interventions may be more effective, and there is no consensus on whether interventions should generally be used on their own or in combination. In general though, the type of intervention selected depends on the type of barrier that needs to be addressed. This section is organized based on the type of barrier that was noted.

5.5.1 Physician Knowledge

When healthcare provider knowledge is identified as a barrier, then provider education is usually required. This could take different forms, including distributing educational materials to healthcare professionals. Studies indicate that this form of education has mixed effects on physician behavior. For instance, guideline implementation strategies have been associated with a median improvement in care processes of around 8 % [18]. In general, continuing medical education, when delivered through a large conference or didactic teaching, has been shown to have minimal effect. Alternatively, providing education in a small group or interactive format has been shown to have a positive effect on practice and possibly clinical outcomes, particularly when there is a reinforcing activity that occurs following the education. Educational outreach by experts and local opinion leaders also has been shown to be particularly effective when the noted gap relates to appropriate physician prescribing [18].

5.5.2 Information Overload, Lack of Awareness of new Evidence, and Lack of Clarity on How to Implement Intervention

Within this subset of knowledge-related barriers, clinical decision support systems have been tested. These may be used in inpatient and outpatient settings, using clinical pathways within electronic medical records or laboratory data sets (for instance, anticoagulation protocols, or antibiotic dosing protocols linked to laboratory data). Clinical decision support systems are most likely to be effective when they are provided: (1) as part of regular clinician workflow, i.e., providing care recommendations within a patient's chart or electronic medical record so that clinicians do not need to seek out recommendations elsewhere; (2) at the time and location of decision-making, i.e., care recommendations provided as chart reminders during a patient encounter, rather than as monthly reports listing all the patients in need of services; or (3) as recommendations rather than a general assessment of the evidence [19]. Clinical decision support systems incorporating all of these elements are likely to be particularly effective.

5.5.3 Strategies Aimed at Other Barriers

Other knowledge implementation strategies that have been used to address a variety of barriers include audit and feedback strategies as well as simple reminders. With audit and feedback strategies, the performance of a physician, group, or organization with respect to a quality indicator is measured, and feedback is provided at the most relevant level, often to the individual provider. This is usually combined with recommendations around how to improve practice since audit and feedback has been shown to be most effective when combined with reminders and education.

Simple reminders, be it verbal to patients or staff (i.e., during the course of regular care) or posters, have been shown to have the largest effects of any of the strategies used on their own [1]. However, there is large variation across studies, which may relate to their use in situations where reminders will not address the most important barrier.

Substitution of tasks has also been shown to be an effective strategy for improving care. For instance, delegating tasks to nurses and pharmacists has been shown in some situations to improve use of guideline recommended treatments, including prescribing and cancer screening [18]. They may be particularly effective in situations where clinical pathways have been developed to guide care. For instance, nurse and/or pharmacist led-anemia protocols have gained popularity in managing anemia in patients with kidney failure requiring erythropoietin since they have been shown to achieve similar or better outcomes with respect to hemoglobin and erythropoietin doses [20, 21].

Finally, patient-mediated interventions, usually reminders or various forms of education, can be effective, particularly for improving preventative care, including vaccinations [18]. Patient decision aids, including paper-based booklets, internet-based tools and videos, are often used to present the risks and benefits of different testing or treatment approaches. While they have been shown to influence patient behavior [1], the impact on other types of health outcomes is less certain.

One of the most effective interventions involving patients as part of the healthcare team is *facilitated relay*, defined as clinical information transmitted by patients to clinicians by means other than the existing medical record [22]. The expectation is that clinicians then act on the information to change patient management. Examples of facilitated relay are patients providing treatment guidelines to providers or sharing the results of home blood pressure readings with providers during a clinic visit.

5.6 Monitor Knowledge Use	After an intervention is undertaken, it is important to assess whether provider and patient behavior is impacted and whether the information targeted within the intervention is being used. Assessing whether knowledge is being used is the first step to evaluating for a change in outcomes. If knowledge has not changed, then it is unlikely that the intervention will impact care and outcomes. There are a variety of frameworks to assess knowledge use that can be used, including whether stakeholders are aware of the target information or whether it has changed behavior. There are many tools that can be used to assess this and readers are directed elsewhere for further information [1].
5.7 Evaluate Outcomes	After assessing knowledge use, it is important to determine whether evidence to practice gaps have been narrowed or healthcare system performance has been affected. Often, this can be done using the same data set that was used to identify the problem—for instance, assessing whether quality indicators have changed, or evidence to care gaps have been closed. In addition to assessing whether practice patterns and care have changed, evaluating whether clinical outcomes have improved is also important, though may not be feasible in all situations.
5.8 Sustaining Knowledge Use	Knowledge translation interventions typically focus on changing patient, provider, or health system behavior at a point in time. However, ensuring that such behavior is maintained requires a different type of intervention. To date, few interventions have incorporated the notion of sustainability, in part because of the ongoing resource requirements of such an intervention [1]. In addition to the barriers and facilitators to consider before implementing an intervention, it is likely that there are different barriers and facilitators to sustaining an intervention and the related practice change over the long term, and these require consideration when determining how best to ensure sustainability.

6 Bringing It All Together: Returning to the Example of Timing of Dialysis Initiation

While dialysis is life saving for patients without any kidney function, starting dialysis in patients without symptoms is intrusive and has a negative impact on quality of life. As noted, the proportion of patients initiating dialysis "early" has increased over the past decade, and there is considerable variation in the proportion of patients initiating dialysis with an eGFR$\geq$10.5 ml/min (approximately 10 % kidney function) in Canada [23], ranging from 20 to 60 % across geographic regions. In 2010, the first randomized trial to clearly inform timing of dialysis initiation was published, suggesting no benefit from early start dialysis [24]. This seminal publication provided needed evidence to inform care in this area. Combined with the noted variability in practice, the impact of dialysis on patient's daily lives, and the fact that the care of patients on hemodialysis costs at least $85,000 per year [25], leaders of Canadian Kidney Care Programs who were surveyed in 2010 by the Canadian Kidney Knowledge Translation and Generation Network (CANN-NET) identified this topic as the top priority area for a new clinical practice guideline and knowledge translation activity [8].

Noting that a current guideline on timing of dialysis initiation was not available, CANN-NET engaged relevant kidney stakeholders, including the Canadian Society of Nephrology Clinical Practice Guidelines group, who established a guideline committee to revisit the cumulative evidence addressing the optimal timing of dialysis by conducting a systematic review addressing the optimal timing of the initiation of dialysis [26]. The review used the approach proposed by Grading of Recommendations Assessment, Development and Evaluation (GRADE) Working group, and adhered to prespecified protocols [27]. Briefly, the committee developed search strategies to identify studies comparing early versus late (as defined in included studies) initiation of dialysis. Mortality, hospitalization, and quality of life were prespecified as critical outcomes, utilization-related measures (time on dialysis, hospitalization, distance traveled for dialysis, and outpatient visits) as important outcomes, and nutritional surrogate markers were noted to be of interest, but not of major importance to decision-making. While 23 studies were identified, only one randomized trial, the Initiating Dialysis Early and Late (IDEAL) study, was found [24]. Timing of dialysis initiation did not affect survival in the IDEAL study, with a hazard ratio of 1.04 (95 % confidence interval [CI]$=0.83$–1.30; $p=0.75$) [24]. The study also noted similar quality of life in both treatment arms, despite a median delay of nearly 6 months in the initiation of dialysis in the late start group. The delay in use of dialysis resulted in lower healthcare costs of nearly CAN$18,000 in the "intent to defer initiation of dialysis" group [28].

To assess barriers to optimal timing of dialysis initiation, a survey of nephrologists in Canada was conducted, which identified some underlying physician beliefs and possible misconceptions about timing of dialysis initiation [29]. Over 40 % of nephrologists felt that initiating dialysis at lower levels of eGFR would negatively impact quality of life and decrease use of peritoneal dialysis. Over half felt uremic symptoms (fatigue and nausea) occurred earlier in older patients or patients with more comorbidity—a view not supported by the IDEAL study [24]. Of importance, only 3 % of nephrologists worked at a facility or institution that had a formal policy regarding dialysis initiation.

Based on the development of the clinical practice guidelines and the survey assessing barriers, several KT interventions are planned for implementation. The survey results on providers' attitudes and the newly developed guidelines were presented in a special interactive forum at the annual Canadian Society of Nephrology meeting in 2013, attended by nearly a third of all Canadian nephrologists. A system of audit and feedback system was implemented in collaboration with the Canadian Organ Replacement Registry (CORR). CORR sends an annual facility-specific report to individual dialysis facilities, which includes a measure indicating the proportion of patients who have been followed by a Nephrologist who started with an eGFR >10.5 ml/min. This was presented alongside blinded information from other facilities in the immediate geographic region and national averages, followed up by communications from CANN-NET describing the relevance and important of this quality indicator. Finally, centers were directed to the recently published guideline, if appropriate.

Since the survey identified knowledge-related barriers for providers, and assuming that knowledge barriers were also relevant for patients, we also created several unique educational materials targeting both patients and healthcare providers. Infographics, a pictorial highlighting the key messages targeting the intended audience, were created to illustrate the key guideline recommendations and emphasize the central role of patient preference and acceptance about when to initiate dialysis therapy (http://www.cann-net.ca/images/Patient-facing_infographic_fro_PRINT_steps_to_planning_for_dialysis-_Mar_17_2014.pdf). These dialysis initiation infographics will be placed in common patient care areas such as clinics, nursing stations, and physician offices. A whiteboard animated video was also developed discussing the state of the evidence, the importance of patient preference and choice, and the role of healthcare providers (e.g., http://youtu.be/mi34xCfmLhw). Finally, an academic detailing visit is planned involving educational outreach by a core group of physicians using standardized educational materials.

The evaluation component will include a pre- and post-intervention time series analysis using available national administrative datasets to look for changes in the proportion of patients initiating dialysis "early." A cluster randomized controlled trial is also planned to evaluate the impact of an expert site visit with standardized educational materials versus passive strategies alone. The outcome of interest will be the proportion of patients initiating dialysis "early." Since it is possible that this strategy may result in excessive delays in dialysis initiation, as a safety outcome, the proportion of patients initiating dialysis as an inpatient will also be tracked.

Utilizing the KTA cycle considerable practice variation regarding the timing of dialysis initiation in Canada was noted. Synthesizing the existing evidence demonstrated no benefit to early dialysis initiation and the adoption of a subsequent "intent-to-defer" strategy. Although the majority of nephrologists followed the existing evidence, key barriers were identified and thus a national knowledge translation strategy was developed to improve care. An evaluation of this strategy is underway.

7   Summary

Knowledge translation is meant to address the evidence to practice gap. This can be facilitated by use of the knowledge to action cycle, integrating policy-makers throughout the research cycle. The knowledge to action cycle begins with the identification of a problem (usually identified as a gap in care provision). After identification of the problem, knowledge creation is undertaken, initially involving knowledge inquiry, followed by synthesis of data into key knowledge products in the form of educational materials, guidelines, decision aids, or clinical pathways. The remaining components of the KTA cycle refer to the action of applying the knowledge that has been created. This includes adapting knowledge to local context, assessing barriers to knowledge use, selecting, tailoring implementing interventions, monitoring knowledge use, evaluating outcomes, and sustaining knowledge use. Involving healthcare decision-makers and key stakeholders at each step increases the likelihood that new information will be incorporated into local practice.

References

1. Straus S, Tetroe J, Graham I (2010) Knowledge translation in health care: moving from evidence to practice. Wiley-Blackwell, West Sussex
2. Graham ID, Logan J, Harrison MB, Straus SE, Tetroe J, Caswell W, Robinson N (2006) Lost in knowledge translation: time for a map? J Contin Educ Health Prof 26:13–24
3. Canadian Institutes of Health Research (2014) More about knowledge translation. http://cihr-irsc.gc.ca/e/39033.html#Definition
4. Baker R, Camosso-Stefinovic J, Gillies C, Shaw EJ, Cheater F, Flottorp S, Robertson N (2010) Tailored interventions to overcome identified barriers to change: effects on professional practice and health care outcomes. Cochrane Database Syst Rev 3, CD005470
5. Improvement IHI (2003) The breakthrough series: IHI's collaborative model for achieving breakthrough improvement. http://www.ihi.org/knowledge/Pages/IHIWhitePapers/

TheBreakthroughSeriesIHIsCollaborative ModelforAchievingBreakthroughImprovement.aspx. Accessed 5 Aug 2012

6. National Kidney Foundation (2002) K/DOQI clinical practice guidelines for chronic kidney disease: evaluation, classification and stratification. Am J Kidney Dis 39:S1–S266

7. Rosansky S, Clark WF, Eggers P, Glassock R (2009) Initiation of dialysis at higher GFRs: is the apparent rising ride of early dialysis harmful or helpful? Kidney Int 76:257–261

8. Manns B, Barrett B, Evan M, Garg A, Hemmelgarn B, Kappel J, Klarenbach S, Madore F, Parfrey P, Samuel S, Soroka SD, Suri R, Tonelli M, Wald R, Walsh M, Zappitelli M, NeTwork FtCKKTaG (2014) Establishing a national knowledge translation and generation network in kidney disease: the CAnadian KidNey KNowledge TraNslation and GEneration NeTwork. Can J Kidney Health Dis 1:2. doi:10.1186/2054-3581-1181-1182

9. Kinsman L, Rotter T, James E, Snow P, Willis J (2010) What is a clinical pathway? Development of a definition to inform the debate. BMC Med 8:31

10. Rotter T, Kinsman L, James E, Machotta A, Gothe H, Willis J, Snow P, Kugler J (2010) Clinical pathways: effects on professional practice, patient outcomes, length of stay and hospital costs. Cochrane Database Syst Rev. CD006632

11. Whittle C, Hewison A (2007) Integrated care pathways: pathways to change in health care? J Health Organ Manag 21:297–306

12. Scott S, Grimshaw J, Klassen T, Nettel-Aguirre A, Johnson D (2011) Understanding implementation processes of clinical pathways and clinical practice guidelines in pediatric contexts: a study protocol. Implement Sci 6:133

13. Allen D, Gillen E, RIxson L (2009) Systematic review of the effectiveness of integrated care pathways: what works, for whom, in which circumstances? Int J Evid Based Healthc 7:61–74

14. Sulch D, Perez I, Melbourn A, Kalra L (2008) Evaluation of an integrated care pathway for stroke unit rehabilitation. Age Ageing 29:87

15. Cunningham S, Logan C, Lockerbie L, Dunn M, McMurray A, Prescott R (2008) Effect of an integrated care pathway on acute asthma/wheeze in children attending hospital: cluster randomized trial. J Pediatr 152:315–320

16. Manns B, Braun T, Edwards A, Grimshaw J, Hemmelgarn B, Husereau D, Ivers N, Johnson J, Long S, McBrien KA, Naugler C, Sargious P, Straus S, Tonelli M, Tricco A, Yu C, For the Alberta Innovates HSICDC (2013) Identifying strategies to improve diabetes care in Alberta,

Canada, using the knowledge-to-action cycle. CMAJ Open 1(4):E142–E150

17. Fervers B, Burgers JS, Haugh MC, Latreille J, Mlika-Cabanne N, Paquet L, Coulombe M, Poirier M, Burnand B (2006) Adaptation of clinical guidelines: a review of methods and experiences. Int J Health Care 18:167–176

18. Grol R, Grimshaw J (2003) From best evidence to best practice: effective implementation of change in patients' care. Lancet 362(9391): 1225–1230

19. Kawamoto K, Houlihan CA, Balas EA, Lobach DF (2005) Improving clinical practice using clinical decision support systems: a systematic review of trials to identify features critical to success. BMJ 330(7494):765–768E

20. Brimble KS, Rabbat CG, McKenna P, Lambert K, Carlisle EJ (2003) Protocolized anemia management with erythropoietin in hemodialysis patients: a randomized controlled trial. J Am Soc Nephrol 14(10):2654–2661

21. To LL, Stoner CP, Stolley SN, Buenviaje JD, Ziegler TW (2001) Effectiveness of a pharmacist-implemented anemia management protocol in an outpatient hemodialysis unit. Am J Health Syst Pharm 58(21):2061–2065

22. Tricco AC, Ivers NM, Grimshaw JM, Moher D, Turner L, Galipeau J, Halperin I, Vachon B, Ramsay T, Manns B, Tonelli M, Shojania K (2012) Effectiveness of quality improvement strategies on the management of diabetes: a systematic review and meta-analysis. Lancet 379(9833):2252–2261

23. Clark WF, Na YB, Rosansky SJ, Sontrop JM, Macnab JJ, Glassock RJ, Eggers PW, Jackson K, Moist L (2011) Association between estimated glomerular filtration rate at initiation of dialysis and mortality. Can Med Assoc J 183: 47–53

24. Cooper BA, Branley P, Bulfone L, Collins JF, Craig JC, Fraenkel MB, Harris A, Johnson DW, Kesselhut J, Li JJ, Luxton G, Pilmore A, Tiller DJ, Harris DC, Pollock CA, Study I (2010) A randomized, controlled trial of early versus late initiation of dialysis. N Engl J Med 363:609–619

25. Lee H, Manns B, Taub K, Ghali WA, Dean S, Johnson D, Donaldson C (2002) Cost analysis of ongoing care of patients with end-stage renal disease: the impact of dialysis modality and dialysis access. Am J Kidney Dis 40(3):611–622

26. Nesrallah GE, Mustafa RA, Clark WF, Bass A, Barnieh L, Hemmelgarn BR, Klarenbach S, Quinn RR, Hiremath S, Ravani P, Sood MM, Moist LM (2012) Canadian Society of Nephrology 2012 Clinical Practice Guidelines for timing the initiation of chronic dialysis. Can Med Assoc J 186:112–117

27. Grading Recommendations Assessment DaEGWG (2012) GRADE Working Group, 2012. http://www.gradeworkinggroup.org/

28. Harris A, Cooper BA, Li JJ, Bulfone L, Branley P, Collins JF, Craig JC, Fraenkel MB, Johnson DW, Kesselhut J, Luxton G, Pilmore A, Rosevear M, Tiller DJ, Pollock CA, Harris DC (2011) Cost-effectiveness of initiating dialysis early: a randomized controlled trial. Am J Kidney Dis 57(5):707–715

29. Mann B, Manns B, Dart A, Kappel J, Molzahn A, Naimark D, Nessim S, Soroka SD, Zappitelli M, Sood M, (CANN-NET) ObotCKKTaGN (2014) An assessment of dialysis provider's attitudes towards timing of dialysis initiation in Canada. Can J Kidney Health Dis 1(3)

Chapter 30

Evidence-Based Decision-Making 8: Health Policy, a Primer for Researchers

Victor Maddalena

Abstract

There is a growing expectation that research will be used to inform decision-making. It is important for researchers to understand how health policy is developed and the different ways they can influence the development of policy.

Public policy is developed to resolve identified problems. Health policy is a subset of public policy and is typically concerned with issues related to the health of populations either from a service delivery perspective or from a broader public health and social determinants of health perspective. The policy planning algorithm is well established and follows the basic decision-making framework: assessment, planning, implementation, and evaluation. A variety of government and nongovernment stakeholders engage in complex debates to identify and resolve policy issues. In this chapter we explore how researchers can use their research to influence the development of health policy. Knowledge translation strategies focused on communicating research to policy-makers require considerable thought and planning.

Key words Health policy, Policy planning algorithm, Decision-making, Knowledge translation

1   Introduction

This chapter will explore health policy and, more specifically, how epidemiological research can inform the development of health policy. While knowledge for knowledge's sake is laudable, there is a growing expectation that research will answer important questions or address issues facing the healthcare system, the health of populations, or society in general. It is therefore useful to understand how the researcher and their research can influence the development of policy.

In this regard I will examine how health policy is developed, the social and political context within which policy is developed, and the ways researchers can be involved in—and influence—the policy process. I will use examples from Canada's health system to illustrate the policy-making process. In particular I will focus on the communication of research results to policy-makers and present

Patrick S. Parfrey and Brendan J. Barrett (eds.), *Clinical Epidemiology: Practice and Methods*, Methods in Molecular Biology, vol. 1281, DOI 10.1007/978-1-4939-2428-8_30, © Springer Science+Business Media New York 2015

some strategies to engage the decision-makers of government. My goal is to present a layperson's guide to policy development as opposed to a theoretical exposition of the intricacies of policy-making. Therefore, my focus and concern will be on practical considerations.

2 What Is Health Policy?

There are various definitions of public policy in the literature. A commonly cited definition of public policy is by Leslie Pal. She states public policy is "…a course of action chosen by public authorities to address a given problem or interrelated set of problems" [1] (p. 2). Others, for example, Lydia Miljan defines policy as "…a conscious choice by governments that lead to deliberate action—the passage of law, the spending of money, an official speech or gesture or some other observable act—or inaction" [2] (p. 3). Silence or nonaction on a particular issue can also be a statement of policy [3]. Deliberate action in the form of policy directives can take the form of the allocation of resources, the enactment of laws or regulations, a publicly stated position, regulations, taxation, and so forth. Public policy is developed within an established framework or process and is generally consistent with social values. Policy can range from the legislation that enables Regional Health Authorities to deliver and monitor a wide range of health services to snow clearing of city streets and sidewalks. While the clearing of snow from streets after a snowstorm may seem far removed from the broad public policy domain, the process of snow removal from city streets is part of a set of broader level policy initiatives related to public safety, healthy cities, and pedestrian-friendly initiatives.

Public policy is often subdivided into governmental or industrial sectors: fisheries policy, economic development policy, agricultural policy, national security policy, resource management policy, environmental policy, social policy, among others. Health policy is merely a subset of public policy and is typically concerned with issues related to the health of the population either from a service delivery perspective or from a broader public health perspective, for example, the treatment or prevention of disease or the promotion of health. These sectors of policy development are not separate and discrete domains and there is often considerable overlap among various policy sectors. Depending on the author and their world view, health policy can be equally concerned with economic development, housing policy, public transit policy, and social policy as much as it is interested in addressing the broader determinants of health (education, employment, social networks, environment, etc.) and service delivery issues in the healthcare system [4].

Within the policy realm there are different levels of policy-making, each with its own process for clarifying purpose and content and protocols for consultation and approval. Macro-level policy-making at the municipal, provincial, national, and international levels generally takes the form of legislation, lawmaking, and establishing regulations. Policies at this level affect larger populations and have broad social implications and legal means of enforcement. The arena for public policy-making at the macro-level occurs within the public domain, in particular municipal councils, provincial legislatures or parliaments, and their supporting infrastructure.

3 Purpose of Public Policy

The general purpose of public policy is to formalize initiatives established by governments and to achieve the overall mission of governments. Policies guide action, establish priorities, and provide the means by which government directives are implemented and monitored. For example, one of the most significant policy statements a government can make is the approval of the annual budget. The budget is a clear statement of priorities, allocating scarce resources to various departments and initiatives to serve the public good. Therefore, public policy should reflect the general needs and values of the population it is serving [2, 3, 5].

The word "policy" conjures up visions of binders on shelves containing policies in public institutions. Here we need to distinguish macro-level health policy from the kinds of institution-specific policy that you find for example in hospitals and other public institutions. Their general purpose is the same but there are some unique differences. Public institutions have a plethora of polices (and accompanying procedures) to govern and direct staff on everything from hiring of staff, procurement of goods or services, and financial management to policies on approvals related to preparing reports on occupational health and safety, human resource policy, protocols for the administration of intravenous drugs, record keeping, and a wide range of other specialized activities that require standardized application. These policies set by administration play an important role in providing consistency and integration of activities within an institution. Institutional policy is developed and approved within the organization and may be unique to the organization or set by industry standards or shaped by legislation and regulatory requirements. The kind of policy we are concerned about in this chapter is macro-level governmental health policy that generally takes the form of legislation or regulations that direct and shape the delivery of health care or other social services.

As an example of macro-level governmental policy-making, let us examine one of Canada's most well-known public policies, the Canada Health Act [6] or Medicare as it is informally known. To understand the Canada Health act, we need to go back in history to examine how federal and provincial powers were established as they relate to health care. In Canada the federal and provincial governments share responsibilities for health care. The Canadian Constitution Act (1867/1982), formerly known as the British North America Act (1867), outlines the structure and operation of the Government of Canada and powers held by the federal and provincial governments [7]. Sections of the Act specifically related to health care include Section 92(7) wherein it states that Provincial governments are responsible for "The Establishment, Maintenance, and Management of Hospitals, Asylums, Charities, and Eleemosynary[1] Institutions in and for the Province, other than Marine Hospitals." The somewhat out-of-date wording reflects the time period when the original act was written in 1867. Simply stated, the Act states that provincial governments can establish their own priorities for health care, manage their own budgets, and plan services to meet the needs of their population—in other words, establish policy.

The Canadian Constitution Act also defines the responsibility of the Federal government as it pertains to health [7]. The Federal government pays some of the costs of health care (further detailed in the provisions of the Canada Health Act (CHA) [6] and the Canada Health Transfer[2] and various health accords that determine levels of funding) and it is responsible for the provision of health care to specific groups, including Aboriginal Canadians, the Royal Canadian Mounted Police (RCMP), prisoners in Federal penitentiaries, refugee claimants, and the Canadian Military [8]. The federal government sets the criteria and conditions that must be met by the provinces to access federal funding under the provisions of the CHA [9].

The Canada Health Act is one of the defining cornerstones of Canadian public policy [6]. The CHA embodies the Canadian values of equity and unity and outlines the principle objective of Canadian health policy which is to "...to protect, promote and restore the physical and mental well-being of residents of Canada and to facilitate reasonable access to health services without financial or other barriers" (CHA Sec.3). The Act ensures "...that all eligible residents of Canada have reasonable access to medically

---

[1] Eleemosynary means relying on charity.

[2] The Canada Health Transfer, or CHT, is the largest transfer of financial resources from the federal government to the provinces and territories. It provides long-term predictable funding for health care and is consistent with the principles of the Canada Health Act. Source: https://www.fin.gc.ca/fedprov/cht-eng.asp

necessary services on a prepaid basis, without charges directly related to the provision of insured health services" [9]. The CHA, as a statement of public policy, outlines the principles and structures that govern Canada's health insurance system. Specifically, those principles are public administration, comprehensiveness, universality, portability, and accessibility. These principles enshrine in legislation the values inherent in Canada's health system [9]. The Canada Health Act is one policy initiative that has served to define a nation and establish the priorities and values associated with the delivery of health care. All other health policy initiatives in Canada are either directly or indirectly influenced by this foundational policy.

It is clear that public policy is a powerful tool that can shape the mission and goals of the public domain. Indeed it is because policy is a powerful way to shape direction that organizations and individuals seek to influence these directions. The process of policy development is very dynamic and takes place in a particular time and place and historical, social, and political context.

4 The Policy Arena

The "policy arena" is a commonly used metaphor for the social and political context within which policy issues are debated and developed. The image of a sports arena with various players or teams competing to "score" points is a reasonably good analogy. Open any daily newspaper or watch the evening news on television and you will see a wide range of public policy issues being debated, refuted, criticized, supported, or examined. On any given issue there are a wide range of stakeholders (individuals or groups) that have an interest in that issue. There are many players or "actors" in the policy arena. The old saying, "You can't tell your players without a program" in the sports context applies equally well to the policy development process.

For example within Canadian provincial governments, there are a host of players involved in the policy process including various levels of junior and senior policy analysts, senior administrators, and of course politicians including Ministers and their support staff. The ruling party in government will have a Premier and a Cabinet comprised of Cabinet Ministers representing various portfolios or departments. The Premier is supported by the Office of the Executive Council and the Office of the Premier. The work of the Cabinet is supported by the Cabinet Secretariat (Privy Council Office at the Federal government level) and a wide range of Standing Committees, senior advisors, and communications personnel [3, 10, 11].

Outside of government there are a wide range of players or actors that have an equally important role to play in the development of public policy including interest groups, lobby groups, nongovernmental organizations, the media, and individual citizens. While there are rare occasions when all stakeholders are in agreement, it is usually the case that there are many divergent opinions on the definition of the problem, the potential solutions, and who ultimately will benefit from the outcomes of a policy issue.

To illustrate the policy arena in action, it may be helpful to cite a specific example. Health human resources (HHR) have been and will likely continue to be a key policy priority for governments, health professional organizations, service delivery organizations, and educational institutions. The ultimate goal of health human resource policy is to ensure reasonable access to the right numbers and mix of health professionals in a reasonable period of time, in an appropriate setting, and at a reasonable cost. On the surface this may seem like a fairly simple problem with an equally simple solution. The challenge in this example, however, is there are many regulated health professional groups (physicians, nurses, physiotherapists, occupational therapists, pharmacists, among others) that have different opinions regarding the optimal number and distribution of health professionals to meet the health needs of the population or insured group.

Health professional organizations at the national and provincial level, the agencies that regulate and license their practice, organizations that represent their professional interests, the educational institutions that train those professionals, and the governments that fund their salaries and the services they provide engage in a complex debate to ensure reasonable access to health care. In addition there are citizen-led public interest groups advocating access to services that require health human resources. Add to this the concerns and interests of those health organizations that utilize the services of health professionals and it is clear the "policy arena" can get crowded and the issues, complex.

In Canada health is a provincial responsibility and therefore each province can make regulations affecting health professions. In this regard the decisions made by one province can have a significant impact on the policies of another province and while there is some degree of standardization across the provinces and territories, there is subtle difference among the provinces. And then there is the issue of health professions seeking to improve their own position vis-à-vis other health professions (also known as professional turf wars). All of these groups and stakeholders have an interest in shaping the problem and identifying solutions. While the debate seeks to ultimately serve the public interest, it is often difficult to distinguish between arguments that purport to serve the public interest versus those that benefit professional interests. At the root of the discussion is the basic problem of resource allocation; unlimited wants and limited resources and the need for governments to make difficult choices!

A policy example is the possible harmful effects of tanning salons and the need to regulate access to tanning beds, particularly for individuals under the age of 19. One side of the debate is advocating that tanning beds are unhealthy because exposure to harmful doses of ultraviolet radiation may lead to the development of skin cancer and they argue that people under 19 years of age should be banned from accessing tanning beds. Proponents of the ban cite research that documents the harmful effects of ultraviolet light that is emitted from the tanning beds. The business owners of tanning salons and their patrons, however, take a slightly different view on the issue. They believe that tanning beds, used properly, are not harmful. They believe the research is inconclusive, that other lifestyle habits in society that are harmful are not banned (so why focus on tanning beds?), that individuals who live in a free society should have the right to access tanning beds, and so forth.

Agencies promoting cancer prevention sell their message to the public, media, politicians, and bureaucrats using research, briefings, meetings with senior officials, and press releases to advocate for a ban on tanning beds for individuals under 19 years of age. They also seek support and endorsement from health professional groups who also hold a similar view. There is strength in numbers. The stronger the argument, the stronger the evidence, the greater likelihood the public and government regulators will agree. The business owners, in turn, also engage in their own social marketing by issuing their side of the story, and they lay out their arguments against the prohibition of tanning beds to individuals under 19. In this policy debate the advocates for a ban on youth tanning appear to have won the argument and a ban has been supported in many jurisdictions.

Public policy debates rarely take place in private. Special interest groups and individual citizens can participate in the policy process through a variety of means including participating in government sponsored consultation processes (e.g., surveys, opinion polls, focus groups), expert consultation processes, legislative hearings, submissions or presentations to Commissions or Special Task Forces, among others. Perhaps the most common form of influencing the policy process is by citizens casting a vote in elections or a referendum. Citizens or interest groups can engage in other forms of policy advocacy including letter-writing, community activism, town hall meetings, and preparing and submitting briefs or position statements to government [3, 5, 12, 13].

The stakeholders (also known as actors) with an interest in an issue seek to promote their views on any given issue. In this regard the media is recognized as a significant player in the public policy process. Policy debates rarely take place in private. Stakeholder groups seek to promote their views using various forms of communication including the popular media. Large and powerful stakeholder groups recognize the importance of effective public relations and communications to promote their views to the public and to government. The media may or may not take an interest in the issue as a possible news story. Both sides of a policy debate will seek to present their perspective to the media to win public and political support [5, 14].

In the middle of the debate, but certainly not a bystander, is the bureaucracy of government. They are usually the recipient of all perspectives on a policy issue. They seek to understand the issues and ensure their government officials and political figures are appropriately briefed on all aspects of the problem and it is their job to examine and bring forth for consideration possible remedies. Each side of the debate will lay out their research and evidence to support their viewpoints. Sometimes this evidence is conflicting and unclear. Influencing the media in a policy debate can be a powerful ally. If an issue can generate significant public interest or even better—outrage—from the public, then governments will usually respond. Power and politics go hand in hand. Well-organized and well-resourced interest groups and stakeholders are at a distinct advantage in a policy debate when compared to unorganized, vulnerable, or marginalized groups that have limited resources.

In the midst of all of this debate, research can play an important role in informing the policy debate on any given issue. And therefore researchers can and should seek to have their research heard.

5   A Policy Planning Algorithm

At a very basic level health policy is concerned with problem-solving [1]. Problems are encountered or identified (current or anticipated) and in response government develops policy to address the problem. The primary objective of policy development is to comprehensively assess the policy issue or problem, identify and implement the most effective and cost-efficient solutions in a manner that is consistent with social values and within existing policy structures and processes. In this regard policy-making is very similar to the kinds of problem-solving that occurs in business or in clinical settings. The difference is in scope of influence.

When a business identifies a problem and devises a solution, the impact is generally limited to that business. When a government identifies a problem and devises a solution, the impacts can be far-reaching and influence large populations. While there are a variety of frameworks and diagrams describing the complexities of policy-making, the basic decision-making algorithm is a circular process and includes assessment, planning, implementation, and evaluation.

5.1 Assessment

Individuals, special interest groups, and political groups seek to have their issue added to the policy agenda. Some groups are very powerful and can easily get the attention of government and the media, for example, the provincial or national physician or nursing associations, or a range of national charitable organizations or groups representing the interests of the pharmaceutical industry. Other groups are less well recognized and their voices may not be as easily heard in the policy arena.

Whenever a policy issue or problem is identified, the first and paramount concern is the need to clearly define the problem and this includes understanding the issue, the context for the issue, and the reasons why it is perceived as a problem. In the assessment phase of policy development, the principle objective is to define and delineate the problem. Key questions need to be answered include for example, what is the nature of the problem? More importantly, who has identified and defined the problem? What are the sources of information to assist you in defining the problem? Is this a new problem? If not a new problem then how have other jurisdictions addressed the issue? If it is a new issue what policy options are available to address the problem? Are these options consistent with prevailing social values? Are the options legal, viable, cost-effective, and publicly acceptable? What is the cost (financial or other) to address (or not address) the problem? What are the longer term implications of the policy options? Are the options being considered consistent with the political views of the government in power? Will these policy options have any unintended effects on particular groups? Who is most affected by this issue and have they been consulted? And perhaps most important, will one of these policy options actually solve the problem! The assessment or problem defining state of policy development is a critical and essential step in the process.

As the problem is being identified and debated, government is receiving letters, presentations, and position papers from individuals, businesses, and stakeholder groups each stating their own views on the subject and trying to influence the policy process by seeking to define the problem (and identify solutions) from their own perspective.

Governments seek to understand the various positions, understand the research behind the positions, and try to determine (a) is this issue worthy of government intervention? (b) if the government did intervene what options are available to formulate a "good policy" response? Because the legislative agenda is so full, policy does not make its way to the floor of a legislature unless it has been identified as a priority.

5.2 Planning

Once the problem has been clearly articulated, all the issues have been identified and discussed and evidence presented, the process of actually planning the policy response take on a more serious tone.

Governments seek to implement policy that will resolve the problem in the most cost-effective manner, with minimal negative consequences and ultimately serving the greatest good for the greatest number of people.

Stakeholder groups, experts, or researchers will often be invited to participate in consultations and planning the policy response because they are often in a position to more fully inform the process and understand the implications and potential outcomes of the initiative. The policy response is often determined by actions that have been implemented in other jurisdictions. Policy analysts in government often develop a network of contacts in other provincial governments in their area of expertise. When a problem arises, they contact their network of colleagues in other jurisdictions with the intent of asking the question, "Have you encountered this problem?" and if so "What did you do about it?" In some cases the problem is unique to a particular situation or context and a new solution must be generated. In these instances the bureaucracy will engage experts inside and outside of government to assist with generating policy options.

5.3 Implementation

As policy initiatives are narrowed down to viable options, a new set of questions are asked including what level of policy intervention is necessary? Does this problem require legislation, regulation, or a lesser form of policy statement from the government? In some instances government may determine that the best role it can play is to act as a broker for industry or among groups to resolve the problems without government intervention.

Once it is determined the government will implement legislation or regulation, it has to go through a series of internal and external vetting procedures. In the case of legislation and regulations, the Minister will need to assess the impact of the policy before implementation. Indeed most government agencies responsible and Cabinet will need to have a detailed process for assessing the impact of a policy option in a variety of domains, for example, economic impact, health impact, social inclusion, costs, monitoring, evaluation, human resources, public relations, impact on other departments in government, and national or international implications.

I will not review the process for implementing legislative and regulations in this chapter; there are several good resources available to describe the detailed and lengthy process of generating legislation and regulations [3, 15].

Suffice to say that once the legislation or regulation or policy has been implemented, there is a process put in place to monitor the outcomes. Politicians and political parties play an important role in policy development and in the implementation of policy. Political parties adopt platforms that, if elected, will form the outline for their policy agenda. When elected, the government in power can create a legislative agenda based on their priorities and create legislation. In the policy arena a large number of interest groups lobby and put forth their ideas of what should be on the policy agenda of governments. From this the government in power together with their bureaucracy sifts through a wide range of concerns identified in government and identified by the public through stakeholders groups.

In some cases, even in the face of overwhelming scientific or research evidence to support a particular policy intervention, governments will decide not to intervene using legislation or regulations. A good example of this is in Canada recently when the Federal government decided to not regulate the food industry in terms of reducing dietary sodium in food products. Instead, while they acknowledge the impact of increased dietary sodium on the health of the population, they decided to not take a firm policy stance on the issue and instead decided to work with the provinces and industry to resolve the problem. They state,

> The federal, provincial and territorial governments are committed to helping create conditions that make the healthier choice the easier choice. Sodium reduction is an important part of healthy living and the governments have been working together towards supporting Canadians in their sodium reduction efforts. The goal is to work towards reducing the average sodium intake of Canadians to 2,300 mg per day by 2016. With this goal in mind, the government is: a) working to increase the awareness and education of Canadians on the issue of sodium as part of healthy eating; b) supporting research related to sodium reduction; c) providing guidance to assist the food industry in lowering the amount of sodium in processed foods. [16]

In this way, the government works with industry to achieve the desired outcome, without the imposition of legislation or strict regulatory constraints.

Ministers of Health (or other portfolios in government) are regularly briefed on a wide range of issues. The legislative agenda is usually very full and only the most pressing legislative concerns rise to the top for action. Governments constantly prioritize the policy issues and decide which among them are a high priority and worthy of immediate attention. Other issues not on the policy agenda are placed in the cue to be dealt with at a later time.

5.4 Evaluation

Due to increased public scrutiny and accountability demands being placed on governments, there is a growing need to evaluate policy initiatives. A wide range of public "watch dog" organizations, non-governmental organizations, the media, and academic or policy think tanks—not to mention the Office of the Auditor General—are also actively engaged in public policy evaluation. Again, the objective is to determine if the policy does what it was supposed to do? Bobby Sui suggests policy-makers should ask the following questions to determine if a policy intervention is "good" policy:

1. Are the interests of stakeholder groups well balanced?

2. Is an accountability framework well articulated?

3. Are the objectives and expected impacts of the public policy explicitly stated?

4. Is the public policy the most cost-effective way to resolve the problem?

5. Is the public policy just to everyone affected by its implementation?

6. Does the public policy balance short- and long-term considerations? [3] (p. 84)

Good policy should reflect the values of society and consistent with the principles of justice and fairness. Evaluation is typically an ongoing process from the time of implementation. Governments typically establish a monitoring process (formal or informal) to track implementation and assess whether the policy has actually solved the problem.

6   Researchers and Policy

The good news is that researchers can play an important role at all stages of policy development. Increasingly governments tend not to take on the role of conducting their own research. The research capacity of many government departments has decreased over the past 20 years. This is due in part to a loss of capacity because of pressures to keep the size of governments small and because the range of issues facing the government at any one time is so significant it is difficult to develop expertise in the full range of issues.

For example in Canada, the Cabinet Secretariat at the provincial level or the Privy Council at the federal level and the general public service provides support to the Premier (provincial), Prime Minister (Federal), and Cabinet and it is their job to ensure the appropriate Minister(s) and Cabinet members understand the full range of options for resolving problems, the impact of each option (financial, political, or other), who is for and against each option, and any risks or mitigating factors. Policy analysts and senior bureaucrats prepare detailed briefings documents and presentations to ensure their political masters fully understand the scope of the problems and options available to them. The Cabinet Secretariat or Privy Council play an important role in coordinating the mass of information that the government in power needs to understand to facilitate the development of good policy decisions [17].

As a researcher you may be drawn into the policy process in one of several ways: either you have done research that you feel can inform policy and you actively seek opportunities to share your research with policy-makers to influence change, or government will approach you to seek your expertise and advice on a subject area because you have done research. A third option is that your research forms part of a body of literature that may inform policy at a later time.

In progressive jurisdictions government and consortiums of health researchers come together to formally collaborate to address pressing policy issues. Programs such as the Contextualized Health Research Synthesis Program (CHRSP) of the Newfoundland and Labrador Centre for Applied Health Research (NLCAHR) are a good example of how researchers collaborate with government to address policy issues. NLCAHR brings together decision-makers in government and researchers to identify important policy questions and to synthesize existing research and contextualize the findings to Newfoundland and Labrador [18]. Specifically, the CHRSP program brings together policy-makers and researchers to:

> "...focus on specific issues, rather than broad research themes; identify issues of concern to health system leaders; use research expertise to formulate researchable questions; synthesize quality research literature (systematic reviews); tailor the syntheses to the local context (challenges, capacities); report research results quickly and in usable formats." [18].

There are various other examples of government-researcher collaborations across Canada that bring together policy-makers and researchers. In some cases government provide funding to these agencies to fund their research projects.

7 Communicating Research Results to Policy-Makers

The first thing you will notice about policy-makers in government is they work on a very different scale of time and second; they are concerned with a different set of priorities. Researchers, even working on the fast track, take a considerable period of time from their idea to the final stage of presenting and publishing their research. Policy-makers on the other hand work with much shorter time frames. When a problem is identified, policy-makers need the research results to inform their policy decision yesterday, or in the best case scenario, today. When researchers and policy-makers work together, this is often the first point of concern. They need information today and it takes time to generate research to answer their very pressing questions. Researchers view their research as a process and policy-makers tend to view research as a product that can inform their policy-making [19].

The second feature—answering to a different set of priorities—focuses on the fact that the primary role of a public servant is to serve the government in power, and through the government they serve the public. Ultimately, policy-makers want to provide the best advice to their senior officials and they have to sift through large amounts of information and navigate through a wide range of stakeholders and special interest groups concerns and issues.

Knowledge translation, the process of translating and communicating research findings to end users for example, industry or decision-makers, is an essential component of the research process. The Canadian Institutes of Health Research define knowledge translation as,

> ...a dynamic and iterative process that includes synthesis, dissemination, exchange and ethically-sound application of knowledge to improve the health of Canadians, provide more effective health services and products and strengthen the health care system. This process takes place within a complex system of interactions between researchers and knowledge users which may vary in intensity, complexity and level of engagement depending on the nature of the research and the findings as well as the needs of the particular knowledge user. [20]

Indeed detailed descriptions of knowledge translation processes are an essential component of many research grant applications. It is also important to engage and involve policy-makers early in the research endeavor and maintain open communication regarding the progress. The earlier and more often policy-makers are involved and the more they are engaged during the research, the greater the likelihood the results of the research will be utilized in the policy process [19].

We are often in the position of being asked to share the results of our research with decision-makers in health organizations or governments. As researchers we are concerned about all aspects of our research. The research process is just as important to us as the outcome. Our training has taught us to be attentive to ethical considerations, research design, and ensuring our methods are appropriately suited to answering our research questions. Rigor, validity, reliability, and generalizability are words that permeate our research conversations. When we present our research in academic settings or at conferences, we carefully describe our process: our research question, our methods for data collection, our methods of analysis and limitations. Findings and conclusions arising from our research are derived from the data and analysis and are generally limited to the scope of the project we have undertaken. As researchers we tend to follow a well-rehearsed script when presenting our research to colleagues and attention to detail is important.

Policy-makers, however, have different concerns in mind when they look to research to inform the policy process. They are less concerned about the procedures of research; rather they are concerned about the outcomes of research. A policy-maker assumes you have done your research according to academic standards and that your data collection and analysis will withstand scrutiny by your peers. Rather they are more concerned with the findings, conclusions, and perhaps more important, the implications of your research as it relates to the issue of concern. This has important implications if you are invited to present your research to government officials. While many senior analysts in government have a background in research, it is generally good practice to repackage your academic presentation and tailor it to your audience. Spend less time explaining the details of your detailed analysis and spend more time explaining what the research "means."

In clinical practice there is an expectation that there is a body of research to warrant a change in clinical practice as opposed to a single study. Similarly in policy-making a single study may or may not serve as the basis for a change in policy. As a researcher, it is not realistic to assume that your single project will be sufficient to change policy. Rather expect that governments will similarly be seeking a body of research to support their decision-making and justify a change in policy. And be aware there are other factors that will be considered in policy decision-making.

The well-known axiom of "research informed policy-making" and "evidence-based decision-making" can quickly become a different kind of exercise known in the field as "decision-based evidence making." In other words, policy-makers may have a particular policy direction in mind and search the research literature to see if there is research to support the policy direction governments are interested in pursuing. This is not to cast a dim light on the integrity of policy-makers, but rather to recognize that the policy process can be very complex and many factors are considered when contemplating a change in direction especially if the policy issue is contentious.

8 Conclusions and a Checklist

Researchers can play an important role in the development of health policy. Indeed there is a growing expectation that research will inform the important decisions faced by health organizations and governments. The health policy development process is complex and involves many governmental and nongovernmental stakeholders. Communicating research to government or NGO policy-makers requires a shift in focus away from attention to the details of the research to a more concise focus on the outcomes. The following checklist may serve as a helpful guide to ensure your research can inform policy decisions.

8.1 Checklist

1. Be aware and keep abreast of the current policy issues related to your field of research.

2. As you conceptualize your research project, identify and build relationships with decision-makers that may have an interest in the outcomes of your research. Apprise them of the goals and aims of your research and keep them updated on your progress.

3. Explore unique knowledge translation opportunities to share the results of your research with potential end users.

4. Try to involve decision-makers in your research as collaborators; if they choose not to be involved, keep the decision-makers apprised of your progress.

5. Seek opportunities to get involved in public consultation sessions on policy issues related to your research.

6. If your research is relevant to a current policy debate, seek opportunities to talk about your research in public media. Radio stations and newspapers are always seeking interesting content on current topics.

7. If invited to present your research to decision-makers, remember a few pointers: understand your audience, stay on topic, keep your messages simple, avoid jargon, if you have any conflicts of interests state them up front, and focus on your results and their policy implications rather than on your methods (no matter how interesting). Finally, provide brief summaries of your research in easy to understand language.

References

1. Pal LA (2006) Beyond policy analysis: public issue management in turbulent times, 3rd edn. Thomson Canada Ltd., Toronto

2. Miljan L (2008) Public policy in Canada: an introduction, 5th edn. Oxford University Press, New York

3. Siu B (2014) Developing public policy: a practical guide. Canadian Scholar's Press, Toronto

4. Shah CP (2003) Public health and preventive medicine in Canada, 5th edn. Elsevier Saunders, Toronto

5. Bryant T (2009) An introduction to health policy. Canadian Scholar's Press Inc., Toronto

6. Canada Health Act (1984). R.S.C. 1985, c. C-6. http://laws-lois.justice.gc.ca/eng/acts/C-6/page-1.html. Accessed 28 Apr 2014

7. Department of Justice (2013) A consolidation of THE CONSTITUTION ACTS 1867 to 1982. DEPARTMENT OF JUSTICE, CANADA. Consolidated as of January 1, 2013. http://laws-lois.justice.gc.ca/PDF/CONST_E.pdf. Accessed 8 May 2014

8. Chenier NM (2004) Federal responsibility for the health care of specific groups. http://publications.gc.ca/collections/Collection-R/LoPBdP/PRB-e/PRB0452-e.pdf. Accessed 28 Apr 2014

9. Government of Canada (2013) Canada Health Act: annual report 2012–2013. http://www.hc-sc.gc.ca/hcs-sss/alt_formats/pdf/pubs/cha-ics/2013-cha-lcs-ar-ra-eng.pdf. Accessed 28 Apr 2014.

10. Government of Newfoundland and Labrador (2010) Introduction to Government. http://www.exec.gov.nl.ca/exec/hrs/onboarding/introduction_government.pdf. Accessed 4 May 2014

11. Marshall CE, Cashaback D (2001) Players, processes, institutions: central agencies in decision-making. Institute on Governance. http://archives.enap.ca/bibliotheques/2008/05/000318487.pdf. Accessed 2 May 2014

12. Dukeshire S, Thurlow J (2002) A brief guide to understanding policy development. Rural Communities Impacting Policy Project. ISBN 0-9780913-0-2

13. Rychetnik L, Carter SM, Abelson J, Thornton H, Barratt A, Entwistle VA, Mackenzie G, Salkeld G, Glasziou P (2013) Enhancing citizen engagement in cancer screening through deliberative democracy. J Natl Cancer Inst 105:380–386

14. Otten AL (1992) The influence of mass media on health policy. Health Aff 11(4):111–118

15. Parliament of Canada (2014) Legislative process. http://www.parl.gc.ca/About/House/

compendium/web-content/c_g_legislative-process-e.htm. Accessed 4 May 2014

16. Health Canada (2014) Sodium in Canada. http://www.hc-sc.gc.ca/fn-an/nutrition/sodium/index-eng.php. Accessed 4 May 2014

17. Government of Canada (2011) The role and structure of the Privy Council Office 2011. http://www.pco-bcp.gc.ca/index.asp?lang=eng&page=information&sub=publications&doc=role/role2013-eng.htm. Accessed 3 May 2014

18. NLCAHR (2014) Contextualized health research synthesis program. http://www.nlcahr.mun.ca/CHRSP/. Accessed 19 Apr 2014

19. Lomas J (2000) Connecting research and policy. ISUMA Spring, pp 140–144

20. Canadian Institutes of Health Research (2014) More about knowledge translation at CIHR. Knowledge translation – definition. http://www.cihr-irsc.gc.ca/e/39033.html. Accessed 14 May 2014

INDEX

A

Accuracy

clinical research data 5, 31

diagnostic tests 39, 42, 46, 219, 289–298

ADAPTE process 491

Address transparency and conflict of interest 447–449

ADL and Barthel index 192

Administrative databases

   advantages 469, 479–481

   creation 470–473

   data linkage 474–475

   definition 469–470

   disadvantages 479–481

   disease definition 473

   example 471–472

   health services research 469–481

   population-based studies 475–479

   sources 470, 474

Alignment of research questions 273–274

Allele-sharing method 353–356

Allocation concealment 8, 162, 261, 390, 392

Allocative efficiency 317–320

Alpha spending 181

Analyses

   biomarkers 207–219, 237, 241

   diagnostic tests 210, 211, 216–220, 289–299, 333

   hypothesis-generating 189

   interim 169, 170, 180–183

   longitudinal studies 64–68, 71–91

   planned 169, 350

   quality of life 261–271

   randomized controlled trials 177–189, 261–271

   subgroup 11, 169

Analysis of covariance (ANCOVA) 234

ANOVA 96, 128, 129

Appraisal of Guidelines, Research, Evaluation (AGREE)
   Collaboration 450

Association studies, for genetic

   identification 359–362, 364

   challenges 362–363

   design 358–361

   interpretation 361–362

   population 360

Audit trail 170, 302

B

Bariatric surgery 388, 460–464

Belmont Report 20

Berlin Code of 1900 19

Bias

   adjustment bias 33, 45

   admission rate bias 32, 35

   aggregation bias 32, 36

   allocation sequence bias 32, 36

   all's well literature bias 32, 35

   apprehension bias 32, 41

   ascertainment bias 11, 55, 147, 335, 336, 392

   assumption bias 33, 45, 47

   attention bias 32, 41

   autopsy series bias 32, 36

   auxiliary hypothesis bias 33, 47

   Bergstrom's bias 32, 35

   bogus control bias 32, 40

   case mix bias 32, 39, 56, 152, 155, 165, 171, 471

   central tendency bias 33, 42

   centripetal bias 32, 36

   channeling bias 32, 36

   cognitive dissonance bias 33, 47

   co-intervention bias 32, 40

   competing death bias 32, 41

   competing risk bias 335–337

   compliance bias 32, 41, 335, 342

   confirmation bias 32, 41

   context bias 33, 41

   correlation bias 33, 47

   culture bias 33, 41

   data capture bias 33, 42

   data completeness bias 33, 45

   data dredging bias 33, 45

   data entry bias 33, 42

   data merging bias 42

   design bias 32, 34

   detection bias 11, 33, 42

   diagnostic access bias 32, 36

   diagnostic bias 335, 341

   diagnostic purity bias 32, 36

   diagnostic review bias 33, 42

   diagnostic suspicion bias 33, 42, 61

   diagnostic vogue bias 32, 36

Patrick S. Parfrey and Brendan J. Barrett (eds.), *Clinical Epidemiology: Practice and Methods*, Methods in Molecular Biology,
vol. 1281, DOI 10.1007/978-1-4939-2428-8, © Springer Science+Business Media New York 2015

Bias (*cont.*)

differential bias 32, 34

distribution assumption bias 33, 45

dose targeting bias 57

drop-out bias 32, 40

ecological fallacy bias 32, 36

end-digit preference bias 33, 42

enquiry unit bias 33, 45

estimator bias...33, 45

expectation bias...33, 42

exposure bias................................ 33, 39, 46, 342–343

exposure suspicion bias 33, 42

faking bad news bias 33, 42

family information bias................................33, 42

forced choice bias...33, 43

foreign language exclusion bias................32, 35

framing bias..33, 43

generalization bias.......................................33, 47

Hawthorne effect...32, 41

healthy worker bias 32, 36, 59

hospital discharge bias 33, 43

hot stuff bias...32, 35

immigrant bias...32, 37

inclusion control bias..................................32, 37

incorporation bias..33, 43

indication bias..33, 43

information bias................................. 32–34, 42, 58, 61,
335, 339–342, 345, 392

insensitive measure bias 33, 43

instrument bias 33, 43

inter-observer variability bias.........................297

interpretation bias.......................................33, 47

intervention bias 335, 342

interviewer bias..33, 43

interview setting bias 33, 43

intra-observer variability bias.........................297

juxtaposed scale bias 33, 43

laboratory data bias.....................................33, 43

latency bias 33, 44

lead time bias................................. 32, 37, 335, 339–341

length time bias 335, 340, 341

literature search bias 32, 34, 35

loss to follow up bias.................32, 37, 335, 337–338, 344

magnitude bias...33, 47

membership bias...32, 37

memory bias 339

migration bias...32, 37

mimicry bias...32, 37

misclassification bias...........................32, 34, 38

missing clinical data bias............................32, 38

mistaken identity bias 33, 47

multiple exposure bias.................................33, 46

Neyman's bias 32, 38, 338

non-contemporaneous control bias......................32, 38

non differential bias 32, 35

non random sampling bias..........................33, 46

non responsive bias 32, 38

non simultaneous comparison bias 32, 38

obsequiousness bias.....................................33, 44

observer effect...32, 41

omitted variable bias...................................33, 46

one-sided reference bias...............................32, 35

outlier handling bias 33, 46

over-diagnosis bias.......................................32, 38

over-matching bias 33, 46, 335, 338

performance bias...............................11, 32, 41

popularity bias 32, 38

positive results bias 32, 35

positive satisfaction bias.............................33, 44

post-hoc significance bias 33, 46

prevalence-incidence bias 32, 38, 335, 338, 344

procedure bias...32, 41

procedure selection bias 32, 38

proficiency bias 32, 41, 335, 342

protopathic bias..33, 44

proxy respondent bias 33, 44

questionnaire bias 33, 44

recall bias 33, 44, 61, 335, 339, 344

record linkage bias 32, 38

referral bias 32, 35, 336

referral filter bias...32, 38

regression to mean bias...............................33, 46

repeated peeks bias 33, 46

reporting bias.................................. 33, 44, 446, 447

response bias.......................................32, 38, 56

response fatigue bias 33, 44

review bias 33, 44

rhetoric bias..32, 35

rumination bias..33, 45

sample size bias..32, 38

sampling bias 7, 16, 32, 39, 61

scale degradation bias 33, 46

scale format bias 33, 44

selection bias................................8, 32, 35, 56, 58,
134–137, 162, 225, 335–338, 343, 346, 392

self-selection bias 32, 39, 337

sensitive question bias.................................33, 44

significance bias 33, 47

solicitation sampling bias...........................32, 39

spatial bias 33, 44

spectrum bias..32, 39

stage bias...32, 39

standard population's bias 33, 46

starting line bias...32, 39

substitution game bias 33, 45

surveillance bias 33, 42, 212, 341

survivor treatment selection bias.............32, 39, 335, 338

susceptibility bias...32, 39

systematic error.......... 5, 6, 31, 32, 34, 35, 42–44, 72, 335
test review bias...33, 45
therapeutic personality bias.............................33, 45
treatment analysis bias.....................................33, 46
unacceptability bias...33, 45
under-exhaustion bias......................................33, 47
unmasking bias 32, 39
verification bias......................................33, 46, 297
volunteer bias....................32, 39, 335, 337, 344
Will Rogers bias 32, 40
withdrawal bias...32, 40
yes-saying bias 33, 45
Biomarkers
cohort study...212, 213
confounding...212, 213
continuous 213, 217–218
C-statistic.................. 147, 150–152, 155, 209, 214, 215
diagnostic............................... 207, 210–212, 216–218
dichotomous 217
generalizability of 219–220
HMG-CoA inhibitors 211
integrated discrimination improvement.............209, 214
in interventional studies...................................211
prognostic cohort study 215–216, 219
reclassification 209, 212, 214–215
risk factors, relationship with..................208–209
sample size.......................................215–216, 219
surrogate outcomes..................................207–223
survival analysis 213
validation 211–220
Biospecimen collection 204
Blinding........................... 5, 11, 25, 41, 44, 61, 164, 217,
345, 361, 392, 403
Blocking 162
Brier score...148
Budgets
development 276–278
direct costs 276–278
indirect costs 278

C

Canadian Agency for Drugs and Technologies in Health
(CADTH) 419, 425
Canadian Health Act (CHA)..............................504, 505
Canadian health care system 274
Canadian hypertension education program.....................451
Canadian Institutes of Health Research
(CIHR)............ 274, 275, 278, 280, 456, 458–462
Canadian Research Ethics Boards....................................21
Candidate surrogate outcomes..9
Case-control design, in association studies........................59
Case-control studies
advantages...60
confounding variables 60

control selection...61
design 61–62
disadvantages...60–61
information bias..61
matching...60, 61
nested case-control study..59–60
sampling bias 61
Case study
diagnostic tests....................................292–293
health technology assessment 433–436
Censoring...................... 105, 106, 110, 118, 122, 123, 125,
126, 128, 147, 183, 205, 213, 251, 252, 257, 258
CHA. *See* Canadian Health Act (CHA)
Children, ethical research on 29
Chronic kidney disease (CKD)
risk prediction models........................ 145, 146, 150–155
TREAT trial...271
Classical test theory...............................204. *See also*
Patient-reported outcomes
Clinical practice guidelines
address transparency....................................447–449
committee........................... 444–445, 447–450
conflict of interest....................................447–449
consultation 449–450
development 443–452
evaluation of 444, 450, 452
evidence grade 443–452
guideline and target audience 444
implementation strategy.....................................449
legal issues 451–452
liability..452
limitations...443–452
reporting 447
revision 451
Clinical relevance.. 3, 13, 334, 347
Clinical research
budget estimation 276–278
cohort study...52–54
funding/grants 171–172, 274–276
goal..5
investigators, travel for......................................277–278
management of....................................279–286
reporting governance in 278–279
staff, training for 279, 282
Clinical studies, precision and accuracy in.........................5
Clinical trials
censoring 183
in economic evaluation 315–329
of end-stage renal disease 269, 303
in ethical research 19–29
financial interest declaration....................................27
of health care costs....................................315, 318
limitations of 160
planning.................. 8, 13, 169, 172, 179, 264, 326–327

Clustered data...94, 110
Cohort studies. *See also* Longitudinal studies
  advantages of..53–54
  ascertainment bias 55
  confounding variables 58
  contamination...55–56
  control group selection................................58–59
  data collection...58
  design 57–59
  disadvantages..54–57
  disease status...58
  dose targeting control 57
  historical controls 53, 54, 57
  matching...58, 60, 61
  period prevalent cohort.................................57
  prevalent *vs.* incident cohorts 57
  prognostic biomarkers..............................52, 53
  selection bias...56
Collaborative health research projects
        (CHRP) program 274
Colorectal cancer 303, 336, 342, 377
Common rule, United States............................21
Competing risk events. *See* Competing risks bias
Competing risks bias 335–337
Complex genetic diseases
  determination of...350
  gene identification strategies 352–364
    association analysis in 350, 357–362
    linkage methods in.........................353–357
  mode of inheritance, determination of...............351–352
Composite outcomes 167, 178, 184, 189, 221
Confidence intervals...................13, 65–67, 72, 91, 97,
        112, 114, 120, 121, 127, 152, 154, 187, 201, 203,
        220, 230, 231, 236, 238, 253, 255, 257, 295, 334,
        390, 393, 399, 405, 406, 411, 496
Confidentiality
  data...21, 280
  privacy and...21–22
Conflict of interest...................................447–449
Confounding bias 11, 32, 34
  minimizing methods......................................11
Confounding biomarkers..................................213
Confounding variables................58, 60, 61, 66, 85,
        212, 338, 343–346
Consolidated Standards of Reporting Trials
        (CONSORT trials) 174, 285
Construct validity................................ 11, 202, 311
Consumables.................................... 172, 276, 277
  individual expenses..277
Contamination
  design 250
  sample size estimate......................................250
  statistical plan 251
  study execution 250–251

Content/face validity...202
Coronary artery stents 433, 434
Correlated data.....................110, 111, 114, 115, 118
Correlation structures.........................114–116, 129
Cost-benefit analysis (CBA) 430
Cost-effectiveness analysis (CEA)
  of health technologies................................433, 434
  in HTA..430
Costs
  of CPG development....................................451
  of diagnostic tests 298
  of health care 315, 318, 323
  minimization analysis 318
Cost-utility analysis (CUA)............................430–432
Cox proportional hazards method...........55, 64, 67, 147, 150
Cox regression model 123, 125, 127, 215, 258
Cox's model
  check for model 110
  coefficient in Cox's regression......................110
  effect (β) of covariate in 109
  variations of 217
Criterion validity...202
Critical appraisal
  causation assessment....................................394
  evidence-based medicine 391
  evidence-based medicine approach..............386
  extrinsic factors..390
  grading of recommendation, assessment, development,
        and evaluation (GRADE)....................388, 390
  levels of scientific evidence 387–390
  meta-analysis 389, 392, 393
  methods...388–390
  Oxford Centre for Evidence-based
        Medicine..388–390
  randomized controlled trials 387, 389, 393
  results applicability 391
  results appraisal..386
  study design 388
  systemic reviews 387, 388, 392
  validity.............................385, 386, 390–392, 394
Critical turning points, in substantive theory 308
Crossover design............................... 15, 164, 171, 185–186
Cross-sectional studies 13, 14, 16, 52, 111,
        344, 387, 388, 393
C-statistic.................................147, 148, 150–152,
        155, 209, 214, 215, 219
CUA. *See* Cost-utility analysis (CUA)
Cumulative index to nursing and allied health
        literature..424

D

Database, bibliographic
  of HTA resources 424
  language and vocabulary used in................ 402, 424, 426

Data collection
    in clinical research 324
    for HTA 428, 429
    in randomized control trial 280, 284–285
Data safety and monitoring committee
    (DSMC) 173, 280
DCCT. *See* Diabetes control and complications trial (DCCT)
DCOR clinical trial,
Decision analysis 323, 324, 333, 420
Decision maker
    cost-utility analysis 318–321
    economic analysis 429–431
    health care 417–419, 432
    health policy 428
    research design..514
Decision trees 431
Derivation set 149, 219
DES. *See* Drug-eluting stents (DES)
Diabetes control and complications trial
    (DCCT) 177–179, 182
Diagnostic odds ratio (DOR)...296
Diagnostic spectrum effect 219
Diagnostic tests
    accuracy 290–298
    assessment of 290–293, 297
    case study...292–293
    choosing tests..298
    continuous measure 296
    costs 298
    diagnostic odds ratio..296
    gold standard 289–291, 296, 297
    likelihood ratio 293–294
    predictive values of..291–292
    randomized trial 298, 299
    receiver operating characteristic curve............294, 295, 297
    reproducibility..297
    research design..298
    sample size..297, 299
    sensitivity and specificity of 290–291
    utility 290, 297, 298
    validity...290
Direct association studies ....358. *See also*
    Gene identification strategies
Direct costs...276, 278
Drop-in 149, 169, 171, 239–241, 249,
    250, 253, 308, 430
Dropout............................ 67, 169–171, 212, 249, 250, 253,
    258, 342, 344, 393
Drug-eluting stents (DES)............................220, 433–436

E

ECONOLIT database, importance of,
Economic analysis
    checklist...431, 432

conducted by path...435
in HTA...429–432
risk reduction...186
Economic evaluation. *See also* Health economics
clinical trials.............................316, 319, 320, 322–324,
    326–327, 329
    conduct...322, 326
    for incremental costs and benefits of
        technology 316, 319, 429
    PATH presentation 434, 436
    planning.. 316, 317, 323, 326–327
    problem 316
    results interpretation..320–322
    strengths 316, 322–323
    types of..317–320
    use by health professionals..................................327–329
    weaknesses 316, 322–323
Economic issues 170
EMBASE and MEDLINE, differences of 426
Endophenotype-based approach, role 359
End-point adjudication committee 173
End-stage renal disease
    clinical trials..220
    cost-effectiveness analysis,
    EVOLVE trial..253–254
    grounded theory study...304
    knowledge translation,
Equipments
    additional,
    required...277
Errors
    accidental...6
    alpha error...9
    effect on study results 6
    measurement.. 11, 203, 339
    random 5, 6, 8, 11, 32, 35, 71, 72, 335, 390
    systematic error................................5–7, 31, 32, 34, 35,
        42–44, 72, 121, 334, 335
    type I and type II, in clinical trial 167
    types of 6, 335
European Regulatory Issues on Quality of Life Assessment
    Group 195
European Union, HRQOL guidelines.....................194–195
Evidence-based decision making
    administrative database utilization....................469–481
    clinical practice guidelines 443–452
    critical appraisal..385–395
    health policy 501–516
    health technology assessment 417–438
    knowledge translation......................................485–498
    meta-analysis...397–412
    systematic review 397–412
    translational research 455–466
Evidence-based research, key elements of.................273–274

Evidence tables, used in CPG 447
Evidence to practice gap................... 485, 491, 493,
        495, 498
Exposed *vs.* unexposed subjects............................55
Extended generalized linear models
    choice of analytical tool 115
    correcting model variance.....................114–116
    fixed effects..112–114
    generalized estimating equations.......................115, 116
    intraclass correlation coefficient....................113
    mixed effect models...114
    panel data layout...111–112
    random effects 113, 114, 120
    variance components, of data........................113
Extended survival models
    correlation among events 117
    correlation in survival times.......................116
    event dependence within subject 116
    ordered events..119–120
    risk set, for survival analysis....................118–120
    shared frailty..117, 121
    time-dependent effects 120
    time-varying covariate 120
    unordered events........................... 118, 123, 126
    unshared frailty..116
External validity 11–12, 57, 58, 149,
        152, 154, 345

F

Factorial designs 15, 163, 169, 185, 242
Final outcome........................... 10, 16, 340
Follow-up
    outcome measures.....................................166
    rate of loss...170–171
    time to complete.......................................165
Food and Drug Administration (FDA), U.S. 166, 194,
        196, 280
Forest plot........................... 121, 404, 405, 407
Foundations. *See also* Funding
    charitable/not-for-profit agencies...........................275
    private and public, for research grants 275
Frailty model 121–122
    generalized linear models........................94–96
Functions, concept of............................72–73
Funding
    agency research theme 273
    for clinical research...........................274–276
    costs...172
    distribution...282
    license required for...........................172
    reporting...335
    sources of...274–276
Funnel plot...403, 405, 406

G

Gene identification strategies
    association analysis in 352
    linkage methods in 352
Generalized linear models
    limitation...94
    members, attributes in 94
    regression coefficients...........................95
    standard link functions and inverses 95
    systematic component of 94
    validity...97
Genetic association study 359–361
    interpretation of...361
Genetic diseases, clinical epidemiologic studies
    ascertainment bias 335, 336
    bias in different designs 13, 343
    bias minimizing methods.......................399
    competing risks bias.......................335–337
    compliance bias...........................335, 342
    confounding,
    confounding minimizing strategies,
    contamination bias...........................335, 342–343
    diagnostic bias 335, 341
    family information bias.......................335, 342
    information bias........................... 335, 339, 342, 345
    intervention bias...........................335, 342
    lead time bias...........................335, 339–340
    length time bias 335, 340, 341
    loss to follow up bias...................335, 337–338, 344
    matching...345
    multivariate modeling.......................345, 346
    non response bias...........................335, 337
    overmatching bias...........................335, 338
    prevalence-incidence bias 335, 344
    proficiency bias...........................335, 342
    recall bias 335, 339, 344
    restriction...345
    selection bias........................... 335–338, 343, 344, 346
    stratification........................... 345, 346, 360–362
    survivor treatment selection bias.......................335, 338
    volunteer bias........................... 335, 337, 344
    Will Rogers phenomenon.......................335, 341
Genetic epidemiology, in complex traits
    allele sharing method.......................353–356
    analysis of linkage studies 355–356
    association analysis 350, 352
    association-based study challenges 357–363
    candidate gene approach.......................358
    complex traits 350–351
    false positive associations.......................361
    genetic risk ratio 364
    genome-wide association study (GWAS)..........358–359,
        361–365

genomic imprinting 352
genotyping technology 358–361, 365
limitations of linkage studies 356–357
linkage methods..353–357
Mendelian patterns of inheritance....................350, 351
mode of inheritance.................................351–352
non Mendelian patterns of inheritance........................352
parametric linkage analysis 353–354
phenotype...349–365
replication studies 355, 356
sample size...................................350, 356, 362–364
segregation analysis...................350, 351, 357
twin studies...350
Genetic equilibrium. *See* Hardy–Weinberg equilibrium
Genetic heterogenicity.................................357
Genetics ELSI (Ethical, Legal, and Social Issues)
biobanks...374–378
budget..379
definition 369–371
deliberative democracy approach 376
GE³LS research 370–374
genetic health literacy 376
history..371–374
interdisciplinary team 370, 372, 378, 379
normative research.......................... 370, 372–274, 379
publication process.......................................379
public engagement.........................371, 373–378
Genetics, Ethical, Economic, Environmental, Legal and
Social Issues (GE³LS). *See* Genetics ELSI
(Ethical, Legal, and Social Issues)
descriptive research 372
integrated research.......................................463
stand-alone research 371, 372
Genome Canada......................... 274, 275, 279,
371, 372
Genomewide association studies 350
Genomic imprinting.......................................352
Good Clinical Practice (GPC) 21
membership guidelines 21
Governance
of ethics review 21
policies..473
reporting..278–279
Grades of recommendation assessment, development and
evaluation (GRADE) 388, 446, 447, 496
Grading, clinical practice guideline 3, 250, 328,
443–452, 461, 491, 496, 497
Grants
budget allocation 278
clinical research..274
review 275
Grey literature 424, 425
Grounded theory methodology....................302–304
Group sequential methods..............................181

H

Hard outcomes 9, 10, 209, 266, 445
Hardy–Weinberg equilibrium...........................361
Hazards proportionality.................................109
Health care
costs...315, 318, 323–325, 478
decision makers.....................................327, 432
funding 274, 322, 327, 328, 463
impact of the therapy on costs of...........315, 322, 323, 326
and medical devices 417, 419
policy...170, 473
problems,
public financing of....................................192
technologies (*see* Health technology assessment)
Health economics. *See also* Economic evaluation
allocative efficiency....................................317–320
cost-benefit study 318
cost-effectiveness study...............................318
cost-minimization analysis 318
cost-utility study...317
decision analysis......................................323, 324
opportunity cost...........................316–317, 320
quality adjusted life year (QALY)......................319–322,
324–326
randomized controlled trials 319
technical efficiency 317, 318, 320
value for money 318, 320, 323, 327, 328
Health outcomes 17, 36, 290, 301, 308, 317,
324, 326, 333, 374, 417, 418, 420, 428–430, 445,
450, 458, 461–464, 475, 476, 490, 495
Health policy
Canada Health Act..............................504, 505
checklist..515–516
communication with policy makers 513–515
definition 502, 506
evaluation..511–512
evidence-based decision making..................501–515
example...............................501–507, 509, 510
implementation 510–511
knowledge translation..................................514
planning..509–510
policy arena.................................505–509, 511
policy problem assessment
public policy.......................... 502–507, 511, 512
public policy purpose 503–505
researcher role.......................................512–513
stakeholders 505–511, 514
Health-related quality of life (HRQOL)
criteria for evaluation...................................196
domains for general measures 198
guidance document, for measurement 196
instruments used for 197
SF-6D and versions.....................................198

Health status 26, 43, 177, 192, 193, 197,
          199, 262, 263, 267, 271, 306–308, 393, 470
Health technology assessment
     basic framework for 419–433
     checklist...431, 432
     cost-benefit analysis in..430
     cost-effectiveness analysis in......................................430
     cost-utility analysis in 430–431
     databases...424–426
     data collection.......................... 428, 429, 435, 437
     decision making framework..434
     definition 418
     dissemination strategies 436
     economic analysis in 429–432
     evidence interpretation in 435
     evidence synthesis...435
     ethical issues 422–423
     examples 419, 423, 427
     findings...432–433, 435
     identifying topics 419–420
     monitoring...433
     problems 434
     recommendations..432
     search strategy 425–426
     social issues...421–422
     sources of evidence..423, 425
     specification..420
Health Utilities Index..319
Healthy years equivalent (HYE)...268
Heart outcomes prevention evaluation
          (HOPE) 163, 173
Helsinki Declaration 20
Hemodialysis, grounded theory study
          for 17, 20, 129, 170, 253, 255, 303–310,
          317, 318, 477, 478, 496
Hereditary nonpolyposis colorectal cancer
          (HNPCC)..303, 357
Heterogeneity test 410
Hierarchy of evidence............................ 13–14, 54, 386, 387
Historical cohort 53, 57, 212
Hosmer–Lemeshow chi square 148
HTA reports..433
Hypothesis-generating analyses 189

I

Identical by descent (IBD) 354
Identity link function..95
Implantable cardioverter-defibrillator 338
Incidence rate ratio...........................80, 85, 89, 90, 103, 110
Incompetence, and ethical research 28, 29
Indirect association studies...358
     identification strategies.....................................352–364
Indirect costs 278, 492
Informed consent 19, 20, 22, 24–29, 160,
          200, 304, 375, 378

Input and output
     possible relationships between 84
     variables measurement......................................55, 82, 83
Intention-to-treat analysis..............................8, 167, 180
Interaction
     coefficient of...85, 87–88
     modeling confounding and...................................85–86
     in multiplicative models.....................................88–90
          hypothetical cardiac events data as IRR...........89, 90
     parameter as measure of...................................82, 87
     statistical meaning 86–87
Interactive parameter estimation 251
Interest phenomenon...6, 202
Interim analyses............................ 169, 170, 180–183
Intermediate (surrogate) response 10
Intermediate variables..9
Internal validity 11–12
Intervention bias..335, 342
Intervention questions, experimental design for..........14–16
Inverse probability of censoring weights...........252, 257–258
Item response theory 193, 204

K

Kaplan–Meier (K–M) analysis 213
Kaplan–Meier method 63, 67, 124, 125
Karnofsky performance status 192
Knowledge to action cycle 459, 460, 486–491, 498
Knowledge translation
     ADAPTE process 491
     barriers... 486, 487, 492–493
     clinical decision support systems 494
     definition 149, 154, 457
     evaluation..460, 498
     evidence to practice gap 491, 493, 495
     example..478, 479, 488, 496, 514
     frameworks 486
     intervention implementation 486, 493, 494
     knowledge products...488–490
     knowledge synthesis 488, 490
     knowledge use sustainability....................................495
     local context...460, 491
     policy maker integration 464, 486
     problem identification 486
     risk prediction models,

L

Lag censoring 251, 257, 258
Latent trait theory...204
Leber's optic atrophy 352
Legal issues
     in CPG development
     in research ethics
Level of evidence
     in diagnostic studies...16
     meta-analysis of randomized controlled trials for.......411

of observational studies................................447
sample sizes and follow up for 184
Level of significance 9, 356
Licensing, for drugs/health technologies...........172
Likelihood
of article being valid 320
based estimation procedures 91, 215, 253
of CKD..8
as function of recombination fraction..........354
and probability...76
ratio 210, 293–294, 353, 392
treatment being successful 322
Linear model. *See also* Generalized linear models
regression coefficients of.........................96, 97
three-dimensional representation 83
Linear predictor.................73, 78, 94, 101, 112, 113
Linear regression 66, 67, 74, 75, 78–80, 86,
96–101, 244, 346
Linear relationship 74, 77, 79
Linkage disequilibrium.................................358
Linkage methods, for genetic identification 352, 353
Literature review. *See also* Systematic review
in clinical trials 4–5
in development of CPG 451
of HTA resources 435
to identify related research...........................4
Living with end-stage renal disease and hemodialysis
(LESRD-H) 306, 307
Logistic function 73, 95, 98–100
Logistic model. *See also* Poisson model, for count, check
for model fail
Coefficient in logistic regression....................79
Dichotomous response 67
vs. linear model
Sigmoid nature and information of error...........73
Structure 98–99
Logit function 95
Longitudinal cohort studies................13, 14, 226,
244–245, 374
Longitudinal data 71, 110, 111, 129
Longitudinal studies. *See also* Cohort studies
analyzing confounders 64
confidence intervals 65–67, 72, 91, 97,
112, 114, 120, 121, 127, 152, 154
confounder identification..............................64
Cox Proportional Hazard Model.....................109
diagnostic test assessment.......................14, 17
log-rank test 63
multivariate models 68, 71–91
odds ratio.............63, 65, 66, 79, 100, 101, 134
power..............................62–64, 68, 81, 84, 97,
106, 115, 119, 166
relative risk 63, 65, 66
risk estimation 65–66
sample size estimation 64
survival data analysis..................................67

M

Markov models.....................................129, 431
Masking.....................................11, 32, 39, 164, 403
Matching
case control studies 60, 61, 65, 134–137, 345, 360
cohort studies...................133, 134, 138, 139
overmatching...338
to reduce confounding...............................134
Maximum likelihood estimation (MLE)..............75, 76, 91,
99, 104, 215. *See also* Likelihood
Memorandum of understanding (MOU).......................283
Memorial University of Newfoundland, research grant
report 276
Memorial University, research ethics board....................462
Mental component summary (MCS)..............................198
Meta-analysis
bias risk...398, 399
data abstraction................... 400, 401, 403–404
evidence matrix.......................................408
flow diagram...404
Forest plot..........................404, 405, 407
Funnel plot 403, 405, 406
heterogeneity test.....................................410
information summary 404–410
information synthesis.........................404–410
limitations............................398, 410–413
meta-regression plot 405–407
protocol......................... 400, 401, 403
publication bias.................. 401, 403, 405, 412
research question 397, 400–402
strengths 410–411
study design 400, 402
study identification 402
Microsatellite markers, advantage of 355
Ministry of Health and Long-Term Care, Ontario..........433
Medical Advisory Secretariat (MAS),
Missing data 11, 15, 16, 54, 129, 164, 205,
261, 263–267, 270
Modifiers...................................... 11, 137, 407, 409
Mortality, clinical outcomes...........................183
Multicollinearity.......................................110
Multiple measurements 93, 111
Multivariable model (R^2 statistics), GFR cohort
study 96
Multivariate analysis
additive models......................................85–88
competing risk model 118
confounding..72, 82–90
Cox regression coefficients 96–97
Cox regression model 127
data transformation 81
exposure–response relationship.......................72, 79–80
extended generalized linear models 111–116
extended survival models 116–128
frailty models 121

Multivariate analysis (*cont.*)
    function 72–77, 79, 80, 82, 84, 85, 87, 88, 90
    generalized linear models...94–96
    general linear model
        coefficients..96–97
            structure...96
            validity..97
    interaction...82–90
    interaction coefficient 87–88
    likelihood...76
    linear predictor......................................73, 78, 94, 112, 113
    logistic model structure..98–100
    logistic regression.......................80, 94, 95, 98–103, 105
    logistic regression coefficients...............................96–97
    Markov chain models 129
    maximum likelihood estimation 75
    model assumption...77, 81
    model choice...78–81
    model random component...78
    model structure...77–78
    multivariate ANOVA 96
    ordinary least squares method.....................................75
    parameter estimates 74, 76, 79, 81, 91
    Poisson model structure..73, 89
    Poisson regression...80, 88, 91
    Poisson regression coefficients....................................80
    probability...76
    propensity score matching 138–139
    random effects model 111
    regression...71–72
    repeated measures ANOVA...............................128, 129
    reporting methods 90–91
    reporting results 91
    risk prediction models...146
    survival analysis methods.................................105–106
    time-dependent effects 120
    time series models...129
    time-to-event data functions 94
    time varying covariates 120
    unordered events marginal model.....................118–119
    variance-corrected models 111, 117, 120, 121
Multivariate ANOVA (MANOVA)..............................129

N

Narrative reviews and systematic review,
        difference of..398
National Health and Medical Research Council
        of Australia 444
National Institute for Clinical Excellence, U.K. 322, 448
National Institutes of Health, U.S. 172, 274
National Library of Medicine (NLM), U.S............. 424, 426
National Research Act (1974) 20
Natural log links 95
Nested case-control studies 59–60

Networking, and clinical research....................................284
Neutral trials..187
Non insulin-dependent diabetes (NIDDM) 173, 357
Non interventional/observational studies 52
Non parametric method. *See* Allele-sharing method
Non participants..56, 404
Normally distributed errors 95
Number needed to treat (NNT)..................... 140, 186–187,
        237, 392, 409
Nuremberg Code...19, 20

O

O'Brien and Fleming method 181, 182
Observational–experimental discrepancy........................188
    Observational studies. *See also* Cohort studies;
        Longitudinal studies
    factors influencing sample size 62–63
    power...62–64
    sample size estimation 62–64
    Sample size for Long-Rank test 63–64
        type I and type II errors..............................63–64
Odds ratio (OR)........................ 45, 63, 65–67, 79, 100, 101,
        134, 209–211, 219, 257, 296, 362, 363, 392, 409
Ontario health care system 434
Ontario Health Technology Advisory Committee...........436
    recommendations...436
Open-label run-in periods, and clinical trials 185
Opportunity costs...316–317, 320

P

Parametric method. *See* Recombinant-based method
Participants
    confirming interpretive summaries.............................47
    in control trial...262
    delaying enrollment 163
    demographic data for identification...........................477
    to enroll eligible..170
    identified based on disease...................................14, 491
    monitoring..169
    quantitative scale...221
    research...25, 26
    selection..7
Patient Perception of Hemodialysis Scale (PPHS)...........309
Patient-reported outcomes
    assessing change...204–205
    characteristics of scales 200–201
    Classical Test Theory...204
    clinically important difference 220
    comparing groups 204–205
    computerized adaptive testing 193, 200, 201, 204
    construct validity 202
    content validity...202
    criterion validity...202
    floor and ceiling effects......................................200, 201

focus groups 199–200, 202
health-related quality of life 192, 195–199
HRQOL claims 193, 195
individualized quality of life 199
individual's observation of experience 193
instrument selection 195
interval consistency reliability 203
item response theory 193, 204
measurement of subjective experience 199
missing data 205
model for assessment 204
professional facilitators 199
PROMIS 199, 204
quality of life domains 199
scale reliability 200–201
scales to discriminate individuals 200
SF-36 197–199
societal level 192
supporting claims of therapeutic benefit 194
test-retest reliability 203
utility 193, 194
validity 202
Patients, interventions, controls, and outcomes 4
Peer-review, of research ethics 412, 459
Personnel
    agreements with department/institution 119
    costs, salary and benefits 22
    training 25
Pharmaceutical manufacturers
    economic evaluation of drugs, role in 324
    licensing of drugs, role in 118
    relationship with guidelines committees 9
Physical Component Summary (PCS) 198
PICO. *See* Patients, interventions, controls, and outcomes
PICO(S) model, for development of search
        strategy 118
Planning
    in clinical trials 184
    of health services 317
    in prognostic biomarker study 211
Poisson distribution 76, 80, 95, 103, 104
Poisson model, for count
    check for model fail 110
    coefficient meaning in 110
    structure of
        likelihood function of l 105
        MLEs of ß parameters 104
        model offset 103
Poisson regression
    goodness-of-fit test for 102, 105
    using Framingham data 105
Policies
    ethical review 19–21
    governance 22

Population
    and clinical trial 24
    and diagnostic test 36
Positional cloning .... 352, 353, 358. *See also* Genetic
        epidemiology, in complex traits
Prader–Willi syndrome 352
Pragmatic trials 241, 428, 438
Precision ratio 91
Predictive values, for diagnostic tests 291
Prentice criterion, to determine surrogate endpoint 223
Privacy data 280
Private industry, clinical research grant 274, 275
Professional organizations, clinical research
        grant 275–276
Programs for assessment of technology in health
        (PATH) 433
Project management
    biospecimen collection 284
    coordinator 281
    data collection 284–285
    ethics 282
    funding distribution 282
    hiring 281
    leadership 279–281
    memorandum of understanding 283
    milestones 282
    networking 284
    organization 279–281
    public relations 284
    reporting 285
    research plan implementation 283–284
    scientific advisory board 280
    team building 279
    training 282
Propensity score matching
    advantages 141
    assessing the balance of covariates 142
    association between exposure and outcome 142
    constructing the score 141
    deriving a score 141
    limitations 141
Proportional hazards model 64, 67, 109, 147–149, 214
Pseudo-R^2 for non linear models 102
Public Health Service, U.S. 20
Public relations, importance of 284
PULSES profile 192
P value 9, 13, 62

Q

Qualitative research
    construct validity 311
    example 304–312
    grounded theory 302–304
    item generation 309–310

Qualitative research (*cont.*)
    methods..301–302
    psychometric analysis..................304, 310–312
    reliability..................................302, 310–312
    scale construction......................304, 309–312
    substantive theory..............................303–307
Quality
    clinical data..262, 280
    clinical evidence..385
    of CPG document......................................450
Quality-adjusted life years (QALYs)
    cost analysis 325
    and CUA 430–431
Quality control 12, 170, 172, 280, 285, 345, 361
Quality of life analysis
    clinically important differences..........268–271
    instruments......................................261–264
    missing data..................................261, 263–267
    multivariate repeated measures model 271
    outcome prespecification 261, 262, 264–267,
        269, 270
    quality adjusted survival..................267–268
    scores 261–271
    SF-36..263
    treatment effect..........................264–265
Quality of life, health-related. *See* Health-related quality of
    life (HRQOL)
Quality of life instrument..310
Quality of Reporting of Meta-Analyses (QUORUM)
    methods..399
Questionnaires..................25, 33, 42, 44, 191, 193, 197–199,
    202, 205, 262, 263, 265, 282–284, 319, 337, 344,
    388, 431, 450

R

Random effect models..................111, 113, 114, 128
Randomized controlled trial analysis
    alpha spending..181
    baseline characteristics..................180, 187–188
    baseline characteristics imbalance..............187–188, 265
    censoring 183
    composite outcomes..................178, 184, 189
    crossover trial..186
    factorial design..............................169, 185
    hypothesis-generating analyses......................189
    intention-to-treat analysis 180
    interim analyses 169, 170, 180–183
    number needed to treat..................186–187
    observational design analyses........................62
    open-label run-in period..........................185
    power..................................187, 225–246
    research questions..................159, 160, 273–274
    stopping rules 181–183, 201, 245
    stratified design 185–186
    two-tailed hypothesis..........................178

Randomized controlled trials design
    adaptive trials..163
    allocation concealment 162
    analysis frequency bias..........................169–170
    audit..162, 170, 172
    bias..171
    blinding 164
    block (*see* Blocking)
    cluster 162
    controlled trial 159–174
    costs..163, 170, 172
    economic issues..170
    end-point adjudication 173
    factorial design..163
    funding 171–172
    imbalanced group 180, 187–188
    loss to follow up..................164, 167, 170–171
    multicenter..................................165, 168
    neutral..179
    non inferiority trials..................................164
    one-tailed, trial design 167
    outcomes..................................166, 170
    parallel-arm trial..15
    planning
        allocations and interventions 165
        inclusion and exclusion criteria..........165
    randomization..................159, 162–163
    recruitment role..........................167–168
    reporting..174
    research question 161
    risk factors 160
    sample size estimation 159, 167
    stratified..................................185–186
    subgroup analyses 169
    subjects, characteristics of 179–180
    surrogate markers of 166
    treatment period 168–169
    trial design 162–166
    trial team 172–173
Random sample..................................7, 8, 220, 225
Random sequences generation..8
Rank preserving structural failure time model
    (RPSFTM)..................................251, 252
Rasch models..204
Recall ratio 425
Receiver operating characteristic (ROC)
    curve 210, 294, 295, 297
Recombinant-based method..........................353, 354
Recombination fraction..................353, 354, 356. *See also*
    Genetic epidemiology, in complex traits
Recruitment rate..167–168
Reference Manager®..426
RefWorks®..426
Regression method of analysis
    estimation purpose....................................74

intercept (β_0) 74
likelihood and probability 76
maximum likelihood estimation (MLE) 75, 76
ordinary least square method 75
parameter estimates 74, 76
Relative risks 45, 54, 63, 65, 66, 89, 101,
    104, 105, 215, 392, 409, 446
Reliability coefficients 203, 204
RENAAL clinical trial 173
Repeated measures 5, 9, 94, 110, 128, 129, 169,
    241, 271, 345
Reporting
    in clinical research 17
    for proper interpretation and evaluation 17
Research design, for diagnostic test 14
Research ethics
    application 29
    application tips 29
    Belmont report 20
    board 22–24, 26, 27, 29, 282
    clinical trials 24, 26
    development 19–21
    governance of 21
    inclusiveness in research 28–29
    informed consent 24–28
    privacy and confidentiality of 21–22
    sample study 20
    study risk, benefit 23–24
Research ethics board (REB)
    composition 22
    functions of 23
    of Memorial University 462
    risks and benefits, review of 23–24
Research participants, ethical
    privacy rights 26
    responsibilities of 26
    withdrawal procedure 27
Research plan, clinical implementation of 279–281
Research question
    accuracy 5, 14
    bias 5–7
    clinical relevance 3, 13
    confounding 6
    construct validity 11
    controls 5–7, 15
    diagnostic test 4, 14, 16, 17
    effectiveness 5, 12, 13, 15, 16
    efficiency 15
    error 3, 5–9, 11, 13, 15
    external validity 11–12
    framing 3–17
    hard end-points 10
    hierarchy of evidence 13–14
    internal validity 11–12
    interventions 14–15

longitudinal studies 17
measurement error 11
measurements 9–11
outcomes 10
patients 4, 16
precision 5–7
random error 6, 8
randomization 5, 8, 13, 17
randomized controlled trials 3, 5, 13, 14
sample size estimation 8–9
sampling 3, 7–8
statistical significance 13
study design 9, 12–14
surrogate markers 10
systematic error 5–7
Restriction, in confounding improvement 58
Review Committees, ethical 21, 22
    Research Ethics Board (REB) 21
Risk factors 4, 14, 34, 44, 51–53, 55–61,
    65, 67, 71, 89, 90, 99, 146, 160, 188, 208–209,
    333, 336, 337, 339, 343, 364, 388, 393, 395, 431,
    458, 477, 478
Risk prediction models
    brier score 148
    calibration 148
    C-statistic 148
    discrimination 147–148
    Hosmer–Lemeshow chi square statistic 148
    index 149
    integrated discrimination improvement 152
    knowledge translation 154
    model development 146–149
    net reclassification index 149, 153–154
    selection of variables 150
    validation cohort 151–152
R^2 statistics 91, 96, 102

S

Safety, in clinical trials 160
    Safety monitoring .... 169, 183. *See also* Data safety and
        monitoring committee
    clinical trial data 169, 183
Sample size
    binary outcomes 231, 240, 241
    biologically plausible effect 238
    calculation 231–235
    clinical trial designs 225–246
    composite end points 226, 243
    confidence intervals 230, 236, 238, 399
    continuous outcomes 231, 299
    diagnostic biomarkers 241
    drop-in 240, 241, 250
    dropout 240, 241
    estimation 8–9, 52, 62–64, 159, 164,
        167, 216, 250, 297

Sample size (*cont.*)
  false negative error............................225, 226
  false positive error.............................225, 226
  infeasible sample size options 241, 242
  longitudinal studies..................226, 244–245
  loss to follow up.......................226, 239–241
  minimum clinically important effect 237, 238
  multiple primary end-points.....................226
  negative predictive value 226, 229
  non adherence...250
  non inferiority trials..........................238–239
  null hypothesis......................63, 64, 166, 227
  pilot studies.....................................236–237
  positive predictive value 230
  power......................................225–246
  pragmatic trials 241
  primary end-point 226, 244
  probability theory 225
  prognostic biomarkers.......................215–216
  publication bias......................................230
  randomized controlled trials 225–246
  random variation 225
  standardized effect size conventions 238
  survival outcomes...................................231
  treatment effect...................237, 240, 241
  treatment effect size estimation 250
  two-group studies....................................226
  type I error............................8, 62, 166
  type II error 9, 15, 166, 167
  underpowered studies 62
  variability of outcome variable.........62, 234, 244
Scale
  characteristics 200–201
  construction, qualitative database in 309–312
  reliability to discriminate individual 200
  utility 430
  validity.......................................311–312
Schedule for the evaluation of individual quality of life
    (SEIQoL) 199
Search strategy, designing........................425–426
SF-6D, derivative measure 198
Short Form-36 (SF-36) Health Survey...........197, 198
Single-nucleotide markers (SNPs) 355
  genotyping for association-based studies...........357–363
SNPs. *See* Single-nucleotide markers (SNPs)
Sponsorship, for guideline development and
    implementation......................................448
Staffing. *See* Personnel
Standardization of training, methods, and protocol 171
Standard link functions and inverses 95
Statements, guideline rules for use of 445
Statistical methods and results, reporting of
  fit component 78
  point estimates..411

special checking, model's requirement 91
  variability in response 77–83
Statistical model
  appropriate model to fit data assumption verification and
      model specification check 79
  components of..78
  critical violations of...................................77
  exposure–response relationship.............79–80
  fit portion of linear model 77
  information gain and residual variance 82
  meanings, model fitted to data 81–82
  multidimensional consequences and inputs 83
  multivariate analysis...........................82–83
  random component of model 80–81
  transformation of data 81
Statistical significance...................3, 13, 46, 47, 62, 188,
    213, 214, 219, 221, 254, 269, 407
Steering committee, for clinical trial management 172
Stopping rules................... 169, 181–183, 201, 245
Stratification, in confounding improvement.....................67
Stratified design
  examples of..185
  structure...109
Study power (1-beta error) 9
Subgroup analysis, of clinical trial 169
Substantive theory generation, grounded
      theory in 304–308
Surrogate outcomes 9, 207–223, 323, 445
Survival analysis
  forms of 108
  key requirements for 105–106
Survival data, study of.................................106
Survival time.......................37, 105, 106, 108, 116, 128,
    147, 252, 253, 340
Systematic review. *See also* Literature review
  advantages...410–411
  conduct..399–401
  in HTA...419, 423
  limitations...............................398, 410–413
  scientific quality................................401–410

T

Target population 4, 5, 7, 11, 34–40, 56,
    61, 155, 216, 263, 310, 347, 388, 411, 444, 450
Technical efficiency 273, 317, 318, 320
Time-to-event data, functions of............106–108
Translational research
  bariatric surgery.................... 460, 461, 463, 464
  Canadian Institutes for Health Research............457–459
  definition 456–457
  evidence-based decision making.................455–466
  evidence-based practice 455, 458
  example..458, 463
  frameworks 457–458

integrated knowledge translation activities 459
integrated knowledge translation team 460–466
knowledge-to-action cycle 459, 460
knowledge translation 457–460
levels 457
phases 457, 458
Treatment effect
   biologically plausible 252
   censoring 252
   clinically important difference 220, 230, 237, 270
   contamination..253
   contamination-adjusted intention-to-treat
      analysis...257
   crossover 249
   design 250
   EVOLVE trial...253, 258
   example...253–258
   intention-to-treat analysis 249, 253
   interactive parameter estimation......................251, 253
   inverse probability of censoring weights 252
   lag censoring..251
   non adherence...253–258
   rank preserving structural failure time
      model...251, 252
   sample size estimation 250
   treatment as received analysis 251
Treatment period..168–169, 186
Treat-to-goal clinical study..51
Tri-Council Policy Statement (TCPS)..................21, 23, 28
   risks and benefits, review of...................................23–24

Trio design, in family association studies.........................360
t Test...64, 96, 97
Tuskegee study 20
Type I error.................. 8, 11, 13, 62, 164, 166, 167, 170, 181
Type II error 9, 15, 43, 62, 166, 167, 187, 227

U

Utility 63, 160, 182, 193, 194, 198, 210, 212,
      214, 231, 262, 267, 268, 290, 297, 298, 317, 319,
      320, 326, 364, 374, 376–378, 386, 430, 431, 458

V

Validation of biomarkers..211–220
Validity of study...11, 17, 27
   external and internal 11–12
Variables
   confounding 58, 60, 61, 65, 66, 85, 212, 338, 343–346
   interacting...85
   types of 60, 137
Variance-corrected models...........120, 121. *See also* Extended
      generalized linear models
Vulnerable populations, in ethical research.........................20

W

Willingness to pay method.............................. 267, 319, 430
Will Rogers phenomenon 32, 40, 335, 341

Z

Z val... 63, 64, 355